THE ENCYCLOPEDIA OF

HIV AND AIDS

Third Edition

THE ENCYCLOPEDIA OF

HIV AND AIDS

Third Edition

Stephen E. Stratton, M.S.L.S., M.A.

Foreword by
Edward A. Morales, M.D.

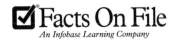

Facts On File
An Infobase Learning Company

The Encyclopedia of HIV and AIDS, Third Edition

Copyright © 2012 by Stephen E. Stratton

Facts On File
An imprint of Infobase Learning, Inc.
132 West 31st Street
New York NY 10001

Library of Congress Cataloging-in-Publication Data
Stratton, Stephen E.
The encyclopedia of HIV and AIDS / Stephen E. Stratton, Evelyn J. Fisher ;
foreword by Edward A. Morales.—3rd ed.
p. cm.—(Library of health and living)
Rev. ed. of: Encyclopedia of HIV and AIDS / Sarah Barbara Watstein, Stephen E. Stratton. 2nd .c2003.
Includes bibliographical references and index.
ISBN-13: 978-0-8160-7723-6 (hardcover : alk. paper)
ISBN-10: 0-8160-7723-1 (hardcover : alk. paper) 1. AIDS (Disease)—Dictionaries. I. Fisher, Evelyn J.
II. Watstein, Sarah. Encyclopedia of HIV and AIDS. III. Title.
RC606.6.W385 2012
362.196'9792003—dc23   2011017597

Facts On File books are available at special discounts when purchased in bulk quantities for businesses, associations, institutions, or sales promotions. Please call our Special Sales Department in New York at (212) 967-8800 or (800) 322-8755.

You can find Facts On File on the World Wide Web at http://www.infobaselearning.com

Text design by Cathy Rincon
Composition by Hermitage Publishing Services
Cover printed by Yurchak Printing, Landisville, Pa.
Book printed and bound by Yurchak Printing, Landisville, Pa.
Date printed: March 2012

Printed in the United States of America

10 9 8 7 6 5 4 3 2 1

This book is printed on acid-free paper.

CONTENTS

ACKNOWLEDGMENTS

Few people write a book alone. Contributing essentially to a work are those who offer time, discussing any number of issues with a writer. There are those who are kind enough to read through the material to make sure it all makes sense, and those who ensure that a spell-check has been performed correctly. Thanks to Guido Núñez-Mujica for discussing biological advances and future treatment for HIV in depth. Thanks to Sarah Watstein for first giving me the opportunity to work with her on the second edition of this book and for giving me the opportunity to attempt this one on my own. Billy Starr, a colleague at the John Spoor Broome Library at California State University Channel Islands (CSUCI), was wonderful enough to check URLs to make sure that these linked up properly. Ronnie Sullivan was good enough to organize the URLs so that they made more sense. Particular thanks must go to Manuel Correia, another CSUCI colleague, who spent his off time this past year reading through the material to check that my language and grammar were correct and understandable. Of course, Dr. Edward Morales also took a great deal of his valuable time to correct any mistakes or misconceptions with regard to medical information. There are also many researchers, educators, nurses, doctors, and caregivers in the field of HIV and AIDS around the world who have contributed to this book through their years of hard work and their efforts to make life easier or even possible for people with HIV. Thanks also to two friends who in particular have been extremely supportive through the years, whatever I decided to do— Frank Kenniston and Jeff Helyer—for just listening to me complain at times. Finally, I want to mention the two men who have shared the ups and downs of life with me, Rodney Blair (1962–91) and Robert Harris (1964–2004). I miss them both, and this book is dedicated to them and the memories of the times I spent with each.

FOREWORD

In the 1980s, when cases of unexplained deaths in previously healthy young adults were first described, the cause of human immunodeficiency virus (HIV) infection and AIDS was unknown. To be sure, all that could be appreciated and described was the rapid pace of illness and death that seemed to afflict previously healthy adults. In 1990, the median time to death following a diagnosis of AIDS was about one year. At that time, the most common presentation of HIV infection was late-stage AIDS. This diagnosis was most often associated with *Pneumocystis* pneumonia, a life-threatening pneumonia that was the cause of a high mortality rate. Even the source and treatment of this pneumonia were poorly understood at that time. Patients who later would be discovered to have HIV infection and AIDS presented to their doctors with these rare diseases or opportunistic infections (OIs) that were associated with unusual complications. At that time, many of these diseases were only sporadically described in medical journals, and little was known about their natural histories and treatments. Eventually, it would take the identification and an understanding of how an infection by a virus, HIV, could severely suppress the defenses of the human body to permit these unusual diseases and their complications to occur.

Now, more than 30 years since the first description of HIV infection and AIDS, knowledge about the cause, treatment, and nuances of this lifelong infection and other associated complications has grown and continues to grow immensely. Where there were only a few medications possibly considered to be useful in the treatment of HIV infection, there are now many alternatives from several classes of medications that have been and continue to be studied with rigorous scientific research. What was once a fast-moving infection with only one drug treatment option and causing rapid deterioration has now become an illness with increasing treatment options and longer survival. While the opportunistic infections still potentially lead to serious complications in HIV infection and AIDS, the experience and treatment options of OIs are better understood. Still, more consequences of living with HIV infection and AIDS continue to be described and studied.

The Encyclopedia of HIV and AIDS is such a resource to facilitate an introduction to and understanding of this rapidly evolving field of research. The main purpose of this book is not to be an end resource but to serve as a useful tool—a key to open the door of what has become a complex disease and even a separate medical specialty. It is hoped that this edition will provide a quick reference with new updates, a starting place to formulate new questions, and updated lists of sources to begin to get answers. By studying and building on our understanding of this infection, we can make a difference in our own lives and the lives of others who are infected with HIV. As Marie Curie noted in a letter to her brother,

"One never notices what has been done; one can only see what remains to be done."

—Edward A. Morales, M.D.
Oxnard, California

INTRODUCTION

In 1981, the U.S. Centers for Disease Control first began collecting information about the appearance of pneumonias and Kaposi's sarcoma in gay men in New York City and Los Angeles. By the time this book is published, 30 years will have passed, and the world has seen the deaths of at least 25 million people from a virus that had not been identified when these initial illnesses were noticed. HIV has changed the world in many ways. Parts of it have seen huge drops in life expectancy. Economic effects on families as well as countries have been enormous. Changes in how health care has been delivered around the world have been enormous. Medical research has made enormous advances in the study of the immune system and the role of viruses in illness because of the money spent trying to understand, prevent, and treat HIV. Yet with all the advances in medical care and the ability of highly active antiretroviral therapy (HAART) medications to control HIV for extended periods, the epidemic continues. Education has made an impact. Statistics in the United States, Western Europe, and Australia showed that clearly stated, properly aimed education and prevention materials can make a difference, as during the first 10 years, infection rates in gay men stabilized and then dropped approximately to their current levels. Recent studies from the United Nations (UN) show that education is making a difference in Africa and in Asia, where new infections have dropped

15 and 25 percent, respectively. Money spent educating people on how to avoid the virus works. For the millions who still live with the virus, the lack of available treatment has been by far the largest challenge, and it has been a stain on Western pharmaceutical companies and the governments that allow these companies to continue to hold drug patents and withhold drugs from people who could benefit immediately from them.

The recent start-up of groups providing treatment through large governmental, multigovernmental, and nongovernmental organizations such as the President's Emergency Plan for AIDS Relief (PEPFAR) and the Global Fund have only just begun to reach the huge numbers of people needing HAART. Even after such assistance has begun, it is now threatened by world recession and governmental hesitancy to continue funding. When this book was last published in 2003, only 7 percent of all HIV-positive people had access to HAART medications. At the end of 2010, according to the World Health Organization (WHO), 36 percent of HIV-positive people had access to HAART. This included 34 percent of people in eastern and southern Africa, but just 22 percent in West and Central Africa. Children who used to fall consistently behind country and region totals for coverage of adults now have better access to medications than adults, with 48 percent of children in West and Central Africa receiving needed HAART medication. In developed countries, the percentage of people receiving needed HAART is higher and treatment has been available longer. The number of deaths in the United States has dropped 69 percent since 1997, when HAART was introduced. Countries that provide needed medications for all people who require them show similar or larger declines in mortality rates. Yet coverage is still needed for more than half of the 33 million HIV-positive people who do not have access to the available drugs, including people in the United States, where state governmental refusal to cover the cost of drugs blocks access to treatment.

This book, which started as a dictionary, has also changed a great deal. It is still a reference source for those who wish to be more knowledgeable about HIV and AIDS. It can be a way for those affected in some manner by HIV and AIDS to understand more about the illness, its prevention, treatment, and social effects. It is not, however, a replacement for consultation with a physician who specializes in HIV or infectious diseases. It is not a replacement for access to needed treatment; nor can it be the latest up-to-date guide, as what is published in medical dictionaries or even on the Internet is often outdated when it is consulted. It can be, however, a guide to basic information about HIV, opportunistic infections, antiretroviral treatments, and social aspects of the illness. It can serve as a guide to Internet sites that can provide more up-to-date statistical data. It can also act as a starting point for conversations with medical providers about particulars for patients and other interested people.

The third edition in your hands has evolved from a collection of short definitions on several hundred terms that made up the first and largely the second editions to an encyclopedia of approximately 150 entries. These entry terms have been chosen to give a broad overview of the virus, the opportunistic infections, treatment, prevention, and a small bit of the social and historic issues of the virus. The evolution of the epidemic has driven the evolution of the book, from scattered bits of information available to researchers to a bigger picture available to general readers. I have attempted to pull together the numerous definitions from the first edition authored by Sarah Watstein and the second edition that we coauthored into overview articles to give the reader a basic understanding of the wide range of information currently known about HIV and AIDS. Writing this edition involved a much different process than the earlier editions. Large portions of the third edition are entirely new, while bits and pieces of the previous editions that have survived editing and rewriting are probably included in newly created larger articles. Material that was outdated and no longer part of the HIV and AIDS literature has been, by and large, removed. As always when the subject is a virus that is transmitted sexually or through injection drug use, many people may consider some of the entries controversial or risqué. I believe I have dealt with the topics fairly and in a balanced manner, trying to represent different viewpoints in some instances. Appendixes have been updated, and the Online Resources list that follows them has been revamped and checked for currency and usefulness. Cross-references and the index should help people locate the material they are seeking. Every effort has been made to ensure the material will be as up-to-date as possible at the time the work is completed. HIV and AIDS research changes rapidly, and though every effort has been made to check accuracy, it is possible some information may be incorrect. I assume responsibility for the work and any mistakes that may be in the text.

I hope that this work helps increase understanding of HIV and the many issues related to it. It is specifically aimed toward an audience of general readers and students. I hope I have been able to reach this group and that the explanations provided have been helpful.

—Stephen E. Stratton

AVERT: AVERTing HIV and AIDS. "History of AIDS Up to 1986." AVERT.org. Available online. URL: http://

www.avert.org/aids-history-86.htm. Accessed April 5, 2011.

———. "Worldwide HIV and AIDS Statistics." AVERT. org. Available online. URL: http://www.avert.org/worldstats.htm. Accessed April 5, 2011.

Joint United Nations Programme on HIV/AIDS. "Eight-Year Trend Shows New HIV Infections Down by 17%—Most Progress Seen in Sub-Saharan Africa." UNAIDS.org. Available online. URL: http://www.unaids.org/en/KnowledgeCentre/Resources/FeatureStories/archive/2009/20091124_pr_Epi Update.asp. Accessed April 5, 2011.

Stover, John, and Lori Bollinger. "The Economic Impact of AIDS." Policyproject.com. Available online. URL: http://www.policyproject.com/pubs/SEImpact/SEImpact_Africa.PDF. Accessed April 5, 2011.

World Health Organization. *Towards Universal Access: Scaling Up Priority HIV/AIDS Interventions in the Health Sector; Progress Report 2010.* Available online. URL: http://libdoc.who.int/publications/2010/9789241500395_eng.pdf. Accessed July 14, 2011.

ENTRIES A TO Z

abacavir Abacavir is one of the NUCLEOSIDE REVERSE TRANSCRIPTASE INHIBITORS (NRTIs); it is manufactured by GlaxoSmithKline under the brand name Ziagen. It is also known as abacavir sulfate and abbreviated ABC. It is always prescribed in conjunction with other antiretrovirals as part of a combination therapy. Abacavir is also found in two combination antiretroviral medications, EPZICOM and TRIZIVIR. It is approved for use in both adults and children. There is a strawberry-banana-flavored liquid formula for infants and people unable to swallow pills.

Dosage
Abacavir is manufactured in 300 mg doses as a yellow-colored tablet. The dosage is either one 300 mg pill twice a day or two 300 mg pills once a day. Abacavir can be taken with or without food. Some abacavir pills are scored, or marked with lines, so they can easily be broken into smaller pieces for dosing with children. The children's dosage is based on the weight of the child; a physician will determine the appropriate amount for a child to take. The amount of the liquid formula of abacavir is also based on weight.

Drug Interactions
Abacavir should never be taken at the same time as the drugs Epzicom and Trizivir, which already contain abacavir. Abacavir decreases the amount of the drug methadone in the body. People taking methadone to manage the symptoms of heroin withdrawal may need to have the dosage of that medication increased by a physician if they must take abacavir. Using any type of alcohol while taking abacavir increases the amount

of abacavir in the body. This can increase the side effects of abacavir and increase the chance a person will suffer one of those side effects.

Side Effects
Between 3 and 8 percent of people who take abacavir have an allergic reaction to the drug. Research into the reaction has shown that this is caused by an inherited genetic marker named *HLA-B*5701*. HLA stands for human leukocyte antigen, and *HLA-B*5701* is one of the numerous genes that play a role in the human immune system, allowing the body to fight off viruses and other pathogens. There is an inexpensive test to determine whether a person carries this genetic marker, and it is recommended for all people who are planning to take abacavir or one of the multidrug combination pills that contain abacavir. If it is determined that someone carries the *HLA-B*5701* marker, he or she will not be prescribed abacavir in any form. The allergic reaction occurs less often among people of African descent.

Signs of an allergic reaction to abacavir can include fever, rash, headache, stomach pain, vomiting, diarrhea, cough, or respiratory illness. People who suspect that they are having a reaction should immediately talk to a physician, as in some cases the reaction can lead to severe illness or death. The reaction most often occurs within the first two weeks of beginning abacavir therapy. If a person is having such a reaction, he or she should never again take abacavir in any form, as the reaction will be more severe the next time a person takes the medication. Some people who have stopped taking abacavir for reasons other than the allergic reaction have suffered the reaction when they restarted abacavir. It is generally recommended that a person who stops taking abacavir for any reason consult a physician before restarting the drug.

Common side effects, not related to the potential allergic reaction, include stomach upset, headache, tiredness, and loss of appetite. These will lessen over time while taking the drug. NRTIs have been implicated in increased fat levels in the blood as well as redistribution of body fat, called LIPODYSTROPHY.

NRTIs have also been shown to cause LACTIC ACIDOSIS and liver disease in a small number of people. Severe pain in the upper abdomen and lower back, as well as severe nausea, can be signs of lactic acidosis. Enlarged spleen, pancreas, or liver can also be a sign of the condition. It is important that all medications be stopped if a physician diagnoses this condition. Liver markers in the blood are always monitored during regular BLOOD WORK/BLOOD TESTS to watch for these conditions, but any symptoms should be reported to a doctor. This reaction to NRTIs is more prevalent among women, obese people, and those who have advanced HIV disease, but its occurrence is unpredictable.

Studies have noted an increase in heart attacks among people taking abacavir, particularly among people already at risk for heart attacks. Those risk factors are being male, having high cholesterol, having high blood pressure, being obese, and smoking.

Abacavir is listed as a pregnancy category C drug. It has been shown to cause death or birth defects in laboratory animals. No studies of abacavir have been done among pregnant WOMEN, and it is unknown whether abacavir causes changes in breast milk for women breast-feeding babies. It is only recommended for pregnant or breast-feeding women if the benefits clearly outweigh the potential risks of the drug.

AIDSmeds. "Atripla (Efavirenz + Tenofovir + Emtricitabine)." AIDSmeds.com. Available online. URL: http://www.aidsmeds.com/archive/Atripla_1577.shtml. Accessed January 24, 2011.

———. "Isentress (Raltegravir)." AIDSmeds.com. Available online. URL: http://www.aidsmeds.com/archive/Isentress_1639.shtml. Accessed January 24, 2011.

———. "Special Issues for Children with HIV: NRTIs." AIDSmeds.com. Available online. URL: http://www.aidsmeds.com/articles/Children_4935.shtml. Accessed January 24, 2011.

AIDS Treatment Data Network. "Ziagen—Abacavir Sulfate." AEGIS.com. Available online. URL: http://ww2.aegis.com/factshts/network/simple/abac.html. Accessed January 24, 2011.

The Body. "HIV/AIDS Medication Basics." TheBody.com. Available online. URL: http://www.thebody.com/content/art40488.html. Accessed January 24, 2011.

Highleyman, Liz. "HLA-B*5701 Screening for Abacavir (Ziagen) Hypersensitivity." HIVandHepatitis.com. Available online. URL: http://www.hivandhepatitis.com/recent/2008/022608_c.html. Accessed January 24, 2011.

United States Department of Health and Human Services. "Abacavir." aidsinfo.nih.gov. Available online. URL: http://www.aidsinfo.nih.gov/DrugsNew/DrugDetailNT.aspx?int_id=257. Accessed January 24, 2011.

abstinence Abstinence is the act of voluntarily giving up something that is seen as pleasurable or intoxicating. It is often used in the sense of giving up or not participating in sexual activity or in the use of alcohol or drugs. Abstinence from sex and injection drugs is seen by many as the one sure way to avoid acquiring HIV, the virus that causes AIDS. In most instances when discussing HIV, the term *abstinence* is used to refer to sexual abstinence.

Sexual abstinence is the method of avoiding HIV, other sexually transmitted infections (STIs), and pregnancy that has been taught by U.S. government funded programs in different forms since 1982. In 1996, expanded funding for abstinence-only sex education programs became law when the U.S. Congress passed welfare reform. Abstinence was also a required part of funding approved under the President's Emergency Plan for AIDS Relief (PEPFAR), which funds

HIV education and treatment programs around the world. The current PEPFAR law requires that the global AIDS coordinator report to Congress when less than 50 percent of funding in a particular country is allocated to abstinence for prevention education.

Initially, abstinence education was funded at low levels and not solely as the only method of sex education. However, when welfare reform was passed, abstinence education funding was increased to $50 million in annual funding. Eventually, annual funding reached $176 million in budget year 2009. In addition, abstinence until marriage became the main, and in some instances the only, government-approved way to educate children, teens, and even unmarried adults about sexuality.

The U.S. government defines abstinence in the Social Security Act of 1996. Section 510(b) of Title V of the law states that an abstinence education program must meet eight points, labeled A–H, to qualify for funding. As stated in the law, an abstinence program:

A. has as its exclusive purpose, teaching the social, psychological, and health gains to be realized by abstaining from sexual activity;
B. teaches abstinence from sexual activity outside marriage as the expected standard for all school-age children;
C. teaches that abstinence from sexual activity is the only certain way to avoid out-of-wedlock pregnancy, sexually transmitted diseases, and other associated health problems;
D. teaches that a mutually faithful monogamous relationship in the context of marriage is the expected standard of human sexual activity;
E. teaches that sexual activity outside the context of marriage is likely to have harmful psychological and physical effects;
F. teaches that bearing children out-of-wedlock is likely to have harmful consequences for the child, the child's parents, and society;
G. teaches young people how to reject sexual advances and how alcohol and drug use increase vulnerability to sexual advances; and

H. teaches the importance of attaining self-sufficiency before engaging in sexual activity.

Youth advocates as well as comprehensive sex education advocates attacked the regulations from the beginning as detrimental to young people. Most argue that young people who choose to be abstinent need to be educated about STIs and the use of various contraceptives for the time when they do become sexually active. They also argue that the inherent bias in the eight points leaves already sexually active youth or gay and lesbian youth alienated and stigmatized for their behavior. Opponents believe that abstinence violates the separation of church and state laws by enacting moral and religious beliefs about sexual behavior and marriage into law. Many states also have constitutional guarantees to health and adequate education; opponents to abstinence education argue these rights are interfered with by these federal regulations which bar the discussion of sexual activity, STIs, and effective ways to avoid them if someone is sexually active.

Studies conducted in 2004 by Representative Henry Waxman and again in 2007 for the U.S. Department of Health and Human Services (HHS) showed that many programs adopted by states and groups receiving federal abstinence education funds were inaccurate or intentionally misleading in the pamphlets, lectures, and videos they provided students. Some students were told that condoms were ineffective in preventing pregnancy in one of every six cases; studies have shown that condoms are 98 percent effective when used properly. Others were informed that a student who could not maintain self-control over sexual activity could not manage to use a condom properly. Other misstatements in the different programs included the assertion that HIV is transmissible through skin-to-skin contact. Another program stated that HIV was transmitted through sweat and tears, which is untrue. Another told students that HIV could not be detected in BLOOD WORK/BLOOD TESTS for 10 years or more after infection. These cited statements have been found in programs produced by using government funds in states such as Colorado, Illinois, South Carolina, and Texas. They have been shown to be untrue through scientific research conducted by both the federal government and private studies. Some of the programs reviewed in the HHS report were found simply to shame students and encourage guilt. Many studies pointed out that these abstinence education materials offered biased opinions on male and female gender roles, abortion, contraceptive use, homosexuality, and reproductive health. Statements made in the materials informed boys that WOMEN expect financial support and that men require constant admiration and have sexual needs that women are expected to fulfill.

Studies of abstinence as a method of birth control and avoidance of STIs have shown poor success rates. A report based on the National Longitudinal Study of Adolescent Health by Bruckner and Bearman reported that among teens who took abstinence-until-marriage or virginity vows, more than 60 percent broke those vows before they were married. The current average age of a first marriage for women is 25 and for men 27. The length of time needed to maintain perfect use of a particular method of birth control or disease prevention is significant; as with any long-term method of prevention, the risk of failure for any number of reasons increases with the length of use. Studies have not shown the reasons teens break abstinence vows or choose to stop using abstinence as a method of disease prevention. The difficulty in supporting abstinence-only programs is that such programs leave individuals ignorant of other methods of birth control or disease prevention. Bruckner and Bearman have shown that students who have been educated in abstinence-only programs have a lower rate of condom use and other birth control methods when they do stop using abstinence as their means of protection. Other studies based on the National Survey of Family Growth and the National Longitudinal Study of Adolescent Health (Finer; Bruckner and Bearman; Trenholm et al.) have also shown that

students in abstinence-only programs do not delay their start of sexual activity, do not have lower rates of STIs, and do not have lower rates of pregnancy than teens in other sex education programs. There has been some success in lowering the rates of STIs and pregnancy when abstinence education is included in a program that also includes education in the full range of options for family planning, including the use of condoms, contraception, and prevention of the spread of HIV and other STIs.

Despite these complaints from educators, the U.S. Congress has renewed funding for abstinence programs each year, and abstinence programs continue to be required in order to receive federal funding for sex education. This led to states' refusing the funds altogether to avoid the federal requirements. California was the first state to do so in 2000, followed by 24 others, including Virginia and Ohio, by 2008. There has also been controversy surrounding the abstinence requirements of the PEPFAR program. HIV education activists believe that it is harmful to require that money be spent solely on abstinence education, ignoring more complete HIV prevention that also includes the message of consistent use of condoms and being monogamous, the other two components of the ABC of HIV prevention. This policy has encouraged some countries to use the U.S. funding solely for abstinence education to ensure the continuation of funding. Removing the discussion of condoms, their use, and their distribution from at least half of HIV education programs funded abroad, the Bush administration began exporting incomplete prevention education and endangering the lives of individuals in those countries.

In May 2009, the Obama administration declared that abstinence-only education would *not* be funded in the U.S. budget that was submitted to Congress. However, the final budget that the U.S. Congress passed was a compromise that allowed states to continue to use federal monies for abstinence-only education but also allowed states to receive federal monies for comprehensive sex education. Some states applied for both types of funding while others chose only comprehensive funding. Minnesota and Virginia were the only states that chose to apply solely for abstinence-only funds. Monies for PEPFAR continue to have requirements for abstinence education, but it is unclear how long these requirements will exist given the lack of effectiveness of these types of programs and the potential benefits of teaching abstinence as one option among others for preventing disease and pregnancy.

AVERT: AVERTing HIV and AIDS. "Abstinence and Sex Education." AVERT.org. Available online. URL: http://www.avert.org/abstinence.htm. Accessed January 24, 2011.

Bruckner, Hannah, and Peter Bearman. "After the Promise: The STD Consequences of Adolescent Virginity Pledges." *Journal of Adolescent Health* 26, no. 4 (2005): 271–278.

Centers for Disease Control and Prevention. "National Survey of Family Growth." CDC.gov. Available online. URL: http://www.cdc.gov/nchs/nsfg.htm. Accessed July 22, 2011.

CHANGE: Center for Health and Gender Equity. "U.S. Foreign Policy & Funding." Genderhealth.org. Available online. URL: http://www.genderhealth. org/the_issues/us_foreign_policy/. Accessed January 24, 2011.

Connolly, Ceci. "Some Abstinence Programs Mislead Teens, Report Says." *Washington Post.* Available online. URL: http://www.washingtonpost.com/wp -dyn/articles/A26623-2004Dec1.html. Accessed January 24, 2011.

Dailard, Cynthia. "Understanding 'Abstinence': Implications for Individuals, Programs and Policies." Guttmacher.org. Available online. URL: http:// www.guttmacher.org/pubs/tgr/06/5/gr060504.pdf. Accessed March 20, 2011.

Finer, Lawrence B. "Trends in Premarital Sex in the United States, 1954–2003." *Public Health Reports* 122, no. 1 (2007): 73–78.

Hanson, Thomas. "Abstinence-Only Sex Education Statistics—Final Nail in the Coffin." Open Education.com. Available online. URL: http://www. openeducation.net/2009/01/05/abstinence-only -sex-education-statistics-final-nail-in-the-coffin/. Accessed January 24, 2011.

Howell, Marcela, and Marilyn Keefe. "The History of Federal Abstinence-Only Funding." Advocatesforyouth.org. Available online. URL: http://www.advocatesforyouth.org/index. php?option=com_content&task=view&id=429&Ite mid=177. Accessed January 24, 2011.

Kliff, Sarah. "The Future of Abstinence." *Newsweek.* Available online. URL: http://www.newsweek. com/id/219818. Accessed January 24, 2011.

PEPFAR Watch. "Abstinence and Fidelity." PEPFARWatch.org. Available online. URL: http:// www.pepfarwatch.org/the_issues/abstinence_and_ fidelity/. Accessed February 28, 2011.

SIECUS: Sexuality Information and Education Council of the United States. "A Brief History: Abstinence-Only-Until-Marriage Funding." Nomoremoney.com. Available online. URL: http://www.nomoremoney. org/index.cfm?pageid=947. Accessed January 24, 2011.

———. "State by State Decisions: The Personal Responsibility Education Program and Title V Abstinence-Only Program." SIECUS.org. Available online. URL: http:// www.siecus.org/index.cfm?fuseaction=Feature. showFeature&FeatureID=1934. Accessed February 28, 2011.

Trenholm, Christopher, Barbara Devaney, Kenneth Fortson, Melissa Clark, Lisa Quay, and Justin Wheeler. "Impacts of Abstinence Education on Teen Sexual Activity, Risk of Pregnancy, and Risk of Sexually Transmitted Diseases." *Journal of Policy Analysis and Management* 27, no. 2 (2008): 255–276.

United States Government Accountability Office. "Global Health: Spending Requirement Presents Challenges for Allocating Prevention Funding under the President's Emergency Plan for AIDS Relief." GAO.gov. Available online. URL: http://www.gao. gov/new.items/d06395.pdf. Accessed January 24, 2011.

University of North Carolina, Carolina Population Center. "National Longitudinal Study of Adolescent Health." CPC.UNC.edu. Available online. URL: http://www.cpc.unc.edu/projects/addhealth. Accessed July 22, 2011.

Africa As of the end of 2010, the United Nations estimated there were more than 33 million cases of HIV in the world, lowered slightly from earlier estimates of closer to 40 million infected people in 2005. This drop in estimated totals resulted from more thorough HIV testing in many countries as well as additional data that became available from some countries for the first time. But whatever the numbers, Africa remains at the center of the HIV epidemic. Of those 33 million people infected, 22.5 million live in sub-Saharan Africa, two-thirds of the total. Of the AIDS deaths counted in 2009, 75 percent occurred in this region. In total, there were 1.3 million people who died of AIDS or HIV-related causes in Africa in 2009. As of 2007, there had been an estimated total of 15 million deaths from HIV-related illnesses in Africa since the epidemic began in the early 1980s. Because the virus tends to affect young adults, who are generally the most sexually active members of any country's population, the virus has left many African countries with large parts of their young adult population dead, leaving older adults to care for children and maintain families and economic stability for households. There are estimated to be more than 11 million orphans in Africa from deaths related to the virus.

In Africa, other issues have often clouded the HIV problem. Cultural norms that make public discussion of sex taboo have made it difficult to talk about sex, particularly about the activities of MEN WHO HAVE SEX WITH MEN (MSM). Leaders have been reluctant to discuss sexual behavior. In Malawi, a small southern African country where 1 million people are now HIV positive, it was illegal to discuss AIDS publicly until 1994. In 2001, Kenya's president, Daniel arap Moi, said it was improper to discuss the usage of condoms, and he simply asked all Kenyans to stop having sex for two years to stem the tide of the disease. In 2001, Swaziland, a small country bordered mostly by South Africa, where more than 25 percent of the adult population had tested positive, King Mswati III ordered all Swazi WOMEN to abstain from sex until the age of 19 and not to wear trousers to avoid encouraging attention from young men. They were to wear a "don't touch" tassel that alerted boys to their vow of chastity. The king also imposed a five-year ban on sex for young women. However, the

king violated his own order, choosing a 17-year-old high school student as his ninth wife shortly after issuing his decree in 2001. He paid the royal fine of one cow for violating the law. The ban was ended by the king a year earlier than set out in his original decree, in 2005; King Mswati III currently has 13 wives.

The disease has been particularly horrific in southern Africa, where large portions of the population are HIV positive and death has taken a large toll on families and economies. In South Africa, the government estimated in 2010 that 18 percent of the population— 5.6 million people— had HIV. More than half of those HIV-positive people lived in two provinces: Mpumalanga, which borders Mozambique and Swaziland, and KwaZulu-Natal, in the eastern part of the country. Recent data suggest that HIV prevalence may be leveling off as testing at maternity clinics has remained level: Approximately 30 percent of all pregnant women tested positive. There was also a decline in the number of new cases among young pregnant women. However, South Africa is one of the few countries in the world where the child mortality rate has increased since the 1990s. According to the Joint United Nations Programme on HIV/AIDS (UNAIDS) report issued in 2008, in government pregnancy clinics 29 percent of all pregnant women tested positive in KwaZulu-Natal. Other provinces showed lower levels of infection: Western Cape, 16 percent; Northern Cape, 15 percent; and Limpopo, 19 percent. An estimated 1.8 million South Africans have died of AIDS-related diseases since the beginning of the epidemic. South Africa has had a particularly difficult time in distributing educational materials as well as medications for HIV. The government of the former prime minister, Thabo Mbeki, even issued denials that HIV was the cause of AIDS. The former health minister, Mantombazana Tshabalala-Msimang, was noted for her insistence that AIDS could be treated with beetroot, garlic, and other vegetables. She was finally dismissed from her post when Mr. Mbeki was removed from office in 2008. Because of the official positions taken by these individuals, South Africa denied antiret-roviral medications to its populace for several years, leading to the death of hundreds of thousands of its citizens. One individual in particular, Zackie Achmat, led a protest of several years, refusing to take antiretrovirals—to which he had access through private insurance—until the government approved the distribution of antiretrovirals for everyone. Mr. Achmat also went abroad to purchase large quantities of the generic versions of the drug to import to South Africa, resulting in his arrest. However, this also led to the availability of these generic drugs in South Africa, after the ensuing publicity forced the pharmacy giant Pfizer to provide the cheaper alternatives to the South African government. In 2003, the South African government finally began providing antiretrovirals for some of the neediest people with HIV infection.

Zimbabwe's current humanitarian crises have been exacerbated by political instability. All systems of government, including education and health, and basic necessities such as food production, became difficult to secure during the last several years. United Nations (UN) estimates put the prevalence of HIV infection at more than 14 percent of people in the country. Although the numbers have leveled off or dropped, it is believed that the reason is simply that people have died. Medical care is currently unavailable to most of the citizenry. Hospitals have closed as a result of lack of funds, lack of medications, and lack of employees because salaries have not been paid. A large outbreak of cholera, a disease spread through poor sanitation and contaminated water, struck the country in late 2008 and killed 2,000 people. Large numbers of people have fled the country for neighboring Botswana and South Africa, creating problems for those governments, including bloody riots in South Africa in 2008 over the numbers of Zimbabwean refugees flooding the country. Testing in clinics before the collapse of the health system in 2008 indicated that new diagnoses were dropping for several reasons. Men in some areas of the country had slowed their rate of sex outside their primary relationship, and condom use had increased in some rural areas of the country. Infection rates for pregnant women vary around the country, from 10 percent in Mashonaland Central province to more than 20 percent in Matabeleland South province. The lack of a stable currency and an unemployment rate of more than 80 percent may be among the reasons for a large drop in the number of men who report having paid for sex between 1999 and 2005. Access to antiretroviral medications is minimal at best, as most are in the possession of wealthy individuals or people who have smuggled in the medications from a neighboring country.

According to 2009 UN data, other countries in southern Africa have a similarly high statistical prevalence of HIV in the population: Botswana, 24.8 percent; Lesotho, 23.6 percent; Malawi, 11.0 percent; Mozambique, 11.5 percent; Namibia, 13.1 percent; and Zambia, 13.5 percent. Lesotho is still showing an increase in the prevalence rates among young women in pregnancy clinics. Parts of Mozambique also still show increasing levels of new HIV cases in pregnant women. Lesotho is a poor country completely surrounded by South Africa. Studies show knowledge of HIV to be very limited, and sexual activity begins young in Lesotho; more than one-quarter of men younger than age 15 say they have already had sex. In this group, however, only 7 percent had used a condom. In Mozambique, education programs, cited in the UN 2007 report, have shown that condom use can be adopted by young adults, as increased participation in safer sex rose to nearly 60 percent of young people surveyed in several areas of the country in 2005, compared to 35 percent prior to educational programs in 2003. Rising levels of infection are consistent across Mozambique again after a leveling off in the early 2000s. Northern areas of the country are less affected, with prevalence rates near 10 percent, while in southern regions, including the capital, Maputo, prevalence rates of 25 percent have been found. The reasons for the differences in regional prevalence in Mozambique are unclear. Male CIRCUM-CISION is performed with more frequency in the North than in the South, and some studies in southern Africa have determined that circumcision can help prevent the transmission of HIV, though questions remain whether these studies are accurate, as cultural reasons may also play a part in the differences.

Botswana has a serious epidemic also. National studies conducted by the UN placed the rate of infection near 25 percent of the adult population (those above 15 years of age) in 2009. In younger people, the rates are higher. At pregnancy clinics, 49 percent of those 30–34 years of age were HIV positive, and 45 percent of those 25–29 years of age tested positive. Among pregnant teenagers, 18 percent tested HIV positive in the most recent national survey. This is, however, a drop in the number of diagnoses from earlier years, which bodes well for stabilization of the infection rates. A survey completed in 2004 among young unmarried men indicated that 95 percent of them used condoms when they had sex. This was an increase from surveys in 2001, in which 81 percent indicated condom use. Education has been good in Botswana with the UN and other nongovernmental organizations pouring extensive resources into the country for education, medical care, and antiretroviral medicines. Treatment of HIV-positive pregnant mothers increased to 75 percent in several areas of the country, decreasing the mother-to-child transmission of the virus. This figure is significantly higher than figures across the region and continent. If a pregnant woman is not treated, there is a 25–45 percent chance that her child will be born HIV positive. In those pregnant women receiving antiretroviral treatment during pregnancy, the rate of mother-to-child transmission is reduced to 2 percent if breast-feeding is also avoided. Changes in life expectancy in Botswana and other similarly affected countries have been dramatic. The median life expectancy has shortened dramatically over the course of the epidemic in southern Africa. Life expectancy in Botswana has now fallen to levels not seen

since 1950. The average person in Botswana can expect to live to the age of 34.9 years according to UN development estimates. Other countries and their life expectancies are Lesotho, 35.2 years; Zimbabwe, 36.6 years; Swaziland, 31.3 years; Zambia, 37.7 years; and Malawi, 39.8 years. These numbers reflect that half the population will die prior to reaching that age and half will live sometime beyond. For comparison, in the United States the life expectancy is 77.5 years, and in Japan it is 82.2 years.

Angola has a comparatively small epidemic for the southern African region. Just 2.1 percent of the population is estimated to be HIV positive. The small percentage may be the result of civil war, which closed large parts of the country to outsiders for many years during the worst of the epidemic. People could not travel to Angola, nor did they want to; and as no HIV sources originated in Angola, few cases were introduced to the country from beyond its borders for many years. Testing at pregnancy clinics does show that rates of HIV infection range higher in the South than in the North. Surveys of health clinics also show high rates of infections among female SEX WORKERS. Namibia is a sparsely populated country where 15 percent of people test HIV positive. UN analysis shows that new diagnoses have stabilized, but the same surveys indicate that little or no behavioral change has occurred with education, as more than 90 percent of young men and 74 percent of young women (ages 15–24) continue to engage in unprotected sexual activity with someone other than their primary spouse.

The island countries of southern Africa have much smaller ongoing epidemics. Madagascar, the largest of the islands, has just a 0.1 percent HIV prevalence rate. The Comoros has a rate of less than 0.1 percent; Seychelles, 0.2 percent; Mauritius, 1.8 percent; and the French colony of Réunion, less than 0.1 percent. The largest of these epidemics is on Mauritius, where INJECTION DRUG USE(R) (IDU) activities are driving the spread of the virus.

Several countries in eastern Africa have large populations of HIV-positive people: Ethiopia, 840,000; Kenya, 1.5 million; Tanzania, 1.4 million; and Uganda, 1.2 million. Other nations, such as Djibouti, Eritrea, and Somalia, have smaller epidemics, but the populations when studied demonstrated little knowledge of HIV or the means to prevent its spread. In most of Africa, the virus is predominantly spread via heterosexual activities. Evidence of changing behavior patterns has led to declining epidemics in Kenya and Uganda. Rates of HIV prevalence are higher among women in both countries. Uganda in particular has had broad success in countrywide education programs about the virus and the ways to prevent the spread. Approximately 6 percent of adults are HIV positive in both countries. Injection drug use is relatively new to Africa and is becoming more evident in the urban areas of eastern Africa. IDUs in Kenya and Mauritius report using already used injection equipment more than 80 percent of the time they inject. In Tanzania's main city, Dar es Salaam, more than 27 percent of male IDUs and 58 percent of female IDUs tested positive for HIV. More than 85 percent of the women in that particular study reported trading sex for injection drugs, a practice that increases the opportunity for the virus to spread. Activity among men who have sex with men (MSM) in Africa has been poorly studied in most cases. MSM activity is illegal in many African countries and popularly believed not to exist or to be an alien problem introduced by tourists or colonizers. However, a study cited in the 2007 UN update conducted in Kenya revealed that there was a population of more than 700 men selling sex to other men in the coastal city of Mombasa, which would indicate a steady population of people purchasing their services. In the few studies that have asked about MSM activity among Africans, it was clear that the majority also engage in regular sex with women. This situation is a possible poorly understood means of the spread of HIV on the continent.

In western Africa, the epidemic is still severe but does not show the same spread as in southern Africa. The virus is largely spread through heterosexual activities and commercial sex workers. The epidemic has leveled off in recent years, with deaths outnumbering new diagnoses. Three countries have shown decline in overall prevalence rates: Côte d'Ivoire, Burkina Faso, and Mali. Surveys in Burkina Faso and Côte d'Ivoire both indicate that women have increased the usage of condoms in their sexual behavior with nonregular partners. Nigeria has the largest epidemic in this region. Although the prevalence rate in Nigeria is only 3.6 percent of adults, it equates to nearly 3 million HIV-positive adults, owing to its large population. Several countries have not measured HIV prevalence with regularity because of civil disturbances. Known HIV prevalence rates in other countries are Central Africa Republic, 4.7 percent; Liberia, 1.5 percent; Sierra Leone, 1.6 percent; and Togo, 3.2 percent. People in some of these countries have just begun to understand the extent of the epidemic there. Rates of infection are highest among female sex workers throughout this large region, followed by pregnant women, then men. Countries with highest prevalence are the Central African Republic and Cameroon; the lowest prevalence is seen in Senegal, Niger, and Mauritania.

Overall, 5 percent of adults in Africa are HIV positive. This is by far the region with the largest number of HIV-positive people in the world. Compounding the statistics is the poverty in the region. Drugs that are available to people living in Western countries are not generally available to Africans, particularly those living in rural areas. Governments in Africa have not had the money to import large quantities of expensive antiretrovirals nor the ability to start up generic drug manufacturing companies to supply the needed medications. The UN and the United States have committed large amounts of money to provide education, medical support, and medications for the people who need assistance in Africa. The economic effect of having a large part of the adult population ill or dying is devastating. Teachers are unable to go to school. Students cannot attend classes because there is not funding to pay teachers, or they lack the time because they need to provide food for themselves and younger siblings. Food harvests have decreased in many parts of southern Africa, in part because farmers are ill or do not have the workers to harvest crops that are grown. Botswana is the first country in Africa to provide antiretrovirals to its population as needed, and is still the only one to administer medications to the majority of its population. South Africa, the richest of African nations, provides HIGHLY ACTIVE ANTIRETROVIRAL THERAPY (HAART) medications to only 28 percent of those who need it. Deaths continue to haunt all of Africa in numbers not seen since the Black Death that plagued medieval Europe. Time will tell whether the education, medications, and funding can help slow and stop the epidemic in Africa.

The Australian. "South Africa's Fatal AIDS Policies Exposed." *Australian.* Available online. URL: http://www.theaustralian.com.au/news/s-africas-fatal-aids-policies-exposed/story-e6frg6uf-1111118153037. Accessed January 24, 2011.

AVERT: AVERTing HIV and AIDS. "The HIV and AIDS Epidemic in Africa." AVERT.org. Available online. URL: http://www.avert.org/aids-hiv-africa.htm. Accessed January 24, 2011.

———. "HIV and AIDS in South Africa." AVERT.org. Available online. URL: http://www.avert.org/aidssouthafrica.htm. Accessed February 28, 2011.

BBC News. "Swazi King Drops Sex-Ban Tassels." BBC. Available online. URL: http://news.bbc.co.uk/2/hi/africa/4165432.stm. Accessed January 24, 2011.

———. "Zimbabwe's Empty Hospitals." BBC. Available online. URL: http://news.bbc.co.uk/2/hi/programmes/from_our_own_correspondent/7829180.stm. Accessed January 24, 2011.

Blomfield, Adrian. "Two-Year Sex Ban Urged in Kenya's War on AIDS." *Telegraph.* Available online. URL: http://www.telegraph.co.uk/news/worldnews/africaandindianocean/kenya/1333850/Two-year-sex-ban-urged-in-Kenyas-war-on-Aids.html. Accessed February 28, 2011.

Freitas, Tamara, Antonio Brehm, and Ana Teresa Fernandes. "Frequency of the *CCR5-Δ32* Mutation in the Atlantic Island Populations of Madeira, the Azores, Cabo Verde, and São Tomé e Príncipe." *Human Biology* 78, no. 6 (December 2006): 697–703.

Global HIV M&E Information. "Regional AIDS Observatories: An Alternative for Small Countries." Available online. URL: http://www.globalhivmeinfo.org/News/Lists/News/DispForm.aspx?ID=1. Accessed January 24, 2011.

McGreal, Chris. "Zackie Achmat: Profile." *Guardian.* Available online. URL: http://www.guardian.co.uk/world/2008/sep/12/matthiasrath.aids. Accessed January 24, 2011.

UNAIDS: Joint United Nations Programme on HIV/AIDS. "Eastern and Southern Africa." UNAIDS.org. Available online. URL: http://www.unaids.org/en/regionscountries/regions/easternandsouthernafrica/. Accessed January 24, 2011.

———. "Global Report: UNAIDS Report on the Global AIDS Epidemic 2010." UNAIDS.org. Available online. URL: http://www.unaids.org/globalreport/Global_report.htm. Accessed February 28, 2011.

———. "West and Central Africa." UNAIDS.org. Available online. URL: http://www.unaids.org/en/regionscountries/regions/westandcentralafrica/. Accessed February 28, 2011.

UNAIDS: Joint United Nations Programme on HIV/AIDS and the World Health Organization. "2007 AIDS Epidemic Update Sub-Saharan Africa." UNAIDS.org. Available online. URL: http://data.unaids.org/pub/Report/2008/jc1526_epibriefs_subsaharanafrica_en.pdf. Accessed March 22, 2011.

United Nations Development Programme. "Human Development Index." In *Human Development Report 2010—20th Anniversary.* Human Development Reports. Available online. URL: http://hdr.undp.org/en/media/HDR_2006_Tables.pdf. Accessed January 24, 2011.

University of California, San Francisco. "Sub-Saharan Africa." HIVInSite. Available online. URL: http://hivinsite.ucsf.edu/global?page=cr09-00-00. Accessed January 24, 2011.

African Americans   The term *African American* refers to people of African descent who live in the United States. The majority of African Americans are direct descendants of immigrants who were forced to enter this country during the 18th and 19th centuries, when their ancestors were forcibly enslaved in Africa and taken to the United States as laborers. Some people who call themselves African American have also arrived in the United States as immigrants from Africa more recently or have immigrated from the Caribbean, South America, or Central America, though they also have African heritage in their genetic makeup. The term encompasses a wide variety of people who have at least some ancestry based in sub-Saharan Africa. Some people prefer to use the term *black American* or *Afro-American*, as opposed to *African American*.

African Americans make up approximately 14 percent of the population of the United States. They are the largest minority group in the United States and are the second-largest racial group in the country after Americans of European or white descent. Although African Americans make up 14 percent of the overall population, they are 48 percent of the total people living with HIV in the United States and make up approximately the same total of new cases of HIV each year, according to statistical data from the U.S. CENTERS FOR DISEASE CONTROL and Prevention (CDC). Of the more than 1.1 million people living with HIV, more than 500,000 are African Americans. This is a huge disparity between the number of African Americans in the general population and the number of HIV-positive people claiming African-American descent.

In some areas of the United States, the disparity is much higher. In Washington, D.C., where HIV is endemic and 3 percent of all people are HIV positive, African Americans make up 76 percent of those totals. Studies in Chicago have shown that 30 percent of African-American MEN WHO HAVE SEX WITH MEN (MSM) are HIV positive. These statistics look closer to numbers found in sub-Saharan Africa. Statistics from most large American cities show high numbers of poor, black men and women suffering disproportionally from HIV. Black people are less likely to know their HIV status. They are less likely to be on HIGHLY ACTIVE ANTIRETROVIRAL THERAPY (HAART) medications. They are likely to have learned about their status late in the ill-

ness, after they had already had OPPORTUNISTIC INFECTIONS (OIs). They live shorter lives after learning of their HIV status. All of these points have led the CDC to explore making HIV testing a regular part of all medical exams, in doctors' offices and in emergency clinic settings, so that people become aware of their HIV status and can receive treatment when needed.

Given the long history of enslavement and economic exploitation that Americans of African descent have faced in the United States, it is not surprising that this group suffers health problems at a greater rate than the majority white population. More black Americans live in poverty than their white counterparts. More black Americans are unemployed or underemployed than white Americans. Because in the United States health insurance is still tied predominantly to being employed full time and receiving health care through private insurance, black Americans are more likely not to have health insurance and to have to pay for medical care on an as-needed basis. Fully 20 percent of African Americans do not have health insurance of any kind, either privately funded through an employer or through government programs such as Medicaid or Medicare. Even when insurance is available, the funding has not kept pace with the need for HIV medications. People are often in need of medications in the United States despite the assertion of the government that everyone is covered for HAART. States, particularly in the South, routinely turn people away from the ADAP (see AIDS DRUG ASSISTANCE PROGRAM), the HIV drug funding program, because the states do not have funds for this. All of this when combined with the strong U.S. funding of medications for people in other countries through the President's Emergency Plan for AIDS relief (PEPFAR) program has drawn anger from many in the African-American community, with calls to heal people in this country before trying to heal those in other countries.

Black Americans also have a distrust of government due to the historic mistreatment they suffered at the hands of the state and federal governments for hundreds of years. As a group, African Americans are less likely to trust government health care than other groups as a result of past government experimentation conducted on black Americans. The Tuskegee "experiment" is the most egregious of the known examples. Beginning in 1932 government health employees used black men in Alabama as living experiments by infecting them with syphilis and then followed how the disease progressed while telling the people involved in the experiment that they were receiving treatment for the illness. This and other known governmental mistreatment cause African Americans to view with skepticism government warnings on HIV. A survey conducted by Oregon State University and published in 2005 showed that fully 48 percent of African Americans believed that HIV was a government-generated virus. More than half of the people in that survey believed that the government had a cure for HIV but was withholding that cure from black and poor people. Smaller but significant percentages believed that HIV was created as part of a plot by the Central Intelligence Agency (CIA) or that the government had created the virus in order to kill black people. Working to educate those who have a long mistrust of the people doing the educating has proven difficult simply because the barriers to overcome are built on proven exploitation in the past.

Since the beginning of the epidemic, African Americans have been affected by HIV and AIDS. Some of the first people affected were Haitian immigrants in New York City as well as black MSM. The first cases of HIV among WOMEN were recorded in 1983, and of two cases that were first recorded one was an African-American woman. Since then African-American women have suffered disproportionally more than other women in the United States with HIV. Today nearly 60 percent of all women living with HIV are black, and black women face an estimated lifetime risk of one in 30 of becoming HIV positive. In comparison, the current lifetime risk for a white woman is one in 588. Black women represent

36 percent of the total cases of HIV among African Americans. This is significantly higher than the 15 percent of the total number of cases that white women represent among white Americans. African-American women are overwhelmingly infected through heterosexual contact: 75 percent. The remaining numbers were predominantly infected through injection drug use (IDU) (see INJECTION DRUG USER. HIV has exacted a heavy toll on black women. It is currently the leading cause of death among black women ages 25–34 in the United States and the third leading cause of death among black women ages 35–44.

African-American MSM are also more likely to be infected than their white MSM counterparts. Surveys have shown extremely high rates of HIV among black MSM in several large cities. Although black MSM do not make up the largest percentage of the epidemic in the black community, nonetheless a large percentage of black MSM are HIV positive. Black gay men face harsh family and community discrimination and condemnation for their behavior. Many studies cite black men who state that they remain hidden from the mainstream gay communities so that they do not appear "gay" to their family and friends. This led to the stories of men on the down low—men who engage in MSM activities but remain married to women—that filled the media in the late 1990s and early 2000s. Studies have shown that there is no more significant amount of men on the down low among black Americans than among white Americans, and that this small portion of the population could not have led to the high numbers of HIV-positive people among the African-American population.

Initially, most HIV research was conducted on white gay males, because this group was predominantly seen as the group affected by HIV and they volunteered to submit to experimental drugs and treatments. As time has gone on, the racial disparity in research trials for HIV treatments and drugs has decreased, and the populations affected, including women and men from all affected groups, are now taking part. Black participants now make up approximately 50 percent of people volunteering in HIV research trials. This has led to some previously unknown findings. One discovery has been that certain HIV antiretrovirals are metabolized more slowly in Americans of African descent. In particular, EFAVIRENZ is absorbed more slowly, and this characteristic can lead to more side effects associated with efavirenz such as the nightmares and other central nervous system issues that are reported among some people. It has also led to the discovery that Americans of African descent carry genetic markers that make them more susceptible to kidney disease than white Americans. Some HIV medications affect the kidneys more than others, and treatment can be adjusted now to match these markers if they become evident through testing.

African Americans are more aware than other groups of the risks and preventive measures needed to fight HIV. They are more likely to have been tested for HIV than other people in the United States, yet the statistics still show how devastating this disease has been in the black community. The reasons are for the most part socioeconomic. Poverty can lead people to avoid medical care altogether to focus on the need for food, shelter, or companionship. Studies conducted among young people in some urban centers have indicated that young black men and women feel very little hope that they will escape the poverty they have grown up with and do not believe they will live long enough to escape the inner city. This creates a ripe environment for HIV spread, as these same youngsters are not concerned about an illness that may or may not eventually kill them, since they see no future. Another factor in the spread of HIV is the fact that one in 20 black men currently spends some period in PRISONS. Prison life is rough and includes extensive drug use and the potential for the spread of HIV among men, who, when released to the community, spread the virus to others. Studies of this phenomenon have been inconclusive. Some claim it is a cause of the spread of HIV; others claim the numbers of HIV positive people in prison were already positive before arriving and that they could not account for the spread continuing on the outside.

Given the numerous socioeconomic reasons that contribute to the spread of HIV and the obvious needs for medications and better access to health care, it is clear that the African-American community has the greatest need for funding, outreach, and education in the future. The stigma of the disease and its causes are something all communities in the United States must discuss, but particularly in the African-American community, where it has been so devastating in its reach.

AVERT: AVERTing HIV and AIDS. "HIV and AIDS among African Americans." AVERT.org. Available online. URL: http://www.avert.org/hiv-african-americans.htm. Accessed March 7, 2011.

Black AIDS Institute. "The Black AIDS Institute." BlackAIDS.org. Available online. URL: http://www.blackaids.org/. Accessed March 11, 2011.

TheBody.com and Kimberly Smith, M.D. "Why There's Such an HIV/AIDS Disparity among U.S. Blacks and Hispanics—and What to Do about It." TheBody.com. Available online. URL: http://www.thebody.com/content/art55578.html?mvg. Accessed March 5, 2011.

Centers for Disease Control and Prevention. "2009 HIV/AIDS Surveillance Report: Vol. 21." CDC.gov. Available online. URL: http://www.cdc.gov/hiv/surveillance/resources/reports/2009report/index.htm. Accessed March 7, 2011.

Charles, Katie. "African-Americans with HIV Are More Susceptible to Type of Kidney Disease Known as HIVAN." *NY Daily News.* Available online. URL: http://www.nydailynews.com/lifestyle/health/2009/07/22/2009-07-22_africanamericans_with_hiv_are_more_susceptible_to_.html. Accessed March 11, 2011.

Fears, Darryl. "Study: Many Blacks Cite AIDS Conspiracy." *Washington Post.* Available online. URL: http://www.washingtonpost.com/wp-dyn/articles/A33695-2005Jan24.html. Accessed March 11, 2011.

Fullilove, Robert E. *African Americans, Health Disparities and HIV/AIDS: Recommendations for Confronting the Epidemic in Black America.* Washington, D.C.: National Minority AIDS Council. November 2006.

Available online. URL: http://www.nmac.org/index/cms-filesystem-action?file=grpp/african%20americans,%20health%20disparities%20and%20hiv/aids.pdf. Accessed July 22, 2011.

Henry J. Kaiser Family Foundation. "HIV/AIDS Policy Fact Sheet: Black Americans and HIV/AIDS." KFF.org. Available online. URL: http://www.kff.org/hivaids/upload/6089-07.pdf. Accessed March 5, 2011.

Thomas, Monifa. "Chicago: 17% of Gay Men Here HIV-Positive, New Stats Confirm." *Chicago Sun-Times,* 27 August 2009. EATG.org. Available online. URL: http://www.eatg.org/eatg/Global-HIV-News/Epidemiology/Chicago-17-of-gay-men-here-HIV-positive-new-stats-confirm. Accessed March 5, 2011.

Vargas, Jose Antonio, and Darryl Fears. "At Least 3 Percent of D.C. Residents Have HIV or AIDS, City Study Finds; Rate Up 22% from 2006." *Washington Post.* Available online. URL: http://www.washingtonpost.com/wp-dyn/content/article/2009/03/14/AR2009031402176.html. Accessed March 5, 2011.

AIDS AIDS is the acronym for acquired immunodeficiency syndrome. A syndrome is a collection of symptoms, characteristics, or phenomena that occur together to make up a particular illness or disease. In Spanish the acronym for the condition is SIDA (*síndrome de inmunodeficiencia adquirida*). AIDS is caused by the HUMAN IMMUNODEFICIENCY VIRUS (HIV) and is the result of the virus's attacking and weakening the immune system so that a variety of OPPORTUNISTIC INFECTIONS (OIs) may then cause illness in a person.

Symptoms and Diagnostic Path

AIDS itself does not have any symptoms because it is a collection of potential illnesses that have a variety of symptoms. Normally these illnesses do not develop in people who have healthy immune systems. Infections in people who have AIDS vary from person to person and depend on variables such as gender, geographic location, and prior exposure to other viruses, parasites, fungi, or bacteria. These OIs are most often controlled in people who have a healthy immune system. In general, systemic signs and symptoms of infection such as fevers, night sweats, swollen lymph glands, chills, weakness, exhaustion, and weight loss can be used to begin a diagnosis for AIDS.

There are three major definitions used in assigning the diagnosis of AIDS in a patient. In the United States, the CENTERS FOR DISEASE CONTROL (CDC) Classification System for HIV Infection provides a case definition for AIDS and for statistical purposes allows the tracking of AIDS case numbers within the country. The WORLD HEALTH ORGANIZATION (WHO) disease staging system for HIV infection and disease and the Bangui definition are used in other parts of the world to define and diagnose a person as having AIDS and for compiling statistics. Both the WHO and the CDC definitions rely on testing for HIV (see HIV TESTS) in the patient's blood. The Bangui definition is based on the systemic signs and the presence of one or more OIs and is generally used in regions where medical testing for HIV is not readily available. Both the WHO and the CDC have different guidelines for the definition and diagnosis of AIDS in children.

The CDC definition identifies a person as having AIDS when he or she tests positive for HIV in the blood and has fewer than 200 CD4 T lymphocytes (CD4) per microliter of blood, or a CD4 T lymphocyte percentage of total lymphocytes of less than 14 percent. A person can also be classified as having AIDS if he or she tests positive for HIV and has any of the more than 20 OIs and other clinical condidtions listed in the CDC case definition. In the United States, once a person has been diagnosed as having AIDS, the diagnosis remains even if the person recovers from the AIDS-defining conditions and his or her CD4 count returns to a number higher than 200 or a CD4 percentage greater than 14.

In the United States, testing centers operate in public health clinics, doctors' offices, and many nonprofit AIDS SERVICE ORGANIZATIONS in urban and rural areas of the country. Being tested for HIV, and indirectly for AIDS, can provide a person with the knowledge needed to treat the syndrome before it becomes dangerous or debilitating. It will also give the person knowledge of the condition to prevent inadvertently exposing others to the virus through the person's activities.

Treatment Options and Outlook

Currently there is no known cure for AIDS. There are numerous medications that can be used to treat HIV and the clinical conditions. If an individual is diagnosed as having AIDS, then treatment is immediately begun to treat any known infections as well as treatment to stop the virus from reproducing in the body. Treatment also to prevent OIs may be started in some cases.

At the start of the epidemic, there were no drugs to treat people diagnosed with AIDS. There was no known cause, and, therefore, nothing to treat it existed. Many thousands of people died before a virus was found to be the cause of the immune system failures. OIs were generally illnesses that were rarely or never seen in such large numbers of patients, and treatment for these illnesses did not exist either. As more was learned about the syndrome, physicians began treating the OIs where that was possible. Pharmaceutical companies began to produce treatments for the various OIs that greatly extended the life expectancy of people who had AIDS. During the nearly 30-year course of the epidemic so far, doctors have learned a great deal both about HIV as well as about the numerous OIs so that treatment is available for most people even if diagnosis of HIV infection is not made until a person becomes ill.

Today there are drugs in several different classes that can combat the virus's ability to reproduce, thereby greatly extending the life expectancy of someone who has been diagnosed with AIDS. NUCLEOSIDE REVERSE TRANSCRIPTASE INHIBITORS (NRTIs), NON-NUCLEOSIDE REVERSE TRANSCRIPTASE INHIBITORS (NNRTIs), PROTEASE INHIBITORS (PIs), NUCLEOTIDE REVERSE TRANSCRIPTASE INHIBITORS (NtRTIs), INTEGRASE INHIBITORS, MATURATION INHIBITORS, ENTRY INHIBITORS, and other classes of drugs have greatly improved the life of an AIDS patient. At the start of the epidemic, it was said that a person diagnosed with AIDS had a life expectancy of two years, if the OIs were treated. Now, access to treatment and a patient's dedication to taking prescribed medications can extend a patient's life far beyond the two years of a generation ago. When the virus can be suppressed to an undetectable level and treatment of the OIs is successful, an AIDS patient can expect to live a fairly normal life.

Risk Factors and Preventive Measures

The greatest risk factor for AIDS is not being treated after testing positive for HIV. Once diagnosed with AIDS, then treatment can both stop the virus from worsening the immune system function and help prevent OIs from taking hold or recurring.

Preventing exposure to HIV can be accomplished by many means. Abstinence is the only known sure preventive for avoiding sexual exposure to HIV but is rarely practiced beyond adolescence by most people in the world. By far the greatest preventive measure is to wear a condom during sexual intercourse, whether vaginal or anal. Oral sex can also spread HIV if a person has any open cuts or sores on the genitals or mouth and gums. Other measures include not reusing dirty or used needles by INJECTION DRUG USE(R)S (IDU) and avoiding direct exposure to blood by health care employees or people who work with people who are bleeding. Using latex or polyurethane gloves and protective goggles and gowns helps protect medical employees when working with any patient who might be bleeding. HIV-positive mothers can prevent the spread of HIV to babies by not BREAST-FEEDING, as HIV is present in mother's milk.

There are many ways an individual can help keep a healthy immune system and encourage the body to fight HIV once exposed to the virus. Exercise, good nutrition, and smoking cessation are three known ways to increase health in general and to keep a person healthy after testing positive for HIV.

National Center for Infectious Diseases. "1993 Revised Classification System for HIV Infection and Expanded Surveillance Case Definition for AIDS among Adolescents and Adults." CDC.gov. Available online. URL: http://www.cdc.gov/mmwr/preview/ mmwrhtml/00018871.htm. Accessed March 5, 2011.

Susman, Ed. "HIV Life Expectancy Now Normal." United Press International in TerraDaily: News about Planet Earth.com. Available online. URL: http:// www.terradaily.com/reports/HIV_Life_Expectancy _Now_Normal_999.html. Accessed March 5, 2011.

World Health Organization. "Interim WHO Clinical Staging of HIV/AIDS and HIV/AIDS Case Definitions for Surveillance." WHO.int. Available online. URL: http://www.who.int/hiv/pub/guidelines/clinical staging.pdf. Accessed March 5, 2011.

AIDS Coalition to Unleash Power (ACT UP)

ACT UP is an AIDS activist organization founded in New York City in March 1987. It was created to draw attention to the AIDS epidemic, because the founders thought that the U.S. government, led by the Reagan administration, was indifferent at best to the mounting crisis. ACT UP formed a week after the author and playwright Larry Kramer challenged those attending a regular speaker series event at the New York Lesbian and Gay Community Services Center to form a political action group to handle the crisis. Kramer was disappointed that the Gay Men's Health Crisis (GMHC), a group he had helped found a few years previously, seemed unable to handle the political aspects of the epidemic and focused instead on social and financial concerns of individuals.

ACT UP quickly became an active force in moving the discussion of AIDS into press and governmental offices, where it had been absent to that point. It was largely made up of young gay men and lesbians who believed that direct action was the answer to the serious lack of funding and services needed in reaction to this epidemic. Initially, meetings were held at the New York Lesbian and Gay Services Center, but interest soon outgrew the space available there. Meetings moved to auditoriums at Cooper Union, a college in Lower Manhattan. Close to 800 people would show up for the weekly meetings, which often included extensive planning of various protest actions as well as sharing enthusiastic energy that kept people excited about the helpful role they were playing in the epidemic. It was often the only enthusiasm people would feel during the ongoing epidemic, as friends, neighbors, and loved ones were dying on a grand scale. ACT UP mobilized the despair and anger of members to be put to effective demonstrations and disruptions that brought about real changes in the course of the epidemic and the nation's response. The ability to mobilize these angry people easily also rested on the fact that many members of ACT UP were people who had HIV or AIDS and considered these actions their only hope to achieve better treatment, access to medications, and health care that they needed.

The first action for ACT UP took place on March 24, 1987, a protest at the intersection of Broadway and Wall Street in Manhattan. Protesters blocked traffic for several hours while handing out flyers describing the need for a policy on HIV treatment from the government, as well as better and quicker access to medications being developed for the treatment of HIV. There were 17 arrests that day. Larry Kramer had published an editorial the previous day in the *New York Times* explaining his anger and the anger of many people against the U.S. FOOD AND DRUG ADMINISTRATION (FDA), the City of New York and Mayor Ed Koch, and the federal government and President Ronald Reagan. Reagan had yet even to mention the term *AIDS* in a speech or public meeting, although 35,000 people had died by this time in the epidemic. ACT UP insisted that HIV-positive people be part of the education, research, and prevention decisions being made in Washington, D.C. They also insisted that potential AIDS drugs be made available immediately, as people were dying at a rate faster than regular governmental approval time frames could combat.

Other well-known protests included an event at Northwest Airlines to denounce their actions in refusing to issue a seat to a man with

AIDS, and a protest of the magazine *Cosmopolitan* in 1988 because an article in the publication stated that heterosexual women need not be concerned about contracting AIDS if they had healthy genitals. More than 150 women picketed the *Cosmopolitan* offices at the Hearst Building, drawing a large media presence to the demonstration. The text of the article was eventually retracted by *Cosmopolitan* for inaccuracies. In October 1988, during the second full display of the AIDS Memorial Quilt, ACT UP members attempted to shut down the FDA and the agency's headquarters in Bethesda, Maryland. Signs resembling tombstones, adorned with such phrases as "I got the placebo" and "I died for the sins of the FDA," were commonly seen in the crowd of approximately 1,000 participants. Activists staged what became known as die-ins, where a person simply lies down and pretends to be dead. Activists did this in front of building doors, in the street, with many holding the tombstones. Traffic was blocked, entrances to the building were effectively obstructed, and media attention from all over the world was drawn to the ACT UP demonstration. More than 150 people were arrested. In 1989, four ACT UP members were arrested for barricading themselves in the Burroughs Wellcome offices in North Carolina. Burroughs Wellcome was the manufacturer of azidothymidine, now zidovudine (AZT), at that time the only drug that had been found to be at all effective in controlling HIV. Burroughs Wellcome was often a target of protests, as the company charged $188 per bottle of 100 pills, or $7,000–$10,000 per person per year for the drug AZT, although most people who had HIV at the time had lost their jobs and medical insurance because of fears and discrimination based on the illness. In December 1989, several thousand ACT UP members and friends went to St. Patrick's Cathedral in Midtown Manhattan during a mass to demonstrate against the Roman Catholic Church's vocal opposition to SAFER SEX education and the use of condoms to protect people from the virus. Many protest-

ers entered the church, eventually disrupting the Communion being given by Cardinal John Joseph O'Connor, and more than 100 people were arrested. In 1992, during another full display of the AIDS quilt, protesters broke through police barricades and dumped the ashes of people who had died of AIDS on the front lawn of the White House.

ACT UP served a variety of purposes, not the least of which was to train a whole generation of activists in a wide range of social change concepts and social advocacy. Members who started in ACT UP went on to form numerous AIDS SERVICE ORGANIZATIONS, as well as work as advisers to government agencies and research groups and to found new groups to serve the community. When ACT UP held their first protest in 1987, the annual budget for HIV and AIDS research was $290 million, and AZT was the only antiretroviral medication approved for the treatment of HIV. In 2009, the proposed budget for AIDS research of all kinds was $3 billion, and there were five classes of antiretrovirals, offering a wide variety of treatment options for patients. When ACT UP started their work, the governmental process for drug approval took seven or eight years, an interval that most ACT UP members and their friends could not afford to wait. The process was generally closed to the public, and the community had no voice with either the drug company or the government in how drug trials or drug development was handled. Now, drug approval can take three years of responsible, successful trials, and a drug can receive advance approval for use. Currently, it is expected that the government will have community members representing the affected communities on advisory boards, research groups, and drug company panels. ACT UP members went from feeling helpless about their situation to feeling empowered that their actions led to changes in the ways both the drug companies and the government were reacting to the disease.

Above all else, ACT UP did exactly what it had set out to do: draw attention to the fact that that tens of thousands of people at that time were sick and dying, and no one was paying any attention because of the communities that were affected. Newspapers began covering the disruptions, the die-ins, the brash interruptions to what was normal, and attention was given to the virus and the people who were affected. The initial demonstrations were so successful that ACT UP groups sprang up in cities across the United States and in Europe. The group itself was set up in a democratic grassroots manner. There was no one person in charge. Meetings often lasted hours, as all were allowed to speak if they chose, and decisions were made on a consensus basis. ACT UP in one city might decide differently how to approach a problem than ACT UP in another city. Protests and actions were rarely coordinated among the different groups, and this often led to infighting among them. One group often tried to outdo another with brash and loud tactics. Bridges were blocked in San Francisco, city council meetings were disrupted across the country, church services were interrupted, Wall Street traffic was closed by marchers, and scientific conventions interrupted. By 1990, it was common to see the ACT UP–created image/words "Silence = Death" plastered on anything that did not move in a city of any reasonable size.

By the late 1990s, most ACT UP groups had disbanded or simply ceased to exist. In part, this was because of the changes to HIV research and funding that the actions had brought about. It was also due to the death of many members who fought for public acknowledgment and discussion but would not live to see the changes they helped create. Other members, as noted, took the energy from the streets to the government and corporate boardrooms, where they were able to provide a voice and a direction to fighting the epidemic that was so badly needed when the group was formed. Other groups such as Queer Nation took the strategies learned from ACT UP and applied them to their own efforts Although often despised by some people and vilified in conservative circles, ACT UP served a specific purpose that was greatly needed and will be remembered for achieving the goals it initially set for itself.

ACT UP: AIDS Coalition to Unleash Power. "ACT UP/New York." ACTUPNY.org. http://www.actupny.org/. Accessed March 5, 2011.

glbtq: an encyclopedia of gay, lesbian, bisexual, transgender, and queer culture. "ACT UP." Glbtq.com. Available online. URL: http://www.glbtq.com/social-sciences/act_up.html. Accessed March 5, 2011.

Kramer, Larry. "The F.D.A.'s Callous Response to AIDS." *New York Times* (23 March 1987), p. A19.

———. "Larry Kramer Gets Angry." POZ.com. Available online. URL: http://www.poz.com/articles/238_1700.shtml. Accessed March 11, 2011.

National Institutes of Health. "Office of AIDS Research Trans-NIH AIDS Research Budget." NIH.gov. Available online. URL: http://www.oar.nih.gov/budget/pdf/OAR10CJ.pdf. Accessed March 11, 2011.

Rimmerman, Craig A. "ACT UP." TheBody.com. Available online. URL: http://www.thebody.com/content/art14001.html. Accessed March 5, 2011.

Wheeler, Lorna. "ACT UP." In *LGBTQ America Today: An Encyclopedia.* Westport, Conn.: Greenwood Press, 2009, 1:10–12.

AIDS dissenters AIDS dissenters are people who do not believe that the HUMAN IMMUNODEFICIENCY VIRUS (HIV) is the cause of AIDS. It has been nearly 30 years since AIDS first began affecting people and nearly 25 years since the virus that causes AIDS was discovered and a test was developed to detect it. Some people, however, remain convinced that HIV has never been proven to be a cause of the symptoms and illnesses of AIDS. They are also known as AIDS denialists.

There are several individuals and groups who have over the years taken the view that AIDS is not caused by HIV. One individual in particular who has always been at the forefront of this view is Peter Duesberg, a virologist at the University of California, Berkeley. He has authored articles and books with another California professor, David Rasnick, espousing their views. Many of the groups in the United States and Europe that deny the HIV connection to AIDS use his work as their main argument. Duesberg had been a well-respected researcher and is a member of the National Academy of Sciences. His ongoing claims regarding HIV and AIDS, however, have provoked derision from almost all other scientists and researchers in the field.

In the early years of AIDS science, there was little information to go on besides reports of the illnesses that were killing people and the connections that could be seen visibly among those individuals. Many "theories" for the cause of AIDS were put forward. Some people believed that AIDS was caused by overuse of recreational drugs. Others thought it was simply a disease or diseases that had been around for thousands of years that were being labeled with a new name. Some viewed the illness as a plot by various governments to rid themselves of a minority population or group that was seen as a threat in some way. Some considered the illness a result of poor nutrition. All of these reasons for denying that HIV causes AIDS continue to be found on many Internet sites maintained by a variety of people and groups.

The most common argument that Duesberg and similar dissidents used, and still use despite evidence to the contrary, was that identifying HIV as the cause of AIDS did not meet Koch's postulates. This is a theory presented in 1876 by a scientist named Robert Koch, which identifies the four steps used to show that a specific pathogen, a germ of some type, definitely causes a particular illness. The four steps are:

1. The same pathogen must be seen in every case of the illness studied.
2. The pathogen must be isolated and grown in the laboratory, away from the person infected.
3. The laboratory-grown pathogen must cause infection in a healthy person injected with the pathogen.
4. The pathogen must then be isolated and grown from the healthy person who was infected by experimental injection.

By 1983, the first two of Koch's postulates were satisfied as scientists in France and the United States isolated HIV from people who were ill and were able eventually to grow the pathogen outside the infected patients. However, satisfying postulates three and four was difficult, as it is unethical to infect another person with a virus that theoretically is deadly with no cure, and there was a lack of animals that could be tested with the virus as the only animals susceptible to HIV proved to be chimpanzees. Chimpanzees are not usually used as laboratory test animals. However, by the late 1990s, these postulates had been satisfied through medical workers who had accidently stuck themselves with needles while conducting experiments with HIV and had become infected. Testing proved that the specific type of the virus they were infected with matched the virus they had been working with when infected. Although Koch's postulates have been met, as shown by several cited sources, some dissenters ignore this fact and continue to cite this reason as denial that HIV causes AIDS.

Other dissenters focus on the high proportion of people who have AIDS and have used recreational drugs during their lifetime. They believe that there is a connection between the constant use of drugs such as amyl nitrate, also known as poppers, and HIV. This theory has been proven untrue, as many people infected with HIV who have had various OPPORTUNISTIC INFECTIONS (OIs) have never used amyl nitrate or other recreational drugs.

South Africa, particularly under the leadership of the former president Thabo Mbeki, encouraged the belief that HIV was caused through poor nutrition or that it was caused by Western governments that were trying to rid the world of Africans. The South African minister of health under Mr. Mbeki, Dr. Mantombazana "Manto" Tshabalala-Msimang, was well known to advocate the use of beetroot and garlic, as well as other natural vegetables and herbs, as a cure for AIDS. For many years, her beliefs and those of Mr. Mbeki prevented South Africa from adopting policies to allow the use of anti-retroviral medications by people in the country receiving government health care. It is believed that these decisions cost the lives of more than 300,000 South Africans from 2000 to 2005. When Mr. Mbeki was replaced as president in 2008, Dr. Tshabalala-Msimang was removed from the post of minister of health.

Other dissenter organizations state that the antiretroviral medications themselves "cause" AIDS and are a plot by multinational pharmaceutical companies to create a market for unneeded medications. Although the initial use of antiretrovirals was not necessarily as successful as some had hoped, it was shown that well-studied, properly used antiretrovirals prevented HIV-positive people from developing OIs over the long term and improved the health of the majority of HIV-positive people when taken properly. Initially, antiretrovirals were taken individually, not as a combination. It has been shown that therapy with only one antiretroviral, known as monotherapy, is not generally helpful except in the prevention of HIV transmission from mother to fetus. Monotherapy allows the virus to mutate, and the drug quickly becomes ineffective against the mutated virus.

There are any number of other reasons cited in dissenters' arguments that HIV does not cause AIDS. None of the reasons or arguments has been shown to be true in the face of scientific studies of the virus, treatment therapies, or causal connections. It has been shown that the continued spread of dissenter myths actually causes unnecessary suffering, continued spread of the virus, and many deaths each year as people ignore facts about the spread of the virus or its treatment.

AIDSTruth.org: The scientific evidence for HIV/AIDS. "HIV/AIDS Science." AIDSTruth.org. Available online. URL: http://www.aidstruth.org/science. Accessed March 11, 2011.

Duesberg, Peter H. "Duesberg on AIDS." Duesberg.com. Available online. URL: http://www.duesberg.com/. Accessed March 11, 2011.

Gallo, Robert C., and Luc Montagnier. "The Discovery of HIV as the Cause of AIDS." NEJM.org. Available online. URL: http://content.nejm.org/cgi/content/full/349/24/2283. Accessed March 11, 2011.

Hemmingsen, Barbara B. "The Odd Claim of the HIV Dissenters: HIV Does Not Cause AIDS; A Critical Evaluation of Their Arguments." *Rational Inquiry* 6, no. 4 (2001). Available online. URL: http://sdari.org/documents/v6n4hiv.html. Accessed March 11, 2011.

Mirken, Bruce. "Answering the AIDS Denialists: Is AIDS Real?" *AIDS Treatment News* 356 (1 December 2000). AEGIS.com. Available online. URL: http://www.aegis.org/pubs/atn/2000/ATN35606.html. Accessed March 11, 2011.

Moroney, Robin. "The Rise of the AIDS Dissenters." *Wall Street Journal,* 4 March 2007. AEGIS.com. Available online. URL: http://www.aegis.org/news/wsj/2007/WJ070301.html. Accessed March 11, 2011.

Nair, Nivashni, and Werner Swart. "Mbeki 'must account for 330,000 deaths.'" *Sunday Times (Johannesburg)* (7 November 2008). AEGIS.com. Available online. URL: http://www.aegis.com/news/suntimes/2008/ST081104.html. Accessed March 11, 2011.

National Institute of Allergy and Infectious Diseases. "The Evidence That HIV Causes AIDS." NIH.gov. Available online. URL: http://www.niaid.nih.gov/topics/hivaids/understanding/howhivcausesaids/pages/hivcausesaids.aspx. Accessed March 11, 2011.

AIDS Drug Assistance Program (ADAP)   ADAP is a federally sponsored program that provides for the prescription medications for low-income individuals who have HIV and do not have the means of paying for their medications. ADAP is a $1.4 billion program that receives both federal and state funding and is nearly one-third of the costs in the current Ryan White CARE (Comprehensive AIDS Resources Emergency) Act, which is the legislation that created ADAP. It is a federally mandated program that each of the 50 states must have and is also available in the District of Columbia and U.S. territories. Approximately 80 percent of ADAP funding is from the federal government, but ADAP is run individually in each state or territory, which must provide the remainder of the ADAP funding.

Each state has its own guidelines to determine who is qualified to receive medications through the program. Each state maintains a list of medications that they will pay for and those that will not be funded. Funding for the states and territories is based on the number of cases of AIDS and HIV in relation to the total number of cases across the country. ADAPs cover not only antiretroviral medications in HIGHLY ACTIVE ANTIRETROVIRAL TREATMENT (HAART), but also antibiotics that are used to treat OPPORTUNISTIC INFECTIONS (OIs), as well as substance abuse and mental health treatments. Some states use their ADAP funds to pay for continuing private insurance for people who are eligible to continue a private insurance prescription plan but may not have the financial means to continue paying the monthly fees.

In 2007, the last year for which statistics are available, 183,000 people across the country were covered under the various ADAP programs. This represents about one-third of all people receiving HIV care in the United States. More than 70 percent of people using ADAP are considered low-income, which is defined as a level of income of 200 percent of the Federal Poverty Level (FPL). FPL varies, depending on the size of a family. In 2009, for a family of one, the poverty level was $10,210. More than 70 percent of the people on ADAP do not have insurance of any kind. Eligibility varies from state to state, and individual states set guidelines for how poor a person must be to receive funding for ADAP benefits. There are seven states that allow a level of income of 500 percent of FPL to qualify for assistance. Both of these numbers are higher than the eligibility for Medicaid coverage, which also will pay for HIV medications if the person is eligible. States pay for drugs in some combination of three ways: through direct purchase, which then requires some manner of distribution; through existing pharmacies or mail order and through paying prescription drug insurance plan costs for individuals, which allows individuals to continue to receive the drugs through their insurance plans; or through rebates, which allow the local pharmacies to handle the paperwork of the ADAP, pay for the drugs directly, and then receive rebates from the pharmaceutical companies.

In addition to funding from Ryan White monies and state support, some funding is derived from rebates from pharmaceutical companies based on purchasing in bulk or through state purchasing mechanisms to save money. More than 20 percent of the 2007 ADAP funding, a significant increase from previous years, was obtained through this method. Despite the cost savings this provided for some states, several states still had waiting lists for people to be eligible for ADAP. What this means is that people in need of medications were unable to pay for them as individuals and did not qualify for ADAP programs because of limits to the available funds in several states. Reports from several states indicated that state ADAPs would have significantly reduced budgets in 2011 and 2012 due to the economic depression the country is currently suffering.

The ADAP program was born out of the AIDS Drug Reimbursement Program, which was started in 1987 when ZIDOVUDINE (AZT) first was approved as a treatment for HIV. The drug was initially priced at $10,000 a year, lowered to $8,000 a year after initial complaints, but still out of reach for most people who had AIDS at the time because most had lost their jobs and insurance as a result of their illness. The funds were provided to all 50 states through the U.S. Health Resources and Services Administration. The funds were transferred in 1990 to be part of the first Ryan White CARE (Comprehensive AIDS Resources Emergency) Act, where it has been funded since. In 1996, as part of the first reauthorization of the Ryan White Act, the U.S. Congress specifically earmarked money to be set aside for funding the ADAP program. In 2006, the most recent reauthorization stated that 75 percent of funding was to be spent on "core medical services," which included medications, outpatient and ambulatory medical services, mental health services, substance abuse services, hospice care, early intervention services, and home health care. The most recent reauthorization for the program took effect in September 2009 and runs for four years.

As the population of HIV-positive people continues to grow by an estimated 50,000 people each year in the United States, according to the CENTERS FOR DISEASE CONTROL and Prevention (CDC), and the extended lifespan that someone with HIV now has because of the available treatment, the cost has risen for ADAP and the need continues to exceed the resources available. Another drawback to ADAP has been that each state can draw up its own formulary, which means the states can decide which drugs they will pay for and which ones they will not. Puerto Rico and 21 states do not make all the current antiretrovirals available for people through ADAP. Rules requiring that ADAPs cover at least one antiretroviral in each drug class were put into place with the 2006 reauthorization of the program. This allowance still does not provide for people who are unable to take particular drugs or whose virus has become resistant to the drugs that a particular ADAP pays for, thus putting them in the situation where they must either use medication that is not fully effective or stop medication altogether.

Another concern for reauthorization of ADAP services is that the CDC is pushing new testing policies they believe will help locate what they estimate to be approximately 230,000 people who are currently HIV positive but do not know they are. If numbers remain consistent, and estimates from the Congressional Budget Office confirm this estimate, then approximately 25 percent of these people will need to use ADAP to receive their medications. This large cost increase will place a burden on the ADAP services at a time when many states are cutting their funding to the program because of budgetary woes. President Obama's health reform plan has some provisions that may help ADAPs in the long run. The proposal being debated in Congress would close the loophole requiring people insured under Medicare to pay out-of-pocket

expenses of more than $4,500, a coverage gap referred to as the donut hole. It will allow people in ADAPs to become eligible for Medicare by allowing ADAPs to pay the cost of the donut hole. It is unclear how the Obama plan will affect the renewal of the Ryan White CARE Act. Forty-five percent of HIV-positive people in the United States live below the FPL, and more than 50 percent do not have medical insurance of any kind. The Obama plan may extend some hope of helping HIV-positive people seek and receive medical care before they become severely disabled and receive medications when needed without a period on a waiting list, as has occurred since the ADAP program began.

Health Resources and Services Administration. "The HIV/AIDS Program: Ryan White Parts A–F." HRSA. gov. Available online. URL: http://hab.hrsa.gov/treatmentmodernization/adap.htm. Accessed March 11, 2011.
Henry J. Kaiser Family Foundation and National Alliance of State and Territorial AIDS Directors. "National ADAP Monitoring Project Annual Report: April 2009." KFF.org. Available online. URL: http://www.kff.org/hivaids/upload/7861.pdf. Accessed March 11, 2011.
McColl, William, and Carl Schmid. "AIDS Drug Assistance Program: Securing HIV/AIDS Drugs for the Nation's Poor and Uninsured." AIDSACTION.org. Available online. URL: http://www.aidsaction.org/attachments/509_aids_drug_assistance_program.pdf. Accessed July 25, 2011.
Scholl, Diana. "Housing Works News & Press: House Health Care Bill Gets Props." HousingWorks.com. Available online. URL: http://www.housingworks.org/news-press/detail/house-health-care-bill-gets-props/. Accessed March 11, 2011.

AIDS service organization (ASO) An AIDS service organization (ASO) is a community-based and -run organization dedicated to serving HIV-positive people in some manner. Some ASOs provide education and prevention services; others provide direct services such as food, medications, medical needs, legal assistance, or housing.

At the beginning of the epidemic in the United States, there was little governmental support or public awareness regarding HIV or the epidemic that was happening in the gay communities across the country. Small, community-based organizations began appearing in larger cities in neighborhoods that had significant gay populations. The first such organization, Gay Men's Health Crisis (GMHC), was founded in 1981 in part by the author Larry Kramer in New York City's Greenwich Village neighborhood. GMHC provided whatever services it could arrange: food, medical services, housing, home care, and support for people who were ill or who had lost jobs because they were sick or discriminated against because they had AIDS or were believed to have AIDS. The GMHC model of services was copied throughout the United States in the initial years of the epidemic, as it provided a wide range of services through its office.

In the initial years of the epidemic, people who had HIV and AIDS were often refused services at organizations that provided these services in general for a variety of reasons. There was a great deal of stigma related to being HIV positive or having AIDS. It was believed by many people that AIDS was caused by sexual deviance, illegal drug use, or illegal sex work. The climate among many social service–providing agencies was that these issues were not ones they wanted to deal with, and so services were not provided. Other people were discriminated against because of the fear that simply being in the same room could spread AIDS from one person to another. Even hospitals had difficulties at times finding nursing staff to work with AIDS patients because of fears that the illness would be spread to them through close contact. For these reasons, gay men, the largest percentage of the people who had HIV for the first decade of the epidemic, often formed groups of volunteers with friends and supporters who created organizations that were solely run to serve people with HIV and AIDS who needed assistance.

One program that in particular drew people into volunteering were the AIDS Buddy programs that sprouted up around the country. People were trained in how to assist individuals with all manner of possible tasks and then were assigned to an individual who needed assistance. Tasks that a buddy helped with ran from simple visitation to becoming the primary caregiver for an individual who could no longer leave the home. Many gay men's families had rejected them and wanted nothing to do with them or their illness. Buddies became the only support many individual HIV and AIDS patients had. Housework, shopping, home health assistance, cooking, and even hospice care often fell to buddies, and to the ASOs. Groups similar to GMHC sprang up in San Francisco, Los Angeles, Houston, Atlanta, Chicago, Miami-Ft. Lauderdale, Dallas, New Orleans, and other cities that had the highest numbers of HIV-positive people.

ASOs quickly became the main institutional method of community, volunteer-based AIDS prevention and education efforts. Funding was initially provided by private foundations or corporations that could be persuaded to support the organizations. Money was raised through parties at people's homes, donation nights at gay bars, and eventually AIDS walks or more public means of fund-raising. Eventually, local funding was supplemented with Ryan White CARE Act monies from the federal government. For the first 15 years of the epidemic, ASOs were the main, and often the only, source of help for people who had HIV and needed assistance. In the mid-1990s, changes in the availability of medication and the outlawing of discrimination against HIV-positive people, based on court decisions and the passage of the Americans with Disabilities Act, resulted in a large drop in clients at many ASOs. Legal issues disappeared in most cases. Health care was no longer refused, and it was illegal for health insurance companies to discriminate the basis of HIV status. People who had been sick for extended periods recovered while taking HIGHLY ACTIVE ANTIRETROVIRAL THERAPY (HAART) medications and no longer needed the various support mechanisms that ASOs had developed. ASOs were forced to adapt to the changing situations, and many organizations failed because they could not. In addition to changes in the health of people they served and in the services needed, the population of the epidemic also changed. Whereas initially the population served and the volunteers were predominantly gay men, the HIV epidemic became more and more an epidemic of poor, minority Americans and injection drug users than solely of gay men.

ASOs today are different in many ways from the early 1980s. Whereas today they have become part of the established grant writing, fund-raising, corporate nonprofit business model, in the early years they were seen as temporary, emergency-funded entities. No one could imagine that they would be needed long term when they were set up. The focus of most ASOs has changed from serving a white gay male clientele to serving clients from all walks of life and all ethnicities. The basic services are the same, but there are some paid staff instead of all volunteers, and federal grants instead of all community dollars.

Andriote, John-Manuel. *Victory Deferred: How AIDS Changed Gay Life in America*. Chicago: University of Chicago Press, 1999.

Brier, Jennifer. "AIDS Service Organizations." In *Encyclopedia of Lesbian, Gay, Bisexual and Transgender History in America*, Vol. 1, edited by Marc Stein. New York: Charles Scribner's Sons, 2003.

Dodd, Sarah-Jane, and William Meezan. "Matching AIDS Service Organizations' Philosophy of Service Provision with a Comparable Style of Program Evaluation." In *Research Methods with Gay, Lesbian, Bisexual, and Transgender Populations*, edited by William Meezon and James I. Martin. London: Routledge, 2003.

alternative treatment Alternative treatment generally refers to any treatment procedures or substances that are not part of traditional Western medicine, which is sometimes referred to as allopathy. Alternative medical treatments have been used by a significant num-

ber of people with HIV, particularly in the early years of the epidemic, often to complement approved treatments from their doctors. Alternative treatment or medicine, also called complementary medicine, can encompass any number of components, ranging from different treatment modes to specific additions to a diet or substances not approved for the treatment of HIV. Some alternative treatments have been investigated in laboratory and observational settings, and some have undergone clinical trials. Other treatments are used though no studies confirm any benefit.

Alternative treatment modes are different types of medicine from the norm. They include ayurvedic medicine, chiropractic, homeopathy, Native American medicine, traditional Chinese medicine, and naturopathy. These modes of treatment, although lumped together as alternative treatment, vary greatly and differ in methods, cost, and philosophy from both Western medicine and one another. One common theme in non-Western medicine is that most of the systems are seen as holistic, meaning they treat the whole person rather than a specific symptom or disease. They are thought to address not only the physical body but the mind and spirit as well. Many of the alternative medical systems believe a person has an innate healing ability, and the goal of treatment is often to restore this system to a proper balance, reinforcing the ability to heal the self. How that is accomplished varies from system to system. These alternative systems have not been well studied in a scientific manner; as a result, allopathic researchers doubt many of the claims made by people practicing or using alternative therapies.

In the initial years of the HIV epidemic, there was no allopathic treatment for the virus. This led people to try any number of methods outside Western medicine to improve their health. Because Western medicine focuses on taking medicines to relieve suffering or improve health, many types of vitamin supplements and natural plant-based products became well known in the HIV community as worth trying since nothing was known to help. There were many rumors and stories of cures effected by taking a particular regimen of vitamins or infusions of a particular plant. None of these stories or rumors has ever been scientifically proven, but the popularity of these products has continued to this day. The same is true for different modes of treatment. Many people believe that traditional Chinese medicine or ayurvedic medicine has kept them healthy with HIV and are adamant about the benefits they feel they receive. Alternative medicine has both supporters and detractors in the HIV community. Some are unyielding in support of various alternative approaches despite research demonstrating otherwise, and some completely reject anything other than traditional Western medicine in spite of positive scientific study findings.

Ayurvedic medicine is the traditional Indian medical system, which involves many therapies, including yoga, meditation, natural herbal medicines, massage, and dietary changes. Traditional Chinese medicine involves similar dietary changes, herbal medicines, and often acupuncture or acupressure. In both ayurvedic and Chinese medicine, dietary changes are important for health. Diets change according to the season, with some foods being recommended based on the changes these systems of thought believe occur in the body during different seasons of the year. According to these beliefs, because some foods are not produced in some seasons, the balance of the body's health can depend on eating the proper food during the proper time of the year. Some studies have looked at the benefits of acupuncture and massage, as well as meditation and yoga, in various illnesses. It is acknowledged by many Western doctors that the mind can play a large role in the health of a person. People who pray, meditate, or otherwise focus their mind on health, or on being well, not only feel better when sick, but believe they can help the process of healing when using Western medicine. Practitioners of both Chinese and ayurvedic medicines believe that there are certain power centers in

the body, and that through releasing "toxins" in these areas, or freeing the movement of energy in and through these areas, the body can begin to heal itself. Acupuncture, acupressure, meditation, massage, and body movement are believed to help free the problems blocking the energy from traveling through the body properly. Tai chi and qi gong are two commonly practiced forms of body movement in China. Yoga is more common in India. All involve some form of meditation in conjunction with physical movements.

Body manipulation, such as acupuncture, massage, or chiropractic, has been popular with HIV-positive people. Other types of body manipulation—including Rolfing (manipulation of the muscles and tendons), osteopathic medicine (bone, joint, and muscle manipulation), shiatsu (traditional Japanese massage), and reflexology (massage or manipulation of the palms of the hands or soles of the feet)—use manipulation of the joints, spine, or muscles and other soft tissue as a way to reduce tension, encourage body energy, and decrease pain in patients. Other types of alternative therapies are based on the belief that the body's energy can be assisted through touch or other means. Electromagnetic therapies uses magnets, sound, light, and/or colors to manipulate the body's "energy fields" to encourage health. Therapeutic touch and Reiki practitioners believe that their hands can change or guide energy in the body to assist a person in healing. Some people also believe that body energy can be manipulated or improved through distance meditation or prayer and will work with someone a great physical distance away from them through these means.

Homeopathy works on the belief that like cures like. What this means in practice is that often the same thing that makes a person ill can cure him or her. Homeopathic medicines use minute amounts of substances, usually plants or herbs, which, in large quantities, may cause illness or certain symptoms such as fever or stomach upset, to treat and cure a person who is exhibiting symptoms similar to those that the substance induces. The substance is diluted in water many times to produce what is called a tincture, which is then given to a patient to relieve symptoms. Research into homeopathy has not proven benefits, but some people remain strong believers in this system of medicine. The National Center for Complementary and Alternative Medicine (NCCAM) is part of the National Institutes of Health. It was formed in 1991, as the Office of Alternative Medicine (OAM) by an act of Congress to study complementary and alternative therapies after it became clear that millions of people were using these means of health care or in addition to regular health care. Reformed as the NCCAM in 1998, the organization provides funding to conduct studies into the use of alternative medicines that evaluate results on the basis of scientific principles. It also trains researchers into alternative medicine and trains people in proven alternative therapies. Alternative medicine is a large-scale business in scope and revenue. People spend millions of dollars a year on these therapies, prompting the government's call for research. As opposed to Western medicine, which is generally covered by medical insurance, the majority of these therapies are not covered by insurance plans. The costs and potential for physical harm to consumers were seen as great, warranting research and a better understanding of their potential benefits and harm.

The largest area of alternative medicine is the market in vitamin, herbal, and plant supplements, which is generally unregulated. HIV-positive people in particular have used any number of supplements and products to try to assist their body in healing. It has also been a market where wild claims of success or benefits are made for a variety of different products. A listing of all the supplements used over the course of the epidemic by HIV-positive people would encompass most products available on the market. Some of the more common ones include folic acid, B vitamins, beta-carotene, St. John's wort, L-lysine, N-acetylcysteine (NAC), selenium, silymarin (milk thistle), iron, coenzyme Q (CoQ-10), and colostrum. Various combinations of herbs packaged in capsule or pill formulations have also been used and recommended by traditional Chinese medicine practitioners. Some of these supplements have been rigorously tested, and some results have become well known. St. John's wort, for instance, has been used in some form by Native American healers for hundreds of years. It has been evaluated in tests for use in the treatment of depression, and some results have been positive for minor depression. However, studies have proven that the use of St. John's wort actually decreases the amount of PROTEASE INHIBITORS (PIs) in the blood and therefore the effectiveness of the drug. Warning labels on such medications as INDINAVIR and other PIs now indicate that fact to consumers. Another well-tested supplement is the mineral selenium. Studies have shown that selenium does help in the treatment of HIV; it actually reduces the viral load of HIV and increases CD4 counts in people who have HIV. It has also been shown that HIV-positive people who have low amounts of selenium in their body are at increased risk for many OPPORTUNISTIC INFECTIONS (OIs). Milk thistle, or silymarin, also has been shown to have benefits. Studies conducted in Europe show drops in HEPATITIS C viral loads when an intravenous formulation of milk thistle is used in conjunction with regular hepatitis C medications. This could potentially be an important extra medication to use when treating people coinfected with HIV and hepatitis C.

Dietary supplements have also been used a great deal by people trying to treat their HIV infection. From outlandish claims by South African governmental officials about the cures provided by eating beet root and garlic to enemas with extracts of bitter melon rind, HIV-positive people have tried all manner of plants and plant extracts in their treatment. Commonly discussed treatments include acemannan, astragalus, bitter melon, blue-green algae, burdock, garlic, ginseng, glycyrrhizin, mulberry roots and seeds, pine cone extracts, shitake mushrooms, and trichosanthin. As with supplements, some of these plant-derived "cures" have been demonstrated to have some validity when tested scientifically, while others have been shown to be ineffective. An extract from the root of the astragalus plant has been shown in recent studies to help the human immune system cells remain active against long-term viruses such as HIV that are not cleared from the body. Astragalus has long been used in traditional Chinese medicine alone or as part of a combination of herbs to treat hepatitis and other liver abnormalities. Another plant, long proposed as a treatment for HIV, is bitter melon, a cucumberlike fruit with wrinkled skin. Extensive research has shown that bitter melon does contain an unusual number of proteins that may have medicinal uses, but, as of this writing, no positive results have been shown with regard to its use against HIV in humans.

Because of the unproven nature of many of the alternative treatments discussed here, it is strongly recommended that a person discuss all supplements and dietary additives as well as alternative treatment modes with a doctor. A complete picture of one's treatment can provide assistance to physicians in diagnosing any changes that may occur, positive or negative, as a result of the use of alternative medicine. Points to keep in mind if a person is considering other treatments outside the norm of Western medicine include obtaining unbiased information about the treatment, side effects, costs, insurance coverage, the training of the person providing the treatment, and discussing the treatment with a person already receiving it to find out about the results that the person has experienced.

AVERT: AVERTing HIV and AIDS. "Alternative, Complementary and Traditional Medicine and HIV." AVERT.org. Available online. URL: http://www.avert.org/alternative-medicine-hiv.htm. Accessed March 11, 2011.

Henry J. Kaiser Family Foundation. "Dietary Supplement Selenium Reduces HIV Viral Load, Increases CD4+ T Cell Count, Study Says." TheBody.com. Available online. URL: http://www.thebody.com/content/art39550.html. Accessed March 11, 2011.

National Institutes of Health. National Center for Complementary and Alternative Medicine (NCCAM). URL: http://nccam.nih.gov/. Accessed March 11, 2011.

National Institutes of Health, Office of Alternative Medicine. "FACT SHEET: HIV/AIDS and Alternative Therapies." AEGIS.com. Available online. URL: http://www.aegis.com/pubs/cdc_fact_sheets/1994/cdc94033.html. Accessed March 11, 2011.

News-Medical. "Astragalus root plant chemical used to fight HIV." News-Medical.net. Available online. URL: http://www.news-medical.net/news/2008/11/11/42761.aspx. Accessed March 11, 2011.

White House Commission on Complementary and Alternative Medicine. "WHCCAMP: Final Report." HHS.gov. Available online. URL: http://whccamp.hhs.gov/. Accessed March 11, 2011.

amprenavir Amprenavir is one of the PROTEASE INHIBITORS (PIs); it is administered as part of a multidrug regimen, used in the treatment of HIV. It is prescribed under the trade name Agenerase, and known by the abbreviation APV. It is no longer manufactured for use in the United States but continues to be used in other countries. It was developed by Vertex Pharmaceuticals and is currently manufactured by GlaxoSmithKline Pharmaceuticals. The U.S. Food and Drug Administration (FDA) originally approved it in 1999.

Dosage

Amprenavir is available in liquid form in some countries. It was also available in pill form prior to its discontinuation. It was one of the early PIs approved by the FDA and each dose required a large number of pills. It was available in 150 mg and 50 mg gel capsules. A single dose was 600 mg twice a day, or four capsules each time the pill was taken. Later dosing was changed to 1,200 mg once a day, or eight capsules. It was taken in conjunction with ritonavir, another PI. Dosing for amprenavir as a liquid was different in the amount used and was based on the weight of an individual. Because it was a liquid, it was often used for children above the age of four.

Drug Interactions

Amprenavir is available in oral liquid and capsules form, both with vitamin E, which helps absorption of the drug. There is no need to consume vitamin E supplements when taking amprenavir, and doing so may cause problems, as the body can build up excessive vitamin E as a result. Another supplement that should be avoided is St. John's wort, which can decrease the amount of PIs in the blood and, therefore, reduce their effectiveness and increase the chance for HIV to build resistance to the drug. Amprenavir is boosted when taking ritonavir, and they are often prescribed together. It may be taken with or without food but should not be taken with high-fat meals, as these can reduce the absorption of the drug. Many other PIs interact with amprenavir, and dosage of amprenavir or other PIs may be adjusted as prescribed at the same time as part of a multidrug HIGHLY ACTIVE ANTIRETROVIRAL THERAPY (HAART) regimen against HIV.

Consumption of alcohol needs to be avoided when using the oral liquid form of amprenavir because it contains propylene glycol, which can cause problems when mixed with alcohol.

Amprenavir interacts with a number of other medications including the cholesterol-lowering drugs simvastatin and lovastatin, antibiotics used to treat infections such as tuberculosis, antidepressant or antipsychotic medications, and calcium channel blockers used in the treatment of heart ailments. It is important that the doctor know and understand all the medications and supplements patients are taking when prescribing amprenavir.

Amprenavir also increases the amount of the drugs sildenafil (Viagra), vardenafil (Levitra), and tadalafil (Cialis)—all erectile dysfunction medications—in the blood, which can cause serious side effects. Lowering the dosage of these medications is recommended to prevent potential complications.

Side Effects

PIs, as a class of drug, often increase the cholesterol and triglyceride levels of patients, and amprenavir does so as well. High lipid levels have been recorded in many patients. This side effect can be managed with appropriate cholesterol-lowering medications. It has also been associated with regimens that can cause LIPODYSTROPHY, or the redistribution of fat within the body. Symptoms are increased fat around the neck area, facial wasting, breast enlargement, and peripheral wasting. Some of these changes disappear when the drug is stopped.

Other side effects include diarrhea, nausea, malaise (feeling tired or exhausted), and headache. About 20 percent of people who take amprenavir develop a skin rash initially. This can generally be managed, as it is mild or moderate in nature. There have been some serious skin reactions or allergies to the drug, so severe rashes should be monitored by a doctor.

Amprenavir is a sulfa drug. People who have allergies to any sulfa drug should not take amprenavir.

AIDSmeds. "Agenerase (Amprenavir)." AIDSmeds.com. Available online. URL: http://www.aidsmeds.com/archive/Agenerase_1069.shtml. Accessed March 11, 2011.
———. "Special Issues for Children with HIV." AIDSmeds.com. Available online. URL: http://www.aidsmeds.com/articles/Children_7566.shtml. Accessed March 11, 2011.
United States Department of Health and Human Services. "Amprenavir." AIDSinfo.NIH.gov. Available online. URL: http://www.aidsinfo.nih.gov/DrugsNew/DrugDetailNT.aspx?int_id=258. Accessed March 11, 2011.

apricitabine   Apricitabine is one of the experimental NUCLEOSIDE REVERSE TRANSCRIPTASE INHIBITORS (NRTIs); it is currently under development by the Australian drug company Avexa. It has received fast track status from the U.S. FOOD AND DRUG ADMINISTRATION (FDA), though it had not been approved for general use as of early 2011. It has been in phase III trials around the world. In late 2009, Avexa announced that the phase III trials were going to be stopped at 24 weeks so that data could be unblinded and evaluated by the company as well as governmental agencies. After evaluating the studies, Avexa then announced in early 2010 that it would cease development of apricitabine. Avexa had failed to find development funds and had failed to sell the rights to the drug, though it could still be purchased as of summer 2011. The company may still be evaluating the use of apricitabine in smaller markets than the United States, where drug approval may be cheaper than the standard U.S. costs for drug development and approval. The chemical structure of apricitabine is similar to that of two other NRTIs, EMTRICITABINE and LAMIVUDINE. The development names for this drug include AVX-301 and SPD-754.

Dosage

Apricitabine was being studied in phase III trials in an 800 mg dose taken twice a day. Earlier drug trials had concluded that this was the optimal dosing for the medication. It will need to be prescribed as part of a combination therapy involving other antiretrovirals active against HIV. Apricitabine is active against lamivudine-resistant virus as well as ZIDOVUDINE-resistant virus and has been shown to develop resistant mutations at a much slower rate than other similar NRTIs.

Drug Interactions

Early results of apricitabine trials have indicated that the drug should not be prescribed at the same time as lamivudine, as lamivudine decreases the amount of apricitabine available inside human cells. It is not believed that apricitabine will have any serious interactions with other HIV medications, as it is not metabolized by the liver and has not been shown to cause any negative interaction with drugs processed through the liver.

Side Effects

No serious side effects have been noted during the drug trials to this point. Common side effects such as headache, diarrhea, and nasal conges-

tion were reported at the outset of taking the medication but decreased as the dosage was continued. No serious incidents have been reported during any of the ongoing trials of the drug.

AIDSmeds. "Apricitabine." AIDSmeds.com Available online. URL: http://www.aidsmeds.com/archive/apricitabine_1593.shtml. Accessed March 11, 2011.
FierceBiotech. "Avexa Closes Apricitabine (ATC) Program." FierceBiotech.com. Available online. URL: http://www.fiercebiotech.com/press-releases/avexa-closes-apricitabine-atc-program. Accessed March 11, 2011.
Medical News Today. "Avexa Closes ATC's Phase III Trial to Evaluate Data." MedicalNewsToday.com. Available online. URL: http://www.medicalnewstoday.com/articles/166087.php. Accessed March 11, 2011.
United States Department of Health and Human Services. "Apricitabine." aidsinfo.nih.gov. Available online. URL: http://www.aidsinfo.nih.gov/DrugsNew/DrugDetailNT.aspx?int_id=415. Accessed March 11, 2011.

Asia   Parts of Asia have been affected heavily by HIV and AIDS, while other parts of the region have managed to survive without high rates of infection and huge numbers of people who have become ill and died. According to Joint United Nations Programme on HIV/AIDS (UNAIDS) statistics in 2010, there were a reported 5 million HIV-positive people living in Asia. This number was less than the UN had projected as an estimate in the mid-2000s, but revised UN statistical tables have decreased the numbers of infected in many areas of the world for the time being. By far the largest number of HIV-positive people in Asia is in India, where it is believed 2.4 million people live with HIV. China is estimated to have 740,000 cases; Thailand, 530,000; Indonesia, Myanmar, and Vietnam, all have between 240,000 and 310,000 people living with HIV. Prevalence rates in Asia vary widely. Although China's prevalence rate is low at 0.1 percent of the population, this represents a large number of people, as China's population is 1.3 billion. India has an HIV prevalence rate of 0.3 percent. Other prevalence rates are Afghanistan, Bangladesh, Japan, Korea, Maldives, North Korea, the Philippines, Sri Lanka, and Timor-Leste at less than 0.1 percent; Mongolia, Bhutan, and Pakistan at 0.1 percent; Indonesia, Iran, Laos, and Singapore at 0.2 percent; Nepal and Vietnam at 0.4 percent; Cambodia and Malaysia at 0.5 percent; Myanmar at 0.6 percent; and Thailand at 1.3 percent of the population.

In Thailand, the government was quick to react to the increasing number of AIDS cases seen in the late 1980s and early 1990s. Thai governmental responses included a large media campaign to increase condom use among SEX WORKERS. They also included broadcast programs about HIV/AIDS that increased awareness in many groups about the illness and ways to prevent its spread. In the 1990s, before the government instituted its 100 percent condom-use plan for sex workers, new infections totaled approximately 140,000 new cases a year. In 2006, that number was 16,000 new cases of HIV infection. Thailand also had an HIV prevalence rate above 2.2 percent, which had fallen to approximately 1.3 percent in the 2010 UN estimates. Despite these huge improvements, UNAIDS reports in 2007 showed that government termination of education funding in the early part of the 21st century had led to slight increases in infection rates for teenagers and for MEN WHO HAVE SEX WITH MEN (MSM). The first group was too young to remember the government campaigns, and studies show a lack of knowledge of HIV and distinct lack of condom use compared to those of other population groups in Thailand. MSM sex workers were never included in the 100 percent condom-use campaign in Thailand, but later, the government began to fund condom campaigns for MSM sex workers. The epidemic was initially spread through sex workers. Sex tourism is a large draw for many people in developed countries and from other Asian countries to Thailand as well as some other countries in Asia. As of 2010, INJECTION DRUG USE(R)S (IDU) and their partners as well as MSM accounted for 20 percent each

of new cases in Thailand. In total, 28 percent of IDUs in Thailand as well as 26 percent of Thai MSM were HIV positive according to recent testing studies.

China first registered a case of AIDS in 1985. The government announced that the virus was introduced to the country by foreigners and was not a problem internally. Laws were passed to ban the entry of HIV-positive people into the country. When later that decade several dozen IDU cases of HIV were detected in the southern provinces, they were again blamed on contact with the West. At that time in China, AIDS was known as *aizibing*, which roughly translates as "loving capitalism disease." Because of the slow acknowledgment of the potential for spread in China, the country was caught off guard in the mid-1990s, when it became clear there were many cases developing among IDUs as well as through contaminated blood in the blood donation system. Several thousand rural Chinese were exposed to HIV via blood and plasma donation methods that reused contaminated needles and that replaced whole blood after plasma had been extracted from donors, from a central blood processing machine, thereby exposing each donor to the blood of all donors at a facility. Many Chinese were paid money for donating blood and plasma during this time and were unaware of HIV because there was no government acknowledgment of the illness or any method in place to prevent its transfer from person to person. Approximately 10 percent of current HIV cases are among former blood donors. Consequently, HIV entered the general population, where it has grown as a heterosexually spread virus because of the numbers of blood donors who were unaware they were infected. Although recent statements by government officials indicate the blood supply is not completely safe, it is now routinely screened and considered much safer than in past years. By the 2000s, China had begun some public education programs to prevent further spread. When the severe acute respiratory syndrome (SARS) epidemic had a great economic impact in 2003, China began spending more on prevention and treatment programs for all public health issues. China began extensive needle exchange and methadone programs after pilot programs showed decreased use of contaminated needles among IDUs and a decrease in drug use and availability. China now has more needle exchange sites and methadone clinics than any Asian country. China's HIV epidemic among sex workers continues to cause concern, as the sex industry has grown enormously with the opening of the Chinese economy. In addition, the growth in sex work is coupled with a culture that does not generally discuss sex. Government programs have been slower to address condom use than needle exchanges. However, some recent trial condom programs have shown good results and may presage expanded education with sex workers and their clients. Just less than half of all HIV cases in China have been spread through heterosexual sex. Male migrant workers who go to the cities for jobs and then return home for vacations are thought to be part of a large clientele for the sex workers, which could further spread HIV through rural regions. MSM sex accounts for a small percentage of cases currently in China. MSM sex is rarely discussed and publicly stigmatized. This could lead to an increase of HIV prevalence in this largely unknown and overlooked group of people. China provides HIGHLY ACTIVE ANTIRETROVIRAL THERAPY (HAART) treatment for approximately 40,000 people, or, according to 2009 UN estimates, about 19 percent of those who need treatment. Medical costs are generally borne by the provincial governments and not the central government. There have been few incentives to spend on treatment of HIV, as the costs must be taken from budgets strained by huge economic growth. Ignorance of HIV remains widespread in China. Surveys show that more than a quarter of medical personnel in China would not serve an HIV-infected patient. Nearly half of people surveyed said mosquitoes could transmit HIV from person to person. Education in China

needs to be a growing concern of the government or even larger numbers of people will be affected by HIV.

Japan, Mongolia, and North and South Korea have small HIV-infected populations. Japan had approximately 10,000 people living with HIV as of 2007, a low prevalence rate given the large population, but 2007 was also the year that showed the largest increase in HIV and AIDS cases to date. Sixty percent of Japan's HIV infections are among MSM. South Korea also has a small number of cases. In South Korea, 98 percent of HIV cases have been brought about by sexual contact. IDUs in Korea can purchase needles cheaply at any pharmacy without a prescription, and this seems to have prevented HIV from entering the IDU community. North Korea currently reports no statistics on HIV.

Indonesia is a large country spread over thousands of islands. Initially, the increase of HIV infection was limited to IDUs living in the large metropolitan areas of the country. However, as in other regions of the world, IDUs are often clients of paid sex workers, leading to the spread of HIV into that community. Studies show that 40 percent of the IDU population in Jakarta, the capital, are HIV positive, and that 25 percent of IDUs in Jakarta partonize paid sex workers. This has led to HIV prevalence rates nearing 20 percent among sex workers in some large cities. MSM sex workers as well as transgender sex workers both show relatively high rates of HIV prevalence. In addition, cultural differences among the islands have caused higher prevalence rates in some locations. West Papua province has prevalence rates of 2.4 percent as a whole and 3.5 percent in the highland regions. Men in that province who have been surveyed indicate that they more frequently use sex workers, frequently have multiple partners, and more often use force when seeking sex than men in other parts of Indonesia. In addition, education programs have not reached this part of Indonesia; very few people know about HIV or the ways to prevent its spread. Inaccessibility to medical clinics, testing facilities, clean needles, and condoms poses high potential for spreading of HIV in Indonesia. Two countries that border Indonesia, Brunei and Timor-Leste, both have small HIV-positive populations. It is unclear, particularly in Timor-Leste—where war and poverty have made HIV education, prevention, and treatment difficult—what prevalence rates exist among high-risk groups such as sex workers and MSM populations. Singapore, also adjacent to Indonesia, is small in area but a populous city. It has been ruled very conservatively for many years. IDU activities, sex work, and MSM behavior are all illegal. HIV has had a small impact, but the country recorded more than 300 new HIV cases in 2006, the largest number yet recorded there. Because many sexual activities are illegal, condom education has been shunned by the government, which has focused education on mother-to-child transmission.

Cambodia had a rapidly growing HIV epidemic largely led by spread in the sex industry in the 1990s. However, a 100 percent condom-use program enforced by the government and nongovernmental organizations led to a leveling off of new cases in recent years. Cambodia still has the highest rate of HIV prevalence in Asia after Thailand. Almost half of those infected by HIV in Cambodia are women, and the second-largest HIV-positive group is infected through mother-to-child transmission. Medical facilities are limited and treatment is not extensive, but education and condom access have driven the sharp decrease in HIV prevalence since the late 1990s. Non-brothel-based sex work has been increasing of late, and government programs to educate the public continue in both licensed and unlicensed brothels. MSM sex workers also show high rates of HIV infection and lower rates of condom use than their female counterparts.

Myanmar's epidemic seems to have peaked at a high in the late 1990s according to the UN, but surveys among high-risk populations and testing in certain cities have not indicated declines in recent years of new HIV-positive cases. In news articles, China's health ministry officials have been quoted as saying Myanmar's HIV numbers

are severe underestimates and do not speak to the true epidemic. It is known that very few of the 240,000 UN-estimated HIV-positive people in Myanmar receive acceptable medical care. In early 2008, Myanmaran officials denied access to relief agencies from around the world when Cyclone Nargis struck the country and left more than 138,000 dead or missing. Similarly, relief, education, and treatment groups involved with HIV have had trouble accessing monies and materials for treatment and education. Very few people in Myanmar have access to HIV medicines, even at the lowered cost of imported generic drugs. The government spends less on HIV relief than those of all similarly affected countries. Rates of infection among IDUs, sex workers, and MSM populations are high, and little is known about regions outside the main cities of Madalay and Yangon, where one in three sex workers and 43 percent of IDUs tested positive in recent studies.

Other Southeast Asian countries show smaller epidemics. The Philippines and Laos both have relatively small prevalence rates. Laos responded quickly with condom campaigns and is believed to have few IDUs and migratory workers, who are high-risk populations, in the region. The Philippines has remained an extremely low-prevalence country. Just 0.8 percent of IDUs tested positive in 2005 and only 0.2 percent of sex workers. No cases of HIV-positive MSM have been recorded in Manila. However, condom use is low in the Philippines and sterile needles are rare, leaving the possibility that the epidemic could take hold quickly given the opportunity.

In Malaysia, the epidemic has been predominantly driven by IDU activity. More than two-thirds of all HIV-positive people report injection drug use. Other cases are, therefore, likely to reflect the sexual partners of IDUs. HIV prevalence rates in the IDU community range from 19 to 40 percent in the large cities, indicating a widespread problem in this community. Currently Malaysia treats IDUs as criminals, and only small pilot projects for opium substitution or needle exchange have been used to stop the spread of the virus or provide education.

Vietnam has a large number of HIV-positive people and a relatively high prevalence rate in the region. Between 2000 and 2005, the HIV-positive population more than doubled, from 122,000 to 260,000. Most of the HIV-positive people reside along the Mekong River and in Ho Chi Minh City, where prevalence rates among the general population exceed 1 percent, but cases have been reported in all provinces. Prevalence rates among IDUs are high; studies show a range from 34 percent to nearly 60 percent in some provinces. UN studies also indicate that nearly 20 percent of IDUs have purchased sex in the past year, indicating a strong chance of spread of the virus into that community. Condom use is low in both the IDU and sex worker communities, though the government has begun some education and distribution programs targeted to this population. In 2005, the government legalized the sale and possession of needles and sterile injection equipment, leading to UN-cited surveys reporting 90 percent use of clean injection equipment among IDUs in the country, which is a promising signal. MSM sex workers are also a concern, as studies have shown a low condom use rate and high HIV prevalence of up to 33 percent in Ho Chi Minh City. General MSM and transgender community prevalence rates range in the area of 7–8 percent.

Some countries in South and West Asia have maintained relatively low HIV epidemics while others have extensive problems with the virus. Bangladesh and Sri Lanka both show very low infection rates of less than 0.1 percent. IDUs in Bangladesh show moderately high prevalence rates below 10 percent, while IDUs in Sri Lanka show very low prevalence rates. Condom use and HIV awareness in both countries are low, patterns that could lead to larger epidemics in the future.

Iran, Pakistan, and Afghanistan show relatively low rates of HIV infection. Iran has had, until recently, a model program for HIV education, prevention, and treatment. The program arose from the work of two physician brothers who had begun treating prisoners who had HIV. Drs. Arash and Kamiar Alaei set up testing facilities, met with the HIV-positive people they could track, and designed a program that was accepted by the government. Clean needles and condoms were distributed in PRISONS and in the communities where HIV was detected. Broad education programs were initiated. However, in 2008, both doctors were arrested and charged with treason and tried in court late in the year for that and other unspecified charges. It is unclear what all the charges were as they were labeled secret, and it is unknown what sentence may be given them. It is also unclear where this leaves the Iranian HIV-infected community, which is largely made up of IDUs and their sexual partners and families. Afghanistan, despite being the largest producer of opium poppies, has a relatively low number of known IDUs. Given the ongoing wars, the extent of HIV infection is unclear in many areas of the country. A cultural history of opium use as well as a community where sexual activity, particularly MSM sexual activity, is not discussed, and large displacement of the population could pave the way for HIV to make inroads there. Reports cited in the 2007 UNAIDS report state that Pakistan has large numbers of IDUs, among whom rates of HIV infection had grown from 1 percent in 2004 to 26 percent in 2006 in the city of Karachi. Similar rates of increase are either confirmed or feared in other large cities. Rates of infection among sex workers remain low, but IDUs often seek out sex workers for services. Condom use is rare and not generally understood as a way to prevent HIV transmission. As an indicator of future HIV spread, surveys of IDUs in Karachi show 80 percent of them were sexually active; 13 percent had purchased sex from females in the past six months, and 8 percent had purchased sex from male sex workers in the same period. The same study in Rawalpindi cited by the UN reported proportions of IDUs purchasing sex, by gender of sex worker, were 28 and 27 percent, respectively.

India has by far the largest HIV epidemic in Asia: An estimated 2.4 million people are HIV-positive. Rates of infection vary widely among states and regions within states. The South and Northeast of India are believed to have the highest concentration of infection. In the northeastern states of Mizoram and Nagaland, which border Myanmar, drug trafficking is heavy and access to sterile injecting equipment is low. IDUs have high rates of infection in these areas as well as in major cities such as Mumbai, Delhi, and Chennai. Prevalence rates range from 30 percent in Mumbai to 40 percent in Chennai. Outside these specific areas, it is believed India's epidemic is a result of spread from the sex industry. Sex workers in all parts of the country have higher rates of infection than the general population. Men from all parts of India who have responded to surveys indicate that paying for sex is not uncommon, particularly among men who work away from home or work in trucking, which is a major form of the transportation of goods in India. Although MSM activities are illegal in India, studies show male sex workers as well as transgender sex workers also have high prevalence rates of HIV. Studies show that 10 percent of unmarried men and 3 percent of married men in several states had engaged in MSM activities in the previous year, and fewer than half of those had used condoms during sex. More than half of the men who stated they had sex with men also stated they had sex with women in the previous six months. Education in India is conducted through a variety of means. The government sponsors HIV prevention education through sex worker collectives as well as in more than 3,600 HIV testing sites around the country. Such education is largely through word of mouth as many of India's sex workers are illiterate, and trafficking in sex workers still occurs in India. India also has large immigrant sex worker communities from EASTERN EUROPE AND CENTRAL ASIA who complicate education efforts, due to language barriers. Brothels are easier to reach in education efforts; however, in some areas of the country, brothels are only a small part of the sex industry, with home-based and street-based work comprising the largest share of the business. Availability of anti-HIV medication is limited in many settings in India. Medical facilities are in poor shape or nonexistent in poorer areas. Many people are unemployed or underpaid and cannot afford even the low cost of generic highly active antiretroviral therapy (HAART). India is one of the larger manufacturers of generic drugs used in HIV treatment, but it exports some of those drugs to other countries, including South Africa.

Asia is also home to the manufacture and distribution of illegal or imitation HIV medications. In 2008, several large internationally led seizures of imitation pharmaceuticals led Interpol and other policing agencies to manufacturing centers in China, Cambodia, and several other countries. In some instances, the seized drugs had no antiretroviral medication in them at all; however, even worse was the finding that some of the seized medications had only small amounts of antiretroviral medication. If the amount of antiretroviral medication in a drug is not of sufficient strength, the virus can build immunity to the medication quickly, causing the person taking the drug to become immune to the positive effects of the medication. Large quantities of illegal drugs of this nature could possibly cause thousands of people to pass on a virus that is untreatable with common generic medications. Interpol reported that more than 16 million pills were seized during the raids in 2008.

Neighboring India is Nepal, where HIV prevalence is higher than in India, but the total number of HIV-infected people is significantly lower. In addition to high rates of infection among the country's IDUs and significant rates of infection among female sex workers, there are between 600,000 and 1 million Nepalese who are migrant workers, most of them working in India. Studies of these male workers show that upward of 8 percent of them return to Nepal HIV positive. In addition, there is significant trafficking in females for sex work in India, and

Nepalese women who have returned to Nepal have HIV prevalence rates nearing 40 percent. Bhutan, a small, mostly closed country sandwiched between China and India, has a very small HIV-positive population. Officials express concern that because the population is becoming more mobile and more open, and because the majority of the population is below the age of 20, there may be an opportunity for HIV to become a larger problem if the government does not make education and prevention a priority. The Maldives have fewer than 100 cases of HIV. Potential risk factors for the small island country include highly mobile migrant workers who run the tourist economy, more than half a million annual visitors to the islands, and an increasing population of IDUs, mainly teenagers or younger adults, who may increase the opportunity for HIV infection to expand here.

Al Jazeera. "Asia Sees Growing AIDS Threat." AlJazeera.net. Available online. URL: http://english.aljazeera.net/news/asia-pacific/2008/12/20081214141191450.html. Accessed March 11, 2011.

Allam, Hannah. "Iran's AIDS-Prevention Program among World's Most Progressive." CommonDreams.org. Available online. URL: http://www.commondreams.org/headlines06/0414-03.htm. Accessed March 11, 2011.

AsiaNews.it. "Myanmar Heading towards Full-Blown AIDS Epidemic." AsiaNews.it. Available online. URL: http://www.asianews.it/index.php?l=en&art=7939. Accessed March 11, 2011.

AVERT: AVERTing HIV and AIDS. "HIV and AIDS in Asia." AVERT.org. Available online. URL: http://www.avert.org/aids-asia.htm. Accessed March 11, 2011.

———. "HIV and AIDS in China." AVERT.org. Available online. URL: http://www.avert.org/aidschina.htm. Accessed March 11, 2011.

———. "South East Asia HIV & AIDS Statistics." AVERT.org. Available online. URL: http://www.avert.org/aids-hiv-south-east-asia.htm. Accessed March 11, 2011.

———. "Who Is Affected by HIV and AIDS in India?" AVERT.org. Available online. URL: http://www.avert.org/hiv-india.htm. Accessed March 11, 2011.

Bennett, Simeon. "SOUTHEAST ASIA: Interpol Seizes $6.65 Million in Counterfeit Drugs." Bloomberg News (17 November 2008). AEGIS.com. Available online. URL: http://www.aegis.com/news/ads/2008/AD082196.html. Accessed March 11, 2011.

Blumenthal, Susan. "AIDS in Asia: An Emerging Frontier in the HIV/AIDS Epidemic." HuffingtonPost.com. Available online. URL: http://www.huffingtonpost.com/susan-blumenthal/aids-in-asia-an-emerging_b_116077.html. Accessed March 11, 2011.

China Daily. "Campaign Targets Unsafe Blood Collection." China.org.cn. Available online. URL: http://www.china.org.cn/english/2004/May/96739.htm. Accessed March 11, 2011.

EATG: European AIDS Treatment Group. "Interpol Seizes $6.65M in Counterfeit HIV/AIDS, Malaria, TB Drugs in Southeast Asia." EATG.org. Available online. URL: http://www.eatg.org/eatg/Global-HIV-News/Access-to-treatment/Interpol-seizes-6.65m-in-counterfeit-HIV-AIDS-malaria-TB-drugs-in-Southeast-Asia. Accessed March 11, 2011.

Iran Free the Docs. "Treating AIDS Is Not a Crime." IranFreeTheDocs.org. Available online. URL: http://iranfreethedocs.org/. Accessed March 11, 2011.

Reuters. "Myanmar Cyclone Toll Rises to 138,000 Dead, Missing." Reuters.com. Available online. URL: http://uk.reuters.com/article/featuredCrisis/idUKBKK15852620080624. Accessed March 11, 2011.

UNAIDS: Joint United Nations Programme on HIV/AIDS. "Asia: Fact Sheet." UNAIDS.org. Available online. URL: http://www.unaids.org/en/media/unaids/contentassets/dataimport/pub/factsheet/2009/20091124_fs_asia_en.pdf. Accessed March 11, 2011.

———. "Global Report: UNAIDS Report on the Global AIDS Epidemic 2010." UNAIDS.org. Available online. URL: http://www.unaids.org/globalreport/Global_report.htm. Accessed February 28, 2011.

UNAIDS: Joint United Nations Programme on HIV/AIDS and the World Health Organization. "2007 AIDS Epidemic Update Asia." UNAIDS.org. Available online. URL: http://data.unaids.org/pub/Report/2008/jc1527_epibriefs_asia_en.pdf. Accessed March 22, 2011.

———. "AIDS Epidemic Update 2009." UNAIDS.org. Available online. URL: http://www.unaids.

org/en/media/unaids/contentassets/dataimport/
pub/report/2009/jc1700_epi_update_2009_en.pdf.
Accessed March 22, 2011.

World Bank. "South Asia—AIDS in South Asia Report."
WorldBank.org. Available online. URL: http://web.
worldbank.org/WBSITE/EXTERNAL/COUNTRIES/
SOUTHASIAEXT/0,,contentMDK:21019386~page
PK:146736~piPK:146830~theSitePK:223547,00.
html. Accessed March 11, 2011.

aspergillosis Aspergillosis is a fungal infection caused by various species of the fungus *Aspergillus*. It is found around the world in both indoor and outdoor locations, making contact with the fungus inevitable. It is vital to the environment, as it helps in the decay of leaf and plant material in the natural world. It is also found in air-conditioning systems as well as carpeting, indoor plants, and ground spices found in most kitchens. There are more than 150 species of *Aspergillus* known to researchers, but just a few of those cause illness. The most common cause is *Aspergillus fumigatus*, though other species including *A. flavus, A. niger,* and *A. terreus* also are known to cause infections in humans.

Infection is caused when a person inhales the spores of the fungus into the lungs. In healthy people, the spore is attacked by the immune system and illness does not generally occur. However, in people who are HIV positive, have previous lung illness such as asthma or cystic fibrosis, or have been using corticosteroids for other illnesses, *Aspergillus* can cause localized lung infections or, in serious cases, invasive aspergillosis.

Symptoms and Diagnostic Path
Some people will develop a lung reaction similar to an allergy to *Aspergillus*. These cases can cause wheezing, worsening asthma attacks, fever, and tiredness. People who have preexisting lung illnesses such as cystic fibrosis or emphysema may contract a form of the disease known as aspergilloma, in which balls of the fungus grow together, forming masses that can cause extreme breathing difficulties, pain, weight loss, and coughing that includes blood in the sputum.

Aspergillus can also cause serious sinus and ear infections that are difficult to eradicate. These cases may appear as simple sinus infections initially but can spread to the central nervous system if left untreated in immunocompromised people. Pain, itching in the ears, and drainage from the ears or sinuses and occasional blood can be symptoms of an *Aspergillus* infection in these areas.

Invasive aspergillosis symptoms include fever, bleeding in the lungs, massive coughing, headache, and chest pain. Diagnosis of any form of *Aspergillus* infection begins with a chest X-ray or a computed tomography (CT) scan that can reveal the fungal balls in the lungs or invasive fungal masses. Skin and blood tests can also reveal antigens to the fungus and lead to a correct diagnosis. Testing on the skin involves either a scratch with or injection under the skin of a small amount of *Aspergillus* antigen. If there is a reaction, a small, hard bump will appear at the site of the scratch or injection, indicating the body already has antibodies to the fungus working to control the infection. Biopsies of tissue, from either the sinus or the lungs, can also determine whether the cause of the infection is *Aspergillus*.

Treatment Options and Outlook
Treatment of aspergillosis in HIV patients has not been studied extensively, so guidelines of treatment are similar to guidelines for HIV-negative people. Aspergillosis occurs most frequently in those who have extremely compromised immune systems. Most HIV-positive people who acquire aspergillosis also have not had HIGHLY ACTIVE ANTIRETROVIRAL THERAPY (HAART) treatment and have had no previous OPPORTUNISTIC INFECTIONS (OIs). Even if a diagnosis can be made, the outlook is not very good for invasive aspergillosis. Studies indicate that even with treatment invasive aspergillosis patients have a median survival time of two to four months. Death often results from aspergillosis that has been uncontrolled through drug treat-

ment. The first step to potential recovery is believed to be successful treatment with HAART, as cases of aspergillosis in HIV-positive patients have become uncommon among those who use HAART to treat HIV infection.

Voriconazole has become the treatment of choice in recent years. It has both oral and intravenous (IV) formulations. It is generally begun as an IV medication and then switched to an oral form after the initial day or two. One study showed a significant difference in treatment outcomes between patients treated with voriconazole and those treated with amphotericin B, which has led to the use of voriconazole in cases of invasive aspergillosis. Amphotericin B has a greater risk of side effects and is not absorbed into the body as readily as voriconazole, though lipid formulations of amphotericin B may have better efficacy in the treatment of aspergillosis. Voriconazole dosing must be adjusted if the HIV-positive person is taking EFAVIRENZ as part of the HAART regimen, as the two drugs used together cause a drop in the availability of voriconazole in the body. Itraconazole or caspofungin can also be used long-term as treatment for invasive aspergillosis.

Allergic *Aspergillus* infections are generally treated with corticosteroids for both HIV-positive and -negative patients, though HAART will be started in those HIV-positive patients not already on the therapy.

Surgical removal of aspergilloma balls or infections may also be undertaken if possible. Sinus, ear, and some lung infections of *Aspergillus* may be treated effectively through removal of the large infections.

Risk Factors and Preventive Measures

As *Aspergillus* is prevalent in most regions of the world, it is next to impossible to prevent exposure to the fungal spores in the air. Avoiding places where the chance of exposure might be relatively higher such as construction or farming areas may decrease the probability of exposure but will not eliminate it entirely. There is currently no prophylactic treatment that works well

over the long term for aspergillosis. HAART is often seen as the best chance to prevent aspergillosis and improve the outlook for healing people who have HIV.

Mayo Clinic Staff. "Aspergillosis." MayoClinic.com. Available online. URL: http://www.mayoclinic.com/health/aspergillosis/DS00950. Accessed March 11, 2011.

MedlinePlus: U.S. National Library of Medicine. "Aspergillosis." NLM.NIH.gov. Available online. URL: http://www.nlm.nih.gov/medlineplus/ency/article/001326.htm. Accessed March 11, 2011.

Merck. "Aspergillosis." MerckManuals.com. Available online. URL: http://www.merck.com/mmhe/sec17/ch197/ch197b.html. Accessed March, 11, 2011.

Phillips, Peter, M.D. "Aspergillus/Aspergillosis Website." Aspergillus.org.uk. Available online. URL: http://www.aspergillus.org.uk/indexhome.htm?secure/articles/asper-aids.html~main. Accessed March 11, 2011.

Sturt, Amy, M.D., and Judith A. Aberg, M.D. "Aspergillosis and HIV." HIVInSite.ucsf.edu. Available online. URL: http://hivinsite.ucsf.edu/InSite?page=kb-05-02-02. Accessed March 11, 2011.

Waknine, Yael. "FDA Safety Changes: Pexeva, Vfend, Suprane." Medscape.com. Available online. URL: http://www.medscape.com/viewarticle/552907. Accessed March 11, 2011.

atazanavir sulfate Atazanavir sulfate is one of the PROTEASE INHIBITORS (PIs); it was developed by Bristol-Myers Squibb and licensed by the U.S. FOOD AND DRUG ADMINISTRATION (FDA) in 2003. It is prescribed under the name Reyataz and also is known by the three-letter acronym ATV. It is commonly called simply atazanavir. The drug used in combination with at least two other medications for the treatment of HIV.

Dosage

Atazanavir is available in pill form in 150, 200, 250, and 300 mg doses. It was the first PI approved for use that could be taken just once a day. The dosage is generally one 300 mg pill once a day for adults. It is most commonly used in combination with another PI, ritonavir, which is given once a day in 100 mg doses. If a patient is sensitive to ritonavir, then the dosage of atazanavir is 400 mg a day, once a day, without ritonavir. Atazanavir has been approved for children above the age of six. The amount given is based on the body weight of the child and will vary as the child grows, starting with the lowest-dose pill. Atazanavir must be taken with food, preferably a full meal, as it requires an acidic stomach in order to be properly absorbed into the body. This is also why it may not be a recommended medication for people who take antacids regularly. Antacids prevent the proper absorption of the drug.

Drug Interactions

As are many medications taken to fight HIV, atazanavir is broken down by the liver once in the body. It can interact with a number of other medications a person may be taking at the same time. Some drugs will raise the level of atazanavir in the body; others will lower the amount. It is important that a doctor know all of the medications that the patient is taking to prevent this from happening.

The most significant interaction takes place with antacids. Long-acting antacids such as omeprazole (Prilosec) or famotidine (Pepcid) that prevent the production of acid in the stomach can generally not be taken concurrently with atazanavir and will not be prescribed at the same time for this reason. There are a number of different types of prescribed antacids, all of which can lower the amount of atazanavir in the blood, and a physician needs to know about these before prescribing this medication. Over-the-counter antacids such as Rolaids, Tums, or Mylanta should be taken at least two hours before or one hour after taking a dose of atazanavir, to prevent poor absorption of the drug.

Atazanavir is not prescribed at the same time as another PI, INDINAVIR. Both drugs can cause hyperbilirubinemia individually, and together they have been noted to cause this side effect.

When atazanavir is administered at the same time as ritonavir, the amount of atazanavir in the body is increased. This is called boosting and is used to increase the amount of atazanavir in the blood, most often because another prescribed medication may be lowering atazanavir below the optimum level. If prescribed at the same time as TENOFOVIR DISOPROXIL FUMARATE, which lowers the amount of atazanavir in the blood, atazanavir must be prescribed with ritonavir and all three pills must be taken with food at the same time. If the HIGHLY ACTIVE ANTIRETROVIRAL THERAPY (HAART) that is prescribed by the doctor includes DIDANOSINE, these two drugs must be taken at least two hours apart to allow each to be absorbed properly.

The drug interacts with a number of other medications including the cholesterol-lowering drugs simvastatin and lovastatin, antibiotics used to treat infections such as tuberculosis, antidepressant medications such as trazadone, herbal supplements such at St. John's wort, and calcium channel blockers used in the treatment of heart ailments.

Atazanavir also can interfere with birth control medications that interrupt the production of hormones in women. It increases the amount of the hormone blockers, and blood levels of the hormones may need to be monitored or dosage adjusted to prevent any negative side effects of the birth control drug. Atazanavir also increases blood levels of the drugs sildenafil (Viagra), vardenafil (Levitra), and tadalafil (Cialis), all erectile dysfunction medications, with serious side effects. Lowering the dosage of these medications is recommended to prevent potential complications.

Side Effects

The most common side effect of atazanavir is the raising of the bilirubin level in the blood, called hyperbilirubinemia, or jaundice. It causes a yellow-brown color of the skin, nails, and the whites of a person's eyes. This has been reported in 4–9 percent of people taking the drug in several studies. Although jaundice can be a sign of liver damage or illness, in these studies no such damage was detected, indicating that this is a cosmetic issue and not a life-threatening condition. However, this is the number-one reason patients stop taking the medication, as they may consider these changes in their appearance unacceptable. Bilirubin levels can fluctuate when a person uses atazanavir, so the hyperbilirubinemia may come and go if a person remains on the drug long term. This side effect disappears when the drug is stopped. The condition occurs more frequently in people coinfected with HEPATITIS B or HEPATITIS C and should be monitored in those instances to prevent any serious liver side effects.

Atazanavir is the first PI that does not cause an increase in triglyceride or cholesterol levels in the blood. Some studies have indicated that it creates an increase in blood levels of high-density lipoprotein (HDL), or what is commonly called the good cholesterol. Common PI side effects such as LIPODYSTROPHY, or redistribution of body fat, are not seen with atazanavir. When atazanavir is prescribed with ritonavir, these side effects may occur, but they have not been recorded to the same degree as with other PI medications.

Other potential side effects include a rash seen in some patients after several weeks of treatment. The rash disappears after a couple of weeks but should be monitored to prevent serious complications such as Stevens-Johnson syndrome, which is a severe allergic reaction to a medication. It can cause an increased risk of bleeding in a hemophiliac and irregular heartbeats in some instances; light-headedness, dizziness, and nausea have also been recorded in some patients. There is an increased risk of kidney stones for patients who are taking atazanavir, though this has not been studied extensively. Increased water intake can help reduce the risk of kidney stones.

AIDS InfoNet. "Atazanavir (Reyataz)." AIDSInfoNet.org. Available online. URL: http://www. aidsinfonet.org/fact_sheets/view/447. Accessed March 11, 2011.

AIDSmeds. "Reyataz (Atazanavir)." AIDSmeds.com. Available online. URL: http://www.aidsmeds.com/ archive/Reyataz_1563.shtml. Accessed March 11, 2011.

———. "Special Issues for Children with HIV." AIDSmeds.com. Available online. URL: http:// www.aidsmeds.com/articles/Children_7566.shtml. Accessed March 11, 2011.

The Body. "Reyataz (Atazanavir)." TheBody.com. Available online. URL: http://www.thebody.com/ index/treat/reyataz.html. Accessed March 11, 2011.

United States Department of Health and Human Services. "Atazanavir." aidsinfo.nih.gov. Available online. URL: http://www.aidsinfo.nih.gov/ DrugsNew/DrugDetailNT.aspx?int_id=314. Accessed March 11, 2011.

Atripla   Atripla is the trade name for a three-drug combination antiretroviral pill. It combines EFAVIRENZ, one of the NON-NUCLEOSIDE REVERSE TRANSCRIPTASE INHIBITORS (NNRTIs) and the NUCLEOSIDE REVERSE TRANSCRIPTASE INHIBITORS (NRTIs) TENOFOVIR DISOPROXIL FUMARATE and EMTRICITABINE. The full common name includes those three drug names, so Atripla is generally the preferred name for the medication. It is the first combination pill to include drugs from two or more classes of antiretrovirals and was approved by the U.S. FOOD AND DRUG ADMINISTRATION (FDA) in 2006. Generic versions of the pill have also been approved for use by the President's Emergency Plan for AIDS Relief (PEPFAR) drug program in areas outside the United States. The Gilead and Bristol-Myers Squibb companies manufacture it jointly. It is considered a complete regimen, meaning no other pills are required in the treatment of HIV, though it can be prescribed with other antiretrovirals if a doctor considers it necessary for some patients.

Dosage

One Atripla tablet a day is the standard prescribed dose. It cannot be adjusted for children or infants, and there is no liquid formula available at this time. Each Atripla tablet contains 600 mg of efavirenz, 300 mg of tenofovir disoproxil fumarate, and 200 mg of emtricitabine. It is generally recommended that the pill be taken on an empty stomach or with a light snack.

Drug Interactions

Atripla should not be taken at the same time that a person is already taking any of the other drugs that make up the combination pill. In addition, LAMIVUDINE and emtricitabine are very similar in nature and should not be combined at any time, as their effectiveness is decreased when they are prescribed together. Any antiretroviral containing lamivudine must be avoided. Drugs that have these characteristics are tenofovir, efavirenz, lamivudine, emtricitabine, COMBIVIR, TRIZIVIR, TRUVADA, and EPZICOM.

Drug interactions that can occur with the individual drugs that are part of Atripla can also occur while using this combination pill.

Tenofovir disoproxil fumarate can cause an increase in the amount of DIDANOSINE, another HIV antiretroviral, in the body. They should be prescribed together only with caution, as this increase can bring about increased risk of didanosine side effects such as pancreatitis and drug-induced neuropathy.

When given at the same time as KALETRA or ATAZANAVIR SULFATE with ritonavir, the amount of tenofovir is increased in the body. Increased signs of tenofovir side effects are possible and require monitoring. At the same time, the amount of atazanavir in the body is decreased when combined with tenofovir, and it should always be given in combination with ritonavir, if this is the preferred combination of anti-HIV medications.

Efavirenz causes the level of most PROTEASE INHIBITORS (PIs) to decrease in a person who is taking both drugs at the same time. Care must be taken in evaluating the amount of drug availability if efavirenz and a PI are prescribed at the same time. However, ritonavir, a PI, taken with efavirenz increases the availability of both drugs in the body.

The efavirenz in Atripla causes a decrease in the amount of methadone available in the body.

Patients who are on methadone treatment to treat an addiction to heroin will need the methadone dosages changed to take this difference into account.

The efavirenz in Atripla also decreases the effectiveness of hormone-based birth control. Women who are taking birth control pills as well as Atripla will need to understand the decreased effectiveness of this combination and seriously consider the use of a condom, diaphragm, or other barrier method to prevent pregnancy. Atripla is not recommended for women who are considering pregnancy because of the drug's potential to cause birth defects.

Atripla has been known to cause some individuals to test positive on drug tests for marijuana or other THC-containing substances. Findings of secondary tests used to confirm the presence of THC in the body have been negative, providing proof that the individual was not consuming THC-containing substances. This situation has caused some people to disclose their HIV status as part of an ongoing job interview process or to indicate it to their employer if required to take drug tests at work.

Several medications used in the treatment of TUBERCULOSIS (TB) can interact with efavirenz, requiring adjustment of the amount of the TB medication or a change in the medication being used to treat TB. A doctor will make an evaluation of this risk when prescribing Atripla. Atripla can also interact negatively with several medications used to treat fungal infections and high blood pressure.

Side Effects

The same side effects that can occur with the individual drugs that are found in Atripla are possible when Atripla is taken. The most common side effects of Atripla include headache, nausea, vomiting, vivid dreams, rash, and insomnia. These generally pass or lessen as the person takes the drug over time.

Patients who are taking efavirenz, one of the three drugs in Atripla, have reported vivid dreams, abnormal thinking, depression, and other neurological symptoms including possible suicidal feelings. Any strong depression or suicidal thoughts must be reported immediately to the physician prescribing the medication, so the patient can be evaluated. Most people taking the drug have reported that after an initial period of vivid dreams, this side effect disappeared.

Atripla can cause a significant increase in levels of liver enzymes and the risk of liver injury due to the efavirenz in Atripla. Baseline liver enzyme levels should be measured before a person starts Atripla and then closely monitored while he or she is taking the drug. In addition, Atripla should not be stopped suddenly by people who also have positive findings for HEPATITIS B, which is treated with tenofovir disoproxil fumarate, one of the other drugs in Atripla. People who have hepatitis B can have rapid rebounds of the disease, and serious liver damage can occur if the medication is stopped quickly without measures including ongoing observation and potential replacement of the hepatitis treatment.

A full listing of side effects and drug interactions can be found in the entries for the individual drugs or at the following Web sites.

AIDS InfoNet. "Atripla (evafirenz + emtricitabine + tenofovir)." AIDSInfoNet.org. Available online. URL: http://www.aidsinfonet.org/fact_sheets/view/439. Accessed March 11, 2011.

AIDSmeds. "Atripla (efavirenz + tenofovir + emtricitabine)." AIDSmeds.com. Available online. URL: http://www.aidsmeds.com/archive/Atripla_1577.shtml. Accessed March 11, 2011.

———. "Special Issues for Children with HIV." AIDSmeds.com. Available online. URL: http://www.aidsmeds.com/articles/Children_7566.shtml. Accessed March 11, 2011.

The Body. "Atripla (Efavirenz/Tenofovir/FTC)." TheBody.com. Available online. URL: http://www.thebody.com/index/treat/atripla.html. Accessed March 11, 2011.

United States Department of Health and Human Services. "Efavirenz/emtricitabine/tenofovir disoproxil fumarate." aidsinfo.nih.gov. Available online. URL: http://www.aidsinfo.nih.gov/DrugsNew/DrugDetailNT.aspx?int_id=424&ClassID=8&TypeID=1. Accessed March 11, 2011.

bacterial enteric infections The term *Enteric* means "of or relating to the intestines." The intestines contain a great variety of bacteria that are a normal part of the human digestive system. However, some bacteria are harmful to the body and can cause many problems through overpopulating the intestines to the detriment of the standard bacteria in the intestines. Many types of bacteria can cause enteric disease in any person; three common enteric infections that cause severe problems for HIV-positive people, particularly in the Western world, are *Shigella*, *Campylobacter*, and *Salmonella*.

All three of these gram-negative bacteria can be found in HIV-positive people at rates 20–100 times the standard incidence rates for the general population. A gram-negative bacterium is one that takes on a particular color during a laboratory staining (Gram stain)test. Gram-negative bacteria typically have a firm outer coat that causes them to be resistant to many antibiotics and increases their chance of becoming resistant to antibiotics used to control an infection. A gram-negative bacterium that commonly causes enteric disease is *Escherichia coli* (*E. coli*). This is common in many less developed parts of the world, but, unlike the other three bacteria, does not cause more deaths in HIV-positive patients than in the general population.

Symptoms and Diagnostic Path

The major symptom of all three of these bacterial infections is gastroenteritis, or inflammation of the intestinal areas. This inflammation causes diarrhea, ranging from mild to heavy; *Shigella* more often causes bloody diarrhea than the other two bacteria discussed. A person who has a compromised immune system can suffer from longer bouts of diarrhea as well as associated fever, weight loss, or vomiting. Bacteremia, which is presence of bacteria in the blood, is also associated more often with these infections in HIV-positive people. Sepsis, an acute inflammatory response throughout the whole body, can also occur in severe cases of enteric bacterial infections.

The weaker the immune system, the greater the risk for complications of these illnesses. In particular, *Salmonella* infection can recur in HIV-positive people even after successful treatment. Recurring *Salmonella* is one of the OPPORTUNISTIC INFECTIONS (OIs) used to define AIDS in an HIV-positive patient.

Diagnosis of any enteric infection begins with stool samples. This can be done through samples gathered over several days, as some bacteria are not easily measured through this type of sampling. In addition, bloody diarrhea and fevers with diarrhea are generally signs that blood infection has occurred and blood samples will also be taken to test for infection. Most blood samples will show evidence of infection by these gram-negative bacteria. On occasion, an endoscopy may be performed to determine the extent of infection. Biopsies of tissue will be taken during the endoscopy. Specific varieties of the bacteria can be determined through cultures of any samples taken by these methods of diagnosis so that the most effective drugs can be used to treat the infection.

Treatment Options and Outlook

Treatment for *Salmonella* infection is generally recommended for HIV-positive patients because of the risk of bacteremia if left untreated. In HIV-negative people, the infection is considered self-limiting and generally will clear itself after a few days. Treatments for individuals who have CD4 T lymphocyte counts above 200 cells/μL will most often last one or two weeks. For patients whose counts are below that CD4 level and patients who have bacteremia, treatment will last longer, often up to six weeks. The most commonly used antibiotic for *Salmonella* infection is ciprofloxacin, a fluoroquinolone. Other fluoroquinolones such as levofloxacin or moxifloxacin could also be used. Trimethoprim/sulfamethoxazole (TMP-SMX) is an alternative treatment, depending on the resistance strain of the bacteria.

People who have low CD4 counts will need to be monitored for *Salmonella* regularly for six months after initial treatment to prevent the return of the bacteria. An ongoing prophylaxis of antibiotics is often given in this case, though resistance to the drugs can occur and will also be monitored.

Treatment for shigellosis (infection by *Shigella* bacteria) is recommended to shorten the length of the infection and to prevent the spread of the illness to others, as it can be easily spread via the oral-fecal route, particularly in children. Fluoroquinolones are the preferred antibiotic; TMP-SMX and azithromycin are also used, depending on bacterial resistance. Most treatments will require a length of three days to one week. A treatment time of two weeks may be recommended for those who have bacteremia.

Infection with *Campylobacter* in HIV-positive or -negative people is problematic because studies have not determined a particular antibiotic to be the best treatment. Resistance to several drugs is common, and a mild case of infection will clear on its own. If infection continues or bacteremia exists, treatment with a fluoroquinolone is the first option. If resistance testing shows such a drug will not work, azithromycin will be used. Patients who have bacteremia will be treated for two weeks. A second drug, from the aminoglycoside family (e.g., amikacin or paromomycin), may also be added in cases of bacteremia.

Risk Factors and Preventive Measures

Enteric bacteria are spread primarily through oral-fecal contact. Regular hand washing will prevent many bacteria from having the opportunity to enter the body, particularly after using a bathroom, diapering a child, having contact with soil, or handling pets; before preparing food; and before and after sex. Unprotected sexual contact can also spread enteric bacteria, so condoms and dental dams are recommended prevention measures.

HIV-positive people should avoid, when possible, raw and undercooked meats and eggs, including seafood, to lessen the possibility of enteric infections. Hands, cooktops, cutting boards, and kitchen utensils should be cleaned after contact with raw and uncooked foods, especially meat.

Listeria monocytogenes, a gram-negative bacterium that causes serious illness in all people regardless of HIV status, also can be avoided by following these procedures. In addition, avoiding soft cheeses such as feta, brie, camembert, and queso fresco; cooking leftovers and precooked foods until steaming hot; avoiding unpasteurized milk and milk products; and avoiding delicatessen foods can lessen the chance of contracting listeriosis.

Travelers to developing countries can lessen their chance of enteric infections by avoiding tap water, ice, uncooked and undercooked foods, raw fruits and vegetables that have not been safely washed or peeled, unpasteurized milk and dairy products, as well as food from street vendors, whose conditions may be less than sanitary. Water can often be treated with iodine or chlorine tablets or can be boiled for at least one minute to reduce enteric infections effectively.

For HIV-positive travelers, a prophylaxis may be prescribed, depending on the level of immune suppression. In these cases, a fluoroquinolone or rifaximin will be given. A patient who is taking TMP-SMX may be considered already to be on a prophylaxis for enteric bacteria.

Food and Agriculture Organization of the United Nations. "HIV Infections and Zoonoses: Enteric

Infection due to *Salmonella* and *Campylobacter.*" FAO. org. Available online. URL: http://www.fao.org/docrep/007/y5516e/y5516e05.htm. Accessed March 11, 2011.

Monrow, Anne. "Gastrointestinal Problems and HIV." TheBody. Available online. URL: http://www.thebody.com/content/art1271.html. Accessed March 11, 2011.

University of California, San Francisco. "Bacterial Enteric Infections." HIVInSite. Available online. URL: http://hivinsite.ucsf.edu/InSite?page=md-agl-bent. Accessed March 11, 2011.

Von Seidlein, Lorenz et al. "Is HIV Infection Associated with an Increased Risk for Cholera? Findings from a Case-Control Study in Mozambique." *Tropical Medicine and International Health* 13, no. 4 (May 2008): 683–688.

bacterial pneumonia Pneumonia is a common cause of HIV-related deaths around the world. It occurs in HIV-positive people with greater frequency than in the HIV-negative population. Some studies have shown that rate to be eight times greater than in the general population. Prior to the availability of HIGHLY ACTIVE ANTI- RETROVIRAL THERAPY (HAART), bacterial pneumonias played a much larger role in developed nations in the death of HIV patients. In developing countries, where HAART is not always regularly available, it continues to be a leading cause of death of HIV-positive individuals. Bacterial pneumonias can affect any person at any CD4 T lymphocyte level and at any stage during HIV illness. It is often the first of the OPPORTU- NISTIC INFECTIONS (OIs) a person contracts and is a primary means of diagnosis of HIV in the developing world.

Pneumonia is an infection of the lungs that causes inflammation of the alveoli as well as fluid buildup. The alveoli are the tiny structures in the lungs that transport oxygen from the air we breathe to the blood system of the body. When the alveoli become blocked or inflamed, a person's breathing becomes more difficult and oxygen does not reach the blood. Although there can be other causes of pneumonia, includ- ing fungi, parasites, and viruses, bacterial pneumonia incidence in HIV-positive people is much higher than the rate in the general population.

Streptococcus pneumoniae and *Haemophilus influenzae* are the two most common causes of bacterial pneumonias in both HIV-positive and HIV-negative people. In HIV-positive people, other varieties of bacterial infection are also seen at much greater rates than in HIV-negative people. *Pseudomonas aeruginosa* and *Staphylococcus aureus* are two varieties of bacteria found at a higher frequency in HIV-positive individuals. Three other varieties that are not as common in HIV-positive people but can be important in evaluating antibiotic treatment are *Legionella pneumophila, Mycoplasma pneumoniae,* and *Chlamydophila* spp.

Symptoms and Diagnostic Path

People who have *Streptococcus* and *Haemophilus* pneumonias generally show signs of acute infection over a three- to five-day period. These symptoms include fever, chills (including shaking), chest pain, highly productive cough with yellow- or green-colored sputum, wheezing, and shortness of breath (dyspnea). White blood cell counts are typically elevated during bacterial pneumonias. An elevated heart rate and drop in blood pressure are also signs of an inflammatory response to the infection.

A chest X-ray will be given to determine the extent of infection. Because of the greater incidence of TUBERCULOSIS (TB) in the HIV-positive community, testing for TB will generally be ordered as well. Sputum, also called phlegm, will also be sampled to determine the type of bacterial infection as well as to look for the presence of *PNEUMOCYSTIS* PNEUMONIA (PCP) and TB bacteria. A bronchoscopy may also be performed to determine the type of bacteria causing the infection, particularly if sputum or blood tests are not conclusive. Determining the variety of bacteria is an important factor in choosing the most effective treatment, as the different forms of pneumonia call for specific medications because of drug resistance and difference in bacteria susceptibility.

HIV-positive people have a higher incidence of bacteremia associated with pneumonia than HIV-negative people. Bacteremia occurs when the infection involved in pneumonia has moved from the lungs to include the blood.

Treatment Options and Outlook

Bacterial pneumonia treatment is the same in both HIV-positive and -negative people. Diagnostic BLOOD WORK/BLOOD TESTS and fluid work will be done prior to antibiotic treatment, but treatment with some medications will be initiated without waiting for diagnostic test results because of the serious nature of the illness.

People treated at home, on an outpatient basis, will receive a combination of drugs. The first choice is usually an oral beta-lactam antibiotic combined with an oral macrolide. Beta-lactam is a type of antibiotic named for its structure. Beta-lactams include penicillin and amoxicillin. Macrolides are another antibiotic family. Azithromycin and clarithromycin are two frequently used drugs for pneumonia from this group of antibiotics. If a person is allergic to penicillin or other drugs in the beta-lactam group, recommendations are to use an oral fluoroquinolone active against respiratory infections, such as moxifloxacin or levofloxacin.

Treatment in a hospital usually includes intravenous (IV) medications. The first line of treatment is an IV beta-lactam and an IV macrolide. Again, if the patient is allergic to beta-lactams, an IV fluoroquinolone will be substituted. Monotherapy alone is no longer recommended for the treatment of bacterial pneumonias because of the increasing incidence of drug-resistant strains of bacteria.

If the diagnostic tests show evidence of *Pseudomonas aeruginosa* bacteria, then the treatment will be a different variety of beta-lactam drugs such as piperacillin-tazobactam or cefepime, which are active against both pneumococcal and *Pseudomonas* pneumonias. Ciprofloxacin or levofloxacin will be added for the two-drug combination. The drug aztreonam will probably be used in place of the beta-lactam if a person is allergic to those drugs.

Other adjustments will be made to medications if the bacterium is a drug-resistant form of *Staphylococcus*.

Risk Factors and Preventive Measures

In areas where HAART is not available, the risk for bacterial pneumonia is greater for those who are HIV-positive and is not limited to people who have specific CD4 T lymphocyte counts. In people who are receiving HAART, bacterial pneumonias are more likely in, though not restricted solely to, people who have CD4 T lymphocyte counts below 200. Studies have shown that the risk for bacterial pneumonias is reduced for people who are receiving PROTEASE INHIBITORS (PIs) in their HAART regimen. An increased risk of bacterial pneumonias was associated in various studies with previous *Pneumocystis jirovicii* infections, injection drug use, and CD4 T lymphocyte cell counts below 200.

There is a vaccine for pneumonia called the 23-valent polysaccharide pneumococcal vaccine (PPV), which has been shown to help protect people against 23 different varieties of the bacteria that can cause pneumonia. A study that followed HIV-positive veterans has shown that the vaccine is effective in the United States for HIV-positive men. However, a study in Uganda showed that PPV was not effective in HIV-positive individuals there. In fact, the cases of pneumonia increased slightly in Uganda immediately after administrating that vaccine, but the mortality rate decreased in this study of the vaccine's effectiveness. The reasons for this are not clear, but it is believed that the varieties of bacteria causing pneumonia are different in African countries than those in the United States. These studies have all been conducted on HIV-positive people who had T cell counts greater than 200. Studies of people with counts below 200 CD4 T cells have not been as conclusive, but HIV specialists generally consider vaccination to be in the interest of the patient. Recommendations also state that the vaccination should be repeated every five years for HIV-positive people.

Physicians also recommend yearly flu vaccines for all HIV-positive individuals, as pneumonia is often associated with the flu. There is no specific medication used as a prophylaxis for bacterial pneumonia, although trimethoprim/sulfamethoxazole (TMP-SMX) can reduce the risk if it is already being taken for PCP risk reduction. Generally, antibiotics are prescribed for bacterial pneumonia prevention, as they can become ineffective for later use in the treatment of the illness.

Despite the effectiveness of HAART in controlling HIV when taken as prescribed, incidences of bacterial pneumonia are still higher among HIV-positive people than among HIV-negative people. Bacterial pneumonias are more common in HIV-positive women than in HIV-positive men. In addition, African Americans are diagnosed more frequently with bacterial pneumonias than Caucasians or Latinos in the United States.

Other factors that have been shown to increase a person's susceptibility to pneumonia include smoking of any substances, INJECTION DRUG USE, and excessive alcohol use. A depressed absolute neutrophil (a type of white blood cell) count, diagnosed through blood work, can also carry an increased risk of pneumonia. An unusual risk factor for pneumonia is the use of the HIV antiretroviral drug ENFUVIRTIDE (T-20), which is believed to occur because it is an injectable medication, which may allow bacteria to enter a person's body during administration of the drug.

AIDSmeds.com. "Bacterial Pneumonia: What Is It?" AIDSmed.com. Available online. URL: http://www.aidsmeds.com/articles/BacterialPneumonia_6703.shtml. Accessed March 12, 2001.

Bernard, Edwin J. "High Incidence of Bacterial Pneumonia Seen in HIV-Positive US Women." NAMaidsmap.com. Available online. URL: http://www.aidsmap.com/en/news/BC74B442-F77E-43AE-A080-3C0C87A8D0EE.asp. Accessed March 12, 2001.

Canadian Lung Association. "Diseases A–Z: Pneumonia; Bacterial Pneumonia." Lung.ca. Available online. URL: http://www.lung.ca/diseases-maladies/a-z/pneumonia-pneumonie/bacterial-bacterienne_e.php. Accessed March 12, 2011.

Kohli, Rakhi, et al. "Bacterial Pneumonia, HIV Therapy, and Disease Progression among HIV-Infected Women in the HIV Epidemiologic Research (HER) Study." *Clinical Infectious Diseases* 43, no. 1 (2006): 90–98. Available online. URL: http://cid.oxfordjournals.org/content/43/1/90.full. Accessed March 23, 2011.

Mayo Clinic Staff. "Pneumonia." MayoClinic.com. Available online. URL: http://www.mayoclinic.com/health/pneumonia/DS00135. Accessed March 12, 2011.

Thaczuk, Derek. "Vaccination for Pneumococcal Pneumonia Effective in HIV-Positive Men." AIDSmap.com. Available online. URL: http://www.aidsmap.com/Vaccination-for-pneumococcal-pneumonia-effective-in-HIV-positive-men/page/1429814/. Accessed March 23, 2011.

United States Department of Health and Human Services. "Enfuvirtide." aidsinfo.nih.gov. Available online. URL: http://www.aidsinfo.nih.gov/DrugsNew/DrugDetailNT.aspx?int_id=306. Accessed March 12, 2001.

bareback *Bareback* is a slang term referring to having sex without condoms. The term is derived from the act of riding a horse without a saddle. Initially, it was a term used by gay men to refer specifically to unprotected anal sex between men, but it has become common among all people as a term for unprotected vaginal or anal sex. The term first came into general use in the late 1990s. Similar terms are *raw sex, natural sex, unprotected sex,* and *uninhibited sex.*

Prior to the late 1990s, infection with the HUMAN IMMUNODEFICIENCY VIRUS (HIV) was seen as an uncontrolled illness. There was no way to stay healthy long term, and so the message that was provided to the gay community as well as people in general was that condoms save lives and it is necessary to use one every time one has sex in order to protect oneself. However, a few things happened in the mid- to late 1990s that changed the message. One was that HIGHLY ACTIVE ANTIRETROVIRAL THERAPY (HAART) became available in the United States and Western Europe. HIV-related deaths dropped dramatically, and so people began to see and experience that it was

possible to live with HIV. This brought about the simplified thinking that HIV was not a death sentence so therefore there was no longer a need to use condoms. The other change that happened in the 1990s was that sex education funding from the U.S. government was curtailed and stopped for condom distribution and discussion of gay male sexual behavior. Money was instead funneled to ABSTINENCE education in schools in the belief that abstinence was the only option regarding sex that should be taught to young people.

Barebacking is a controversial topic in the gay male community. There are many people who become extremely angry when discussion turns to the topic of any man's having anal sex with another man without a condom. On the other side are men who state that their intimacy is no place for regulations, and as long as they tell their spouse or partner their HIV status, whether or not they then have unprotected anal sex is not anyone's business. The discussion takes place among friends as well as in the community of gay men and HIV educators all around the world. People on both sides of the debate are adamant about their position.

On one side of the discussion is the view that anyone who has sex without a condom is endangering his own health as well as potentially the health of others. This side holds that people who engage in unprotected sex are highly likely to infect themselves or others with a number of potential illnesses in addition to HIV. The discussion also usually includes condemnations of such people for then spreading those illnesses to others knowingly or unknowingly. This side believes people are fooling themselves if they believe they know that their partner(s) is uninfected with HIV or some other illness.

The opposite side of the discussion includes several different arguments. Proponents argue that they are negative and only have sex with their partner, who is negative for HIV. They believe that as adults they can make judgements about their situation and are forthright about the risks to themselves or others. Some of these individuals are already positive and believe there is

no harm in having bareback sex with other positive people. This activity of negotiation between partners and choosing only partners of the same HIV status is known as serosorting. Some people believe serosorting ensures safety in barebacking. Some people feel a greater intimacy exists between a couple if no condom is involved, and some men claim that they are unable to sustain an erection if they wear a condom.

These discussions have also moved to a somewhat more public arena, that of pornography. For many years, beginning in the mid-1980s, all gay male pornography that was produced involved the use of condoms, though this was not practiced in heterosexual pornography. At the time that bareback sex first began receiving attention, marketers for the pornography companies began producing films with gay male actors who did not use condoms. Many educators believe this added to a growing culture of glorifying bareback sex. In addition, Internet sites that seek to eroticize barebacking have appeared. Videos displaying the behavior are widely available on these sites, and conversations among people on these sites indicate that there is a community of people who engage in barebacking behavior regularly and purposefully. Specific slang terms that are associated with barebacking explain what individuals are discussing. The *bug* or the *gift* refers to HIV. A *bug chaser* is someone who is seeking to be infected with HIV. A *gift giver* is someone willing to infect a bug chaser. Barebacking parties are group sex parties where condoms are not allowed. *Bug brothers* are a group of men infected with HIV.

Some gay men believe that testing positive is an inescapable fact given that they are engaging in sex with a population that has a high rate of infection: Currently around 20 percent of MEN WHO HAVE SEX WITH MEN (MSM) in the United States are HIV positive. Other men seek to feel wanted or to be part of a group, and being HIV positive is one way that they believe they can join and be welcomed by a particular group of men. The self-esteem of some gay men is low enough that the idea of joining any group is appealing. Some people seek a thrill of engaging in bareback sex much as they seek a thrill from any dangerous activity. Living on the edge is seen as a life choice, and sex is part of that. Other men simply are willfully ignorant and believe that if neither they nor their sex partner mention the virus, then their sex partner is HIV negative. Drugs and alcohol also encourage barebacking as people forget to follow SAFER SEX guidelines or simply become caught up in the heat of the moment and think that one night of barebacking is not going to affect them.

The reality of the situation, as is often the case in situations painted in black and white, is that there is a great deal of gray, or middle ground, negotiated and discussed between the two different viewpoints. Whether or not governmental leaders or foundations that fund education programs wish to acknowledge it, people are going to have sex without using a condom in many situations. In some countries, the cost of condoms places them outside the reach of many people. In other locations, some men do not allow their women or male sexual partners the option of using a condom. These situations alone account for a large percentage of unprotected sex of any variety. In places where condoms are readily available and within the financial reach of most people, education needs to address the issue that some people are not going to engage in protected sex at every encounter.

Among gay men, a population that has been well studied, several factors seem to emerge as reasons for engaging in barebacking. Improvements in the treatment of HIV are seen as a major part of this issue. Many men, particularly younger men, think that HIV is treatable and not deadly, as it once was viewed by their older counterparts. Younger men and women both have not had the advantage of a strong prevention education program. Abstinence simply teaches not to have sex but does not teach how to avoid illnesses that are a possibility every time people have sex. Fatigue from practicing safer sex is also a cause of potential barebacking

among some people. Years of messages aimed at preventing HIV in some cases are now ignored in the gay male community. In addition, two areas of concern among researchers have been the rise of available sex partners through the Internet and the ongoing use of recreational drugs in many communities. Both of these factors that contribute to the ongoing practice of unprotected sex are cited in several studies of barebacking.

Recent studies about the sexual behavior of teenagers show that teens remain sexually active despite abstinence education. A 2009 study published in the *American Journal of Public Health* also showed an increase in behavior other than vaginal intercourse, including oral sex and anal sex, among heterosexuals. Teens report that these activities do not constitute "real sex" and that they maintain their virginity despite having engaged in these types of sexual activity. This idea has led to the creation of the slang term *saddlebacking* by the sexuality columnist Dan Savage. The term is derived from the Saddleback Church, a Protestant church whose minister has been a political advocate of abstinence education. It refers to heterosexual teens' engaging in bareback sex believing there are no consequences of their activity.

As studies cited here have demonstrated, both gay and heterosexual individuals choose to have sex without condoms. As studies by the U.S. government have shown, abstinence is not an effective tool if it is not combined with education about the use of condoms and the potential for pregnancy and infections when engaging in unprotected sex. In a book released in 2002, Ann O'Leary, a researcher at the CENTERS FOR DISEASE CONTROL (CDC) and prevention, argued that as opposed to an all-or-nothing message from prevention educators, a more realistic message needs to be adopted to reach more people in regard to safer sex. A method of harm reduction education must take place to reach those engaging in unprotected sex. An honest assessment of the possibilities of infection resulting from various sexual activities is needed.

Sexually transmitted infections (STIs) affect a person's viral load negatively and can cause complications if left untreated in HIV-positive as well as -negative people. Discussion with HIV-positive people must make it clear that they can be infected with other strains or types of HIV as well as numerous other STIs. Urban legends exist that only people in the receptive role of intercourse are susceptible to HIV infection and other STIs. These need to be countered with honesty and statistics discussing the very real chance for someone in the insertive role to contract and spread illnesses. Responsibility for decision making needs to be addressed in all populations. As noted by O'Leary, strategies for prevention of HIV transmission need to be offered individually and cannot solely rely on the use of a condom.

ACT: AIDS Committee of Toronto. "Bareback Sex and You." ACToronto.org. Available online. URL: http://www.actoronto.org/home.nsf/Pages/bareback. Accessed March 12, 2011.

Berg, Rigmor C. "Barebacking among MSM Internet Users." *AIDS and Behavior* 12, no. 5 (September 2008): 822–833.

Centers for Disease Control. "Trends in HIV/AIDS Diagnoses among Men Who Have Sex with Men—33 States, 2001–2006." *MMWR* 57, no. 25 (27 July 2008): 681–686. Available online. URL: http://www.cdc.gov/mmwr/preview/mmwrhtml/mm5725a2.htm. Accessed March 12, 2011.

Graham, Judith. "HIV/AIDS Diagnoses Up for Gay Men; Tomorrow's Testing Day." *Chicago Tribune.* Available online. URL: http://newsblogs.chicagotribune.com/triage/2008/06/hivaids-diagnos.html. Accessed March 12, 2011.

Guttmacher Institute. "Facts on American Teens' Sexual and Reproductive Health." Guttmacher.org. http://www.guttmacher.org/pubs/FB-ATSRH.html. Accessed March 12, 2011.

Lescano, Celia M. et al. "Correlates of Heterosexual Anal Intercourse among At-Risk Adolescents and Young Adults." *American Journal of Public Health* 99, no. 6 (June 2009): 1131–1136.

Markham, Christine M., Melissa Fleschler Peskin, Robert C. Addy, Elizabeth R. Baumler, and Susan R. Tortolero. "Patterns of Vaginal, Oral, and Anal Sexual Intercourse in an Urban Seventh-Grade Population." *Journal of School Health* 79, no. 4 (April 2009): 193–200.

O'Leary, Ann, ed. *Beyond Condoms: Alternative Approaches to HIV Prevention.* New York: Kluwer, 2002.

Pardini, Priscilla. "Federal Law Mandates 'Abstinence-Only' Sex Ed." *Rethinking Schools* 12, no. 4 (Summer 1998). Available online. URL: http://www.rethinkingschools.org/archive/12_04/sexmain.shtml. Accessed March 12, 2011.

Robb, Amanda. "Abstinence 1, S-Chip 0." *New York Times* (13 October 2007). Available online. URL: http://www.nytimes.com/2007/10/18/opinion/18robb.html. Accessed March 12, 2011.

Rofes, Eric. "Barebacking and the New AIDS Hysteria." TheStranger.com. Available online. URL: http://www.thestranger.com/seattle/barebacking-and-the-new-aids-hysteria/Content?oid=688. Accessed March 12, 2011.

Savage, Dan. "Savage Love: Saddlebacked!" TheStranger.com. Available online. URL: http://www.thestranger.com/seattle/SavageLove?oid=1031968. Accessed March 12, 2011.

Sowadsky, Rick. "Barebacking in the Gay Community." TheBody.com. Available online. URL: http://www.thebody.com/content/art2276.html. Accessed March 12, 2011.

Tanne, Janice Hopkins. "US State Rejects Federal Funding for Abstinence-Only Sex Education." BMJ.com. Available online. URL: http://www.bmj.com/cgi/content/full/331/7519/715-a. Accessed March 12, 2011.

Tomso, Gregory. "Bug Chasing, Barebacking, and the Risks of Care." *Literature and Medicine* 23, no. 1 (Spring 2004): 88–111.

Wolitski, Richard J. "The Emergence of Barebacking among Gay and Bisexual Men in the United States: A Public Health Perspective." *Journal of Gay & Lesbian Psychotherapy* 9, no. 3/4 (October 2005): 9–34. Available online. URL: http://www.informaworld.com/smpp/content~db=all~content=a904562388. Accessed March 12, 2011.

bartonellosis   Bartonellosis is the name given to infections caused by bacteria within the *Bartonella* species. There are currently 23 known varieties of *Bartonella* bacteria. The most commonly known illnesses are cat-scratch fever, which is caused by the bacteria *Bartonella henselae,* and trench fever, which is caused by *Bartonella quintana.*

Cat-scratch disease is so named because it was thought to be transmitted to humans via scratches by cats. In reality, the bacteria is spread through the feces of the fleas living on cats, and cats pass on the bacteria to humans via their claws after scratching areas infested by the fleas. Trench fever is associated with body lice infestation and is seen in homeless populations with greater frequency than in the general population.

One other illness, Carrión's disease, is known to be caused by *Bartonella* bacteria. Although extremely serious, it is endemic only in Peru, Ecuador, and Colombia, and is no more common in HIV-positive patients than in the general population. There is still significant research being done into the *Bartonella* species, and there may be other infections as yet unassociated with *Bartonella* that are discovered to arise from this type of bacteria.

Symptoms and Diagnostic Path

Cat-scratch disease is a self-limiting illness in a person who is HIV negative and has a healthy immune system. Cat-scratch disease symptoms include swollen lymph nodes, fever, backache, headache, and exhaustion. Symptoms of trench fever include high fever, severe headache, eye pain, soreness of the muscles of the legs and back, and pain in the lower legs. Although trench fever can last a month and symptoms are sporadic during the illness, it too is generally a self-limiting illness that the body can fight off with a healthy immune system.

Bartonella infection is most commonly noticed in HIV-positive patients when the immune system has become severely compromised. Most infections among HIV patients are seen when the CD4 T lymphocyte cell count has fallen below 50 cells/μL.

The main manifestations of bartonellosis are bacilliary angiomatosis (BA), which resembles Kaposi's sarcoma, as large red to purple lesions on or just below the skin, and peliosis hepatis, an illness characterized by random large blood-filled lesions on the liver and occasionally other organs of the body. *B. henselae* causes peliosis hepatis; both *B. henselae* and *B. quintana* can cause BA. Other symptoms of ongoing bartonellosis infection include a persistent fever, night sweats, weight loss, and BA. Systemic bartonellosis is possible, with lesions affecting all major organ systems, and bacteremia (bacterial infection of the blood) causing major problems. Endocarditis (infection of the lining of the heart) and osteomyelitis (infection of the bone or bone marrow) are also possible in bartonellosis.

Treatment Options and Outlook

Treatment for bartonellosis, though often lengthy, is generally successful. Erythromycin and doxycycline have been used to treat all manifestations of bartonellosis. Treatment with these medications generally lasts for a period of three months. Other drugs that could be used in treatment are azithromycin, tetracycline, and clarithromycin. If central nervous system infection is detected, treatment with doxycycline is recommended.

Relapse of the illness can occur after treatment has been completed; it is not common. Manifestations such as BA and peliosis hepatis gradually disappear as recovery from the infection occurs.

Risk Factors and Preventive Measures

Homeless people or people who may be marginally homeless need to be educated on the dangers of body lice infestations, particularly if they are HIV positive. Eradicating the lice as well as maintaining a clean state free of lice can protect an individual from trench fever.

People who own cats should be aware that cats that are outside can contract fleas, which can potentially carry bartonellosis into the home. Cats should receive ongoing flea prevention treatment from a veterinarian. Rough play with a cat or interaction with stray cats can occasionally result in scratches that should be thoroughly washed and cleaned to prevent the possible spread of the bacteria.

There is no general prophylactic treatment for bartonellosis, although people who have been treated for the disease who have CD4 T cell counts below 200 may be kept on ongoing doxycycline treatment until their counts rise above 200.

Hammoud, Kassem A., M.D. "Bartonellosis." emedicine.com. Available online. URL: http://www.emedicine.com/MED/topic212.htm. Accessed March 12, 2011.

Koehler, Jane E., M.D. "Bartonella-Associated Infections in HIV-Infected Patients—AIDS Clinical Care." *JournalWATCH Specialties.* Available online. URL: http://aids-clinical-care.jwatch.org/cgi/content/full/1995/1201/1. Accessed March 12, 2011.

———. "HIV and *Bartonella:* Bacillary Angiomatosis and Peliosis." HIVInSite.ucsf.edu. Available online. URL: http://hivinsite.ucsf.edu/InSite?page=kb-05-01-03. Accessed March 12, 2011.

Schwartz, Robert A. "Bacillary Angiomatosis." emedicine.com. Available online. URL: http://www.emedicine.com/DERM/topic44.htm. Accessed March 12, 2011.

bevirimat Bevirimat dimeglumine is an anti-HIV drug currently in phase IIb trials in the United States. It is also referred to by the drug identifiers PA-457 and MPC-4326. Bevirimat was initially developed by Panacos Pharmaceuticals. In 2009, the rights to the drug were purchased by Myriad Pharmaceuticals, hence the change in drug identifier. Bevirimat was initially derived from a betulinic acid found in the Chinese herb *Syzigium claviflorum,* derived from a tree in Southeast Asia and Australia.

Bevirimat is one of the MATURATION INHIBITORS. It is the first drug in this class of potential HIV antiretrovirals. Maturation inhibitors work against the virus during the phase of viral reproduction, when the virus assembles the proteins needed to create new viral particles to send out to infect other cells. Specifically, bevirimat interferes with the virus as it begins to use the host cell's membrane to form its own viral coating, or envelope, to protect itself and bud from the cell as a new viral particle. This is approximately the same point of development that PROTEASE INHIBITORS (PIs) are designed to target to work against the virus. Instead of interfering with the protease, maturation inhibitors interfere with gag (group-specific antigen) protein development, preventing the virus from infecting other cells. Development of bevirimat has been slow but encouraging. It would put a new class of drugs on the table in the fight to control HIV. Bevirimat received fast-track status from the U.S. FOOD AND DRUG ADMINISTRATION (FDA) in 2005. In 2010, the company making bevirimat stopped all development to focus solely on cancer-treating chemicals.

Dosage

Bevirimat is available as a liquid and as a pill. It is currently being tested as a 100 mg pill taken twice daily. Development of the drug has proven difficult, as the original pill formulations did not deliver the same amount of the drug into the body as the liquid formulation. Initially, a 50 mg pill had been tested, but a new formulation of the drug has proven more effective than the initial formulation that had been undergoing testing. Probably bevirimat will be prescribed in addition to other antiretrovirals; however, it is unknown at this time which antiretrovirals may work well with it.

Drug Interactions

It is possible that bevirimat may interact with other HIV medications, but studies thus far have not focused on this issue. Bevirimat is known to be more effective in some people than in others. Approximately 40 percent of people who have HIV have a type of virus that has specific mutations that do not allow bevirimat to work against it. BLOOD WORK/BLOOD TESTS can determine whether a person's virus will be susceptible to bevirimat. In the most recent studies, bevirimat was very effective against the viruses that allowed it to work, whereas it was not effective in people who had those specific viral mutations. It is believed that some previous resistance to protease inhibitors may interfere with the genetic structure that bevirimat targets in order to work well in the body.

Side Effects

Side effects in tests have been mild. Headache and gastrointestinal discomfort have been reported. Both diarrhea and constipation were reported by approximately 15 percent of the participants in the study.

AIDSmeds. "Bevirimat (PA-457)." AIDSmeds.com. Available online. URL: http://www.aidsmeds.com/archive/bevirimat_1897.shtml. Accessed March 12, 2011.

Highleyman, Liz. 2009. "Maturation Inhibitor Bevirimat Is Well Tolerated and Effective in Predicted Responders." *NAMaidsmap* (18 September 2009). Available online. URL: http://www.aidsmap.com/Maturation-inhibitor-bevirimat-is-well-tolerated-and-effective-in-predicted-responders/page/1436071/. Accessed March 12, 2011.

———. "Myriad Halts Development of HIV Maturation Inhibitor Bevirimat." HIVandHepatitis.com. Available online. URL: http://www.hivandhepatitis.com/recent/2010/0611_2010_c.html. Accessed March 12, 2011.

United States Department of Health and Human Services. "Bevirimat." aidsinfo.nih.gov. Available online. URL: http://www.aidsinfo.nih.gov/DrugsNew/DrugDetailNT.aspx?MenuItem=Drugs&Search=On&int_id=414. Accessed March 12, 2011.

blood work/blood tests People who have the HUMAN IMMUNODEFICIENCY VIRUS (HIV) or AIDS often speak about blood work and the results of blood work. The term *blood work* refers in general to various laboratory tests performed on a person's blood to determine his or her health, potential problems in standard measures of the properties of the blood, and the presence of virus in the blood. Tests including viral load, CD4 T cell counts, and complete blood counts are generally run every three to four months at a minimum for HIV-positive people. Other tests such as liver and kidney function, lipids, and electrolytes may not be measured so often but will be measured at least once a year to maintain a good record of how well a person with HIV is progressing.

Viral Load and CD4 Counts

After a person has tested positive for HIV with an approved HIV test, a doctor will ask that several other blood tests be performed. The two considered most important and the two that most people are familiar with are the viral load test and the CD4 count. These two tests with a number of others can allow a doctor to get a better understanding of how healthy a person with HIV is and how advanced his or her illness has become.

The CD4 count measures the number of CD4 T cells in a person's blood. A CD4 T cell is a type of white blood cell (a lymphocyte). When a person's CD4 T cells are measured, other types of lymphocytes are also measured: CD8 T cells, B cells, and NK cells. White blood cell counts help to determine the health of the immune system. CD4 T cells are the cells that HIV infects and uses to reproduce. Over time, the number of CD4 T cells declines in a person infected with HIV. CD8 T cells help to identify and kill cells that have been infected with viruses or bacteria. B cells work to kill infections that are in the body but outside cells. NK cells help to fight cancers and infections in cells. They are part of the innate immune system and are larger than T or B cells. NK stands for *natural killer* because the cells have chemicals in them that destroy infected cells on contact.

Typically, in an HIV-negative person, CD4 T cell counts range from 500 to 1,500/mm^3 (cubic millimeter, or microliter). CD8 T cell counts normally range from 300 to 800/mm^3. There are generally two CD4 T cells for every one CD8 T cell in a person who has a normal immune system. In HIV-positive people, that ratio is often reversed. HIV-positive people often have fewer than 500 CD4 T cells/mm^3. Recommendations for patients to start treatment now reflect that people who have fewer than 500 CD4 T cells/mm^3 should be on treatment with antiretroviral drugs. Another value that is measured at the same time as the various lymphocyte counts is the percentage count of CD4 T cells among all lymphocytes. The normal range for HIV-negative people is 28–58 percent. HIV-positive people often have percentage readings much lower than 28 percent.

The other standard blood test is the viral load count. This blood test measures the amount of virus that can be detected in a milliliter of blood, approximately a teaspoon. When a person has this measured prior to treatment, it can range anywhere up to 1 million or more copies of the virus per milliliter. A high viral load indicates that the virus is actively reproducing, and the virus can progress rapidly with that many copies. If treatment with antiretrovirals is working properly, then the viral load will be undetectable. This means the amount of virus is less than what the test can measure, which, depending on the test used, can be either fewer than 500 copies or fewer than 40 copies per milliliter of blood. It does not mean that a person is cured. When viral load climbs to 5,000–10,000 copies per milliliter, most physicians will recommend a change of treatment, as this can indicate that the HIGHLY ACTIVE ANTIRETROVIRAL THERAPY (HAART) regimen is not working as well as possible.

Complete Blood Count

Viral load and CD4 counts are generally run concurrently with a complete blood count (CBC). A CBC can indicate many things about the health of a patient. It measures the number of white blood cells (lymphocytes, neutrophils, eosinophils, basophils, and monocytes), number and quantity of red blood cells (hemoglobin, hematocrit, mean corpuscular volume, and mean corpuscular hemoglobin), and number of platelets.

Red blood cells are produced in bone marrow, the interior areas of the bones. They carry oxygen and carbon dioxide to the blood. The raw number reported in a CBC shows how many red blood cells a person has in a cubic millimeter (μL or mm^3) of blood. Differences exist in the normal ranges of red blood cells between men and women. Ranges can be 4.0–5.3 μL for women and 4.5–6.1 μL for men. People who have HIV often have slightly lower numbers of red blood cells, as some HIV antiretrovirals cause the bone marrow production to be suppressed. Significantly lower numbers can indicate anemia. This can be treated with iron supplements, other medications, or, if serious enough, a blood transfusion.

Hematocrit measures the amount of red blood cells in relation to the percentage of other cells in the blood. Higher numbers indicate higher levels of red blood cells. It can also be used to determine anemia. Hemoglobin is a red blood cell protein that carries oxygen. Normal levels of hemoglobin in the blood are different for men and women. Normal ranges for men are 14–18 grams per deciliter (g/dL). Levels in women range from 12 to 16 g/dL.

Other measures are mean corpuscular volume and mean corpuscular hemoglobin. These measure the size of the red blood cells. People who have low mean corpuscular volume generally have a deficiency in iron or have a chronic disease. Some B vitamin deficiencies or even use of ZIDOVUDINE may cause higher than normal values on this test. Mean corpuscular hemoglobin is used at times to determine whether a person has an anemia; some leukemias are detected through this test, which measures the weight of hemoglobin in a red blood cell.

White blood cells are also produced in the bone marrow by stem cells located there. There are five main types of white blood cells. A lowered amount of white blood cells in general is known as leukopenia because white blood cells are also known as leukocytes. In addition to lymphocytes, discussed earlier, there are eosinophils, basophils, and neutrophils, known collectively as granulocytes. Granulocytes typically fight bacterial or parasitic infections. They constitute 50–80 percent of all white blood cells. Eosinophils are responsible for fighting allergens, and their numbers increase dramatically during an allergic reaction or asthma attack. Some HIV drugs can lower granulocyte levels in the blood, in particular of neutrophils. *Neutropenia* is the term for lowered numbers of neutrophils in the blood. Monocytes are short-lived white blood cells. They typically move into the tissues, where they become cells known as macrophages, which consume bacteria and other foreign matter in the tissues.

White blood cells generally are represented in blood in stable percentages. During an allergy attack, eosinophils increase in number. During an infection of some type, neutrophils increase. A large increase in immature or small white blood cells can indicate a blood disease of some type.

Platelets allow the blood to clot and allow healing of external injuries. A person who has a lowered number of platelets may have an increased incidence of bleeding or bruising. A normal platelet count range is 150,000–400,000 cells/μL. Anything below 150,000 cells/mm^3 is not within the normal range. Decreased platelet count may cause problems with bruising or bleeding. At this point, a doctor may change the HAART dosage as a result of the drop in platelets it may be causing or suggest a blood transfusion to increase the platelet count. Thrombocytopenia is the condition of lowered numbers of platelets. One secondary problem that occurs in some HIV-positive people is idiopathic thrombocytopenic purpura (ITP). This name indicates that the reason for the lowered platelets is unknown and the condition will cause bruising or purpling in areas of the body.

Liver and Kidney Function

Other blood work that is commonly ordered for HIV-positive people can measure liver and kidney functions. This is important because the antiretrovirals that people take to treat HIV are typically filtered out of the body through the kidney and the liver. Some of the drugs are known to cause stress on the liver or kidneys, particularly if a person has another illness that already affects these organs.

Liver panels, or liver function tests, measure several different enzymes and proteins that can help determine liver health and proper function. It is not unusual for someone who has HIV or is having HAART to have abnormal liver function test results. One of the tests measures the levels of bilirubin. Bilirubin is the yellow pigment produced by the remains of dead blood cells that are collected and disposed of by the liver. It is also the product that gives bruises a yellowing color as they heal. When a person has severe HEPATITIS B or HEPATITIS C, it causes yellowed skin and eyes, known as jaundice. High bilirubin levels can indicate liver or bile duct malfunction because the liver is unable to remove the bilirubin from the body. In HIV-positive people, both ATAZANAVIR SULFATE and INDINAVIR can cause elevated bilirubin levels, also called hyperbilirubinemia. Some people stop taking those two drugs if the bilirubin levels become too high and they report yellow eyes and yellowing skin color. Yellowing is not a sign of illness in and of itself, as the bilirubin levels do not in this case indicate liver problems and do not occur with everyone.

Three enzymes are also measured on most liver panel tests: ALT, AST, and ALP. ALT, or alanine aminotransferase, is an enzyme found in the liver; elevated levels are a good indication of liver disease, particularly hepatitis. AST, or aspartate aminotransferase, is an enzyme found in the liver and some muscles, including the heart. ALP, or alkaline phosphatase, is an enzyme that indicates bile duct blockage or illness. These three enzymes, when measured together and compared to each other, can help determine whether liver dysfunction is occurring.

Albumin is a protein made by the liver. Low levels of albumin can indicate liver disease. Low albumin levels may also indicate a kidney problem, malnutrition, or shock. High levels of albumin are generally seen in a person who is dehydrated.

There are two main kidney function tests that a doctor may order. Blood urea nitrogen (BUN) and creatinine both can indicate impaired kidney function. Creatinine and BUN measure the way the kidney is processing these substances and removing them from the body. Some HIV drugs or HIV itself can cause kidney function to decrease or cause kidney failure in rare instances.

Resistance Testing

Resistance testing is becoming more routine for HIV-positive people who are taking antiretroviral medications. It can be used to determine the type of HIV that a person has, as well as particular mutations that will make the virus resistant to particular medications or classes of medications.

HIV genotypic testing requires up to three weeks to obtain results. This testing looks at the genotype, or genes, of the virus. It examines the ribonucleic acid (RNA) and determines which mutation markers the virus displays. Each mutation of the virus appears on the RNA and allows a researcher to see which medications are likely to work well against the virus.

Phenotypic testing, or assay, takes longer for a lab to return to the doctor. This assay looks at how the virus responds to different medications. The virus is grown at the laboratory among the different antiretrovirals to see which of the drugs kill the virus and which do not. This test requires at least a month before results are known. Both genotypic and phenotypic assays require that a person be taking some type of HAART regimen so the tests can determine why the virus is or is not susceptible to the antiretrovirals.

Another blood test the doctor may decide to order is called the tropism assay. This looks at the virus and determines which of the two proteins HIV uses to enter the cells of the body. CXCR4 and CCR5 are the two proteins that HIV needs to adhere to in order to enter the cell. Some HIV uses one or the other, and some viruses, particularly when the diagnosis is AIDS, use both proteins to adhere to cells. There are particular medications—MARAVIROC, for instance—that are designed for use only against the virus that uses CCR5 to enter the cell.

Lipid Panels

Lipid panels measure the cholesterol and triglyceride levels in the blood. Some HIV antiretrovirals are known to raise cholesterol and triglyceride levels. This blood test requires that a person fast for at least 12 hours prior to having the blood drawn. A desirable cholesterol level is one that is below 200 milligrams per deciliter (mg/dL) for total cholesterol. Cholesterol is made up of two parts, high-density lipoprotein (HDL, or good cholesterol) and low-density lipoprotein (LDL, or bad cholesterol). HDL levels of 50–60 mg/dL are considered good. An amount higher than 60 mg/dL can provide some protection against heart disease. An HDL lower than 40 mg/dL increases the risk of heart disease. For LDL, the lower the number, the better off a person is. Anything lower than 120 mg/dL is considered optimal or near-optimal. Anything above that is less than optimal, and an LDL above 190 mg/dL is extremely high. Triglyceride is a type of fat that is generally related to a person's lifestyle. A good triglyceride level is 150 mg/dL or less. Anything above 200 mg/dL is considered high. A person who smokes, is obese or overweight, does not engage in any physical activity, eats a diet high in carbohydrates, or drinks excessive amounts of alcohol is more likely to have high triglyceride levels, although some illnesses and drugs can raise the level of triglycerides. A doctor will measure both a person's cholesterol and triglyceride levels before initiating HAART, as some of these medicines can cause the levels of triglycerides or cholesterol to increase, raising a person's risk for heart disease and stroke.

Electrolytes

Electrolytes are chemicals in the body that are in a general state of balance. Each of the chemicals is required for the proper functioning of some part of the human body. Most commonly measured during a blood test of electrolytes (sometimes called a chemistry screen) are sodium, potassium, magnesium, chloride, calcium, and two hydrogen compounds, hydrogen phosphate and hydrogen carbonate. The body requires that they be in balance for the electrical stimulus that controls muscles and nerves, blood pH, and proper hydration (water content). If a person has electrolytes that are not in balance, overhydration or dehydration can occur, muscles and neurons do not work properly, and eventually, if fluids and electrolyte balance are not restored, a medical emergency can occur. HIV-positive people can sometimes have electrolyte imbalances caused by the different medications they take, through improper kidney or liver functioning or other potential causes. A test of electrolytes is generally administered on a regular yearly basis.

American Association for Clinical Chemistry. "HIV Viral Load: The Test." LabTestsOnline.org. Available online. URL: http://www.labtestsonline.org/understanding/analytes/viral_load/test.html. Accessed March 12, 2011.
———. "Human Immunodeficiency Virus." LabTestsOnline.org. Available online. URL: http://www.labtestsonline.org/understanding/conditions/hiv-2.html. Accessed March 12, 2011.
Project Inform. "Blood Work: A Complete Guide for Monitoring HIV." ProjectInform.org. Available online. URL: http://www.projectinform.org/info/bloodwork/index.shtml. Accessed March 12, 2011.
Zachary, James A., M.D. "Understanding Lab Tests in HIV Treatment." HIVInfo.us. Available online. URL: http://www.hivinfo.us/labtest.html. Accessed March 12, 2011.

breast-feeding Breast-feeding is the act of nursing a baby from a human breast. Breast-feeding is the way all babies had been fed in human history until more recent times, when baby formula was created and used in many resource-rich countries as an alternative to breast-feeding. Breast-feeding is generally done by the mother of the child, but in historical times in Western countries, wet nurses—women who were lactating—would be employed to provide breast milk to babies whose mothers had died in childbirth or could not for some reason produce breast milk. In some cultures, notably parts of AFRICA, communal breast-feeding, or breast-

feeding of all children in a village or area by all women who are lactating in the village, is still a common occurrence.

Exclusive breast-feeding is giving the baby only milk from the breast. Replacement feeding or formula feeding, is giving the baby food, usually in the form of a milklike liquid, generally made with a powdered formula mixed with water from whatever source the mother has. Mixed feeding is the term used to describe feeding a baby a combination of formula and breast milk.

Breast-fed babies have been shown in studies to be healthier babies, even in resource-rich countries. Breast milk from a healthy woman contains all the nutrients and food a baby needs in the first months of its life. Breast milk also contains HUMAN IMMUNE SYSTEM stimulants that can help protect a baby against early childhood illnesses such as diarrhea and respiratory infections. However, breast-feeding can also pass on to the baby some drugs or alcohol that the mother has consumed. It is also a way diseases can be spread, especially HIV, as well as TUBERCULOSIS (TB). This is why counseling a woman prior to delivery of her baby is important so that the potential benefits and dangers of breast-feeding to her and her child can be discussed.

Breast-feeding has been a poorly understood and often ignored means by which HIV can be passed to children. It was discovered in the mid-1980s that several mothers who became infected with HIV while breast-feeding had passed the virus to their children. The WORLD HEALTH ORGANIZATION (WHO) issued guidelines stating that it was possible to transmit HIV in this manner but that it did not view breast milk as a major issue in the TRANSMISSION of the virus. However, by the early 1990s, studies conducted predominantly in sub-Saharan Africa were showing that the rates of infection for children who were breast-fed were significantly higher than for babies who were formula fed. Further studies in the late 1990s suggested that babies breast-fed for longer periods were more susceptible to transmission of HIV than those breast-fed for shorter duration. Studies early in the current decade showed that babies raised with mixed feeding were at higher risk for HIV transmission through breast-feeding than either babies who were exclusively breast-fed or those who were formula fed. A study completed in 2006 in Botswana determined that during an outbreak of diarrhea in the country, babies of HIV-positive mothers who were breast-fed survived at a higher rate than did formula-fed babies of HIV-positive mothers. A study completed in 2008 highlighted the potential for a lactobacillus found in yogurt to prevent the spread of HIV by binding to the virus and preventing transmission. A study is currently under way in Tanzania to test this possibility.

Current WHO guidelines leave the choice to the mother but strongly encourage counseling prior to initiation of breast-feeding. The only sure, and completely safe, method to ensure HIV is not spread to a baby through feeding is to use formula for the entirety of the process. WHO guidelines are expressed with the acronym AFASS, which stands for *acceptability, feasibility, affordability, sustainability,* and *safety. Acceptability* is important because in most cultures breast-feeding is the norm and expected. If a woman decides to formula feed, people in her family or community may assume she is HIV positive, and she, her child, or other family members may face discrimination and isolation. If formula feeding is not acceptable in her community, then it may not be practiced properly, and this will harm the baby more than not doing it at all. *Feasibility* refers to the time, skills, and knowledge required to formula feed. It takes a good amount of time to build a charcoal fire, heat the formula, allow it to cool, and follow the guidelines of the formula manufacturer to store the mixed formula properly. Mixed formula can only be stored for two hours in any condition without a refrigerator. A mother must be able to handle these various tasks that involve large quantities of her time to ensure proper feeding using formula. *Affordability* refers to the cost of the fuel, either wood or bottled gas, to have a fire; the cost of the formula itself; and the cost of water to allow the mother

to make the formula properly. In most countries, the cost of formula exceeds the minimum wage of the family and must be supplemented through programs that pay for the formula. *Sustainability* refers to the ability to maintain access to the water and formula for six months, as the baby needs this period on formula to develop properly. Any disruption to the water supply or availability of formula can have serious consequences for the baby. *Safety* speaks to the need for a safe, secure water supply. It also refers to the need to boil the water and the utensils used in the preparation of the formula to prevent any germs from causing illness in the baby. This is one of the most important issues in formula preparation in resource-poor areas of the world.

Mixed feeding has been shown to be the more dangerous of the three options available to women. This is because the formula is not as gentle on the baby's stomach and intestines and can cause irritation to the lining of these digestive organs. It is possible that the HIV in the mother's breast milk more readily enters the baby's immune system in these cases as the baby is switched from formula to breast milk to other foods. Studies have shown that babies who are mixed fed have higher rates of HIV infection than those either exclusively breast-fed or formula fed.

Recommendations currently specify that if breast-feeding is the option that is chosen, it be limited to the first six months of the baby's life. At that point, the benefits of breast-feeding have been acquired by the baby, and it is probably safer to wean the baby and introduce other foods and formula. Extending the breast-feeding increases the risk of HIV transmission. Babies who are breast-fed more than 18–24 months potentially have a 10–20 percent higher risk of HIV than babies infected in utero or during delivery.

Another way to decrease the risk of HIV transmission during breast-feeding is keeping the mother aware of her own health. Higher rates of HIV transmission occur in the first few weeks of HIV infection as well as when a person's immune system is weakening. Viral load is a measure of the viral activity in a person. Higher viral loads as well as lower CD4 counts are both indicators that the baby is at higher risk of receiving HIV through the mother's breast milk. Breast inflammation of any kind is also a sign that a baby's risk of acquiring HIV may be higher. Nipple abscesses, mastitis, or even chapped and cracked nipples can offer ways for the virus to pass much more easily to the baby. If the use of antiretrovirals is available to a mother, the risk of transmission is lower. A woman being treated successfully for HIV will have a lower viral load and generally higher CD4 count, so that her chance of passing the virus on is lessened. A mother can also be aware of her baby's health. If a baby has sores or lesions on the inside of the mouth or is suffering with a case of thrush, this could theoretically increase the baby's chance of acquiring HIV during breast-feeding. Treatment of the baby with antiretrovirals during the six months of breast-feeding has also been shown to reduce the transmission of HIV.

Breast-feeding remains a vital part of the lives of most children in the world. The purpose of the WHO recommendations is to recognize the importance of breast-feeding while making the process as safe as possible for both the baby and the mother. Research continues to make headway into the topic, as it has been poorly understood through much of the HIV epidemic.

AVERT: AVERTing HIV and AIDS. "Introduction to HIV and Breastfeeding." AVERT.org. Available online. URL: http://www.avert.org/hiv-breastfeeding.htm. Accessed March 12, 2001.

Creek, Tracy et al. "A Large Outbreak of Diarrhea among Non-Breastfed Children in Botswana, 2006." RetroConference.org. Available online. URL: http://www.retroconference.org/2007/Abstracts/30582.htm. Accessed March 12, 2011.

Linkages. "Reducing Mother-to-Child Transmission of HIV among Women Who Breastfeed—Rehydration Project." Rehydrate.org. Available online. URL: http://rehydrate.org/breastfeed/breastfeeding-hiv-pmtct.htm. Accessed March 12, 2011.

ScienceDaily. "New System Blocks HIV Transmission via Breastfeeding." ScienceDaily.com. Available online. URL: http://www.sciencedaily.com/releases/2008/07/080703125224.htm. Accessed March 12, 2011.

Swanminathan, Nikhil. "Strange but True: Males Can Lactate." *Scientific American.* Available online. URL: http://www.scientificamerican.com/article.cfm?id=strange-but-true-males-can-lactate&sc=rss. Accessed March 12, 2011.

World Health Organization. "HIV Transmission through Breastfeeding." UNFPA.org. Available online. URL: http://www.unfpa.org/webdav/site/global/shared/documents/publications/2004/hiv_transmission.pdf. Accessed March 12, 2011.

candidiasis Candidiasis is a fungal infection caused by the overgrowth of the fungus *Candida,* which occurs naturally in the human body. It can be found on the skin and in the stomach and gastrointestinal (GI) tract, colon, rectum, vagina, mouth, and throat. For most of a person's life *Candida* is harmless and does not cause problems. It actually helps to control bacteria that enter the body through the GI tract. However, under certain conditions, *Candida* grows uncontrollably, causing problems.

The species *C. albicans* is most often the cause of the infection, though other varieties can cause similar problems. Resistance to drugs used to treat *Candida albicans* has caused *Candida glabrata* to appear more often in some individuals. Candidiasis is also called a yeast infection. It can affect the skin, nails, and mucous membranes of the mouth, esophagus, lungs, GI tract, and vagina.

Symptoms and Diagnostic Path

Oral candidiasis, also known as thrush, appears in the mouth as white, creamy bumps that are easily removed if disturbed or small lesions or patches that cannot be removed. Thrush is often seen in babies or young children as they build their immune system but rarely seen in adults unless their immune system is not functioning properly. The bumps can be found on the tongue, inner lips, roof or sides of the mouth, and under the tongue. The thrush can cause a burning sensation or a change in the taste of food. It can also cause difficulty in swallowing because of the sensations and pain. Thrush can be distinguished from the similar-appearing hairy leukoplakia because the white patches are easily dislodged when scraped.

Vaginal candidiasis may also be known as a yeast infection or vaginitis. Symptoms include a yellow-white, thick, aromatic discharge from the vagina that closely resembles cottage cheese. It can cause burning or itching in and around the labia (outer lips of the vagina). Urination can be painful. Up to 75 percent of adult women will have vaginitis during their lives, so it is not an unusual condition; however, because of the compromised immune system of HIV-positive women, recurrent frequent cases can cause problems. Pregnancy and diabetes also seem to increase the chance of a *Candida* outbreak. Diagnosis other than by observation may be done to differentiate the symptoms from a urinary tract infection. A sample of the vaginal secretions is taken for lab observation and confirmation of *Candida.*

Candidiasis of the esophagus, leads to inflammation of the lining of the esophagus, or esophagitis, which can be seen by a doctor by looking into the mouth and down the throat. It can cause chest pain and swallowing difficulties. Weight loss may occur as patients report not being hungry or having trouble eating and swallowing. An endoscopy may be performed if tests on oral lesions are inconclusive or if esophagitis is believed to be present. An endoscopy is an examination done through inserting a small tube, which contains a small camera to view the lining of the organ, into the throat and esophagus. At times, oral candidiasis may not be evident at the same time as esophagitis, necessitating an endoscopy.

If not kept in control by the immune system or medication, *Candida* can also spread to infect other parts of the body such as the lungs, the circulatory system, and the brain if the person's immune system is especially weakened. Invasive candidiasis is usually a problem only when the HUMAN IMMUNE SYSTEM has become very weakened. HIV-positive people are most likely to face problems with *Candida* when their CD4 T lymphocyte cell count falls to below 200 cells/μL. Once the CD4 T cell count falls below 100, OPPORTUNISTIC INFECTIONS (OIs) may be frequent and can recur even after successful treatment. *Candida* is often the first illness an HIV-positive person will have.

Treatment Options and Outlook

Treatment for candidiasis can be topical, meaning applied to the surface where the infection occurs, such as on the skin, in the vagina, or in the mouth. A treatment can also be systemic, meaning it is active throughout the body. The type of medication taken depends on the symptoms and diagnosis. Treatment is generally successful for oral, vaginal, and muscosal candidiasis. It can be more difficult for esophageal or invasive infection.

Initially, candidiasis can be treated effectively with oral fluconazole. It is a once-daily pill that is taken for two to three weeks, depending on the symptoms. It is relatively easily tolerated by most people and has been proven very effective at controlling *Candida*. Oral ketoconazole and itraconazole have been proven less effective in controlling oral candidiasis and are not recommended by the government treatment guidelines because of their varying rates of absorption.

Oral nystatin is administered in the form of an oral rinse, or mouthwash. It is swished around the mouth several times and then swallowed. This procedure is followed at least four times a day for a period of several days. This drug has proven effective in controlling simple thrush outbreaks, particularly for people who have difficulty swallowing or tender mouths from the candidiasis. Lozenges, also known as troches, of either nystatin or clotrimazole, can also be

prescribed for oral candidiasis. These are taken several times a day and sucked on, not chewed or swallowed whole.

Creams or ointments can be used to treat vaginal candidiasis. Clotrimazole, miconazole, tioconazole, as well as other azole medications are effective in controlling vaginitis. Oral tablets such as fluconazole can also be used. Medications are taken or applied for a period of at least seven days. Suppositories, caplets inserted into the vagina, can also be used to treat vaginal candidiasis.

Esophageal candidiasis can be treated effectively with fluconazole, as well as several varieties of echinocandin drugs. Echinocandins are antifungal medications that must be taken intravenously (IV). Caspofungin and micafungin are two echinocandins that are typically used in treating esophageal candidiasis. Other IV drugs may also be used.

Systemic or invasive infection with candidiasis is treated with an IV antifungal or oral tablets. Again, fluconazole is the treatment of choice. Other options include amphotericin B, voriconazole, caspofungin, micafungin, and anidulafungin. All of these treatments may also be used in cases of fluconazole-resistant *Candida*. Systemic candidiasis is difficult to treat, and success rates are poor. Patients generally have very low T cell counts and have difficulty fighting the infection even with proper medication.

Risk Factors and Preventive Measures

HIV-positive and HIV-negative people can both develop candidiasis. Stress, poor diet, and sleeping problems can lead to disruptions in body function and encourage *Candida* growth. In addition, people who are on antibiotics for long periods can develop *Candida* infections in the mouth or vagina. Inhaled steroids, such as those taken for the treatment or prevention of asthma, can also lead to candidiasis. Other activities that have been linked with candidiasis development in the mouth are smoking, excessive drinking, and intake of large quantities of sugar.

Vaginal candidiasis can be a recurrent problem for women who are HIV positive. Spread of yeast infections via sexual contact can occur during heterosexual activity; the man notices a burning sensation of the urethra and development of a red, inflamed head of the penis within a few hours of unprotected intercourse with a woman who has candidiasis.

Prophylaxis for candidiasis can be given to patients who have experienced previous episodes of infection and whose CD4 T cell counts have fallen below 200. However, fluconazole-resistant strains of *Candida albicans* as well as other *Candida* species that are not susceptible to fluconazole can make candidiasis a very dangerous illness for an HIV-positive person.

Centers for Disease Control. "Candidiasis." CDC.gov. Available online. URL: http://www.cdc.gov/nczved/divisions/dfbmd/diseases/candidiasis/index.html. Accessed March 12, 2011.

———. "Guidelines for Prevention and Treatment of Opportunistic Infections in HIV-Infected Adults and Adolescents." National Institutes of Health Web site. Available online. URL: http://aidsinfo.nih.gov/contentfiles/Adult_OI_041009.pdf. Accessed March 12, 2011.

Fichtenbaum, Carol J., M.D., and Judith A. Aberg, M.D. "Candidiasis and HIV." HIVInSite.UCSF.edu. Available online. URL: http://hivinsite.ucsf.edu/InSite?page=kb-05&doc=kb-05-02-03. Accessed March 12, 2011.

Miller, Karl E. "Does Vaginal Candidiasis Affect Genital HIV Shedding?" *American Family Physician* 72, no. 10 (15 November 2005): 2087–2124.

Project Inform. "Systemic Candidiasis and HIV Disease." TheBody.com. Available online. URL: http://img.thebody.com/legacyAssets/49/77/candidiasis.pdf. Accessed March 12, 2011.

Caribbean Outside sub-Saharan AFRICA, the Caribbean region has a higher percentage of its population who are HIV positive than any other place in the world. The Caribbean, as defined in the United Nations (UN) reports on AIDS, consists of the island nations of the Caribbean Sea, Bermuda in the central Atlantic Ocean, Belize in Central America, and Suriname, Guyana, and the French overseas department of Guiana on the South American continent. The countries that are not islands are linked culturally and historically more often with the Caribbean than with the Spanish- or Portuguese-speaking countries that are covered in reports on LATIN AMERICA. Numbers cited in this article are drawn from several Joint United Nations Programme on HIV/AIDS (UNAIDS) reports.

HIV was first seen in Haiti in the very early 1980s and then was quickly diagnosed in most of the other island countries by the mid-1980s. There is an overall prevalence rate of 1.0 percent in the Caribbean. HIV/AIDS is the leading cause of death in the region for people between the ages of 15 and 44 and HIV/AIDS totaled 14,000 deaths in the region in 2007. It is estimated that 230,000 people are currently living with HIV in the Caribbean. The following are the prevalence rates for specific areas: Bahamas, 3.1 percent; Barbados, 1.2 percent; Cuba, 0.1 percent; Dominican Republic, 0.9 percent; Guyana, 1.2 percent; Haiti, 1.9 percent; Jamaica, 1.7 percent; Puerto Rico, 1.2 percent; Suriname, 2.4 percent; and Trinidad and Tobago, 1.5 percent. Rates of infection have declined in some countries, most notably Haiti, Dominican Republic, the Bahamas, and Barbados.

Haiti was one of the first countries that diagnosed AIDS cases and was initially associated with AIDS because of media hysteria about the disease before much was known about HIV. Newspapers characterized the epidemic with the four Hs: Homosexuals, hemophiliacs, heroin users, and Haitians were the initial groups who could be identified as suffering from the same symptoms and the same unusual illnesses, and for a while the tag was applied. Since then, Haiti has lost more than 300,000 people to AIDS-related illnesses, and approximately 120,000 people were HIV positive as of 2010. AIDS-related illnesses cause the death of more than 7,000 Haitians each year now. Because of the consistently poor economy and poor government structure, many Haitians seek employment outside the country, and this route is believed to have been the way HIV initially entered Haiti, taken back by workers who had been in Africa in the 1970s. HIV prevalence has fallen in recent years in the capital among pregnant women who are tested at clinics, from more than 5 percent to 3 percent. Studies also show a drop in mean numbers of sexual partners on a regular basis, and condom use has increased. However, in the rural areas, condoms are rarely available, and studies show people do not use them with any regularity. Treatment improvement has occurred in Haiti, as approximately 40 percent of those needing HIGHLY ACTIVE ANTIRETROVIRAL THERAPY (HAART) receive it through various nongovernmental agencies working on the island. HIV-positive pregnant WOMEN are one group among whom such progress has lagged, as only 12 percent of HIV-positive women have received antiretroviral treatments of any kind. It is unclear how the earthquake of 2010 in Haiti affected delivery of HIV medications or the overall transmission rates of HIV. The severe disruptions it caused in terms of health care and living situations may not be known for several years.

The Dominican Republic shares the island of Hispaniola with Haiti, and the epidemic there seems to have slowed. The commercial sex industry is the main mechanism of spread of the virus. SEX WORKERS in the capital show a prevalence rate of above 3 percent. Condom distribution as well as prevention education have increased condom use levels to near 100 percent in parts of the capital, Santo Domingo. Migrant workers, many from Haiti, work in sugarcane fields in the Dominican Republic, and these camps have consistently shown high rates of HIV in studies. Again, HIV-positive women do not receive the necessary treatment to prevent mother-to-child TRANSMISSION; and these rates remain unnecessarily high given that most CHILDREN are born in government hospitals.

Cuba's epidemic began in the early 1980s in soldiers who returned from duty in Africa. It's initial policy was to segregate all HIV-positive people at hospitals or areas where they did not mix with the general population. Cuba began screening blood and blood products in 1986,

prior to most other countries in the region. The government provided and continues to provide all food and living spaces free to this population, which has also encouraged some self-segregation by HIV-positive people, even after enforced quarantine was removed, because all basic needs are met by the government. Cuba is the only country in the Caribbean that has 100 percent distribution of antiretroviral medications. It is also the only country in the region that tests all pregnant women and provides antiretrovirals to prevent mother-to-child transmission of the virus. Only 28 cases of mother-to-child HIV have ever been recorded on the island. The distribution of medication is sustainable because of the low number of HIV-positive people on the island. Of concern, however, is the fact that 20 percent more HIV cases were detected in 2006 than in the previous year. Women accounted for 10 percent of those new cases, a 30 percent jump from the previous year. Men account for more than 80 percent of all HIV-positive people in Cuba. MEN WHO HAVE SEX WITH MEN (MSM) activity is the main cause of the spread of HIV on the island.

Puerto Rico has twice the rate of HIV infections of the mainland United States. INJECTION DRUG USE(R)s remain the main source of HIV spread on the island. If Puerto Rico were one of the U.S. states, it would rank ninth for the number of HIV-positive people, but it ranks only 27th in total population among states. Concerns over the availability of HIV medical care and antiretrovirals have plagued Puerto Rico recently. Many patients have gone without care or medications as a result of poor funding from the federal government and mismanagement of the funds that have been received in the territory. These phenomena spell future deaths and a worsening of the already high rate of infection on the island.

Jamaica's epidemic has been fairly steady for several years. It is predominantly spread through sexual activity, both heterosexual and homosexual. The rate of HIV prevalence among Jamaica's sex workers is currently 9 percent. Although education has been good in recent years and the majority of women and men understand how

HIV is spread and how to prevent the spread, studies show Jamaicans report high numbers of sexual partners and unprotected sexual activities. Discrimination and stigma in Jamaica toward high-risk groups, especially MSM, are high and continue to prevent effective education outreach in some populations. Provision of testing to pregnant mothers as well as antiretroviral treatment to these women has slowed the mother-to-child transmission.

The countries that are not islands—Belize, French Guiana, Guyana, and Suriname—all have epidemics that are significantly higher than those of countries surrounding them in Central and South America. Guyana's epidemic is predominantly spread through sexual activity. Sex workers test HIV positive at a rate of 30 percent in some areas. MSM test positive in the capital region at a rate of 21 percent, and 80 percent of MSM in Guyana also report recent sex with women. Guyana has recently expanded their mother-to-child prevention program to counter rises in that HIV-positive population. Further education to counter widespread prevention myths and discrimination against MSM and HIV-positive people may help to slow the epidemic. Belize has the highest rate of HIV prevalence in Central America and the fourth-highest rate in the Caribbean. It is double the rate of infection of its neighbor Guatemala and eight times the rate of infection of its other neighbor, Mexico. Spread is predominately sexual, as men report multiple sex partners and infrequent condom use. Partonage of paid sex workers is also commonplace in the country. Suriname also has a relatively large population of HIV-positive people. Rates of infection are higher among women than men. Again, the virus is predominately spread through sexual contact. A 2005 survey of sex workers done in the capital, Paramaibo, by the Pan-American Health Organization and cited in United Nations (UN) reports indicated that 21 percent of female sex workers and 36 percent of male sex workers tested HIV positive. Although late in getting started, Suriname now provides free condom distribution, education in

schools, and sex worker education programs. It will be some time before results of these efforts can be realized. French Guiana is an overseas department of France, and statistics are represented in French totals. Other French overseas departments in the Caribbean—Saint Martin, Guadeloupe, and Martinque—all have higher prevalence rates than any regions of mainland France. French Guiana shares many of the same problems as its neighbors Suriname and Guyana, a population that is sexually active and uncommitted to practicing SAFER SEX on a regular basis.

Other island nations in the Caribbean have HIV epidemics that are for the most part spread through heterosexual and homosexual sex. Bermuda is the main exception; injection drug use is the main cause of infection there. Most nations report high sexual activity rates in the young populations and a lack of knowledge about the spread of HIV and ways to prevent infection. Extended access to education for HIV-positive people in the region has helped improve health and reduce deaths, particularly in the Bahamas and Trinidad and Tobago. In the Bahamas, mother-to-child transmission rates dropped from 25 percent of pregnancies in 1997 to below 5 percent of pregnancies in 2003.

AVERT: AVERTing HIV and AIDS. "HIV and AIDS in the Caribbean." AVERT.org. Available online. URL: http://www.avert.org/aids-caribbean.htm. Accessed March 12, 2011.

Cohen, John. "Special Online Collection: HIV/AIDS—Latin America and Caribbean." *Science*. Available online. URL: http://www.sciencemag.org/sciext/aidsamericas/. Accessed March 12, 2011.

Conseil National du SIDA. "The Epidemic of HIV in French Guiana: A Political Problem." CNS.sante. fr. Available online. URL: http://www.cns.sante.fr/spip.php?article287&lang=en. Accessed March 12, 2011.

Eckholm, Erik. "Puerto Rico's AIDS Care in Disarray over Funds." *New York Times* (5 June 2007). Available online. URL: http://www.nytimes.com/2007/06/05/health/05puerto.html. Accessed March 12, 2011.

Henry J. Kaiser Family Foundation. "HIV/AIDS Policy Fact Sheet: The HIV/AIDS Epidemic in the Caribbean." KFF.org. Available online. URL: http://www.kff.org/hivaids/7505.cfm. Accessed March 12, 2011.

Joseph, Emma. "Caribbean Nations See HIV Success." BBC. Available online. URL: http://news.bbc.co.uk/2/hi/americas/7764990.stm. Accessed March 11, 2011.

KPBS News. "Cultural Factors Contribute to High HIV Prevalence in Belize, KPBS Reports." KaiserHealthNews.org. Available online. URL: http://www.kaiserhealthnews.org/daily-reports/2006/february/22/dr00035568.aspx?referrer=search. Accessed March 12, 2011.

Mulot, Stephanie. "Antilles et Guyane françaises: Une épidémie à part." Pistes.fr. Available online. URL: http://www.pistes.fr/transcriptases/125_494.htm. Accessed March 12, 2011.

PANCAP: Pan Caribbean Partnership against HIV AIDS. "HIV AIDS in the Caribbean." PANCAP.org. Available online. URL: http://www.pancap.org/index.php. Accessed March 12, 2011.

Sullivan, Mark P. "AIDS in the Caribbean and Central America." *Congressional Research Service.* Available online. URL: http://fpc.state.gov/documents/organization/62680.pdf. Accessed March 12, 2011.

UNAIDS: Joint United Nations Programme on HIV/AIDS. "Caribbean." UNAIDS.org. Available online. URL: http://www.unaids.org/en/regionscountries/regions/caribbean/. Accessed March 12, 2011.

———. "UNGASS Country Progress Report Belize." UNAIDS.org. Available online. URL: http://www.unaids.org/en/dataanalysis/monitoringcountryprogress/2010progressreportssubmittedbycountries/belize_2010_country_progress_report_en.pdf. Accessed March 12, 2011.

UNAIDS: Joint United Nations Programme on HIV/AIDS and the World Health Organization. "2007 AIDS Epidemic Update Caribbean." UNAIDS.org. Available online. URL: http://data.unaids.org/pub/Report/2008/jc1528_epibriefs_caribbean_en.pdf. Accessed March 22, 2011.

———. "AIDS Epidemic Update 2009." UNAIDS.org. Available online. URL: http://www.unaids.org/en/media/unaids/contentassets/dataimport/pub/report/2009/jc1700_epi_update_2009_en.pdf. Accessed March 22, 2011.

Centers for Disease Control (CDC) The Centers for Disease Control and Prevention (CDC) is one of the 13 main agencies of the U.S. Department of Health and Human Services. It was founded in 1946 after World War II ended, primarily as a MALARIA control agency of the federal government. It is headquartered in Atlanta, Georgia, near the campus of Emory University. Atlanta was at one time a center for malaria in the United States. The original name of the agency was the Communicable Disease Center. The focus of the agency has grown over time to include all public health concerns, including communicable diseases, sexually transmitted infections, environmental health, disaster preparedness, birth defects, immunizations, and technical assistance in these areas to communities and agencies in the United States and around the world. The CDC maintains large quantities of epidemiological data so that they can track illnesses as they occur as well as historic outbreaks of illnesses for use in future decision making. The public mission of the CDC "is to collaborate to create the expertise, information, and tools that people and communities need to protect their health—through health promotion, prevention of disease, injury and disability, and preparedness for new health threats."

In June 1981, the CDC published a report by a physician at the University of California Los Angeles of five MEN WHO HAD SEX WITH MEN (MSM) in Los Angeles who had all been treated for a rare pneumonia, *PNEUMOCYSTIS carinii* PNEUMONIA (PCP), between October 1980 and May 1981. In addition to the PCP, the men had all been diagnosed at some point with CYTOMEGALOVIRUS (CMV), and they all had CANDIDIASIS. This was the first mention in medical literature of any type about what would eventually be labeled *acquired immunodeficiency syndrome* (AIDS). The publication was the *Morbidity and Mortality Weekly Report* (MMWR), a CDC publication that is used to this day to track early outbreaks of contagious illnesses, reports of unusual or rare illnesses seen in groupings, or any information deemed vital that the CDC receives that doctors, hospitals, and city and state public health clinics are required to report to them.

The next month, another article appeared in the *MMWR* that related several cases of PCP and a rare cancer called Kaposi's sarcoma (see HUMAN HERPES VIRUS 8). In the 30 months prior to the July publication, 20 young men who had been engaged in MSM sexual activity in New York City had been diagnosed with Kaposi's sarcoma, a disease that had been diagnosed only three times among men of this age group in New York City since 1960 prior to these cases. Another six cases had been recorded in the same age group in California over the same period. When the men were admitted to the hospital for care, it was also seen that many had pneumonias, and some had TOXOPLASMOSIS, candidiasis, and disseminated herpes infections. The story also reported that in the month since the first report of PCP, another 10 gay men had been identified with PCP in California, some in San Francisco and the rest again in Los Angeles. It was noted that all of these illnesses were generally only seen in people who had severe HUMAN IMMUNE SYSTEM dysfunction. These noted patients all had immune systems that seemed not to be working properly. The editors of the *MMWR* at the CDC cautioned that doctors should be on the lookout for MSM displaying these illnesses who had immune suppression. After these articles, another 70 cases of similar illnesses in the gay community were reported to the CDC, by August 1981.

In the months and years that followed, the CDC was the lead government agency in tracking the cases of what they initially labeled gay-related immune disorder, or GRID. The name was used because at that time no one outside this population and no women had been reported with these conditions. This name was changed in July 1982 to acquired immunodeficiency syndrome (AIDS) after researchers and doctors began reporting the same illnesses and immune suppression in other groups. The public press seized on the classes of people and began referring to them as the four Hs: homosexuals, Haitians, hemophiliacs, and heroin users. Again, reports in the *MMWR* would soon add children and people who had received blood transfusions.

The CDC was involved in meeting with doctors around the country to discuss the cases; take medical, sexual, and life histories of the currently living patients; and try to find commonalities among all of them. Randy Shilts in his book *And the Band Played On* details the role the CDC played in tracking and documenting the illness. The CDC quickly formed a task force and became the early funder and organizer for research into the unknown illness, with no increases in funding to handle the suddenly huge workload to track a problem that was quickly becoming widespread. At the same July 1982 meeting, the CDC believed it had enough information about the illnesses to issue precautions and warnings to medical workers on how to work with AIDS patients. It began warning blood agencies, such as the International Red Cross, that there was a potential for a new blood-borne illness to be spread through these particular groups. Despite such early warnings, blood banks ignored the CDC and caused countless people to be infected via blood transfusions and clotting factor made from blood that was used by people who had hemophilia. Blood banks did not alter their donation practices until 1985.

Despite the accolades of different authors regarding the hard work many at the CDC put in to learn about the new illness, there were also scathing reports about the lack of budget allocated for AIDS in the early years. Funding was slow to arrive, and administrators appointed by the Reagan administration did little to allocate funding through the CDC to address the problem. In relation to the number of deaths AIDS caused, very little was allocated to the problem when comparing the government funding available when Legionnaire's disease caused a few deaths in the late 1970s and the amount spent to determine the cause of Tylenol poisonings in 1982, which far outstripped the money spent that year for AIDS work.

The CDC was often criticized in the early days of the epidemic, not just for lack of funding, but for their conservative approach to education as well as the initial public health warnings, which were often seen as insensitive and unhelpful to many people in the public. The CDC often refused to fund or cancelled funding for brochures, videos, or educational training materials that were deemed too risqué or too explicit for Americans. At the same time, the CDC was at the forefront of trying to close all public bathhouses in large cities, where men often went to have anonymous sex. Both of these measures were seen as the government's unwillingness to work with the gay male community or even to discuss gay sexuality issues. The CDC has had to fight internally conservative policies with proper public health action to prevent the spread of HIV. It has been a difficult struggle for the agency to balance through the years of the epidemic.

The CDC Web site states, "As a part of its overall public health mission, CDC provides leadership in helping control the HIV/AIDS epidemic by working with community, state, national, and international partners in surveillance, research, and prevention and evaluation activities." The CDC is still the lead government agency in funding prevention programs, and maintains constantly updated estimates and case numbers for HIV infection and AIDS.

Centers for Disease Control and Prevention. "About CDC." CDC.gov. Available online. URL: http://www.cdc.gov/about/. Accessed March 12, 2011.
———. "Kaposi's Sarcoma and *Pneumocystis* Pneumonia among Homosexual Men—New York City and California." *Morbidity and Mortality Weekly Report* (4 July 1981). AEGIS.com. Available online. URL: http://www.aegis.com/files/mmwr/1981/MMWR04JUL81.pdf. Accessed March 12, 2011.
———. "MMWR: Past Volumes (1982–2010)." *Morbidity and Mortality Weekly Report*. Available online. URL: http://www.cdc.gov/mmwr/mmwr_wk/wk_pvol.html.
———. "*Pneumocystis* Pneumonia—Los Angeles." *Morbidity and Mortality Weekly Report* (5 June 1981). AEGIS.com. Available online. URL: http://www.aegis.com/files/mmwr/1981/MMWR05JUN81.pdf. Accessed March 12, 2011.
Graham, Jeff. "1981–1986: In the Beginning." TheBody.com. Available online. URL: http://www.thebody.com/content/whatis/art32414.html. Accessed March 12, 2011.
National Institutes of Health. Office of NIH History. "In Their Own Words." NIH.gov. Available online. URL: http://history.nih.gov/NIHInOwnWords/index.html. Accessed March 12, 2011.

Chagas disease   Chagas (pronounced SHA-gus) disease is an illness caused by the parasite *Trypanozoma cruzi*. It is found only in the Western Hemisphere, with highest incidences in Brazil, Mexico, and Central America, but is on occasion seen as far north as the southern United States and as far south as southern Chile and Argentina. It is believed to affect 10 million people in the Americas. The CENTERS FOR DISEASE CONTROL and Prevention (CDC) believes 100,000 people in the United States may carry the disease, most of them immigrants from endemic areas. As there is no natural vector (the triatomine bug) of the disease in most of the United States, spreading the disease through this means is unusual in this country.

The parasite is spread through the feces of the triatomine bug, also known as the assassin bug or the kissing bug. The triatomine bug becomes infected through biting a person or animal that is already infected with the parasite. The insect feeds on animal and human blood. It then passes on the parasite by excreting on the person or animal it bites; when the person scratches the bite, he or she becomes infected with the parasite as it enters the bloodstream through the insect bite. It is also possible to pass on the parasite through blood transfusion, BREAST-FEEDING, and contaminated food. The triatomine bug most often lives in the cracks of mud or adobe homes and homes with grass or stick roofing, emerging at night to feed. Use of lime, a building product made from crushed limestone, in the preparation of the mud or adobe has been shown to reduce the infestation of the bugs, thereby lowering infection rates in some endemic areas.

Chagas disease can have both acute and chronic forms. Acute forms can cause exhaustion, fever, aches and pains, and a swelling at the site of infection called a chagoma. In 90 percent of cases, the symptoms clear up, but the parasite remains in the body unless the person is treated. Chronic infection occurs in about 25 percent of people, who carry the infection over the course of several years. The most common problems include heart disease, arrythmias that can cause sudden death, intestinal disease that leads to malnutrition and difficulties eating, and central nervous system inflammation and lesions in the brain.

Symptoms and Diagnostic Path

In HIV-positive people, the disease can be reactivated after many years in individuals who have chronic disease and a weakened immune system. They can also develop acute Chagas disease symptoms from a recent exposure if their immune system is not functioning well. Because the disease is limited currently to a particular geographic region, the illness may not be seen regularly in many parts of the world or be mistaken for other illnesses that an HIV-positive person may suffer. Recent travelers to areas of endemic Chagas disease need to make their doctors aware of any recent travel if they become ill afterward.

Chagas symptoms, when they are reactivated in an HIV-positive person, generally involve the brain. Swelling can occur in the lining of the brain, the meninges, and lesions can be detected by scans. Signs can be similar to results seen in TOXOPLASMOSIS scans, so it can be difficult to determine what may be causing the problems without blood testing for the parasite. Both BLOOD WORK/BLOOD TESTS and cerebrospinal fluid testing can detect the parasite during an acute or reactivated disease. In people who are chronically infected, these tests are not always accurate, and blood antibody tests for the parasite are used to determine whether a person has been infected. Other tests that may be performed include brain biopsy to determine the extent of the infection if other means cannot yield conclusive results.

Treatment Options and Outlook

For treatment in HIV-positive people, two drugs are commonly used. Neither is licensed for use in the United States, but they are available through the CDC. Benznidazole is the drug of choice given over a one- to two-month period. Nifurtimox is the other drug that is generally given, for a three- to four-month period. Neither drug will clear the parasite from a person's body, but both reduce the amount of the parasite in the body and prevent the clinical symptoms of the disease. The studies that have been done in HIV-positive patients show that early recognition and diagnosis increase the survival rate and success of treatment. Approximately half of all people treated during an acute infection with these medications will successfully clear the parasite from their system, although it is unknown whether HIV-positive people respond with the same success rate. Both medications can be toxic to some people, and monitoring the patient will be required during their use.

HIGHLY ACTIVE ANTIRETROVIRAL THERAPY (HAART) is believed to prevent both acute phases of the disease as well as reactivation of chronic forms of the illness in HIV-positive people. It is important to start a patient on HAART if he or she is not currently using anti-HIV medications when diagnosed with Chagas disease to help prevent the illness from reactivating.

Risk Factors and Preventive Measures

There is no preventive drug or medication for Chagas disease at this time. Prevention when traveling to endemic areas involves the use of mosquito netting when sleeping in homes that are likely to house the insect and the use of insect repellents to prevent them from biting. Because the parasite is in the blood of a chronically infected person, it is more likely that Chagas disease will be passed through blood transfusions, ORGAN TRANSPLANTATION, injection drug use, or mother-to-child transmission during pregnancy. It was only in 2007 that the American Red Cross began testing their blood products for T. cruzi, so transfusions prior to this time may have some risk of carrying the parasite.

Centers for Disease Control and Prevention. "Parasites—American Trypanosomiasis (also known as Chagas Disease)." CDC.gov. Available online. URL: http://www.cdc.gov/parasites/chagas/. Accessed March 12, 2011.

Kaminstein, David M. "Chagas' Disease." In *The Encyclopedia of Medicine,* edited by Donna Olendorf et al. Detroit: Gale, 1999.

Kirchhoff, Louis D. "Chagas Disease (American Trypanosomiasis)." eMedicine.com. Available online. URL: http://www.emedicine.com/med/TOPIC327.HTM. Accessed March 12, 2011.

Powderly, William G. "Management of Chagas' Disease in an HIV-Infected Patient." Medscape. Available online. URL: http://www.medscape.com/viewarticle/413279. Accessed March 12, 2011.

Ramos-Filho, C. F. "Chagas' Disease in HIV Infection." *AIDS: Official Journal of the International AIDS Society* 8, suppl. 4 (November 1994): S17.

children   AIDS was first diagnosed in children in 1982, a year after the syndrome was first identified in adults. By 1992, HIV was the seventh leading cause of death among children younger than four years of age in the United States. Today, in Western countries, early diagnosis and antiretroviral treatment and use of preventive treatment for OPPORTUNISTIC INFECTIONS (OI) have allowed infection rates in children to drop dramatically from the 1980s and have extended the lives of children infected with HIV.

The term used to describe acquisition of HIV by children during a pregnancy, during birth, or through BREAST-FEEDING is *perinatal TRANSMISSION.* This is also referred to as vertical transmission or mother-to-child transmission (MTCT). Statistics in the United States show that between 100 and 200 children are infected perinatally each year. There were, in 2005, more than 6,000 children living with HIV in the United States who had been infected perinatally. Minority children are at a higher risk of perinatal transmission, as 20 percent of perinatal transmission occurs in LATINO/A AMERICANS and 66 percent in AFRICAN AMERICANS. These numbers highlight both the need for greater education and outreach to these communities and the lack of early-pregnancy medical care and early testing available to these mothers. Of the nearly 8,500 people diagnosed with AIDS through perinatal transmission during the epidemic, approximately 57 percent have died.

Unfortunately, around the world, HIV affects more than 2 million children. In 2007, according to United Nations (UN) statistics, more than 370,000 children were born HIV positive. One of every seven people who died of HIV complications in 2007 was a child. Nine of every 10 children living with HIV live in sub-Saharan AFRICA. Large numbers of HIV-positive children also live in the CARIBBEAN, LATIN AMERICA, and South or Southeast ASIA. Smaller numbers live in WESTERN AND CENTRAL EUROPE and NORTH AMERICA. Nearly 90 percent of these children acquired their HIV from their mother during pregnancy, birth, or breast-feeding. This is the most common way for children to become HIV positive. At the beginning of the epidemic, some children acquired HIV through untested blood received in transfusions or through blood products such as clotting factor, which is used to treat hemophilia, a bleeding disorder. This manner of transmission has generally been eliminated in most Western countries. Testing of blood from donations and the use of genetically engineered clotting factor have eliminated these sources of transmission. However, resource-poor countries do not often have the ability to test all blood donations, particularly in emergency settings. There is also generally not enough funding in many countries to pay for proper resterilization of needles used for immunizations, lack of which can cause the spread of the virus. In addition, sexual transmission of the virus in children does occur. In many countries, sexual activity starts young; for example, 16 percent of young women and 12 percent of young men have sex before the age of 15 in sub-Saharan Africa. Also, in some parts of southern Africa, it is believed that sex with a virgin will kill the virus, so some men will rape, or force sex on, much younger children in the false belief that they can cure AIDS through this act.

All children born to HIV-positive mothers test HIV positive at birth by the standard HIV antibody test. This is because all babies receive their immune system cells initially from their mother, so if the mother has antibodies to a particular virus, the baby will also. The mother's immune system cells can remain in the baby for several months after birth. Testing for antibodies to HIV will not take place until at least 18 months after the child is born. HIV TESTS are generally given shortly after birth, at one to two months of age and again at four to six months of age. The tests look for the virus itself and not the antibodies. U.S. federal guidelines suggest that if the baby tests negative on at least two of these occasions, then an HIV antibody test should be run around 18 months of age to determine whether the baby is indeed HIV negative. If the baby tests positive on at least two of the tests, then a positive HIV antibody test will show the baby is HIV positive. By 18 months, a baby will have lost the antibodies given by its mother and developed its own immune system cells and antibodies.

HIV affects children differently than it affects adults. It immediately impairs a child's immune system at birth. The reason for this is that the immune system in an HIV-positive child is not able to build itself naturally as an HIV-negative child's immune system would. As a baby is exposed to various bacteria, viruses, and other illnesses, a normal immune system strengthens itself and builds immunity to these infections. When HIV impairs the formation of an immune system, the child's body has no way to recognize and fight off illnesses such as chicken pox and other common problems such as ear or nasal infections. Unlike adults, who become HIV-positive later in life, children do not have immune system memory cells that can recognize various types of illness and respond quickly to an infection. Illnesses such as CYTOMEGALOVIRUS (CMV) or *Pneumocystis* PNEUMONIA (PCP) in adults require memory cells that children do

not possess to help fight the infection. Also, in children born to mothers who have used alcohol or drugs heavily during a pregnancy, the baby may have to fight the effects of withdrawal from these substances in addition to HIV. One clear effect of HIV in babies is that the viral load in babies and children is higher than it is in adults. This makes it especially important that babies, as do adults, receive antiretroviral therapy as soon as possible to reduce the effects of HIV on their immune system. Children who have HIV suffer from opportunistic infections (OIs) just as adults with HIV disease do. However, some OIs seen in adults, such as TOXOPLASMOSIS and HUMAN HERPES VIRUS 8, are seen much less frequently in children. Pneumonias are more common in children who have HIV. *Pneumocystis* pneumonia and lymphocytic interstitial pneumonitis, the latter rarely seen in adults, are common. Yeast infections, such as CANDIDIASIS, are also common in children.

About 25 percent of all children born to women who have AIDS will become HIV positive if there is no intervention during or just after the pregnancy. This is true across all countries and in all general populations. Studies throughout the epidemic of MTCT as well as women and children who have HIV have shown that women who are HIV positive and have low viral load counts and CD4 T cell counts above $200/\mu L$ have a lower chance of passing the virus to their baby, approximately 8 percent. Studies in the United States also have proven that mothers who are aware of their HIV status and are receiving proper HIV and pregnancy care have an even lower chance of passing HIV to the babies, approximately 1 percent.

Because of this research, prevention of MTCT has been a priority in most HIV education and outreach programs in the United States as well as in all other countries with such programs. In 1997, a study conducted in Uganda showed that a single dose of the drug NEVIRAPINE, one of the NON-NUCLEOSIDE REVERSE TRANSCRIPTASE INHIBITORS (NNRTIs), given to the mother when she began labor and a single dose given to the baby after birth prevented HIV transmission in half of the study participants as compared to the known rate for mothers who did not receive the treatment. Nevirapine is a relatively inexpensive drug and because it is given only once to the mother and once to the child has proven effective even in resource-poor countries where the cost of treatment makes antiretroviral therapy unavailable to most people. Over time, there have been some concerns about resistance to future treatment of HIV because of the single-dose regimen. There has been evidence that both mother and child do develop some RESISTANCE to the use of nevirapine in future drug regimens. Because the drug is taken only once, the virus has time to recognize the medication and overcome the method the drug uses to stop viral replication. This can cause problems especially if the baby is breast-fed by the mother, as the baby may become infected with a nevirapine-resistant virus in that manner. This resistance to nevirapine also makes the virus resistant to the drug EFAVIRENZ.

The WORLD HEALTH ORGANIZATION (WHO) guidelines specify that prevention treatment for MTCT of HIV in resource-poor countries be done with a combination of ZIDOVUDINE and nevirapine. This has been tested in various settings and has proven the most effective therapy in preventing the spread of HIV to babies and the treatment least likely to lead to resistance in either mother or child. The treatment with zidovudine is recommended to start at 28 weeks of pregnancy—or earlier, if possible—for the mother. Then, a dose of nevirapine should be administered at the time labor starts. After delivery, a mother should receive a seven-day course of zidovudine plus a seven-day course of LAMIVUDINE. The WHO recommends a single dose of nevirapine for the baby as soon after birth as possible followed by a seven-day course of treatment with zidovudine. This treatment regimen is, of course, more difficult to manage in resource-poor countries and requires much more dedication to and understanding of the task of following the regimen of the mother, but it is also much more successful in preventing HIV transmission during birth. If a mother receives less than four weeks of zidovudine treatment, WHO guidelines call for the child to receive four weeks of zidovudine rather than one week, as recommended when the mother had begun treatment. Resistance to zidovudine does not usually develop, even in a single-drug regimen, until several weeks after the medicine is started. It is believed that these guidelines should be safe for the majority of women and not promote long-term resistance to treatment options with other antiretroviral drugs.

Children provided some of the many images of HIV patients in the early years of the epidemic. Ryan White became a well-known child in the United States in the late 1980s. At age 14, he was forced into the media spotlight in 1984 after becoming ill with pneumonia as a result of HIV complications, in his hometown of Kokomo, Indiana. Local officials barred him from attending school, as they feared that he would spread HIV to other people by breathing on them or using the same cafeteria silverware or similar means. Although eventually the local school board was forced by the courts to admit Ryan to classes, more than half of the students in the school he attended were withdrawn from school by their parents because of hysteria created by rumors about how HIV was spread. Ryan White was victorious in court, but the school system forced him to use a separate bathroom, and he had to eat with disposable plates and silverware at the school. Eventually, his family left Kokomo when unknown assailants shot at their home. The family moved to nearby Cicero, Indiana, where they were accepted by the community, and AIDS education programs helped people to understand there was nothing to fear being around a person with HIV. Ryan White somewhat reluctantly became a national spokesperson for people who had HIV. He had acquired the virus through blood product transfusions used to treat his hemophilia, and had become well known because of the way he was treated by others in his community. Yet he made the most of his speaking abilities, winning friends across the globe including the singers Michael Jackson and Elton John. He testified before the U.S. Congress about the discrimination he had faced. Shortly after White died in 1990 at the age of 18, the United States finally passed a comprehensive care law that provided funding for the treatment of people with HIV who had no insurance. The Ryan White CARE (Comprehensive AIDS Resources Emergency) Act continues to be funded today as a means of providing HIV care for those unable to afford it.

Other children who became well known in the United States were the Ray brothers, Ricky, Robert, and Randy. They were also hemophiliacs who had acquired HIV through blood products. They too were banned from attending school in their hometown of Arcadia, Florida. When they attempted to fight that discriminatory act, the school board ordered their removal from school, and unknown people in the community burned their home to the ground. Like Ryan White, they became spokespeople for people with HIV, working to provide education to political leaders as well as various news and media personalities. Randy was the only brother still alive as of 2011.

Hydeia Broadbent is now a well-known AIDS activist. She was born HIV positive to a drug-addicted woman in 1985 and has lived her whole life with the virus. She was abandoned at birth in Las Vegas, Nevada, and was adopted early in life. She was not diagnosed with HIV until she became seriously ill at three years of age. Hydeia began speaking publicly about HIV when she was six years old. By the time she was 12, she was traveling around the country speaking about HIV prevention and treatment. Hydeia, whose name means "gift" in Swahili, and her mother, authored a book, *You Get Past the Tears,* which details the struggles they faced learning about and dealing with HIV. Hydeia may be most remembered for her speech before the Republican National Convention in 1996, where she said, "I am the future and I have AIDS." These children all added a dimension to the HIV epidemic that was generally invisible when the only images seen were of gay men or

Africans who were dying. They played an important role in educating the public about the virus and were seen in the media by large numbers of people who may not have received any AIDS information otherwise.

One of the most moving events early in the epidemic was the plight of Romanian children in the late 1980s. A testament to the difficulties of a resource-poor country and the policies of the former dictator, Romania had 10,000 children who were HIV positive by 1992. Birth control and abortions were illegal in Romania unless a woman had already had at least five children. Unwanted babies were left at government offices or hospitals anonymously, creating large orphanages in the country. Policies in the orphanages and government care centers for these children were to provide injections of whole blood to the children to help boost their immunity. However, because Romania was such a resource-poor country, often the blood was untested for viruses, and care centers had few needles for the injections. This led to the problem of thousands of sick children in state-run orphanages that the new government was left to face when the dictator Nicolae Ceausescu was overthrown in a coup in 1989. Previously, the Romanian government had denied that HIV was a concern for their country. By the year 2000, more than 60 percent of all pediatric HIV cases in Europe were in Romania, the vast majority of those living in state-run institutions. Since this initial epidemic among children, Romania has developed strong programs in HIV treatment and in HIV care for children. The model of care developed there has been used in southern Africa, where there are also large numbers of HIV-positive children living in orphanages.

Treatment of HIV in children has always lagged behind the treatment for adults. New drugs are tested initially in adult populations. Most of the time, new drug CLINICAL TRIALS are not done in children until after the government has approved the drug for use in adults. Guidelines for use of some HIV medications in children are based solely on word of mouth and experimentation with dosage levels because optimal levels of many drugs in small children have not yet been determined.

Some drugs have liquid alternatives that can be used in infants who are unable to swallow pills, but these are few. Treatment in older children, though easier because they can swallow pills, can be difficult because often children need to be supervised to assure that they have taken their pills. Just as in adults, maintaining a schedule for taking antiretroviral medications is important to their success. Missed doses can lead the virus to become immune to the effects of the drugs. When used as directed, HAART in children has been successful in reducing illness, increasing life span, reducing viral load levels, and increasing CD4 counts, just as it has in adults.

Absolute CD4 counts in children below six years of age are not as telling a measure of the health of the immune system as they are in adults, although falling CD4 counts over time can be taken as a measure of the immune system's decline. Children's CD4 counts fluctuate more when they are young and tend to be much higher than those of adults. Children less than six years of age can benefit from percentage CD4 cell counts, which measure the CD4 cells in relation to other types of lymphocytes. The normal percentage of CD4 helper T cells in people is anywhere from 28 to 68 percent of their total lymphocytes. A count lower than 21 percent is considered abnormally low. This number tends to remain fairly constant, whereas the absolute CD4 count can often go up or down over the course of several months. A falling CD4 percentage is a sign the immune system is failing.

The WHO recommends antiretroviral treatment for children below the age of five regardless of their CD4 percentages, absolute CD4 count, or viral load count. The U.S. federal treatment guidelines for children also now recommend the same course. Studies conducted in South Africa by the WHO showed that infants who began HAART regardless of their immune system indicators fared much better than chil-

dren who did not receive treatment until their immune system was viewed as failing. Previous studies have shown that children on HAART have fewer cases of TUBERCULOSIS as well as other serious illnesses. They also have demonstrated that once a child has reached five years of age, disease progression is similar to that in adults with HIV. Treatment for young children after five years of age and teens should be similar in approach to that for adults.

Children known or believed to have HIV are often given prophylactic antibiotics to help prevent illness, particularly in resource-poor countries where antiretroviral access is limited. Trimethoprim/sulfamethoxazole (TMP-SMX or cotrimoxazole) is a standard antibiotic that is used for HIV patients to prevent *Pneumocystis carinii* pneumonia, tuberculosis, and other bacterial infections. HIV-positive children treated with TMP-SMX had fewer hospital stays and fewer bacterial infections than HIV-positive children who did not receive the drug as infants. The cost of this drug is significantly lower in most areas of the world than the cost of antiretroviral treatment.

Across the world, access to testing for pregnant women and infants continues to be a barrier to both prevention and treatment of HIV. Hospitals, clinics, and testing sites in resource-poor countries tend to be few and far between. Cost barriers to antiretrovirals remain significant in many areas. Although there have been considerable cost reductions in the provision of antiretrovirals, particularly in AFRICA, access remains difficult in some locations. Indian pharmaceutical companies have negotiated contracts to provide HAART medications at a fraction of the cost of American or European companies. The United Nations (UN) as well as some nongovernmental organizations (NGOs) that provide antiretroviral medications in resource-poor areas have worked with the Indian companies to provide relatively inexpensive access to these drugs since 2006. UN studies show costs have fallen significantly during that time. As only 4 percent of children worldwide who needed HAART were able to receive it according to estimates made in 2005, any increase in access is a step toward better medical care for children who have HIV.

The need for better medical care in general as well as for better access to treatment in resource-poor countries will continue to be a problem for HIV-positive children. Prevention of HIV remains the best hope for reducing the number of HIV-positive children around the world. Fear, shame, and stigma associated with an HIV-positive diagnosis remain the major threats to prevention in many countries. Until the basic medical care and basic access to medication are available, HIV will be a devastating illness in many resource-poor areas of the world.

AIDSmeds.com. "Special Issues for Children with HIV: Introduction." AIDSmeds.com. Available online. URL: http://www.aidsmeds.com/articles/Children _7566.shtml. Accessed March 12, 2011.

AVERT: AVERTing HIV and AIDS. "HIV & AIDS Treatment for Children." AVERT.org. Available online. URL: http://www.avert.org/hiv-children.htm. Accessed March 12, 2011.

———. "Preventing Mother-to-Child Transmission (PMTCT) of HIV." AVERT.org. Available online. URL: http://www.avert.org/motherchild.htm. Accessed March 12, 2011.

Broadbent, Hydeia. "The Official Hydeia L. Broadbent Page." HydeiaBroadbent.com. Available online. URL: http://www.hydeiabroadbent.com/. Accessed March 12, 2011.

Centers for Disease Control and Prevention. "Mother-to-Child (Perinatal) HIV Transmission and Prevention." CDC.gov. Available online. URL: http://www. cdc.gov/hiv/topics/perinatal/resources/factsheets/ perinatal.htm. Accessed March 12, 2011.

Dente, Karen, M.D., and Jamie Hess III. "Pediatric AIDS in Romania." Medscape.com. Available online. URL: http://www.medscape.com/ viewarticle/528693. Accessed March 12, 2011.

National Pediatric AIDS Network. "NPAN: The National Pediatric AIDS Network." NPAN.org. Available online. URL: http://www.npan.org/default. asp?anchor=Home. Accessed March 12, 2011.

NYU Center for AIDS Research. "Children and HIV." HIVInfoSource.org. Available online. URL: http:// www.hivinfosource.org/hivis/hivbasics/children/. Accessed March 12, 2011.

United States Department of Health and Human Services. "HIV during Pregnancy, Labor and Delivery, and after Birth: Health Information for HIV Positive Pregnant Women." aidsinfo.nih.gov. Available online. URL: http://aidsinfo.nih.gov/contentfiles/ Perinatal_FS_en.pdf. Accessed March 12, 2011.

———, Working Group on Antiretroviral Therapy and Medical Management of HIV-Infected Children. "Guidelines for the Use of Antiretroviral Agents in Pediatric HIV Infection." aidsinfo.nih. gov. Available online. URL: http://aidsinfo.nih. gov/contentfiles/PediatricGuidelines.pdf. Accessed March 12, 2011.

World Health Organization, Interagency Task Team on Prevention of HIV Infection in Pregnant Women, Mothers and Their Children. "Guidance on Global Scale-up of the Prevention of Mother-to-Child Transmission of HIV." WHO. int. Available online. URL: http://whqlibdoc.who. int/publications/2007/9789241596015_eng.pdf. Accessed March 12, 2011.

circumcision Circumcision is the removal of the foreskin, the double fold of skin that covers the glans, or head, of the penis. It is performed for cultural and/or religious reasons in many regions of the world. In some cultures and religions, the circumcision is performed at birth or shortly thereafter, while other cultures wait until the child reaches adulthood or age of sexual activity, and it is part of the rites of passage that boys undertake to be declared men.

Circumcision is generally practiced in the Jewish and Islamic faiths and is generally not the norm in the Catholic faith. Protestant Christianity does not have particular religious requirements about circumcision. The highest rates of circumcision are in the MIDDLE EAST AND NORTH AFRICA, Southeast ASIA, and the United States. The lowest rates of circumcision in the general population are found in Europe. In the United States, approximately 70 percent of the males are circumcised; the percentage is higher among white Americans and lower among black Americans. Canada has a much lower circumcision rate of approximately 30 percent.

Attitudes in the United States toward circumcision began to change in the late 1800s and early 1900s. Before this time, circumcision was not a common practice among most Americans. Writers about medicine and sexuality in the Victorian era began to discuss the ability of circumcision to cure all manner of bad habits and increase the healthiness of men. Circumcision began to be linked to the overall movement toward cleanliness that occurred at this time. In a period of a couple decades, circumcision went from being a rarely performed surgery in the United States to a generally accepted routine to do everything from increase the energy of a child to prevent illness and masturbation. Studies claimed that diseases ranging from syphilis to mental illness could be prevented or cured through circumcision. It became part of the American habit and was generally unquestioned as the proper thing to do for a child. It represented modern, clean, and forward-thinking parents, and young men who remained uncircumcised were assumed to be the poor, minorities, and unclean.

However, despite the assumed medical benefits of circumcision, there was very little literature that supported the health benefits of the operation. Some studies over the years have indicated that there is a lessened chance of penile cancers among circumcised men, but other studies show that the rates of this rare cancer are lower than the rate of botched circumcisions that cause more problems for the individual being circumcised. In 2000, the American Medical Association (AMA) stated that circumcision is a nontherapeutic operation with no demonstrated benefit. This acknowledgment put the AMA in line with most of the large medical associations around the world in stating that circumcision was of a cultural or religious nature and not demonstrated to benefit health.

In recent years, discussion of circumcision as a medical procedure has increased as opponents of the operation have become more numerous. These advocates, including the medical group Doctors Opposing Circumcision, state that male circumcision is no different from female circumcision in that it involves the forced removal of intact body tissue from a child without his or her permission. They cite numerous studies over the years that show that there is no justification for the procedure on medical grounds. They also have examined historical documents from the time that the rate of circumcision increased in the United States that demonstrate that the reasons given for male circumcision were the same as those given at the time for female circumcision, but that practice was ended while male circumcision became a standard operation. The reasoning for both procedures from that time frame is similar to the justification given in cultures that today still practice female circumcision.

The question of circumcision as a preventive surgery for HIV infection had long been debated during the HIV epidemic. Many of the same arguments that were used to argue for circumcision for HIV prevention were arguments that had been used for circumcision as a preventive for SYPHILIS and other sexually transmitted infections (STIs). Studies suggested to American doctors and policymakers of the time that circumcision might provide a way to decrease the risk of HIV spread. Although there are several studies that draw different conclusions on both sides of the argument, both the U.S. government and the WORLD HEALTH ORGANIZATION (WHO) have begun programs that fund the circumcision of children and adult men in areas of high HIV prevalence.

Doctors and opponents of circumcision point to the statistics that disprove the belief that circumcision is beneficial in preventing the spread of HIV. In such countries as Malawi, Ghana, Cameroon, and Swaziland, the percentage of circumcised men who are HIV positive is larger than the percentage of uncircumcised men who are HIV positive. The United States, which has a significantly higher population of circumcised men, also has a significantly higher percentage of HIV-positive people as compared to WESTERN AND CENTRAL EUROPE, where circumcision is not generally practiced. Spain, the European country with the lowest number of circumcised men, is the country whose HIV-positive rates are most similar to those in the United States, leading some observers to draw the conclusion that circumcision has no correlation to preventing the spread of HIV.

Circumcision advocates cite trials being carried out in Kisumu, Kenya, and Rakai District, Uganda, that revealed at least a 53 percent and 51 percent reduction in the risk of acquiring HIV infection, respectively. They believe that these findings support those published in 2005 by the South Africa Orange Farm Intervention Trial, sponsored by the French National Agency for Research on AIDS, which demonstrated at least a 60 percent reduction in HIV infection among men who were circumcised. They cite a range of protection of 1 to 2 percent better in the circumcised group, which translates to a 50 percent better rate of noninfection. The advocates have been successful in having several circumcision programs funded in African countries on the basis of those numbers. Activists against circumcision—or, as some prefer to be known, intactivists—believe that the statistics do not reflect the bias inherent in the studies. These activists believe bias based on providing education provided to the circumcised men in how to use condoms that was not provided to the uncircumcised men could have influenced the study. Other bias may have been introduced through recruitment of circumcision volunteers from church groups in the countries studied, as church members may be more inclined not to participate in sexual activities outside marriage and be more willing to be circumcised. Close evaluations of all studies have revealed few data to support widespread circumcision, particularly as it is known that HIV prevalence rates in the United States and Western Europe show no differences between circumcised and uncircumcised men. These studies, however, have led the WHO to endorse circumcision as a significant tool in the fight to reduce the spread of HIV. There is strong encouragement from both the WHO and U.S. government programs to make

circumcision a regular part of the HIV prevention programs in all countries where programs are funded by these agencies.

One of the forgotten points in the whole discussion of whether to circumcise or not is that education in how to use condoms and the availability of condoms are far better approaches and far less costly than circumcising in any part of the world. All HIV activists in Africa and elsewhere are concerned that the news trumpeting the studies may translate to a message that circumcision prevents AIDS, whereas, of course, it does not. Focus on the actual prevention of transmission of HIV and the treatment of the illness in those affected is likely to do more to prevent the spread of the virus than an elective surgery.

Two recent studies on the foreskin and circumcision speak to the need for further understanding of the transmission route of HIV and the perceived need or desire to circumcise. Kigozi and colleagues in 2009 showed that the size of a man's foreskin correlated to the risk of acquiring HIV during sexual encounters; the more area of mucosal tissue that existed on the foreskin, the greater the opportunity to acquire HIV. Price and associates in 2010 evaluated the bacterial composition of the foreskin mucosa. This study showed that bacterial composition changed after circumcision. The changes in the bacterial composition led to a less anaerobic environment that involved fewer inflammatory response–related cells in the area of the penis. By reducing the inflammatory response, the opportunity for HIV to infect immune cells is reduced, thereby making circumcision a potential benefit in the reduction of the spread of HIV. The same researchers indicated that the study of penile mucosa could be used to find ways of reducing the anaerobic bacteria in the penile mucosa through the development of MICROBICIDES to produce a safer mucosal state on the penis, without the loss of the foreskin, which would allow men in areas where retaining the foreskin is a cultural or religious norm to avoid circumcision.

Anonymous. "Circumcision and HIV." circumstitions.com. Available online. URL: http://www.circumstitions.com/HIV.html. Accessed March 12, 2011.

Centers for Disease Control and Prevention. "Male Circumcision and Risk for HIV Transmission: Implications for the United States." CDC.gov. Available online. URL: http://www.cdc.gov/hiv/resources/factsheets/circumcision.htm. Accessed March 12, 2011.

Doctors Opposing Circumcision. "The Use of Male Circumcision to Prevent HIV Infection." Available online. URL: http://www.doctorsopposingcircumcision.org/info/HIVStatement.html. Accessed March 12, 2011.

Family Health International. "Clearinghouse on Male Circumcision for HIV Prevention." Available online. URL: http://www.malecircumcision.org/. Accessed March 12, 2011.

Gollaher, David L. "From Ritual to Science: The Medical Transformation of Circumcision in America." *Journal of Social History* 28, no. 1 (Fall 1994): 5–36.

Juncosa, Barbara. "Fact or Fiction: Does Circumcision Help Prevent HIV Infection?" *Scientific American*. Available online. URL: http://www.scientificamerican.com/article.cfm?id=circumcision-and-aids. Accessed March 12, 2011.

Kigozi, Godfrey et al. "Foreskin Surface Area and HIV Acquisition in Rakai, Uganda (Size Matters)." *AIDS: The Official Journal of the International AIDS Society* 23, no. 16 (23 October 2009): 2209–2213.

Price, Lance B. et al. "PLoS ONE: The Effects of Circumcision on the Penis Microbiome." PLoSone.org. Available online. URL: http://www.plosone.org/article/info%3Adoi%2F10.1371%2Fjournal.pone.0008422. Accessed March 12, 2011.

Reuters. "Circumcision May Not Cut HIV Spread among Gay Men." Reuters.com. Available online. URL: http://www.reuters.com/article/2010/03/09/us-circumcision-gay-idUSTRE6283Z820100309. Accessed March 12, 2011.

VanHowe, R. S., M.D. "Circumcision and HIV Infection: Review of the Literature and Meta-Analysis." *International Journal of STD and AIDS* 10 (January 1999): 8–16.

Williams, N., and L. Kapila. "Complications of Circumcision." *British Journal of Surgery* 80 (October 1993): 1231–1236. CIRP.org. Available online. URL: http://www.cirp.org/library/complications/williams-kapila/. Accessed March 22, 2011.

Wilton, David. "Male Circumcision and HIV." circumcisionandhiv.com. Available online. URL: http://www.circumcisionandhiv.com/. Accessed March 12, 2011.

Xu, F., L. Markowitz, M. Sternberg, and S. Aral. "International AIDS Society—Abstract—2193307." iasociety.org. Available online. URL: http://www.iasociety.org/Default.aspx?pageId=11&abstractId=2193307. Accessed March 12, 2011.

clinical trials A clinical trial is the process of testing one or more medications or medical interventions on humans. The results of the testing are recorded, analyzed, and used to determine best treatment options or whether to move forward in the production of a particular medication or device. All drugs used in treating people for any illness must go through a series of clinical trials testing their effectiveness and determining the proper dosage. It is often stated, as a reason to explain a drug's cost to patients, that only one of every 1,000 substances that is evaluated by a drug company progresses to the point of being in a clinical trial and only one of five of those in a clinical trial will eventually make it to the market.

Clinical trials are conducted in research organizations that are generally based at universities, hospitals, or community organizations set up to conduct trials. Drug companies also conduct trials of new substances they hope to market. All clinical trials are supervised by a group of specialists, usually doctors or other health care professionals, and interested citizens who form an Institutional Review Board (IRB) that ensures that the clinical trial follows required legal practices and proper regulations for the treatment of people participating in the trial. IRBs can be found at most universities, hospitals, and government agencies, as well as many community organizations that are performing any type of research involving human subjects. The IRB approves and monitors the design and structure of the study as well as the ongoing findings of the research at times.

Currently, the length of time a substance undergoes laboratory testing before even entering a clinical trial process averages three and a half years. At that point, it can take another eight years on average and many millions of dollars to receive approval by the U.S. FOOD AND DRUG ADMINISTRATION (FDA). The length of time involved has drawn extensive criticism, particularly in the early years of the HIV epidemic, as thousands of people were dying and no drugs had been approved for the treatment of HIV or the numerous OPPORTUNISTIC INFECTIONS (OIs) that people who had AIDS suffered during this time. The activist group ACTUP organized large protests at the offices of the FDA that brought about changes in the approval process that actually shortened the average time to market for some drugs and eventually accelerated the approval process for drugs that were intended for emergency need. The FDA also approved what are called compassionate use guidelines, which allow an experimental drug to be used by people who are sick when there are no other options available for them, while the drug undergoes continued testing in clinical trials prior to full approval.

In the United States, the FDA has the ability to approve or reject all medications intended to be sold as prescriptions as well as many medical instruments and devices that can be used for treating different illnesses. FDA approval for new medications is not granted until a sequence of clinical trials has been conducted to show that the proposed new drug or device has gone through extensive testing to prove that it is safe and useful for its intended purpose for sale to the public. In the European Union, the European Medicines Agency holds a similar role in approval and marketing of drugs, though some countries, such as the United Kingdom and Germany, maintain their own approval agencies that existed prior to European integration. The Canadian Health Products and Food Branch serves a similar role in Canada. Some countries base their approval process on these larger boards, while others maintain independent approval boards.

A clinical trial is typically designed as a double-blind study. This means that neither the researcher nor the persons participating in the trial know who is receiving the actual treatment and who is receiving a placebo, a fake medication meant to be similar to the drug being tested. It is the responsibility of the outside review boards to monitor such research studies to protect the health of all people involved. Many clinical trials of treatments and medications in Western countries involve payment to individuals for their participation in the program. This may vary from a few dollars each time the person enters the study for evaluation to free medical treatment and monitoring for the length of the study. Study participants are recruited from the community to represent as broad a group as possible. In the case of HIV drugs, clinical trials actively seek people of color, men, WOMEN, INJECTION DRUG USE(R)s, and all people who would potentially take the medication were it on the market. Understanding how it works in a variety of people helps to understand how it will work overall.

Before a drug goes to a clinical trial, many hours of laboratory time are spent evaluating a potential substance for possible use. Substances are first tested in vitro, which means "in glass." It is the term used to mean tested in a laboratory. Simply because a substance has worked in vitro does not mean it will work in vivo, or "in the body." If studies have shown the substance to be successful in vitro, it will then be tested in animal models, meaning live animals will be used to test the safety, strength, and effectiveness, if possible, of the substance against the particular illness that the researchers are trying to cure or prevent. Animals typically used initially are mice or rats; then potentially rabbits or dogs; and finally primates such as macaques may be used to test particular drugs before any substance is ever tested in humans.

In the United States, there is a four-tier process of clinical trials in humans, three of which must be completed before the drug is approved and one that must be completed after drug approval to monitor incidents in the general public after the drug has been prescribed. These tiers are called phases, and studies conducted on humans are referred to as phases I, II, III, and IV.

Phase I trials of drugs are conducted domestically and internationally with people who are healthy and generally have no relation to the illness that the drug may be used to treat. Phase I trials have a small number of participants, usually fewer than 50 people. These studies test vaccines, drugs, and medical devices for safety and what is known as pharmacokinetics. Pharmacokinetics is the study of how a drug is absorbed, processed, and eliminated from the body. A phase I trial also tests different amounts of a substance in different people to determine what might be an effective amount of the substance for treatment purposes. If there are any side effects or serious problems with administration of the substance, this is generally when it is learned. A phase I trial usually last just a few days or weeks at most. It is not intended to test how well the drug performs in treating someone but is concerned with the safety and potential dosing levels of the drug.

After phase I studies have determined that there are no significant safety concerns about the drug or device, phase II trials can be started. These trials generally involved 50–500 people. These people may be at any point along the continuum of wellness to illness with whatever condition the drug is eventually intended to treat. Phase II studies are conducted at a large number of U.S. and international sites. Phase II trials are meant to begin testing how well the drug performs its intended function. Often phase II is broken down into two different stages, known as phase IIa and phase IIb. Phase IIa is generally a pilot study, a small study with just a few people to test the process of working with the drug, or getting people adjusted to taking the drug. Phase IIb is called a small controlled study; phase II trials usually last about two years.

Phase III trials are conducted on a large scale, often with thousands of participants at many sites, often around the world, though they can be conducted in just a few sites. Participants include people with a variety of class, race, and ethnic backgrounds, and of both genders to include the widest spectrum of people who have a particular illness in testing a potential treatment. The purpose of phase III trials is to determine efficacy (how well or efficiently a vaccine or drug works) and what type of immune response occurs, in the case of HIV medications. Phase III trials generally last at least two years or longer in some cases, depending on what is being evaluated. Generally, these are the toughest of the trials, and researchers learn much more about the drug through the high number of volunteers and the greater length of the study.

The final part of clinical trials is phase IV, which consists of after-market approval testing of the drug. These studies look at people who are regularly taking the drug as prescribed and study the long-term effect of the drug on them. Some side effects or interactions of drugs cannot be found in the relatively small number of people tested in the premarket phases. Sometimes the side effects of drugs are unknown unless studied through the people who use them regularly. It was this sort of study of the COX-2 inhibitors, pain relievers already approved by the FDA, that led to their removal from the market after phase IV studies showed they also increased the risk of heart attacks and strokes significantly.

The most strenuous type of study is a double-blind, randomized, controlled trial. These terms all define some aspect of the study. *Double-blind* means that neither the person taking the drug nor the person giving out the drug knows who is receiving the experimental treatment and who is not. If, for instance, drug A is being tested, then some people will receive drug A and other people will not receive drug A, so what they are taking is called a placebo. A placebo is a false treatment designed to resemble whatever drug or treatment is being tested so that no one can tell the difference. A *randomized trial* means that neither the patient nor the researcher can decide in which part of the study he or she will participate. If there are two parts, or arms, of a study, the study participant effectively flips a coin and is randomly assigned to a particular arm. A *controlled trial* means that one part of the study is receiving the drug under study and the other part of the study is not. This allows researchers to compare what, if anything, happens when randomly assigned people who have similar characteristics take the drug and others do not. Clinical trials can often have multiple arms studying many different characteristics while still maintaining a randomized, controlled, double-blind study.

Every clinical trial has some guidelines about who is eligible to participate in the study. Some studies may limit participation to particular groups of people, as the intended use of the drug is solely aimed at them. For instance, clinical trials for a vaccine aimed to prevent cervical cancer will probably admit only women, since men generally do not have cervixes. Generally, however, studies are looking for the widest range of participants. There may be some requirements regarding general overall health, including no ongoing opportunistic infections, which is a common requirement. Many early HIV medication trials were conducted only on gay men, and the majority of those who participated were white. Since those initial trials, most studies have sought as wide and diverse a pool of participants as possible. Some studies have shown that differences do exist at times among different people and particular drugs. Some AFRICAN AMERICANS, for instance, absorb the drug EFAVIRENZ at a slower rate, but the amount of the drug reaches higher levels in their bodies than in most other people. In this instance, they may have more side effects such as the vivid dreaming that can accompany the use of efavirenz.

Before joining a clinical trial, a potential participant must be informed of all the risks and of his or her responsibilities as a participant. Informed consent requires the participant's signed agreement to participate in the trial. Before signing any documents, participants are asked whether they understand and accept every component of the trial. A written description of the study, along with the opportunity to ask questions, are always provided to a potential volunteer before the trial begins. A volunteer may say no to participating at any time and may drop out of the trial at any time.

IRBs, data monitoring committees, FDA inspections, and community advisory boards (CABs) provide four means of protection for volunteers. Scientists, doctors, and others from the local community, including laypersons, serve on IRBs to review and monitor a hospital's or research institution's medical research involving people. They monitor studies to help make sure that there is the least possible risk to volunteers and that the risks are reasonable in relation to the expected benefits. IRBs make sure that volunteer selection is fair and that informed consent is obtained correctly.

Data monitoring committees are used mainly when one treatment is being compared with another and in studies in which treatments are selected for patients at random. These committees are particularly important in double-blind studies of treatments for serious or life-threatening diseases. These experts review information from studies to make sure they are being done in a way that is safest for the volunteers. During a study, if the committee finds that the treatment is harmful or of no benefit, it stops the study. If there is evidence that one treatment gives a greater benefit than another, the committee stops the study, and all volunteers are offered the better treatment. CABs are made up of members of the community affected by the illness under study. These became very important in HIV clinical trials, as these community-run boards provided assistance and guidance to researchers in the best ways to reach people to participate in studies and to reach out to members of the HIV community. They also advised researchers on issues that were being raised by the community about clinical trials that were ongoing in the community. Researchers initially found it difficult to work with communities affected by HIV for a number of reasons. Ultimately, CABs have provided a way for the community to be more involved in the research study and for the researchers to interact more with the community.

There have been several groups involved with HIV clinical trials in the past 30 years. AIDS Clinical Trial Group (ACTG), AIDS Community Research Initiative of America (ACRIA), Community Programs for Clinical Research on AIDS (CPCRA), HIV Vaccine Trials Network (HVTN), and International AIDS Vaccine Initiative (IAVI) are some of the larger groups that have been involved with HIV clinical trials. These research groups are somewhat like associations in that they involve researchers in different areas of the United States and the world in the same study, thereby involving a large number of people from many walks of life in HIV research. Currently, the U.S. National Institutes of Health funds six clinical trial groups that focus on HIV and AIDS. They are:

1. AIDS Clinical Trial Group (ACTG)
2. HIV Vaccines Trial Network (HVTN)
3. HIV Prevention Trials Network (HPTN)
4. International Maternal Pediatric Adolescent AIDS Clinical Trials (IMPACT)
5. International Network for Strategic Initiatives in Global HIV Trials (INSIGHT)
6. Microbicide Trials Network (MTN).

Those six organizations are currently the coordinating groups that oversee all the HIV clinical trials funded by the U.S. government. The U.S. Department of Health and Human Services' funding for clinical trials in HIV was changed dramatically during the most recent decade. Whereas most clinical trials were traditionally done in the United States, now much more effort is put into drug trials for the FDA that are done in conjunction with other nations. Clinical trials for vaccines, new drugs, as well as treatment regimens are now often done in multicountry settings. All rules of the FDA and the safety mechanisms of U.S.-based clinical trials must be met in overseas locations. This often proves challenging, but it is now considered part of the process of conducting new trials.

U.S. drug clinical trials and the drug approval process are often seen as bureaucratic processes that take much longer than necessary. Some HIV activists claim that many people die while waiting for drugs or treatments to be approved. Some FDA critics believe that approval for drugs and treatment ought to be done across developed countries. Many European countries run their own approval processes and clinical trials, and Canada has its own agency for drug approvals. Some business and economic writers argue that as long as one government agency in the developed world has approved a particular drug for use in humans, then the U.S. government should accept that approval and do likewise. They argue that costs to corporations would be lowered by eliminating duplication of approval processes in many different political entities. This in turn would lower the cost of drugs to the developed world, as a treatment or drug approved in Europe or Canada would be available in the United States, and vice versa. Whether this will occur anytime soon depends on political policy and pressure that corporate or patient advocates bring to bear on the FDA and whether American citizens are willing to allow decisions about drugs they use to be made in places outside the United States.

Clinical trials can be beneficial to patients but at the same time pose some risk to the participants in the trials. The risk lies in the knowledge that the clinical trial is an experiment, the purpose of which is to determine whether or not a particular treatment strategy or new drug is beneficial. If the drug is *not* beneficial, then there is the potential that people in the trial may suffer for not having treatment with a substance or treatment that is known to be effective. There is also the potential that the substance does not help and may actually make a person more ill. These detriments to participating in a clinical trial are balanced by the knowledge that a person may be receiving a potentially successful new treatment or drug. People who may not have other options may be able to receive new medications, or at least participate in a study that will help them or others like them in the future through the knowledge gained in the study.

AIDS Clinical Trial Group. "About ACTG–AIDS Clinical Trials Group Network." ACTGnetwork.org. Available online. URL: https://actgnetwork.org/about-actg. Accessed March 13, 2011.

AVERT: AVERTing HIV and AIDS. "The History of HIV and AIDS in America." AVERT.org. Available online. URL: http://www.avert.org/aids-history-america.htm. Accessed March 13, 2011.

The Body. "HIV/AIDS Clinical Trials." TheBody.com. Available online. URL: http://www.thebody.com/index/treat/clintri.html. Accessed March 13, 2011.

European Medicines Agency. "Regulatory—Human Medicines." EMA.europa.eu. Available online. URL: http://www.ema.europa.eu/ema/index.jsp?curl=pages/regulation/landing/human_medicines_regulatory.jsp&murl=menus/regulations/regulations.jsp&mid=WC0b01ac058001 ff89. Accessed March 12, 2011.

Highleyman, Liz. "A Guide to Clinical Trials: Part 1. Understanding Clinical Studies." *BETA: Bulletin of Experimental Treatments for AIDS* 17, no. 4 (Summer 2005): 42–49.

Homedes, Nuria, and Antonio Ugalde. "Multisource Drug Policies in Latin America: Survey of 10 Countries." *Bulletin of the World Health Organization.* SciELO.org. Available online. URL: http://www.scielosp.org/scielo.php?script=sci_arttext&pid=S0042-96862005000100016. Accessed March 13, 2011.

Klein, Daniel B. "Drug-Approval Denationalization: Library of Economics and Liberty." EconLib.org. Available online. URL: http://www.econlib.org/library/Columns/y2009/Kleindrugapproval.html#. Accessed March 13, 2011.

National Institutes of Health. ClinicalTrials.gov. Available online. URL: http://clinicaltrials.gov/. Accessed March 13, 2011.

coccidioidomycosis Coccidioidomycosis is a respiratory illness caused by two species of the fungus *Coccidioides: C. immitis,* found in the San Joaquin Valley of California and in other desert locations of the southwestern United States and northern Mexico; and *C. posadasii,* found in the desert of the southwestern United States, Mexico, and parts of Central and South America. Until 2002, there was only one recognized species of *Coccidioides,* so research on the fungus prior to that time refers only to the one species.

The fungus grows only in areas of low rainfall, high temperatures, and low elevation. The illness is also known as valley fever, San Joaquin Valley fever, Arizona lung, or desert fever in various parts of the United States. The fungus lives in the soil of these areas and is easily disturbed through various activities such as walking, riding vehicles through the area, farming, construction, or other activities that cause soil to become airborne. The spores of the fungus are inhaled and cause illness once they are in the lung. Coccidioidomycosis can also infect cows, dogs, and a variety of other mammals.

Symptoms and Diagnostic Path
The majority of people who inhale the spores of the fungus will not suffer any noticeable illness. Their body's immune system will function well against the spores, and they will develop immunity to reinfection. Then there is a group of people who will become infected with a lung infection that can cause fever, weight loss, coughing, and other flulike symptoms. Approximately 40 percent of people fall into this category. The infection will eventually clear on its own in most cases.

Approximately 2 percent of people exposed to the fungus will develop a chronic invasive form of the disease requiring treatment. The fungus forms nodes of infection in the lungs that can be observed with an X-ray or computed tomography (CT) scan. These people can also be at risk for the infection's disseminating to other parts of the body, including the spleen, liver, kidneys, bones, and brain. If the meninges, the lining around the brain, becomes infected, the illness can require years of treatment to cure and prevent it from recurring, and in some cases it can lead to death.

In HIV-positive people, the chance of developing the disseminated form of the illness is greater than in the general population. Although the disease is relatively common, and up to 50 percent of people in the endemic areas have been exposed to the fungus, many doctors are unaware of the illness if they do not practice in the regions where it is found. Travelers to these areas may become ill weeks to months after their initial exposure to the fungus, and should make their physicians aware that they have lived or traveled in endemic regions. Disseminated disease can have several symptoms. Meningitis, pneumonia, swollen liver, and swollen lymph nodes are common in disseminated illness.

Skin testing to observe whether there is an immune system response to antigen for the fungus, injected under the skin, can be used to determine whether a patient has been exposed at some point to the fungus. However, most HIV-positive people who have disseminated coccidioidomycosis do not generate enough of an immune response to react positively to the skin test. Cerebral spinal fluid (CSF) and blood can be drawn to test for antibodies to the fungus, but again, these tests are not very reliable in HIV-positive individuals. Diagnosis in most HIV-positive people must rely on the growth of the fungus from tissue samples or the observation of the spherules of the fungus through staining of samples. The fungus will grow from blood samples or tissue from infection sites, such as a bone or skin lesion, or from a biopsy of lung tissue, in three to five days.

Treatment Options and Outlook

People who have a mild infection or local lung involvement can be treated with an azole antifungal drug. The recommended dose is 400 mg a day of fluconazole or itraconazole orally. Other possible drugs include posaconazole, voriconazole, or caspofungin.

Amphotericin B is the recommended medication for people who are severely ill or those who have a disseminated infection. Although all studies that have been done were completed with standard amphotericin B, lipid formulations of the drug can theoretically be used and

may have fewer side effects. In HIV patients who have CD4 T lymphocyte cell counts below 200 cells/μL, treatment guidelines recommend some form of medication, whatever variety of the infection has developed. On occasion, some physicians will treat a patient with both amphotericin B and an azole antifungal. Once a patient has responded to the amphotericin B, an oral antifungal will be continued for at least a year.

Outcomes for HIV-positive people who have disseminated coccidioidomycosis are poor. Studies report a death rate of approximately 70 percent over follow-up periods of six months. Success rates in treating localized lung infections in HIV-positive people are much better, as only 10 percent die in the first six months.

Risk Factors and Preventive Measures

Prevention of the disease in endemic areas is difficult, if not impossible. Between 10 and 50 percent of people living in endemic areas will be exposed to the fungus during their lifetime. Avoidance of activities such as farming, landscaping, or construction will decrease exposure to disturbed soil. There is no current method to eliminate the fungus from soil.

Infection with the fungus can lead to disseminated illness in AFRICAN AMERICANS at 10 times the rate for non-Hispanic white Americans. People of Asian descent, in particular Filipinos, also have a greater susceptibility to the disseminated form of the disease. In Filipinos, the chance of disseminated illness is 150 times greater than in non-Hispanic whites. Some research has indicated that there is a genetic predisposition that causes these higher rates that is possibly tied to a person's blood type, but there is no conclusive study as of yet to pinpoint a particular reason. Pregnant WOMEN also run a higher risk of contracting the pulmonary form of the disease.

Maintaining good health is the best way to prevent coccidioidomycosis. People who are HIV positive should maintain their health as much as possible, including starting HIGHLY ACTIVE ANTIRETROVIRAL THERAPY (HAART) when advised by their physician. This may help prevent the disseminated forms of the illness from taking hold in the body. There is no current preventive medication, but HIV-positive people will probably use a suppressive medication if they have had a coccidioidomycosis infection previously until their CD4 T lymphocyte count is above 200 cells/μL. Those treated for disseminated infection will probably use an oral antifungal for the rest of their life to prevent recurrence.

There have been VACCINES AGAINST HIV/AIDS previously tested in humans to prevent infection from the *Coccidioides* fungus, but none has proven effective, and there is no vaccine currently approved for use.

Aberg, Judith A., M.D. "Coccidioidomycosis and HIV." HIVInSite.ucsf.edu. Available online. URL: http://hivinsite.ucsf.edu/InSite?page=kb-00&doc=kb-05-02-04. Accessed March 13, 2011.

Chatterjee, Archana. "Pediatric Coccidioidomycosis." eMedicine.com. Available online. URL: http://www.emedicine.com/PED/topic423.htm. Accessed March 13, 2011.

Doctor Fungus. "Coccidioidomycosis." DoctorFungus.org. Available online. URL: http://www.doctorfungus.org/mycoses/human/cocci/coccidioidomycosis.php. Accessed March 13, 2011.

Kirkland, Theo N., M.D., and Joshua Fierer, M.D. "Coccidioidomycosis: A Reemerging Infectious Disease." *Emerging Infectious Diseases* 2, no. 3 (July–September 1996): 192–199. Available online. URL: http://www.cdc.gov/ncidod/EID/vol2no3/kirkland.htm. Accessed March 13, 2011.

Merck. "Coccidioidomycosis." *Merck Manuals Online Medical Library.* Available online. URL: http://www.merck.com/mmhe/sec17/ch197/ch197e.html. Accessed March 13, 2011.

United States National Library of Medicine. "Coccidioidomycosis." MedlinePlus. Available online. URL: http://www.nlm.nih.gov/medlineplus/ency/article/001322.htm#Alternative%20Names. Accessed March 13, 2011.

Combivir (zidovudine + lamivudine) Combivir is the trade name for a combination pill consisting of two NUCLEOSIDE REVERSE TRANSCRIPTASE INHIBITORS (NRTIs), ZIDOVUDINE and LAMIVUDINE. It was first approved by the U.S. FOOD AND DRUG ADMINISTRATION (FDA) in 1997 for use in combination therapy with other HIV antiretrovirals. Combivir was the first combination drug marketed in the United States. It helped greatly reduce the number of pills that an HIV patient had to take during the day, significantly increasing adherence to taking the pills regularly. Prior to combination pills, HIV-positive people often had to take many pills on a particular schedule to obtain the correct dosage of medications.

Combivir is used frequently by women who are pregnant. The majority of studies involving vertical TRANSMISSION of HIV have been undertaken with zidovudine. Although it is listed as a drug *not* to use during pregnancy because it is believed to have a potential for birth defects, as shown in tests on animals, its use in developing countries immediately prior to delivery of a child has been shown to be beneficial to mother and child. The benefits probably outweigh the risks in such short-term use of the drug.

Dosage
The dosage cannot be modified because this is a combination pill. Because the dosages are preset in the pill, and it cannot be divided, it is not approved for use for children below the age of 12 or people who need dosages to be adjusted for medical reasons. It contains 300 mg of zidovudine (AZT) and 150 mg of lamivudine (3TC). The dose is one pill, two times a day. It can be taken with or without food, as absorption is not affected by food.

Drug Interactions
Drug interactions with Combivir are similar to the interactions that can occur if a person is taking both drugs individually. Combivir should not be prescribed at the same time as ZALCITABINE, as they interact to prevent optimal concentrations of both drugs in the body.

Combivir should not be taken at the same time as any other medication containing lamivudine or zidovudine. In addition to the individual drugs, this includes the combination pills EPZICOM, TRIOMUNE, and TRIZIVIR. Lamivudine is very close in structure to the antiretroviral drug EMTRICITABINE, and they act in the same manner against HIV. It is recommended that the two medications not be prescribed together, as this combination may not confer any added benefit to treatment. Emtricitabine is also found in the combination pills TRUVADA and ATRIPLA.

Combivir should not be taken at the same time as ribavirin, a drug used in the treatment of HEPATITIS C. The zidovudine in Combivir interacts with ribavirin and causes a decrease in the availability of zidovudine in the body while increasing potentially dangerous side effects of zidovudine. Methadone can cause an increase in the amount of zidovudine in the body, thereby increasing side effects of the drug. People taking some medications for the treatment of TUBERCULOSIS (TB) and *MYCOBACTERIUM AVIUM* COMPLEX (MAC) as well as other antibacterial medications may need to switch HIV antiretrovirals, as the amount of zidovudine in the body can be lowered below levels optimal for controlling HIV.

Combivir should not be taken at the same time as STAVUDINE. The drug zidovudine in Combivir and stavudine are antagonistic, meaning they do not work together in the body and can cause more side effects when combined. There are also some PROTEASE INHIBITORS (PIs) that can cause zidovudine to drop to lower levels in the body. The FDA has not made recommendations on dosage adjustments in some of these instances, but a doctor can weigh the benefits of potential HIGHLY ACTIVE ANTIRETROVIRAL THERAPY (HAART) combinations to use with Combivir.

Lamivudine can increase in concentration in the body when taken with trimethoprim/sulfamethoxazole (TMP-SMX), a common antibiotic used to treat *PNEUMOCYSTIS* PNEUMONIA. Dosages do not generally need to be adjusted, though a doctor may end the use of Combivir if there is a concern about this interaction. Lamivudine is also approved by the FDA for the treatment of chronic HEPATITIS B. If a doctor needs to change a patient's HAART medications and Combivir is one of the drugs that is changed, the doctor may continue lamivudine as part of the regimen if

the patient has a positive test for result hepatitis B. Anytime that hepatitis B treatment is stopped, there remains a chance that the hepatitis B will flare up, potentially causing damage to the liver. The physicians will probably monitor liver function BLOOD WORK/BLOOD TESTS to assure this does not happen.

Side Effects

Combivir, as a combination pill, will cause the same side effects at the two drugs lamivudine and zidovudine when taken individually. Lamivudine is generally well tolerated on its own with very few day-to-day side effects. It has been associated with anemia in some people.

Zidovudine causes a host of side effects, including cramps, diarrhea, headache, tiredness, gas, trouble sleeping, and rash. Long-term use of zidovudine has been associated with the development of myopathy, a weakness of the muscles including the heart. Symptoms include general weakness of muscles, particularly those closest to the trunk of the body. Bone marrow problems can also occur with the long-term use of zidovudine, resulting in the decreased production of red or white blood cells. This occurs more frequently in people who are taking certain antibiotics such as ganciclovir and TMP/SMX.

As Combivir is made of two NRTIs, it has all the problems associated with NRTI use. Several potential serious side effects can occur with NRTI use, which has been linked to LIPODYSTROPHY, the loss of fat from some areas of the body and the accumulation of fat in others. NRTI use can also cause a rise in cholesterol and triglyceride levels.

LACTIC ACIDOSIS, an excess of lactic acid in the bloodstream, has also been linked to NRTI use. It is a rare condition but can occur with greater frequency in women and obese individuals. Lactic acidosis is a very dangerous condition and should be monitored closely. Hyperlactemia, higher than normal levels of lactate in the blood, can be a way to identify someone who may be at risk for severe lactic acidosis. If symptoms of nausea, stomach pain, shortness of breath, irregular heartbeat, vomiting, weakness, and tiredness occur while taking Combivir, consult a doctor immediately. Although other NRTIs are more often associated with lactic acidosis, zidovudine has been believed to be the cause of some cases of this condition.

AIDSmeds. "Combivir (Zidovudine + Lamivudine)." AIDSmeds.com. Available online. URL: http://www.aidsmeds.com/archive/Combivir_1083.shtml. Accessed March 13, 2011.
———. "Special Issues for Children with HIV: NRTIs." AIDSmeds.com. Available online. URL: http://www.aidsmeds.com/articles/Children_4935.shtml. Accessed March 13, 2011.
The Body. "Combivir." TheBody.com. Available online. URL: http://www.thebody.com/content/treat/art1312.html. Accessed March 13, 2011.
New Mexico AIDS Education and Training Center. "Combivir (Zidovudine + Lamivudine)." AIDSInfoNet.org. Available online. URL: http://www.aidsinfonet.org/fact_sheets/view/417. Accessed March 13, 2011.
United States Department of Health and Human Servides. "Lamivudine/Zidovudine." AIDSInfo.nih.gov. Available online. URL: http://www.aidsinfo.nih.gov/DrugsNew/DrugDetailNT.aspx?MenuItem=Drugs&Search=On&int_id=285. Accessed March 13, 2011.

cryptococcosis Cryptococcosis is an infection most often caused by the fungus *Cryptococcus neoformans* and on rare occasions by *C. gattii*. Cryptococcus spores are found in soil, especially in areas of bird droppings, throughout the world. *C. gattii* has been isolated from various species of eucalyptus (or gum) trees in tropical and subtropical areas as well as parts of the Pacific Northwest in the United States and British Columbia, Canada. Although the trees have been implicated in the dispersal of the fungus, recent studies suggest it may be dispersed through human activities as well.

Cryptococcosis is found more often in AFRICA and ASIA than in the Americas or Europe. It has also become less prevalent among HIV-positive people since the advent of HIGHLY ACTIVE ANTIRETROVIRAL THERAPY (HAART) in the late 1990s.

Prior to HAART, cryptococcosis affected between 5 and 8 percent of all HIV-positive patients in the United States. The majority of cases are now seen in HIV-positive patients who have a CD4 T lymphocyte count of less than 50 cells/μL.

The fungus passes to humans when soil or trees are disturbed in some manner and the spores are inhaled into the lungs. In people who have healthy immune systems, the fungus is contained in the lungs and eliminated. In HIV-positive people who have weakened immune systems, the fungus spreads from the lungs to the rest of the body, causing problems with several organs and the central nervous system (CNS).

Symptoms and Diagnostic Path

Cryptococcal infection in the lungs can produce symptoms of pneumonia including coughing, shortness of breath, and fever. In cryptococcus infection of the CNS, the symptoms are the same as those of meningitis: fever, severe headache, stiff neck, and tiredness. Cryptococcosis can also cause vague symptoms such as fatigue, weight loss, memory loss, or disorientation. Also in disseminated infections, skin lesions or eruptions that look like small warts can be seen.

In order to diagnose cryptococcosis properly, a spinal tap must be performed to measure the virus in the cerebral spinal fluid. Although blood testing can also be used to detect the infection, antigen to the fungus may not appear in the blood of some patients who have disseminated infection. It is not known how long after exposure to *C. neoformans* illness begins to appear.

Treatment Options and Outlook

The treatment standard is intravenous (IV) amphotericin B given several times a day over the course of at least two weeks in combination with oral flucytosine. That will be followed up by eight weeks of treatment with fluconazole, another antifungal. Because of the difficulty in clearing the fungus from the CNS and the body, no single-drug treatment is recommended. Amphotericin B can have many side effects, especially involving the kidneys. Monitoring the CNS and BLOOD WORK/BLOOD TESTS will ensure that the fungus is controlled and that there are no serious side effects.

Because HIV-positive people tend to contract this infection when their immune system is already functioning poorly, treatment is not successful approximately 10 percent of the time. Most deaths occur within the first two weeks of treatment. Treatment failure with standard medicines can occur, and there are no drugs that have been tested extensively for treatment against cryptococcosis.

Risk Factors and Preventive Measures

There is no specific way to avoid exposure to *Cryptococcus,* as it is ubiquitous in the environment. There is no prophylactic medication used to prevent cryptococcosis from developing because of the fear that a person may become immune to the effects of the medicine, thereby making it ineffective if an infection does develop. However, a person who has been treated for cryptococcosis and whose immune system is highly compromised may be placed on a maintenance dose of medication to prevent the infection from recurring. The maintenance dosing may be halted when a person's immune system has returned to a level of at least 200 CD4 T lymphocytes/µL.

Aberg, Judith A., M.D., and William G. Powderly, M.D. "Cryptococcosis and HIV." HIVInSite.ucsf. edu. Available online. URL: http://hivinsite.ucsf. edu/InSite?page=kb-05-02-05. Accessed March 13, 2011.

Centers for Disease Control and Prevention. "Cryptococcus (Cryptococcosis)." CDC.gov. Available online. URL: http://www.cdc.gov/nczved/divisions/dfbmd/diseases/cryptococcus/. Accessed March 13, 2011.

King, John W. "Cryptococcosis." eMedicine.com. Available online. URL: http://emedicine.medscape.com/article/215354-overview. Accessed March 13, 2011.

University of Adelaide. "Cryptococcosis." *Mycology Online.* Available online. URL: http://www.mycology.adelaide.edu.au/Mycoses/Opportunistic/Cryptococcosis/. Accessed March 13, 2011.

cryptosporidiosis   Cryptosporidiosis (also commonly called crypto) is a highly contagious infection caused by the protozoan *Cryptosporidium*. It is found in human and animal feces and can contaminate public water supplies and rivers and streams. There are several different species of *Cryptosporidium* that infect humans, including *Cryptosporidium hominis,* found only in humans, and *Cryptosporidium parvum,* found in both cattle and humans. The spores (oocysts) of the parasite are not killed through freezing or through standard chlorination processes found in most public water systems. It can be spread from human to human through oral-fecal contact. Approximately 30 percent of adults in the United States test positive for antigens to *Cryptosporidium*. The protozoan infects the small intestine most frequently, but HIV-positive people will also experience infection of the large intestine and possibly the pancreas and biliary ducts.

Symptoms and Diagnostic Path

Cryptosporidium causes severe diarrhea in all people whom it infects. It is quite common in children and can last up to a couple of weeks before it becomes manageable in people with healthy immune systems. Standard symptoms include cramping, nausea, fever, vomiting, abdominal pain, and persistent diarrhea.

To diagnose cryptosporidiosis, a sample of the patient's feces is tested for antigens to the parasite. Another approach is to examine stool under a microscope, but several stool samples over a several-day period may be needed to find the parasite in either case.

Treatment Options and Outlook

There is no current treatment for cryptosporidiosis in HIV-positive people. The only method of controlling a *Cryptosporidium* infection in an HIV-positive person has been to restore the immune system function through HIGHLY ACTIVE ANTIRETROVIRAL THERAPY (HAART), which then allows the body to control the infection on its own. This, along with rehydration and management of the diarrhea, is the mainstay of treatment to this day.

In less serious cases, nitrazoxanide, which has a broad action against numerous protozoa, helminths, and bacteria, has been approved for treatment of *Cryptosporidium parvum* in both children and adults. One 500 mg tablet given twice a day over three days will clear most oocysts from stool samples, allowing a person to recover. Studies have shown that in HIV-positive people a 14-day treatment course of 500–1,000 mg twice daily has been somewhat clinically helpful in clearing oocysts from the stools of a patient, but will not cure the infection completely.

Risk Factors and Preventive Measures

HIV-positive people can prevent the spread of *Cryptosporidium* through several measures. Hands should always be washed after contact with any feces such as diapering babies, handling pets or other animals, gardening, and before eating and preparing food. HIV-positive people must refrain from drinking water from lakes, rivers, streams, ponds, or oceans and be aware that contamination has occurred from drinking fountains and public water parks. Drinking water while traveling abroad can also increase the risk of contracting cryptosporidiosis. Boiling water for several minutes can kill the parasite and should be done if no reliable water is available. In the home, reverse osmosis filtering systems can remove the parasite from all drinking water. Swimming in contaminated pools can also spread cryptosporidiosis. Avoid any oral-anal contact during sex without protection, i.e., condoms or dental dams. People should also avoid eating raw oysters, because testing of oysters has shown that *Cryptosporidium* can survive in an oyster for up to two months, and the organism has been found in commercial oyster-growing grounds.

Centers for Disease Control and Prevention. "Parasites—Cryptosporidiosis (also known as crypto)." CDC.gov. Available online. URL: http://www.cdc.gov/crypto/. Accessed March 13, 2011.

Merck. "Cryptosporidiosis." Merck.com. Available online. URL: http://www.merckmanuals.com/home/sec17/ch196/ch196f.html. Accessed March 13, 2011.

White, A. Clinton, Jr. "Cryptosporidiosis." eMedicine.com. Available online. URL: http://emedicine.medscape.com/article/215490-overview. Accessed March 13, 2011.

cytomegalovirus Cytomegalovirus (CMV) is a member of the human herpes family of viruses. It can cause severe illness in immunocompromised people, small babies, and a pregnant woman's unborn child. It is also called human herpes virus 5 (HHV-5). Between 50 and 80 percent of adults have been exposed to CMV by the time they are 40 years old. It is found in all parts of the world and appears in all types of people regardless of race, class, or gender. Most people are exposed to CMV when they are infants or children. Typically, it causes no symptoms and presents no problems for a healthy immune system. MEN WHO HAVE SEX WITH MEN (MSM) and the INJECTION DRUG USE(R) (IDU) population have higher rates of CMV infection than the general population, indicating that the spread of the virus occurs through the same means as the spread of HIV.

It is spread through body fluid contact with someone who already has CMV. Routine testing for the virus shows that adults as well as children shed the virus from their body fluid well after they have been exposed to it. Detectable amounts of CMV can be found in blood, urine, breast milk, saliva, vaginal secretions, tears, and semen. Once a person has been exposed to CMV, it will stay in his or her body for life, possibly reactivating in later life when the person is elderly or has a compromised immune system such as after ORGAN TRANSPLANTATION or when a person has HIV.

In WOMEN who are pregnant and exposed to CMV for the first time, their child is at high risk for developing birth defects. In babies, some signs of congenital CMV infection are jaundice (yellowed skin), purple spotting on the skin, pneumonia, enlarged liver or spleen, and seizures. CMV is now the second most common cause of mental retardation in children after Down syndrome. Other birth defects that can develop in the fetus of a mother exposed to CMV during her pregnancy include blindness, deafness, autism, a smaller head, and thrombocytopenia. Death occurs in a small percentage of affected fetuses. This does not occur in infants of women who have previously been exposed to the virus, but only in those of women who first become ill while they are pregnant.

Symptoms and Diagnostic Path

In HIV-positive people, CMV becomes reactivated as the immune system becomes weaker. Many different organs can be affected by CMV when a person's immune system is weakened. The most common sign of an infection in HIV-positive people is CMV retinitis, a progressive inflammation and destruction of the retina, the part of the eye responsible for receiving and transmitting light. Symptoms indicating retinitis can include blurred field of vision, peripheral vision blurring, and white spots in the vision that are called floaters, as they seem to float in the person's field of vision. Examination of the eye will show white or yellow cottony patches that are lesions on the retina, bleeding in the eye, with limited inflammation in most cases. The course of retinitis is always progressive, and if it is not treated, blindness will result within a period of two to three weeks, most often in one eye, though it can occur simultaneously in both eyes.

Other forms of CMV can also occur. Infection of the intestines occurs in 5 to 10 percent of cases. Symptoms include painful diarrhea, tiredness, fever, weight loss, and abdominal pain. CMV can also occur in the esophagus, causing fever, nausea, swelling, and discomfort during eating. Involvement in the central nervous system (CNS) can cause a variety of symptoms, including dementia (see HIV ENCEPHALOPATHY), disease of the heart ventricles, disease of the spine causing partial paralysis, and numbness in

the legs. These various infections occur in people with CMV who have extremely low CD4 counts and are not on HIGHLY ACTIVE ANTIRETROVIRAL THERAPY (HAART). Prior to HAART, approximately 30 percent of all AIDS patients would be diagnosed with CMV during their illness.

The virus can be detected in blood samples through antigen tests or culturing for the virus. Although a positive antibody test result does not necessarily determine active disease, the lack of antibodies can eliminate CMV as a cause of any unknown illness. Biopsy of tissue from the lung, esophagus, or colon can also determine whether CMV illness is present.

Treatment Options and Outlook

Oral valacyclovir, intravenous (IV) ganciclovir, IV ganciclovir followed by oral valganciclovir, IV foscarnet, IV cidofovir, or the ganciclovir intraocular implant combined with valgonciclovir can all can be used to treat CMV retinitis. The itracocular implant is a small device surgically placed in the eye that releases medicine slowly over the course of several months. Eventually, the device will need to be removed and replaced by another implant. The intraocular implant is recommended to treat immediate serious lesions in the eye. Recommendations may also include an intravitreous injection (an injection in the eye) of ganciclovir to start medication of the eye immediately until surgery can be scheduled for the implant.

Because of the many locations in the body where CMV can occur, as well as the low level of immune function in people who have CMV infection, different combinations of these medications may be used to bring the infection under control. If the HIV-positive person has not begun HAART, that will also be started because of the known benefits of reconstituting the immune system in dealing with CMV infection. Some patients may experience what is known as IMMUNE RECONSTITUTION INFLAMMATORY SYNDROME (IRIS) when they start HAART while still receiving treatment for an active CMV infection. Several of these treatments can cause other problems, including drug toxicity and drug compliance issues because of the number of pills required, so these factors will be weighed in the decision to determine which medications will be used to treat the CMV.

Treatment of HIV-positive pregnant women is handled in the same manner as if they were not HIV positive. Most studies have shown that CMV infection in the fetus is related to an active CMV infection in the mother that occurs during a pregnancy rather than to exposure to CMV antibodies in the mother's body. Therefore, HIV-positive women who become pregnant do not need any prophylaxis against CMV to protect the fetus. Those HIV-positive women who test negative for CMV antibodies simply need to maintain good hygiene and avoid instances of possible infection.

Risk Factors and Preventive Measures

As CMV is present in a large percentage of the population, it is difficult to prevent the illness from becoming a problem if a person's CD4 T lymphocyte count falls below 100 cells/µL. Use of HAART by HIV-positive people can help maintain a person's immune system and prevent the opportunity for CMV disease to begin. Treatment with oral valganciclovir to prevent CMV is not recommended because of cost and the ease with which CMV can become resistant to the medication, and studies have shown no long-term effect of such treatment.

Families who have small CHILDREN are more at risk to acquire a new case of CMV, as people generally catch the virus early in life. Hand washing and careful cleaning of dishes and kitchen surfaces can help stop the spread of the virus, though not completely prevent it. HIV-positive children in day care facilities or HIV-positive adults who work in such settings must take extra precautions to prevent exposure to CMV if they have not already been exposed. Testing for antibodies for CMV can determine whether a person has been previously exposed to CMV.

AIDS.org. "Cytomegalovirus (CMV)." AIDS.org. Available online. URL: http://www.aids.org/topics/cytomegalovirus-cmv. Accessed March 13, 2011.

Centers for Disease Control and Prevention. "Cytomegalovirus (CMV) and Congenital CMV Disease." CDC.gov. Available online. URL: http://www.cdc.gov/cmv/overview.html. Accessed March 13, 2011.

Drew, W. Lawrence, M.D., and Jacob P. Lalezari, M.D. "Cytomegalovirus and HIV." HIVInSite.ucsf.edu. Available online. URL: http://hivinsite.ucsf.edu/InSite?page=kb-05-03-03#S1X. Accessed March 13, 2011.

Mayo Clinic. "Cytomegalovirus (CMV) Infection." MayoClinic.com. Available online. URL: http://www.mayoclinic.com/health/cmv/DS00938/DSECTION=symptoms. Accessed July 24, 2011.

Wong, Derek. "Cytomegalovirus." Virology-Online.com. Available online. URL: http://virology-online.com/viruses/CMV.htm. Accessed March 13, 2011.

D

darunavir Darunavir, one of the PROTEASE INHIBITORS (PIs), is made by Tibotec Therapeutics and sold under the name Prezista in the United States. It is abbreviated as DRV. It was approved for use in 2006 for adults and for children older than age six in 2008. It is always prescribed for use in conjunction with ritonavir and as part of a multidrug combination of antiretrovirals for use in the treatment of HIV. It is active against both wild-type HUMAN IMMUNODEFICIENCY VIRUS (HIV) and varieties that are resistant to other drugs.

Dosage

In treatment-experienced people, that is, people who have previously taken antiretroviral medications for HIV, the dosage is one 600 mg tablet twice a day combined with one 100 mg ritonavir capsule each time darunavir is taken. For people who are treatment naïve (those who have not taken HIV antiretrovirals before), the dosage is 800 mg (two 400 mg pills) once a day with one 100 mg ritonavir capsule at the same time. Darunavir and ritonavir must be taken with food. Whether it be a snack or a full meal is not important as long as some food is eaten when taking the medication.

Drug Interactions

As many PIs do, darunavir interacts with the medications it is taken with and can cause increases or decreases in the amount of the drug available in the body. Darunavir is not generally administered with SAQUINAVIR, as this combination causes a drop in the amount of darunivair active in the body. It also is not prescribed at the same time as lopinavir, as tests indicate that the combination significantly decreases the amount of darunavir in test patients. Similarly, if darunavir is administered with INDINAVIR, another PI, both drugs' availability is increased in the body. It is unclear what dosing recommendations should be made in this instance.

Darunavir interacts with a number of other medications, including the cholesterol-lowering drugs simvastatin and lovastatin, antibiotics used to treat infections such as TUBERCULOSIS, antidepressant and antipsychotic medications, and medications for arrhythmias of the heart. It is important that a doctor know and understand all the medications and supplements a patient is taking when prescribing darunavir.

Darunavir also increases the amount of the drugs sildenafil (Viagra), vardenafil (Levitra), and tadalafil (Cialis)—all erectile dysfunction medications—in the blood, which can cause serious side effects. Lowering the dosage of these medications is recommended to prevent potential complications.

Estrogen-based birth control methods will be less effective when taking darunavir. Women using these forms of birth control may seek to use a barrier protection method such as condoms while using darunavir.

Methadone levels in the body decrease substantially while a person is taking darunavir. Individuals who are prescribed methadone for the treatment of opiate addiction should have dosages adjusted and monitored by a doctor.

Antifungal medications such as ketoconazole, itraconazole, and voriconazole are affected by darunavir and ritonavir. Amounts of ketoconazole and itraconazole are decreased in the blood while the quantity of voriconazole is increased. Caution is required in prescribing these antifungals to determine the proper dosage to treat the fungal infection while not causing harm to the person taking darunavir.

St. John's wort, an herbal supplement, should never be taken with a PI, as it has been shown to reduce the amount of PI in the body greatly.

Increased levels of fluticasone, an inhaled steroidal allergy or asthma treatment, may occur while taking darunavir. Patients should be monitored for any changes due to this interaction.

Side Effects

Darunavir seems to have fewer short-term effects and has not been shown to cause as many cholesterol and triglyceride problems as some other PIs. However, the most common side effects of darunavir are similar to those of other PIs. Some patients report diarrhea, headache, nausea, and sinus infections.

Darunavir can cause an increase in bleeding in patients who have HEMOPHILIA AND HIV.

Interactions when darunavir is taken with some cholesterol-lowering medications have included facial swelling and rhabdomyolisis, the breakdown of muscle tissue, which is passed into the bloodstream, causing potential kidney damage if not observed early in the event. Prescribing darunavir with some cholesterol-reducing medications necessitates close monitoring.

Protease inhibitors, as a class of drug, often increase the cholesterol and triglyceride levels of patients. High lipid levels have been recorded in some darunavir patients. This side effect can be managed with appropriate cholesterol-lowering medications. Darunavir has also been associated with treatment regimens that can cause LIPODYS-TROPHY, or the redistribution of fat within the body. Symptoms are increased fat around the neck and stomach area, facial wasting, breast enlargement, and peripheral wasting in the arms and legs. Some of these changes disappear when the drug is stopped.

Some people who use darunavir develop a skin rash initially. This can generally be managed, as it is mild or moderate in nature. There have been some serious skin reactions, or allergies, to the drug, so a doctor should monitor severe rashes.

Darunavir has been associated with higher liver enzyme levels and liver stress in some people. This was seen in the clinical trials of darunavir, and was more frequent in people who already had damaged livers through chronic HEPATITIS B, HEPATITIS C, or cirrhosis. Liver function should be checked prior to prescribing darunavir, and liver enzymes need to be monitored regularly for people who are already at risk of liver problems.

Darunavir is a sulfa drug. People who have allergies to any sulfa drug should not use darunavir.

AIDS InfoNet. "Darunavir (Prezista)." AIDSInfoNet. org. Available online. URL: http://www.aidsinfonet. org/fact_sheets/view/450. Accessed March 11, 2011.

AIDSmeds. "Prezista (Darunavir)." AIDSmeds.com. Available online. URL: http://www.aidsmeds.com/archive/Prezista_1562.shtml. Accessed March 11, 2011.

———. "Special Issues for Children with HIV." AIDSmeds.com. Available online. URL: http://www.aidsmeds.com/articles/Children_7566.shtml. Accessed March 11, 2011.

The Body. "Prezista (Darunavir, TMC114)." TheBody.com. Available online. URL: http://www.thebody.com/index/treat/tmc114.html. Accessed March 11, 2011.

United States Department of Health and Human Services. "Darunavir." aidsinfo.nih.gov. Available online. URL: http://www.aidsinfo.nih.gov/DrugsNew/DrugDetailNT.aspx?int_id=397&ClassID=1&TypeID=1. Accessed March 11, 2011.

delavirdine Delavirdine is one of the NON-NUCLEOSIDE REVERSE TRANSCRIPTASE INHIBITORS (NNRTIs); it was approved in 1997 for use in the treatment of HIV. It is always used in conjunction with at least two other antiretrovirals to form a combination therapy. Delavirdine is manufactured by Pfizer, Inc., and is sold under the trade name Rescriptor. It is not commonly prescribed because of the high number of pills that must be taken.

Dosage

Delavirdine is available in 100 mg tablets and 200 mg capsules. The 100 mg tablets can be dissolved in water so that those who have problems taking pills can more easily swallow them. The dosing is pill heavy—400 mg three times a day, amounting to four 100 mg tablets three times a day, or two 200 mg capsules three times a day. Delavirdine may be taken with or without food; however, because delavirdine requires acid in the stomach to be absorbed properly, patients should not take any antacid one hour before or after taking delavirdine. An acidic juice such as orange or cranberry juice may help absorption.

Because the level of the drug in the body is important with antiretrovirals, it is necessary to take the three doses of delavirdine approximately eight hours apart each day. When delavirdine was introduced, the pill burden (the number of pills a person has to take daily) was not an issue because there were no options. Since that time, other HIGHLY ACTIVE ANTIRETROVIRAL THERAPY (HAART) regimens that require fewer pills have become more appealing to most people. Delavirdine is not approved for use by people below the age of 16. Pregnant women can take delavirdine, but there have been no studies measuring whether the drug is passed to infants through breast milk.

Drug Interactions

There are many drug interactions with delavirdine. It is processed through the body by the liver, so other drugs that are processed in the same manner can be affected by delavirdine. The amount of delavirdine can be increased or decreased, depending on which drugs the person is currently taking. Because DIDANOSINE tablets have a stomach buffer as part of the tablet, delavirdine and didanosine should be taken at least one hour apart. Delavirdine should not be

administered as a regimen with FOSAMPRENAVIR, which is one of the PROTEASE INHIBITORS (PIs). That combination may cause a mutation that prevents delavirdine from acting in the body.

All potential PIs that can be combined with delavirdine will have increased levels in the body caused by interaction with delavirdine. Dosage of PIs may need to be lowered to account for the increases caused by mixing them with delavirdine. The only exception to this rule is ATAZANAVIR SULFATE, whose level in the body is lowered if it is administered with delavirdine.

Delavirdine will increase the amount of methadone in the body. If a person is taking methadone as part of a program to withdraw from heroin use, dosage of methadone may need to be adjusted.

Statin drugs, which are taken to lower cholesterol levels, interact strongly with delavirdine. Two statins, simvastatin and lovastatin, should never be taken with delavirdine, as this increases the amount of the statins in the body to dangerous levels. Two other statins, atorvastatin and rosuvastatin, may be combined with delavirdine, but in the lowest possible doses until levels of the drugs in the body can be determined. Two other statins have been shown to work best with delavirdine: pravastatin and fluvastatin.

The herbal supplement St. John's wort lowers the levels of NNRTIs in the blood. St. John's wort should not be taken at the same time as delavirdine. Ergot medications, which are used to treat some migraine headaches, should also not be taken at the same time as delavirdine.

Some antibiotics used to treat infections such as TUBERCULOSIS and *Mycobacterium avium* COMPLEX infections, which can occur in HIV-positive people, should not be mixed with delavirdine. Rifampin, rifabutin, and clarithromycin levels are increased sharply while delavirdine levels are generally decreased, prohibiting combined usage.

Astemizole, an antihistamine, should not be mixed with delavirdine. Some antifungal medications used to treat some infections in HIV-positive people are also not to be used in combination with delavirdine. These drugs can increase the levels of delavirdine above the necessary amount in the body. A doctor will have a full list of medications that can and cannot be taken at the same time as delavirdine.

Side Effects

Some common side effects reported with delavirdine include headache, diarrhea, nausea, and fatigue. These disappear or lessen over time while on the medication.

A skin rash reaction is common to all the NNRTI class drugs. About 25 percent of people who use delavirdine report such a rash upon beginning the drug. The rash can be lessened or avoided if the drug is started gradually. Some people can develop a serious rash that involves blistering, lesions around the mouth, and redness and swelling of the eyes (conjunctivitis). These are symptoms of a serious rash reaction that can be fatal if left untreated. The rash generally appears within one to three weeks after starting delavirdine. If such a skin reaction occurs in a patient who has stopped taking delavirdine, the person should not begin taking delavirdine again as the skin rash and reaction will be more serious. Liver abnormalities can also occur, particularly if a person taking the drug already has a liver condition. Elevated liver enzyme levels can provide a measure of potential liver damage and be a sign that the drug should not be continued.

AIDS InfoNet. "Delavirdine (Rescriptor)." AIDSInfoNet.org. Available online. URL: http://www.aidsinfonet.org/fact_sheets/view/433. Accessed March 11, 2011.

AIDSmeds. "Rescriptor (Delavirdine)." AIDSmeds.com. Available online. URL: http://www.aidsmeds.com/archive/Rescriptor_1614.shtml. Accessed March 11, 2011.

———. "Special Issues for Children with HIV." AIDSmeds.com. Available online. URL: http://www.aidsmeds.com/articles/Children_7566.shtml. Accessed March 11, 2011.

The Body. "Rescriptor (Delavirdine)." TheBody.com. Available online. URL: http://www.thebody.com/index/treat/rescriptor.html. Accessed March 11, 2011.

United States Department of Health and Human Services. "Atazanavir." aidsinfo.com.nih.gov. Available online. URL: http://www.aidsinfo.nih.gov/DrugsNew/DrugDetailNT.aspx?int_id=166. Accessed March 11, 2011.

didanosine Didanosine was first approved by the U.S. FOOD AND DRUG ADMINISTRATION (FDA) in 1991, the second antiretroviral approved for the treatment of HIV. It was approved as a capsule form in 2000 and then as a generic pill in 2004. It is known by the trade name Videx or Videx EC, which is manufactured by Bristol-Myers Squibb, as well as by the letters *ddI*, an abbreviation of the full chemical name dideoxyinosine. Didanosine is one of the NUCLEOSIDE REVERSE TRANSCRIPTASE INHIBITORS (NRTIs), a class of drugs with several known side effects. For the first few years after it was approved, didanosine was used for treatment as a monotherapy. After studies showed that treatment with more than one antiretroviral was much more effective, this was stopped. Didanosine must be part of a multidrug prescription of antiretrovirals to stop HIV from reproducing in the body. Initially, didanosine was available only in large chewable tablets. These were similar in consistency to an antacid tablet, very chalky and thick. The manufacturer discontinued these tablets in 2006 after the availability of capsules caused the use of the chewable tablets to drop dramatically.

Dosage

Didanosine is now available in a variety of formulations, the most common of which are capsules in both generic and trade formulations, which are the same drug and interchangeable in use. The standard dosage is one 400 mg capsule a day. Because didanosine interacts with several other HIV medications, an adjustment may be required when different combinations of HIGHLY ACTIVE ANTIRETROVIRAL THERAPY (HAART) are prescribed. There are also 125 mg, 200 mg, and 250 mg capsules available for these purposes.

Adults or adolescents weighing less than 130 pounds will be prescribed one of the lower dose capsules.

The drug is also available in powder that can be mixed with water to make an oral solution. The amount of powder will be determined by the age and weight of the patient. A doctor will make the determination and provide the proper instructions for use of the didanosine powder.

Didanosine must always be taken on an empty stomach. It deteriorates quickly in the stomach when too much acid is present. This is why it was initially available only in chewable tablets with an antacid as part of the drug. Generally, the written material available with the drug recommends that the drug be taken one hour before or two hours after a meal. This has always been difficult to mix into a regular drug routine for many people. Even the newer capsule and the oral liquid forms of the drug require taking didanosine on an empty stomach.

Drug Interactions

Didanosine interacts with several drugs because of the requirement that it be taken on an empty stomach and because of the side effect profile of the drug. A patient must always notify a doctor of other prescription drugs that are currently being taken so that the proper medications can be added to those. Didanosine, when taken in combination with EFAVIRENZ or NEVIRAPINE, has been shown to cause an increased likelihood of early treatment failure, requiring a new HAART combination sooner than normally expected. TENOFOVIR DISOPROXIL FUMARATE can cause the amount of didanosine in the body to increase to six times the normal amount that is recommended, thereby increasing the chance of side effects associated with didanosine. A doctor will adjust the dosage to decrease the chance of side effects.

Some medications perform better when taken on an acid stomach, the opposite of didanosine. These drugs should not be taken at the same time as didanosine. Usually a break of two hours before or after taking didanosine is recommended when taking dapsone, itraconazole, and ketoconazole. PROTEASE INHIBITORS (PIs), particularly those that must be taken with food, should be taken at least two hours before or after a person takes didanosine.

Didanosine should not be prescribed at the same time as STAVUDINE, another NRTI, which has been linked to an increased risk of NEUROPATHY and pancreatitis. This combination may increase the risk of both conditions. Other drugs that cause an increased risk of pancreatitis include trimethoprim/sulfamethoxazole (TMP-SMX) and pentamidine, which are used in the treatment of some HIV-related OPPORTUNISTIC INFECTIONS (OIs).

Methadone, a drug used to treat heroin addiction, causes a significant decrease of the amount of didanosine in the body. This can lead to treatment failure. The amount of didanosine must be monitored closely if the two drugs must be administered together.

The use of ganciclovir and valganciclovir causes an increase in the amount of didanosine in the body. These drugs are often used in the treatment of recurring CYTOMEGALOVIRUS (CMV) in HIV patients.

Side Effects

Didanosine is an NRTI, a class of drugs that can cause several serious side effects. NRTI use has been linked to LIPODYSTROPHY, the loss of fat from some areas of the body and the accumulation of fat in others. NRTIs can also cause a rise in cholesterol and triglyceride levels. Although didanosine has not been directly linked to these conditions, it is part of the class of drugs that have been associated with these side effects. An increase in the rate of heart attacks was discovered during a long-term drug study involving the use of didanosine with ABACAVIR. Any such use with abacavir or abacavir-containing combination pills (EPZICOM and TRIZIVIR) should include monitoring of cholesterol levels, triglyceride levels, and cardiac function.

LACTIC ACIDOSIS has also been linked to NRTI use. It is a rare condition and can occur with greater frequency in WOMEN, obese individuals, and people who have been using NRTIs for an extended period. It is a very dangerous condition involving elevated levels of lactic acid in the blood, and it should be monitored closely. Hyperlactatemia, higher than normal levels of lactate in the blood, can be an indication that someone might be at risk for the more serious lactic acidosis. If symptoms of nausea, stomach pain, shortness of breath, irregular heartbeat, vomiting, weakness, and tiredness occur while taking didanosine, the patient should consult a doctor immediately. Didanosine use should be stopped immediately if lactic acidosis is detected, and the drug should not be restarted.

Peripheral neuropathy, a burning, tingling, painful deadening of the nerves in the extremities, has been linked to didanosine. If it is discovered early, the symptoms can end eventually; if it is not detected, it can be debilitating and extremely painful. Because of the increased incidence of neuropathy in people who are coadministered stavudine for HIV, the two drugs are not prescribed at the same time. In general, people who have previous episodes of pancreatitis, peripheral neuropathy, or a history of alcoholism should not be prescribed didanosine, as the risk for recurring pancreatitis or neuropathy would increase significant for the person while taking didanosine.

Some cases of portal hypertension have been reported with didanosine use, particularly over time. Portal hypertension is high blood pressure of the portal vein, which drains blood from the intestines and spleen to the liver. Symptoms include elevated liver enzyme levels as well as swollen spleen and bleeding of the esophagus. The results, if not discovered early, can lead to death or require liver transplantation. Individuals who use large amounts of alcohol may be at higher risk for developing portal hypertension when using didanosine.

AIDS InfoNet. "Didanosine (Videx, ddI)." AIDSInfoNet. org. Available online. URL: http://www.aidsinfonet. org/fact_sheets/view/413. Accessed March 11, 2011.

AIDSmeds. "Special Issues for Children with HIV." AIDSmeds.com. Available online. URL: http:// www.aidsmeds.com/articles/Children_7566.shtml. Accessed March 11, 2011.

———. "Videx EC (Didanosine, ddI)." AIDSmeds. com. Available online. URL: http://www.aidsmeds. com/archive/Videx_1585.shtml. Accessed March 11, 2011.

The Body. "Videx (Didanosine, ddI)." TheBody.com. Available online. URL: http://www.thebody.com/ index/treat/ddi.html. Accessed March 11, 2011.

United States Department of Health and Human Services. "Didanosine." aidsinfo.nih.gov. Available online. URL: http://www.aidsinfo.nih.gov/DrugsNew/Drug DetailNT.aspx?int_id=16. Accessed March 11, 2011.

discrimination Discrimination is overt or subtle unequal treatment or denial of opportunities to individuals or groups. The stigma attached to HIV and AIDS has in the past prompted and continues to cause a wide range of individual and social reactions to persons who have AIDS or who are HIV positive. HIV-positive people have the same civil and social rights as noninfected people. Examples of these rights include access to justice; public benefits such as Social Security or Social Security Disability Income (SSDI); medical confidentiality; educational rights, such as the right to attend regular classroom schools; employment, the right to work if they are able as well as the right to seek employment in all fields; free speech, such as the right to publish and distribute AIDS educational materials; and housing, insurance, immigration, professional licensure, and public accommodation.

Since the outbreak of the HIV epidemic, people in all walks of life and in many different settings have reported discriminatory practices. Many people were immediately fired from jobs in the early 1980s when they either disclosed the fact that they were HIV positive or had to use sick days for an illness that was known to be AIDS related. Initially, there was no way for these people to receive protection under antidiscrimination laws. Most people quietly sought to receive Social Security or SSDI payments so that they did not have to face situations in which they could be fired again. Health insurance companies often denied coverage to HIV-positive people once their status was known. Life insurance companies would not sell insurance to HIV-positive people. Some school systems did not allow children who had HIV to attend regular classroom school. Some towns burned down homes of people who were HIV positive to chase them out of town when their status became known. There was a great deal of stigma and shame attached to HIV and AIDS. To this day, that stigma continues in many places in the United States and around the globe. The United Nations cited a study in their 2008 report on AIDS that said that 27 percent of Americans would prefer not to work with a woman who was HIV positive.

Perhaps the most striking conclusion to be drawn from the stories of discrimination reported in newspapers or read on the Internet is that HIV and AIDS generate tremendous fear around the world because it is unknown or not understood well. TRANSMISSION of the virus remains poorly understood by many people. When it was a new disease in the early 1980s, no one knew what caused AIDS or how it was transmitted. Since it has been linked to a virus, people have had a difficult time understanding that it is not a virus like influenza that can be spread through coughing or hand-to-hand touching. Whether this is a result of poor education efforts by governments or media, many people remain unaware that HIV is difficult to spread in most situations. In addition, HIV is spread through activities such as sex and injection drug use (see INJECTION DRUG USE(R)) that already carry strong social taboos. Many people view HIV as a punishment for immoral or illegal behavior, whether sex or drug use. HIV is seen as a crime and HIV-positive people are considered victims, though sometimes innocent ones. It has been portrayed as something that happens to other people, whether a poor mother in South Africa or a gay man in San

Francisco, and it is kept apart from the mainstream of life. Sex already carries many highly charged emotions in most countries, and HIV-positive people have been portrayed as promiscuous, immoral, and deviant because the virus can be acquired through sexual activity. WOMEN in particular have been demonized in ASIA and AFRICA, accused of promiscuity and portrayed as prostitutes, although men play at least an equal role in the spread of the virus in these regions.

One result of the fear and stigmatization of people with HIV is that many people are unwilling to be tested for the virus or to seek health care if they are sick. In some countries, just going to a clinic that provides testing and antiretroviral medications can lead a person to be branded as immoral or promiscuous. People fear the potential loss of employment opportunities, loss of marriage and childbearing potential, loss of support from family and friends, and feelings of hopelessness and insecurity, particularly in places where health care is difficult to receive, expensive to obtain, or simply unavailable. Because people are afraid to be tested or treated, many people learn they are HIV positive late in the disease process, when they are ill and there is a stronger likelihood of dying because of the extreme weakness of their immune system. This hesitation also allows the virus to continue to be spread easily, as people do not protect themselves or others when they are unaware they have the virus. This simply furthers the sense of shame and discrimination already associated with HIV.

Discrimination laws provide a legal foundation for the rights of people with HIV and AIDS. In the United States, the Americans with Disabilities Act, passed in 1990, was the first law that allowed HIV-positive people to protect themselves from discrimination. This law was passed and courts have applied and upheld the interpretation that HIV is a medical disability and individuals cannot be discriminated against on the basis of their medical condition. When the law was updated and rewritten in 2008, the phrase "functions of the immune system" was listed as one of the "major life activities" that are adversely affected by a disability. The law covers all processes of employment, from seeking a job to retirement; public accommodations, meaning services and transportation available to the public; and public services, including health care. The law applies broadly to businesses and individuals providing goods and services to the public, including private employers of 15 or more people and federal and state agencies. In 1990, the law had the immediate effect of allowing people with HIV to seek legal assistance against discrimination.

Despite these legal assurances, cases of discrimination occur on a regular basis. Cirque du Soleil was sued by an employee in 2003 for terminating employment because of the fear that HIV could be transmitted in the work setting. The case eventually was settled after the federal Equal Employment Opportunity Commission (EEOC) determined the issues in the suit in favor of the employee. In 2008, the Transportation Security Administration (TSA) was sued by a retired military man who had applied for a job as a baggage inspector but was denied a position because of the TSA's belief that his health would be substantially put at risk by the potential illnesses he might encounter working at an airport. This case is currently being handled through an appeals process within the government agency to reverse the TSA decision.

In other areas, HIV-positive people face discrimination on a regular basis. Several countries bar anyone who has HIV from receiving a visa or gaining entry to the country. Until recently, the United States was one of those countries. Restrictions on people visiting the United States and potential HIV-positive permanent residents were lifted on January 4, 2010. Other countries with discriminatory bans include the United Arab Emirates, Singapore, and South Korea. Around the world, discrimination can be seen in school accommodations, employment, medical settings, and even the community in general. One well-known example was the South African woman Gugu Dhlamini, who was stoned and beaten to death by her neighbors after appearing at a UN-sponsored World AIDS Day event and speaking openly about being HIV positive.

Until the denial and fear that surround HIV and AIDS lessen, the discrimination that many HIV-positive people suffer will continue. Working to eliminate the fear of the virus through education, increasing the availability of medications so all can receive treatment, and providing assistance to those who face discriminatory actions can help HIV-positive people to be as safe and respected as people who are not HIV positive.

Aggleton, Peter, Kate Wood, Anne Malcolm, and Richard Parker. *HIV-Related Stigma, Discrimination and Human Rights Violations: Case Studies of Successful Programmes.* UNAIDS.org. Available online. URL: http://data.unaids.org/publications/irc-pub06/JC999-HumRightsViol_en.pdf. Accessed March 13, 2011.

American Association for World Health. "Fact Sheets: Discrimination & HIV/AIDS." TheBody.com. Available online. URL: http://www.thebody.com/content/art33117.html. Accessed March 13, 2011.

American Civil Liberties Union. "HIV/AIDS Discrimination." ACLU.org. Available online. URL: http://www.aclu.org/hiv-aids/hivaids-discrimination. Accessed March 13, 2011.

AVERT: AVERTing HIV and AIDS. "HIV and AIDS Stigma and Discrimination." AVERT.org. Available online. URL: http://www.avert.org/aidsstigma.htm. Accessed March 13, 2011.

The Body. "HIV/AIDS-Related Discrimination Cases." TheBody.com. Available online. URL: http://www.thebody.com/index/legal/discrimination.html. Accessed July 24, 2011.

Gorenberg, Hayley. "Confronting HIV Discrimination in the Workplace: A Case Study." *Human Rights Magazine* 31, no. 4 (Fall 2004): 16–19. ABAnet.org. Available online. URL: http://www.americanbar.org/publications/human_rights_magazine_home/irr_hr_fall04_casestudy.html. Accessed March 13, 2011.

UNAIDS: Joint United Nations Programme on HIV/AIDS. "UNAIDS Report on the Global AIDS Epidemic 2010." UNAIDS.org. Available online. URL: http://www.unaids.org/globalreport/Global_report.htm. Accessed March 13, 2011.

United States Congress. "Americans with Disabilities Act of 1990, as Amended." ADA.gov. Available online. URL: http://www.ada.gov/pubs/ada.htm. Accessed March 13, 2011.

drug patents and pricing When the first AIDS drug went on the market in 1989, the price was so high that many people who suffered from HIV and AIDS could not afford the medication because they had lost their jobs and health insurance. ZIDOVUDINE, the first antiretroviral, was initially priced at $7,000–$10,000 per person a year. As the cost of this drug was so high, U.S. Representative Henry Waxman held hearings about the cost of zidovudine. Representative Waxman pointed out in hearings that zidovudine was largely paid for through government-funded research many years prior to its current usage. He also pointed out that zidovudine development was covered by the Orphan Drug Act, which approved government funds to pay for more than 70 percent of the costs of the development of this drug. The Orphan Drug Act covers medicines developed for illnesses that affect so few people that drug companies would not generally fund their production because of the lack of return on investment of research and development.

Despite the U.S. congressional hearings and the protests of AIDS activists, the cost of zidovudine remained high, generating an estimated $225 million in sales. The government eventually addressed the need for funding by creating ADAP (see AIDS DRUG ASSISTANCE PROGRAM), to help those people who could not afford the medication to pay for it. In addition, a black market for zidovudine was quickly created as people who would not or could not take their medication provided it to those who could take it but could not afford it. Community-based drug exchanges popped up in major cities with large HIV-positive populations because of the high costs of HIV medications and the inability of ADAP to cover everybody who needed the drugs. Drugs were recycled; if someone died,

any leftover pills were passed on to the drug exchange and sent back into the community. If someone switched medications, pills were funneled to the drug exchanges.

As time went on and various drugs were added to the antiretroviral arsenal against HIV, the monthly cost of prescriptions increased. The typical cost for a patient on HIGHLY ACTIVE ANTIRETROVIRAL THERAPY (HAART) initially ran $12,000–$15,000 a year in the United States. HIV activists held numerous protests against pharmaceutical companies' pricing strategies, but for the most part few or no changes were made to the costs of the drugs. In Europe, prices were 25–40 percent lower than in the United States because the government-run health care programs there can purchase drugs in larger quantities for the whole country, negotiating lower prices, whereas U.S. pharmacies and hospitals do not buy in such volume. As HIV spread around the world, calls for access to medications in developing countries were added to the voices of U.S. activists. Millions of people in countries such as Brazil, India, South Africa, and Uganda needed antiretrovirals, too, and the costs placed them beyond what individuals or nations could afford. Many nations, particularly in AFRICA, have neither the government-run health care systems available in Western Europe nor the hospital, insurance, and pharmacy networks that are available in the United States. People in many countries may receive health care if they can reach a government-run health care facility, but the costs of prescriptions after seeing a medical specialist must be paid from their own funds. If a person needs a prescription, he or she will pay for that medication.

Throughout the epidemic, pharmaceutical companies have made large profits while people in the United States and overseas have died because of the lack of access to medications that existed to treat them owing to the excessive costs of the drugs. HIV drugs are not the only medications that are excessively priced as drugs for many other illnesses can also be extremely expensive. The pharmaceutical companies earn large profits, even in lean times, as can be noted in industrial surveys and statistics. Links to industrial statistics and individual company numbers can be found on Yahoo or any stock market Web site. Pharmaceutical companies often explain high prices in terms of the amount of money they expend on research and development (R&D) of new drugs. However, articles by Donald Light and Rebecca Warburton and by the Congressional Budget Office indicated lower costs of R&D than the pharmaceutical industry lobby claims. Many of the drugs used in the treatment of HIV and AIDS were originally developed under U.S. government-funded research and then later licensed to various drug companies for production, thereby negating the companies' arguments about the costs of R&D. In addition to zidovudine, DIDANOSINE, ZALCITABINE, STAVUDINE, and SAQUINAVIR were paid for almost entirely throughout the research and development and clinical trial process by the U.S. government through grants to researchers. In addition to paying for the cost of R&D in many cases, the U.S. government provides pharmaceutical companies with a large tax credit that equals 35 percent of the amount expended on R&D. An additional 20 percent tax credit is given on expenditures above a base dollar amount. In addition, pharmaceutical companies are granted extended tax credits for building plants in tax zones (specially designated areas granted tax exemption) around the country, adding to cost savings that Light and Warburton believe create a situation allowing pharmaceutical companies great profit margins while charging consumers, particularly American consumers and their insurance companies, large sums for medicines.

When a pharmaceutical company develops a new drug, it can patent that drug for a period of 20 years. This means that in the United States no other company can manufacture or profit from this drug. In general, all industrialized countries have agreements that allow a patent in one country to be equal to a patent in another country, so if a Dutch or English company patents a product in their home country, they also are granted a patent in the United States. In

developing countries, this has not been true. Although the United States has been successful in negotiating some trade agreements on patent recognition with developing countries—for example, Guatemala—other developing countries have refused to agree to these demands in trade negotiations. The results of these agreements show the disparity that occurs when the United States forces a country to purchase only patented medicines. Guatemala provides access to medication to just 1 percent of its population through government agencies. All others on medications must be supported through donations from nongovernmental organizations (NGOs). Activists claim that this simply pulls money from individuals in Western countries to support the private corporate benefits that pharmaceutical companies receive from favored trade status. Requiring the corporations to provide the drugs at a lower cost, or allowing the production of generic drugs—medications made from the same formula as the expensive, brand name drug but sold at a competitive price and without the patent attached—would make the necessary medicines affordable in countries such as Guatemala.

The World Trade Organization (WTO) is the international agency that regulates trade among the majority of countries in the world. It was created in 1995 and was the successor organization to the General Agreement of Tariffs and Trade (GATT), which was a trade agreement, but not an organization itself. One section of the WTO agreement was the Trade-Related Aspects of Intellectual Property Rights (TRIPS). TRIPS requires each member of the WTO to adopt, among other things, rules establishing 20-year patent recognition on pharmaceuticals. There were two exceptions given for TRIPS rules. One group of exceptions granted several years to developing countries to begin compliance with the regulations. For some countries, this rule would last until 2000, for others longer. It has since been extended to 2016 for the poorest countries. This provision allowed countries to produce generic versions of medicines patented elsewhere, until they were required to bring their country's rules in line with the WTO. A second exception allowed compulsory licensing, which permitted a country to allow generic manufacture of a patented drug, as long as the drug patent holder was paid a percentage of the profit derived from the sale of the generic drug. Under this exception, generic drugs could be manufactured in a developing country or imported from another country.

These exceptions have given generic manufacturers the opportunity to increase competition among drug makers and have allowed the price of antiretroviral medications to fall dramatically in some developing countries. While prices in the United States remain at close to $10,000 a year, in parts of Africa the price for antiretrovirals may be $130 a year. India first began manufacturing generic antiretrovirals before all of the WTO regulations applied to their country in 2001. This allowed India to begin exporting generic drugs to other nations, an opportunity it took advantage of to begin shipping drugs to Africa. Brazil also began manufacturing antiretrovirals, and the government was soon providing HAART to all HIV-positive people who wanted to receive it. South Africa was unable to manufacture drugs under the WTO agreements to which they were a partner. When the South African government passed a law allowing patent circumvention to meet the needs of the largest HIV population in the world, 39 pharmaceutical companies joined to file legal challenges against the government's attempt to provide generic drugs for dying people. This created much bad publicity for the giant drug companies. However, it was not until 2001 that the pharmaceutical companies stood down and stopped their legal filings in South Africa. WTO negotiations in Doha, Qatar, gave countries the right to use compulsory licensing in situations of their own choice, to be used to support drug access and public health benefits in those countries. In addition, U.S. president Bill Clinton issued an executive order that drug companies in the United States not pressure African countries to abide by WTO drug regula-

tions. By 2001, the Indian generic drug company Cipla was beginning exports of many antiretrovirals to South Africa.

By 2005, India and Brazil were to begin participating fully in WTO and the various TRIPS regulations. However, both countries refused the granting of patents for specific drugs, using different mechanisms to invalidate the patent requests filed by pharmaceutical companies. This situation has led to continued manufacture of many generic drugs and exporting of the drugs by these countries. So although prices for antiretrovirals are low in some countries because of the use of generics, prices remain extraordinarily high in the United States, as generic drugs cannot be manufactured there during the 20-year patent window. At this time, only zidovudine is beyond patent in the United States. Several other generic antiretrovirals have been tentatively approved in the United States, but these are for participation in the PEPFAR program, which funds drugs for patients in other countries. The situation that has arisen in the past few years as WTO windows of compliance pass and more countries are expected to meet trade guidelines is that countries ignore or break these rules to guarantee inexpensive access to their HIV-positive population. Pharmaceutical companies, despite profits of more than 20 percent even during the current economic recession, press the U.S. government hard for stricter enforcement of international trade agreements. Pharmaceutical companies in the European Union (EU) also pressure the EU governing agencies to enforce regulations. In early 2011, the EU was pressing India to stop the manufacture of HIV medications (among other drugs) to fall in line with WTO regulations. The *British Medical Journal* (*BMJ*), a leading medical research journal, issued an editorial against the maneuvering of the EU. If successful, the trade agreement being pushed by the EU would eliminate the largest center of generic drug production and possibly drive HAART costs back to the excessive levels seen only in the United States.

This situation in which neither governments nor patients were benefiting from prices, patents, and delays in getting medicines to HIV-positive people led to the founding of UNITAID by five countries (Brazil, Chile, France, Norway, and the United Kingdom). UNITAID acts as a buyer for drugs from all sources available, such as pharmaceutical companies, governments, and products of generics to fund antiretrovirals for use in developing countries. The initial funding mechanism was an airline tax levied in member countries, though other levies and funding are used to fund the purchase of drugs. The United States and Canada are not currently UNITAID members. UNITAID is not an acronym, but the name for the organization, whose offices are housed at the World Health Organization (WHO) in Switzerland.

UNITAID recently proposed what it is terming a patent pool that encourages pharmaceutical companies to join and voluntarily give up the patent rights to their drugs in middle- and low-income countries in exchange for licensing their drugs to generic manufacturers to increase access and lower costs. Although the program is supported by many countries and organizations, as of yet no drug companies have agreed to participate. UNITAID has been successful in inducing drug companies to agree to tiered pricing based on the standard income of people in countries participating in UNITAID. There seems to be some interest among the drug companies in allowing the use of their patented drugs, as pressure from governments and individuals to provide broader access to the lifesaving antiretrovirals has been high.

As UNITAID continues to work with companies for greater, less expensive access to drugs, companies continue to raise prices for antiretrovirals in the United States. While drug companies generally win the court battles in the United States over price increases and patent protections, in other countries, they often do not win these battles. Indian courts in particular have favored rights of access to generic drugs, and patent applications have been rejected for drugs already patented in Western countries. Courts in other countries such as Brazil, South Africa, and Thailand have also granted local companies the right to produce generic drugs over the arguments of pharmaceutical giants.

Drug pricing both in the United States and in developing countries remains a highly contentious issue. Drug companies continue to press governments for extended patent rights, tax credits, and tax exemptions, as well as funding for R&D. Patient advocates continue to push for access to needed medications for all the HIV-positive individuals struggling to afford medications in the United States and abroad. Currently, the U.S. government funds ADAP (see AIDS DRUG ASSISTANCE PROGRAM) programs partially in all the states and territories to support pharmaceutical company pricing. How long this will continue is unknown, as both states and the federal government are under pressure to reduce costs across the board during the ongoing recession. Although many activists continue to fight high drug costs here and across the globe, it is unclear whether they will be able to cause a drop in costs or encourage pharmaceutical companies to find other means of maintaining profits and patent protections for extended periods at the cost of human lives.

One other concern talked about by both the pharmaceutical companies and activists is the lack of new drugs taken to the U.S. FOOD AND DRUG ADMINISTRATION for approval. It has been longer than three years since the last new HIV medication was approved in 2008. Activists express concern that the drug companies are not motivated to advance new drugs in the pipeline because these newer medications would perhaps cause a drop in profits of established medications the companies presently have on the market. Drug companies counter that argument by restating that the costs involved make new medications simply too difficult to bring to the current market, that current drugs work so well, and that the R&D costs for such drugs simply exceed the ability to make a profit. With numerous conflicting demands for profit, for new medications, and for potential cures, the discussions in this area of public policy remain highly important for all HIV-positive people as well as drug companies and governments around the world.

Alcorn, Keith. "Brazil Rejects Tenofovir Patent." aidsmap.com. Available online. URL: http://www.aidsmap.com/Brazil-rejects-tenofovir-patent/page/1431528/. Accessed March 13, 2011.

AVERT: AVERTing HIV and AIDS. "AIDS, Drug Prices and Generic Drugs." AVERT.org. Available online. URL: http://www.avert.org/generic.htm. Accessed March 13, 2011.

Congress of the United States, Congressional Budget Office. "Research and Development in the Pharmaceutical Industry." Washington, D.C.: U.S. Congressional Budget Office, 2006. Available online. URL: http://www.cbo.gov/ftpdocs/76xx/doc7615/10-02-DrugR-D.pdf. Accessed March 25, 2011.

Consumer Project on Technology. "Additional Notes on Government Role in the Development of HIV/AIDS Drugs." CPTech.org. Available online. URL: http://www.cptech.org/ip/health/aids/gov-role.html. Accessed March 25, 2011.

Gladwell, Malcolm. "High Prices: How to Think about Prescription Drugs." New Yorker (25 October 2004). NewYorker.com. Available online. URL: http://www.newyorker.com/archive/2004/10/25/041025crat_atlarge. Accessed March 13, 2011.

Guha, Anne Mira. "Prices for Abbott's Norvir (Generic Name Ritonavir) as a Standalone Product in 2010." KEIOnline.org. Available online. URL: http://www.keionline.org/prices/ritonavir. Accessed March 13, 2011.

Hari, Johann. "The Horrifying Hidden Story behind Drug Company Profits." HuffingtonPost.com. Available online. URL: http://www.huffingtonpost.com/johann-hari/the-horrifying-hidden-sto_b_251365.html. Accessed March 13, 2011.

Hawai'i Department of the Attorney General. "News Release: Hawai'i Reaches $82 Million Settlement with Pharmaceutical Companies." Hawaii.gov. Available online. URL: http://hawaii.gov/ag/main/press_releases/2010/2010-21.pdf. Accessed March 13, 2011.

Housing Works. "The Price Isn't Right." TheBody.com. Available online. URL: http://www.thebody.com/content/policy/art44897.html. Accessed March 13, 2011.

Huff, Bob. "Paying for Life." TheBody.com. Available online. URL: http://www.thebody.com/content/policy/art2597.html. Accessed March 13, 2011.

Khwankhom, Arthit. "Thailand to Break HIV Drug Patent." Nation (Bangkok, Thailand). NationMultimedia.com. Available online. URL: http://www.nationmultimedia.com/2006/11/30/headlines/headlines_30020346.php. Accessed March 13, 2011.

Leung, Rebecca. "Prescriptions and Profit." CBS News. Available online. URL: http://www.cbsnews.com/stories/2004/03/12/60minutes/main605700.shtml. Accessed March 13, 2011.

Light, Donald W., and Rebecca Warburton. "Demythologizing the High Costs of Pharmaceutical Research." BioSocieties 6, no. 1 (2011): 34–50. Available online. URL: http://www.pharmamyths.net/files/Biosocieties_2011_Myths_of_High_Drug_Research_Cos ts.pdf. Accessed March 24, 2011.

Love, James. "The Production of Generic Drugs in India." BMJ: British Medical Journal 342, no. d1694 (22 March 2011). BMJ.com. Available online. URL: http://www.bmj.com/content/342/bmj.d1694.full. Accessed March 25, 2011.

Morris, Kelly. "HIV Drug Patents in the Spotlight." Lancet Infectious Diseases 9, no. 11 (November 2009): 660–661.

OECD: Organisation for Economic Co-operation and Development. "OECD Health Data 2010—Frequently Requested Data." OECD.org. Available online. URL: http://www.oecd.org/document/16/0,3746,en_2649_37407_2085200_1_1_1_37407,00.html. Accessed March 13, 2011.

Project Inform. "Shape-Shifting: The Art of Drug Pricing." TheBody.com. Available online. URL: http://www.thebody.com/content/policy/art43415.html. Accessed March 13, 2011.

UNITAID. "UNITAID Approves Patent Pool." UNITAID.eu. Available online. URL: http://www.unitaid.eu/en/resources/news/237-unitaid-approves-patent-pool.html. Accessed March 12, 2011.

Weissman, Robert. "Free Trade, Expensive Drugs." TheBody.com. Available online. URL: http://www.thebody.com/content/policy/art38430.html. Accessed March 13, 2011.

Willis, Andrew. "Something 'Rotten' in EU Pharmaceutical Sector, Says Croes." EUObserver.com. Available online. URL: http://euobserver.com/867/28430. Accessed March 13, 2011.

Yahoo! Finance. "Industry Browser—Healthcare—Drug Manufacturers—Major—Company List." Yahoo.com. Available online. URL: http://biz.yahoo.com/p/510qpmd.html. Accessed March 13, 2011.

———. "Industry Summary." Yahoo.com. Available online. URL: http://biz.yahoo.com/p/sum_qpmd.html. Accessed March 13, 2011.

Yarchoan, Mark. "The Story of AZT: Partnership and Conflict." Scribd.com. Available online. URL: http://www.scribd.com/doc/1049/The-History-of-Zidovudine-AZT. Accessed February 28, 2011.

E

Eastern Europe and Central Asia These two regions are grouped together because they make up the majority of what was at one time the Soviet Union and communist bloc countries. There are many common characteristics to the epidemic in these countries despite the wide range of culture, language, and religion among them. The data cited in this article are found predominately in United Nations (UN) reports listed in the references. The HIV epidemic did not manifest itself as early in this region as in AFRICA or WESTERN AND CENTRAL EUROPE. The first cases of HIV in Russia were seen in the mid-1980s. As stated by Grisin and Wallander, it is believed that it first entered the country with soldiers returning from duty in Africa. In one instance, a soldier was directly implicated in infecting at least 15 other people through sex with other bisexual soldiers. The soldiers then passed the virus to their spouses through sex; in one instance, a soldier passed it to several people through blood transfusions he provided after returning to the Soviet Union. Although the initial reaction of the Soviet government was one of denial, the most rapid spread was seen in the same populations where the spread occurred in the West: SEX WORKERS, people who engaged in unprotected sexual activities, the INJECTION DRUG USE(R) (IDU) community, and those who received blood and blood products.

Initially, Soviet law and policy made education about the virus difficult. Official statements were that the virus was a Western problem probably created by the U.S. government and not a problem for the virtuous Soviet system. Statements from the medical community in the old

Soviet Union also made it difficult for patients, as many doctors refused to treat them, believing that not treating these patients would allow the virus to die out naturally and rid society of unwanted social ills. Laws passed made it illegal for a person who was HIV positive to travel in the Soviet Union, and mandatory terms in PRISONS were given to those who were accused of attempting to spread the virus after they had been infected. The laws allowed fear and mistrust to spread, keeping potentially HIV-positive people from being tested and helping the virus to spread through misinformation and denial.

Another large factor in the spread of HIV in this region was the Soviet policy in Afghanistan, which the Soviets occupied in the late 1970s and into the 1980s. Large numbers of troops from the Soviet Union became IDUs while in Afghanistan. When the Soviet system ended and troops were withdrawn, they took their drug use home to the various Soviet republics that became independent countries in the 1990s. The collapse of the economies and huge unemployment in this region after the Soviet collapse provided a breeding ground for an increase in the use of heroin, which was easily accessible to the region owing to the suddenly open markets created during the occupation of Afghanistan. The opening up of Soviet borders also allowed access to those markets. IDU became and remains the number one way that HIV has been spread in Russia, Ukraine, Estonia, as well as the other countries in this region. Rates of infection among some IDUs are among the highest seen in the world. Up to 70 percent of IDUs are HIV positive in some urban areas of Russia and Ukraine.

Measuring the epidemic in this region has also been difficult because of the late acknowledgment that the virus is a problem and the lack of government infrastructure to measure the volume and record the incidence of infection. Up until 1999, Estonia recorded only 12 cases of HIV in the country, but after record keeping began, within two years, 1,500 cases had been recorded. Similar jumps in the number of HIV-positive people were recorded in Ukraine, Russia, and Kazakhstan during this period. Since official acknowledgment of the epidemic in the early part of the 21st century, the numbers of new HIV-positive cases have dropped annually in the Baltic countries of Latvia, Lithuania, and Estonia. However, new diagnoses continue to rise in the rest of the region, including Azerbaijan, Georgia, Kazakhstan, Kyrgyzstan, Moldova, Tajikistan, and Uzbekistan, which now has the largest number of HIV-positive people after Russia and Ukraine. This region is currently considered by the United Nations (UN) to have the most rapidly expanding epidemic in the world.

By 2009, there were approximately 1.5 million people who had HIV infection in this region. By far the largest numbers of HIV-positive people are in Russia with approximately 850,000, followed by Ukraine with 350,000. In terms of prevalence among the adult population, defined as those above the age of 15, Ukraine has a prevalence of 1.5 percent of the population. Estonia's prevalence rate is 1.2 percent, and Russia's is 1.0 percent of the adult population. Other prevalence rates are as follows: Armenia, 0.1 percent; Azerbaijan, 0.1 percent: Belarus, 0.3 percent; Georgia, 0.1 percent; Kazakhstan, 0.1 percent; Kyrgyzstan, 0.3 percent; Latvia, 0.7 percent; Lithuania, 0.1 percent; Moldova, 0.4 percent; Tajikistan, 0.2 percent; and Uzbekistan, 0.1 percent. Little is known about the HIV epidemic in Turkmenistan, as the country does not provide data to the UN on cases or incidence.

In Russia, the epidemic is compounded by the vast territory and the lack of funding of education and treatment. Lack of medical facilities in remote areas of central and eastern Russia also hampers education and treatment. The epidemic is largely contained within the IDU community and their sexual partners. There are upward of 2 million IDUs in Russia according to the UN. Despite the large number of IDUs, there are only 69 centers for the exchange of needles in Russia, most located in the largest urban areas. The UN estimates that this covers only 5 percent of Russia's IDUs, thereby leaving many users without access to education about the spread of HIV or access to clean needles. Substitution therapy—the use of methadone or buprenorphine, both legal opiates, to replace the addictive heroin so a user does not have to use injecting equipment—does not exist in Russia. Ukraine has a well-developed program of IDU education as well as an extensive needle exchange program that issues clean injecting equipment to IDUs at a higher rate than other countries in the region. Opiate substitution programs also exist in Ukraine, though there is some concern regarding their use by the police to harass IDUs, which may deter their extensive use, has been raised in UN reports. Needle exchanges and opiate substitution are few and far between in the Central Asian states but some funding has begun at least in large urban areas. Much easier access to these programs exists in the Baltic countries. The Caucasus republics—Armenia, Azerbaijan, and Georgia—all have relatively small but growing numbers of IDUs as well as a growing HIV epidemic. Access to needle exchange programs or opiate substitution is extremely limited.

Sex workers are the other main cause of the spread of the virus in Russia and the rest of the region. Incidence rates are higher than in the general population, reaching rates of 30 percent in some major cities both in Russia and in Central Asian countries. Unprotected sex and multiple partners remain the standard for sex workers throughout the region. Education is unavailable or inadequate, and less than 35 percent of Russian sex workers understand the risk behaviors that can lead to HIV exposure. Sex workers are also often IDUs who trade for injection drugs, leading to multiple ways to acquire HIV. Sex workers in the Caucasus region are also showing large jumps in HIV prevalence rates in the last few years, indicating a burgeoning problem.

Testing of blood and blood products is a reasonably established procedure in the Baltic countries as it is in most of Russia, but is lacking in remote regions of Russia as well as in Central Asian countries. Outbreaks of HIV that have been traced to blood donations have been reported in Tajikistan, as well as Kyrgyzstan and Kazakhstan.

Neither Russia nor the other countries in this region make HIGHLY ACTIVE ANTIRETROVIRAL THERAPY (HAART) medications available routinely to HIV-positive people. Uzbekistan, Kazakhstan, and Moldova are the three countries of this area that make medications available to at least 20 percent of their HIV-positive population. The other countries fall far short of this percentage, below countries such as Zambia and Botswana, where far greater percentages of the population are HIV positive. Russia and the other countries of this region also do not manufacture generic drugs as India and Brazil do, thereby reducing costs on the medical systems and patients for the medicines in these two countries. Costs are very high for all medications in Eastern Europe and Central Asia. Russia and the Baltic countries have also had large epidemics of TUBERCULOSIS among their IDU populations, further stressing the medical system as well as increasing chances of the population's susceptibility to HIV.

Because Russia and the neighboring countries first began to observe cases of HIV in the late 1990s and early 21st century, it is believed that they will suffer the largest number of deaths from the disease within the next five years. The lack of education, prevention, medical treatment, and IDU treatment facilities may at that time be better addressed as thousands of people from this region fall ill and die of the effects of HIV.

AVERT: AVERTing HIV and AIDS. "HIV and AIDS in Russia, Eastern Europe and Central Asia." AVERT. org. Available online. URL: http://www.avert.org/ aids-russia.htm. Accessed March 13, 2011.

Grisin, Sarah A., and Celeste Wallander. "Russia's HIV/AIDS Crisis: Confronting the Present and Facing the Future." Heart-Intl.net. Available online. URL: http://www.heart-intl.net/HEART/092504/ RussiasHIVAIDSCrisis.pdf. Accessed March 25, 2011.

Moran, Dominique, and Jacob A. Jordaan. "HIV/AIDS in Russia: Determinants of Regional Prevalence." *International Journal of Health Geographics* 6, no. 22 (6 June 2007). Available online. URL: http:// www.ij-healthgeographics.com/content/6/1/22. Accessed March 13, 2011.

Twigg, Judyth L., ed. *HIV/AIDS in Russia and Eurasia, Volume 1.* 2 vols. New York: Palgrave Macmillan, 2006.

UNAIDS: Joint United Nations Programme on HIV/ AIDS. "The Changing HIV/AIDS Epidemic in Europe and Central Asia." UNAIDS.org. Available online. URL: http://data.unaids.org/Publications/ IRC-pub06/jc1038-changingepidemic_en.pdf. Accessed July 24, 2011.

———. "Eastern Europe and Central Asia." UNAIDS. org. Available online. URL: http://www.unaids.org/ en/regionscountries/regions/easterneuropeand centralasia/. Accessed March 13, 2011.

———. "UNAIDS Report on the Global AIDS Epidemic 2010." UNAIDS.com. Available online. URL: http:// www.unaids.org/globalreport/Global_report.htm. Accessed March 13, 2011.

UNAIDS: Joint United Nations Programme on HIV/ AIDS and the World Health Organization. "2007 AIDS Epidemic Update Eastern Europe and Central Asia." UNAIDS.org. Available online. URL: http:// data.unaids.org/pub/report/2008/jc1529_epibriefs _eeurope_casia_en.pdf. Accessed March 22, 2011.

———. "AIDS Epidemic Update 2009." UNAIDS.org. Available online. URL: http://www.unaids.org/ en/media/unaids/contentassets/dataimport/pub/ report/2 009/ jc1700_epi_update_2009_en.pdf. Accessed March 22, 2011.

World Bank. "Blood Services in Central Asian Health Systems." WorldBank.org. Available online. URL: http://siteresources.worldbank.org/INTECAREG TOPHEANUT/Resources/cabloodbankstudy.pdf. Accessed March 13, 2011.

efavirenz Efavirenz is one of the NON-NUCLEO-SIDE REVERSE TRANSCRIPTASE INHIBITORS (NNRTIs); it is manufactured by Bristol-Myers Squibb in

NORTH AMERICA and some European countries, under the trade name Sustiva. It was approved for use in the United States in 1998. It is also known commonly as EFV. In much of Europe and the rest of the world, Merck manufactures efavirenz and it is sold under the name Stocrin.

Dosage

Efavirenz is available in tablets and capsules. It is generally taken as one tablet of 600 mg once a day. It is recommended that it be taken just prior to bed with a light snack or on an empty stomach. It should not be taken with high-fat meals, as they can cause an unneeded increase in the amount of efavirenz in the body. Efavirenz also is available in 200 mg and 50 mg capsules. These lesser amounts are intended for CHILDREN. A doctor will prescribe the proper amount of efavirenz, which is based on the weight of the child. It has not been approved for use by infants or newborns.

Efavirenz must be taken in combination with other antiretrovirals to make up a full HIGHLY ACTIVE ANTIRETROVIRAL THERAPY (HAART) regimen. It is also part of the triple drug combination ATRIPLA.

Drug Interactions

There are several drugs that should not be taken with efavirenz. One is Atripla, as this is a combination antiretroviral that already contains efavirenz. Efavirenz should not be taken with ETRAVIRINE, another NNRTI. It causes levels of etravirine in the blood to drop, making it less effective. It can cause lowered levels of several of the PROTEASE INHIBITORS (PIs). ATAZANAVIR SULFATE, SAQUINAVIR, FOSAMPRENAVIR, KALETRA, and AMPRENAVIR may have to be boosted with the drug ritonavir to raise the levels of the drugs to maximum effectiveness.

Efavirenz can cause a decrease in the amount of sildenafil and varenafil in the body. These are two erectile dysfunction medications. Anyone taking these should consult a doctor regarding the recommended dose of these medications. Efavirenz can also interfere with birth control pills taken by WOMEN. If a woman is using birth control pills, she should also use a barrier method of some type to prevent pregnancies when taking efavirenz. Efavirenz is also known to cause birth defects. Women who wish to become pregnant or are already into a pregnancy should not take efavirenz or Atripla.

Efavirenz will interact with some medications used to treat bacterial OPPORTUNISTIC INFECTIONS (OIs) such as TUBERCULOSIS and *Mycobacterium avium* COMPLEX infections. Its effects on individual drugs vary: Some interactions cause the levels of efavirenz to drop, and other drugs cause drops in the level of the antibiotic. Doses may need to be adjusted, depending on which drug is prescribed.

The drug can cause a drop in the level of calcium channel blockers, which are taken to control high blood pressure or chest pains or to regulate an irregular heartbeat. Certain migraine medicines cannot be combined with efavirenz.

The drug should not be taken with cisparide, which is used to control heartburn and acid reflux disease. In addition, the herbal supplement St. John's wort will cause the levels of efavirenz in the body to drop, thereby making it ineffective. Efavirenz can also interact with medications used to treat fungal infections in HIV-positive people.

Efavirenz is eliminated slowly from the body, often remaining present two weeks or more after a person has stopped taking the drug, much longer than most antiretrovirals. If a person is taking efavirenz and switches antiretrovirals or stops taking medications to clear the system, it is important that he or she continue taking some antiretrovirals for the entire two weeks, allowing it to clear the body. If not, the virus can develop a mutation to the drug efavirenz, as it is the only drug present during the time it takes to clear the body. Developing a mutation that prevents efavirenz from working against HIV also will probably prevent any antiretroviral in the NNRTI class from being effective against the virus. Studies have shown that approximately 20 percent of AFRICAN AMERICANS process efavirenz more slowly than other people, but it is not clearly understood why. Therefore, clearing the drug may take even longer in this population.

Side Effects

The major side effect that people complain about with efavirenz is the result of one of the benefits of the drug. Some HIV antiretrovirals do not cross the blood-brain barrier, which generally stops many medications from entering the brain area. However, efavirenz crosses that barrier, allowing it to fight the virus in the brain. Because of this, more than 50 percent of patients in clinical trials have reported some central nervous system (CNS) side effects. These can range from mild dizziness to sleeplessness, vivid or scary dreams, sleepiness, headache, and, in some instances, euphoria, depression, or hallucinations. It is strongly suggested that efavirenz be taken just before bedtime so that some or all of these symptoms are lessened as a person sleeps. These symptoms generally lessen or disappear within a month of when the drug is started.

Some people have had major problems with CNS symptoms when taking efavirenz. Suicide, major depression, and symptoms of angry or violent behavior have been reported. This has occurred more often in people who have a history of mental illness. It occurs in approximately 1 percent of the people taking efavirenz. The drug has been shown to cause an increase of seizures if someone suffers from seizures or has been known to have seizures at some point in his or her medical history. A rash can occur in about 25 percent of people when starting the drug. The majority of people recover from the rash without stopping the drug, but approximately 1 percent have a serious rash with ulcers, blistering, and seeping. People who have such a severe rash should stop taking efavirenz under advice from a doctor. Rashes are more common among children beginning efavirenz than among adults.

Efavirenz can cause people to test positive for marijuana use in testing for illegal drugs. Some-one who has to take a urine test for drug use will need to inform the laboratory taking the urine sample that he or she is using efavirenz. This will allow them to use a more sensitive test to avoid a false positive test result.

AIDSInfoNet. "Efavirenz (Sustiva, Stocrin)." AIDS InfoNet.org. Available online. URL: http://www.aidsinfonet.org/fact_sheets/view/432. Accessed March 15, 2011.

AIDSmeds. "Special Issues for Children with HIV." AIDSmeds.com. Available online. URL: http://www.aidsmeds.com/articles/Children_7566.shtml. Accessed March 11, 2011.

———. "Sustiva (Efavirenz)." AIDSmeds.com. Available online. URL: http://www.aidsmeds.com/archive/Sustiva_1615.shtml. Accessed March 15, 2011.

The Body. "Sustiva (Efavirenz, Stocrin)." TheBody.com. Available online. URL: http://www.thebody.com/index/treat/sustiva.html. Accessed March 11, 2011.

United States Department of Health and Human Services. "Efavirenz." aidsinfo.nih.gov. Available online. URL: http://www.aidsinfo.nih.gov/DrugsNew/DrugDetailNT.aspx?int_id=269. Accessed March 11, 2011.

elvitegravir Elvitegravir is an experimental HIV INTEGRASE INHIBITOR that is currently undergoing phase III drug testing in humans. The drug is manufactured by Gilead Sciences. It is referred to as GS-9137 in research reports. It has not been given a trade name, and the U.S. FOOD AND DRUG ADMINISTRATION (FDA) has not approved it as of this writing. Elvitegravir is the second integrase inhibitor drug to enter phase III testing. The phase III trial was extended, in early 2011, to run 96 weeks instead of 48 weeks, to explore the long-term safety and effectiveness of the drug. Early analysis of the study results show elvitegravir to be as effective as the other integrase inhibitor on the market, raltegravir.

Elvitegravir is a modified quinolone antibiotic, so it may have interactions similar to those of other quinolone drugs such as levofloxacin or ciprofloxacin. As an integrase inhibitor it works against HIV in a way that is different from the way most other medications currently available on the market do. RALTEGRAVIR is the only other currently available integrase inhibitor.

Already Gilead Sciences has announced that it is beginning to test elvitegravir with an as-yet-unnamed boosting agent that is different from ritonavir. It has announced plans to produce a four-drug pill combining elvitegravir, the boosting agent (known as GS-9350 in research studies), TENOFOVIR DISOPROXIL FUMARATE, and EMTRICITABINE; that would make another one-pill-a-day anti-HIV treatment available for patients.

Dosage

Elvitegravir is currently being tested in a variety of dosages, and a specific dosing pattern has not been established. It is being tested for use in conjunction with ritonavir, which in earlier studies boosted the efficiency of the drug. Phase III studies are using 85 mg and 150 mg tablets, depending on which other HIV medications are being taken by the study participant. It is currently thought that a dose of one pill twice a day is sufficient.

Drug Interactions

Elvitegravir is known to have increased absorption into the body when used with ATAZANAVIR SULFATE boosted with ritonavir and when used with KALETRA. Study participants taking these medications will receive a lowered dose of elvitegravir to test proper dosing of the medication. Early studies of elvitegravir show a higher rate of absorption when taken with food.

Side Effects

The most common side effect reported in early trials has been headache. It is expected that as the drug is boosted currently in trials with ritonavir there may be increased levels of cholesterol and triglycerides, as is seen with treatments based on PROTEASE INHIBITORS (PIs). Phase III trials have revealed such side effects as diarrhea, nausea, headache, back pain, and upper respiratory infections. Side effects were in the similar range as those experienced when taking raltegravir.

AIDSmeds. "Elvitegravir (GS-9137)." AIDSmeds.com. Available online. URL: http://www.aidsmeds.com/archive/GS-9137_1638.shtml. Accessed March 15, 2011.

"AIDSmeds.com—Special Issues for Children with HIV: Introduction." Available online. URL: http://www.aidsmeds.com/articles/Children_7566.shtml. Accessed March 15, 2011.

The Body. "Antiretroviral Medications in the Pipeline." GMHC Treatment Issues, September 2010. Available online. URL: http://www.thebody.com/content/art40488.html. Accessed March 15, 2011.

Hitt, Emma. "Elvitegravir Noninferior to Raltegravir." Medscape.com. Available online. URL: http://www.medscape.com/viewarticle/746786. Accessed July 24, 2011.

United States Department of Health and Human Services. "Elvitegravir." aidsinfo.nih.gov. Available online. URL: http://www.aidsinfo.nih.gov/DrugsNew/DrugDetailNT.aspx?int_id=421&ClassID=7&TypeID=2. Accessed March 15, 2011.

United States National Institutes of Health. "A Phase 2 Study of the Safety of Ritonavir-Boosted GS-9137 (GS-9137/r) Administered in Combination with Other Antiretroviral Agents for the Treatment of HIV-1 Infected Subject." ClinicalTrials.gov. Available online. URL: http://clinicaltrials.gov/ct2/show/NCT00445146?term=gs+9137&rank=1. Accessed July 24, 2011.

emtricitabine   Emtricitabine, one of the NUCLEOSIDE REVERSE TRANSCRIPTASE INHIBITORS (NRTIs), is used in the treatment and control of HIV. It is sold under the trade name Emtriva and also commonly called FTC or coviracil. The U.S. FOOD AND DRUG ADMINISTRATION (FDA) approved it in 2003. It is similar in design to LAMIVUDINE, and if HIV becomes resistant to one of these two drugs, it is generally resistant to both of them. It is manufactured by Gilead Sciences.

Dosage

The drug is available in a 200 mg capsule that is taken once a day. It is also available in a liquid formula for babies, young CHILDREN, and those who have difficulty swallowing pills. The dosages for the liquid are based upon weight and start at 6 mg of liquid for each kilogram of body weight, up to a 240 mg dose for adults.

Emtricitabine can be taken with or without a meal, though high-fat meals may reduce the concentrations of the drug in the body. Emtricitabine is removed from the body through the kidneys. If a person already has decreased kidney function, lowered doses of the drug may be needed.

Emtricitabine has also been shown to be effective, as has lamivudine, against HEPATITIS B (HBV). Because of this, individuals who are both HIV- and HBV-positive need to be monitored if the drug is stopped for any reason. Stopping emtricitabine may cause a flare-up in symptoms of HBV, which could be dangerous for liver function.

Drug Interactions

Emtricitabine should not be taken at the same time as any pill that contains the drug as part of combination therapy. These pills are TRUVADA and ATRIPLA. It should also not be taken at the same time as lamivudine, as these two drugs are very similar and have no benefit for the patient when taken at the same time. Any combination pill that contains lamivudine will also not be prescribed at the same time as emtricitabine. Those pills are EPZICOM, TRIZIVIR, TRIOMUNE, and COMBIVIR.

When prescribed at the same time as TENOFOVIR DISOPROXIL FUMARATE, the amount of emtricitabine in the body is raised. It is possible that other drug interactions can occur, though none has been noted as severe in studies. As with lamivudine, when the common mutation in the virus M184V appears to be due to emtricitabine use, it actually improves the activity of ZIDOVUDINE and tenofovir against the virus.

Side Effects

NRTIs can potentially cause several serious side effects, though emtricitabine is generally well tolerated. General side effects that have been reported include headache, diarrhea, nausea, and rash. They have not lasted long nor have they been serious in most people. Skin pigmentation, the creation of freckles, has been noted in some people who use emtricitabine. This has been reported more often in children than adults. It may also cause a darkening of the palms of the hands or soles of the feet. It is also believed to occur more frequently among AFRICAN AMERICANS.

On rare occasions, NRTIs can cause a severe disorder called LACTIC ACIDOSIS. This is a buildup of lactate in the blood, which needs to be addressed immediately by a doctor. Symptoms of lactic acidosis include sharp pains in the abdomen near the liver, or in the lower back; vomiting, difficulty breathing, extreme tiredness and muscle weakness; and headache. Hyperlactatemia, which can be measured through BLOOD WORK/BLOOD TESTS, can provide a measure of elevated lactate levels and may give some indication of whether this condition is likely to occur. Though rare, it does occur more often among WOMEN, obese individuals, and people who have been on NRTIs for extended periods.

AIDS InfoNet. "Emtricitabine (Emtriva)." AIDSInfo Net.org. Available online. URL: http://www.aidsinfo net.org/fact_sheets/view/420. Accessed March 11, 2011.

AIDSmeds. "Emtriva (Emtricitabine)." AIDSmeds. com. Available online. URL: http://www.aidsmeds. com/archive/Emtriva_1578.shtml. Accessed March 11, 2011.

———. "Special Issues for Children with HIV." AIDS meds.com. Available online. URL: http://www.aids meds.com/articles/Children_7566.shtml. Accessed March 11, 2011.

The Body. "Reyataz (Atazanavir)." TheBody.com. Available online. URL: http://www.thebody.com/ index/treat/emtricitabine.html. Accessed March 11, 2011.

United States Department of Health and Human Services. "Emtricitabine." aidsinfo.nih.gov. Available online. URL: http://www.aidsinfo.nih.gov/DrugsNew/Drug DetailNT.aspx?int_id=314. Accessed March 11, 2011.

enfuvirtide Enfuvirtide is one of the fusion inhibitors, or ENTRY INHIBITORS, and is used in the treatment of HIV. It is always prescribed as part of a multidrug combination of medications. Enfuvirtide is an injection drug that is taken subcutaneously, just below the skin. It is not available in pill or liquid form for ingestion. It was approved by the U.S. FOOD AND DRUG ADMINISTRATION (FDA) in 2003 for use in treatment-experienced individuals. The drug has not been approved for use in treatment-naïve HIV-positive people. It was the first entry inhibitor–class drug approved by the FDA.

Enfuvirtide is most commonly called T-20 and is sold under the trade name Fuzeon. T-20 was the product number assigned to the chemical by the company that originally discovered the drug, Trimeris; it is currently owned by Trimeris and by Roche Pharmaceuticals and is abbreviated ENF. It is difficult to use, as it is dispensed in a powder form in small vials and must be mixed with sterile water, also provided in small vials, before use. It cannot be shaken, as it will foam, but must be rolled around in the mixing container instead. It can be refrigerated once it is mixed if it is used before 24 hours have passed. After mixing, it must then be taken into the needle, taking care that no crystals of the powder are unmixed. Even in the world of antiretrovirals, T-20 is expensive, at close to $3,000 a month. It is seen as a last-chance salvage drug for people for whom other antiretroviral combinations have failed.

Dosage

T-20 is injected below the skin twice a day. The dose is one milliliter. Instructions suggest that the patient pinch an inch of skin and use this method to make sure the drug is below the skin but not into a muscle. The preferred injection sites are the upper arm, upper legs, and abdomen. It is recommended that after an injection, the individual massage the area of the injection or use a massaging device to do so. This can help prevent or lessen any injection area reactions.

Smaller dosages are recommended for CHILDREN ages six to 16. T-20 has not been approved for use by people below the age of six.

Drug Interactions

There are no known drug interactions for T-20. It acts in conjunction with other antiretrovirals.

Side Effects

The major side effect of T-20 is a postinjection site reaction. These reactions can include burning, itching, swelling, redness, pain, slightly hardened skin at the injection site, and formation of a small bump. Most people report some injection site reactions, but they are not consistent and may not always occur. The reaction may be worse if the injections are given repeatedly in the same spot or if the injection goes too deep, as into a muscle. A skin reaction usually lasts for less than seven days. Reactions lasting longer may be infected and require further care by a doctor.

Individuals who have HEMOPHILIA AND HIV or take blood-thinning medication may experience some bleeding when taking this medication.

During clinical trials, people taking T-20 were more susceptible to BACTERIAL PNEUMONIA than other people in the studies. If patients develop a cough, fever, and trouble breathing they should contact a doctor immediately.

Rarely, an allergic reaction has been seen in T-20 patients. This reaction includes rash, fever, shaking, nausea, vomiting, and breathing difficulties. If the drug is restarted after such an allergic reaction, the condition will be worse.

Other side effects include peripheral NEUROPATHY, insomnia, decreased appetite, and muscle pain. Because T-20 is considered a salvage drug, patients may be more susceptible to IMMUNE RECONSTITUTION INFLAMMATORY SYNDROME responses as their immune system begins to recover T cells and the HIV viral load decreases.

AIDS InfoNet. "Enfuvirtide (Fuzeon)." AIDSInfoNet. org. Available online. URL: http://www.aidsinfo net.org/fact_sheets/view/461. Accessed March 11, 2011.

AIDSmeds. "Fuzeon (Enfuvirtide, T-20)." AIDSmeds.
com. Available online. URL: http://www.aidsmeds.
com/archive/Fuzeon_1628.shtml. Accessed March
11, 2011.
———. "Special Issues for Children with HIV." AIDS
meds.com. Available online. URL: http://www.aids
meds.com/articles/Children_7566.shtml. Accessed
March 11, 2011.
The Body. "Fuzeon (Enfuvirtide, T-20)." TheBody.
com. Available online. URL: http://www.thebody.
com/index/treat/fuzeon.html. Accessed March 11,
2011.
United States Department of Health and Human Services.
"Enfuvirtide." aidsinfo.nih.gov. Available online. URL:
http://www.aidsinfo.nih.gov/DrugsNew/Drug
DetailNT.aspx?int_id=306&ClassID=4&TypeID=1.
Accessed March 11, 2011.

entry inhibitors   Entry inhibitors work to prevent the entry of HUMAN IMMUNODEFICIENCY VIRUS (HIV) into human cells, where they transform and become part of the cells' genetic code, reproducing as the cells reproduce. There are several steps in the process of entry into the cell, and drugs are being developed to interfere with the process at each of those steps. Although these drugs may work in different ways, they are classed together as entry inhibitors.

HIV is a virus; all viruses need to find a host, that is, a place to live. HIV uses the HUMAN IMMUNE SYSTEM cells as its place to live and reproduce. It infects the cells of the immune system, predominantly the CD4 T cells, but also macrophages and microglial cells. To do this, HIV uses several small proteins first to attach themselves, and then it inserts its genetic code into the cell, forcing the cell to produce more viral particles, which then can infect other immune cells.

The first step in the process occurs when the HIV finds a T cell. HIV has on its outer wall a protein called gp120. The *gp* stands for glycoprotein. This glycoprotein matches up with a protein receptor, called a CD4 receptor, on the T cell. The virus and the T cell have matched receptors, they become bound, and it is possible for the virus to take the next step in attaching itself to the cell.

At this point, the virus must take a second step and look for a different kind of receptor of the T cell. Depending on the type of HIV in the body, this is either a CCR5 receptor or a CXCR4 receptor. CXCR4, also sometimes called fusin, is a specific binding protein found on many immune system cells in the body. HIV that uses this receptor is called CXCR4 tropic. CCR5 is another binding protein found on T cells. It is the most common binding protein that HIV uses to attach itself to a cell. Most HIV is CCR5 tropic, meaning it can only attach using the CCR5 receptor; CXCR4 tropic virus is much less common. One entry inhibitor drug called MARAVIROC interferes with the attachment of the virus to the CCR5 receptor, preventing HIV from attaching itself to cells. Maraviroc is also called a chemokine receptor antagonist or a CCR5 inhibitor.

In the third step in the process, after binding and matching receptors, another glycoprotein, called gp41, inserts itself into the cell, causing the virus and the cell to fuse, or join, much more closely together. This then allows the virus to insert its genetic information into the cell, which will later allow viral reproduction. Drugs that interfere with this portion of the process are called fusion inhibitors. They prevent the virus from fusing to the T cell. The fusion inhibitor currently available to treat HIV infection is called ENFUVIRTIDE. Enfuvirtide interferes with gp41 and prevents the fusing of the virus and the cell.

Work on developing new entry inhibitors continues. Preventing the HIV from entering the cell at all is seen as a way to prevent HIV from ever fully infecting a person. Entry inhibitors have generally been well-tolerated drugs. There are some side effects because, as a class of drug, they work in several different ways to block the entry of HIV to the cells. Although enfuvirtide has few side effects as a medication, administering it intramuscularly can cause some discomfort. People who take maraviroc report some side effects such as dizziness and some upper respiratory problems, such as cough. These medications must be taken as a combination therapy as must all antiretrovirals in order to have several places where the virus replication can be stopped. Entry inhibitors currently in some phase of development include ibalizumab (TNX-355) from TaiMed Biologics, SP01A from Samaritan Pharmaceuticals, and PRO-140 from Progenics.

AIDSInfoNet. "Attachment and Fusion Inhibitors under Development." AIDSInfoNet.com. Available online. URL: http://www.aidsinfonet.org/fact_sheets/view/460. Accessed March 25, 2011.

AIDSmeds.com "Entry Inhibitors (including Fusion Inhibitors)." AIDSmeds.com. Available online. URL: http://www.aidsmeds.com/archive/EIs_1627.shtml. Accessed March 15, 2011.

The Body. "Fuzeon: In a Class by Itself." TheBody.com. Available online. URL: http://www.thebody.com/content/art13791.html. Accessed March 15, 2011.

Esté, José A., and Amalio Telenti. "HIV Entry Inhibitors." Lancet 370, no. 9581 (7 July 2007): 81–88.

Highleyman, Liz. "Novel Entry Inhibitor VIR-576 Shows Promise in Early Study." HIVandHepatitis.com. Available online. URL: http://www.hivandhepatitis.com/recent/2011/0107_2011_b.html. Accessed March 16, 2011.

Tibotec/Virco. "HIV Animations." Tibotec/Virco.com. Available online. URL: http://www.tibotec-hiv.com/bgdisplay.jhtml?itemname=hivmovies. Accessed April 5, 2011.

Epzicom   Epzicom is the trade name for a multidrug combination antiretroviral pill. It is composed of two other antiretrovirals: LAMIVUDINE and ABACAVIR. Both of these drugs are NUCLEOSIDE REVERSE TRANSCRIPTASE INHIBITORS (NRTIs), and, therefore, Epzicom is also an NRTI. It is manufactured by GlaxoSmithKline and was approved by the U.S. FOOD AND DRUG ADMINISTRATION (FDA) in 2004. It is also marketed under the trade name Kivexa in the United Kingdom and other countries.

Dosage

Epzicom combines 600 mg of abacavir and 300 mg of lamivudine in one tablet. It is taken orally once daily. Because it is a fixed dose tablet, it is not recommended for CHILDREN or patients who need to adjust dosages because of weight or drug interactions. Epzicom is always combined with at least one other antiretroviral, usually one of the PROTEASE INHIBITORS (PIs).

Drug Interactions

Epzicom has the same drug interactions that lamivudine and abacavir have individually. Epzicom is never prescribed with lamivudine, abacavir, or TRIZIVIR. Because Epzicom is a combination of lamivudine and abacavir, it would be dangerous to increase the doses of either drug. Trizivir is a combination drug that also contains abacavir and lamivudine and would not be prescribed at the same time for the same reasons. The drugs EMTRICITABINE and TRUVADA, which contains emtricitabine, are not generally prescribed at the same time as lamivudine as these drugs are very similar, and prescribing them at the same time is not believed to offer any benefit to the patient.

Abacavir decreases the amount of the drug methadone in the body. People who are taking methadone to manage the symptoms of heroin withdrawal may need to have the dosage of that medication increased by a physician while using Epzicom. Using any type of alcohol while taking Epzicom increases the amount of abacavir in the body. This can increase the side effects of abacavir and increase the chance of having the side effects.

Lamivudine increases in concentration in the body of a person who is taking trimethoprim/sulfamethoxazole (TMP-SMX), an antibiotic used for prevention and treatment of PNEUMOCYSTIS PNEUMONIA (PCP). Patients who are taking Epzicom may need to adjust the dosage of TMP-SMX if their doctor believes this could cause problems.

Side Effects

Epzicom contains abacavir. Between 3 and 8 percent of people who take abacavir have an allergic reaction to the drug. Research into the reaction has shown that this is caused by an inherited genetic marker named *HLA-B*5701*. There is an inexpensive test that is recommended for all people who are planning to take abacavir or one of the multidrug combination pills that contain abacavir, such as Epzicom. This test will determine whether a person carries this genetic marker. A person who is determined to carry the *HLA-B*5701* marker will not be prescribed abacavir in any form. *HLA-B*5701* is one of the numerous genes that play a role in the HUMAN IMMUNE SYSTEM, allowing the body to fight off viruses and other pathogens. HLA stands for human leukocyte antigen. The allergic reaction occurs less often among men and people of African descent. Signs of an allergic reaction to Epzicom can include fever, rash, headache, stomach pain, vomiting, diarrhea, cough, or respiratory illness. People who suspect that they are having a reaction should immediately talk to a physician about their suspected symptoms, as in some cases the reaction can lead to severe illness or death. The reaction most often occurs within the first two weeks of beginning Epzicom. A person who has such a reaction should never again take abacavir in any form, as the reaction will be more severe. Some people who have stopped taking Epzicom for reasons other than the allergic reaction have suffered the reaction when they restarted the pill. It is generally recommended that if a person stops taking Epzicom for any reason, he or she consult a physician before restarting the drug.

Common side effects, not related to the potential allergic reaction, include stomach upset, headache, tiredness, and loss of appetite. These will lessen over time while the person is taking the drug. NRTIs have been implicated in increased fat levels in the blood as well as changes in the distribution of fat in the body, LIPODYSTROPHY.

NRTIs have also been shown to cause LACTIC ACIDOSIS and liver disease in a small number of people. Severe pain in the upper abdomen and lower back, as well as severe nausea, can be signs of lactic acidosis, which is elevated levels

of lactic acid in the blood. Enlarged spleen, pancreas, or liver can also be a sign of the condition. It is important that all medications be stopped if a physician diagnoses this condition. Liver markers in the blood are always monitored during regular BLOOD WORK/BLOOD TESTS to watch for these conditions, but any symptoms should be reported to a doctor. This reaction to NRTIs is more prevalent among WOMEN, obese people, and people who have advanced HIV disease, and can occur at any time.

An increase in heart attacks among people taking abacavir in studies has also been noted, particularly among people already at risk for heart attacks; those risk factors are being male, having a high cholesterol level and high blood pressure, being obese, and smoking. People taking Epzicom should be monitored for heart ailments.

Abacavir is listed as a pregnancy category C drug. It has been shown to cause death or birth defects in laboratory animals. No studies of abacavir have been done among pregnant women, and it is unknown whether abacavir causes changes in breast milk for women who are BREAST-FEEDING babies. It is only recommended for pregnant women or those who are breast-feeding if the benefits clearly outweigh the potential risks of the drug.

AIDS InfoNet. "Epzicom/Kivexa (Abacavir + Lamivudine)." AIDSInfoNet.org. Available online. URL: http://www.aidsinfonet.org/fact_sheets/view/422. Accessed March 11, 2011.

AIDSmeds. "Epzicom (Abacavir + Lamivudine)." AIDSmeds.com. Available online. URL: http://www.aidsmeds.com/archive/Epzicom_1580.shtml. Accessed March 11, 2011.

———. "Special Issues for Children with HIV." AIDS meds.com. Available online. URL: http://www.aids meds.com/articles/Children_7566.shtml. Accessed March 11, 2011.

The Body. "Epzicom (Abacavir/3TC, Kivexa)." The Body.com. Available online. URL: http://www.thebody.com/index/treat/epzicom.html. Accessed March 11, 2011.

Highleyman, Liz. "HLA-B*5701 Screening for Abacavir (Ziagen) Hypersensitivity." HIVandHepatitis.com.

Available online. URL: http://www.hivandhepatitis.com/recent/2008/022608_c.html. Accessed March 16, 2011.

United States Department of Health and Human Services. "Abacavir/Lamivudine." aidsinfo.nih.gov. Available online. URL: http://www.aidsinfo.nih.gov/Drugs New/DrugDetailNT.aspx?int_id=407. Accessed March 11, 2011.

etravirine   Etravirine was the first of the NON-NUCLEOSIDE REVERSE TRANSCRIPTASE INHIBITORS (NNRTIs) approved by the U.S. FOOD AND DRUG ADMINISTRATION (FDA) in more than 10 years, when it became available in 2008. It is sold under the trade name Intelence. It is manufactured by Tibotec Pharmaceuticals, which is wholly owned by the company Johnson & Johnson.

Etravirine is effective in the treatment of HIV that is resistant to treatment by other NNRTI drugs. Etravirine is not currently approved for use by HIV-positive people who are *not* treatment experienced. It is approved only as a second-line treatment in combination with other antiretroviral drugs.

Dosage

Etravirine is available in 100 mg tablets. The standard dose is two 100 mg tablets twice a day. The tablets can be dissolved in water by those people who have trouble swallowing pills. Etravirine needs to be taken immediately after eating a full meal. It should never be taken on an empty stomach. Absorption into the body at necessary levels is only successful when food is present in the stomach.

Pregnant WOMEN may take etravirine, and no birth defects have been associated with its use in animals or humans. It is unknown whether etravirine passes to an infant through BREAST-FEEDING. Etravirine has not been approved for use in CHILDREN below the age of 16.

Drug Interactions

Etravirine interacts with several other HIV anti-retroviral medications. It should not be taken with any of the other NNRTI class drugs. When it is mixed with boosted or unboosted PROTEASE INHIBITORS (PIs), etravirine levels in the blood can be either increased or decreased. For these reasons, it should not be taken with boosted ritonavir. It should also not be taken with TIPRANAVIR, ATAZANAVIR SULFATE, or FOSAMPRENAVIR. It can be taken in regular dosing regimens with boosted DARUNAVIR and SAQUINAVIR.

Etravirine interacts with several antibiotic medications used to treat TUBERCULOSIS and *Mycobacterium avium* COMPLEX infections. Rifampin, rifabutin, and clarithromycin should not be taken at the same time as etravirine.

Etravirine can interfere with the proper dosing of antifungal medicines used to treat CANDIDIASIS infections. Dosage adjustments to lesser amounts of such drugs as fluconazole may be necessary to maintain proper levels of the antifungal in the body. In addition, anticonvulsant drugs should not be used with etravirine.

Cholesterol-lowering statins interact in different ways with etravirine. Simvastatin and lovastatin levels in the body are lowered with etravirine. Atorvastatin levels may be lowered, and dose adjustments may be necessary. Fluvastatin levels will increase. It is believed that rosuvastatin and pravastatin levels are not affected by etravirine, and they may be safely prescribed at the same time.

Levels of the erectile dysfunction medications sildenafil, vardenafil, and tadalafil will be lowered in the blood during use with etravirine, and dosage may be adjusted upward to achieve the necessary levels for proper functioning.

The herbal supplement St. John's wort lowers the level of etravirine in the body significantly and should not be taken by a person who is using etravirine.

Side Effects

Headache, diarrhea, and nausea were the most common side effects reported with etravirine in clinical trials. These side effects lessened over time.

NNRTIs are known to cause a rash reaction in some people when they begin treatment. A rash affected approximately 15 percent of all people starting etravirine in one study. In some cases, this rash was severe and included sores around the mouth, blistering, and redness and swelling around the eyes. If these symptoms occur while taking etravirine, a doctor must be consulted immediately. It is a sign of a serious but uncommon reaction that could be life threatening. A person who stops taking etravirine because of this allergic rash reaction should never start the drug again. The rash typically appears within one to three weeks after starting etravirine. The rash will generally end shortly afterward in most people.

AIDS InfoNet. "Etravirine (Intelence)." AIDSInfoNet. org. Available online. URL: http://www.aidsinfonet. org/fact_sheets/view/434. Accessed March 11, 2011.

AIDSmeds. "Reyataz (Etravirine, ETV, TMC-125)." AIDS meds.com. Available online. URL: http://www.aid smeds.com/archive/intelence_1618.shtml. Accessed March 11, 2011.

———. "Special Issues for Children with HIV." AIDS meds.com. Available online. URL: http://www.aids meds.com/articles/Children_7566.shtml. Accessed March 11, 2011.

The Body. "Intelence." TheBody.com. Available online. URL: http://www.thebody.com/content/ treat/art39381.html. March 15. 2011.

United States Department of Health and Human Services. "Etravirine." aidsinfo.nih.gov. Available online. URL: http://aidsinfo.nih.gov/DrugsNew/ DrugDetailT.aspx?MenuItem=Drugs&int_id=398& Search=Off&ClassID=0&TypeID=0. Accessed March 11, 2011.

Food and Drug Administration (FDA) The United States Food and Drug Administration (FDA) is the agency of the federal government that is "responsible for protecting the public health by assuring the safety, efficacy, and security of human and veterinary drugs, biological products, medical devices, our nation's food supply, cosmetics, and products that emit radiation," according to the agency's Web site. It recently became the agency responsible for managing tobacco when Congress passed a law declaring tobacco a drug that needed to be regulated. The FDA is part of the Department of Health and Human Services and consists of several smaller offices that function within the FDA.

The FDA has responsibility within the United States to regulate the testing, sale, and promotion of pharmaceutical drugs and food products. It also approves new medical procedures for marketing on the basis of evidence of efficacy and safety. Early in the AIDS crisis, when the epidemic's disastrous scope was barely imagined, AIDS activists pressed the FDA for a faster and more humane response to this public health emergency. Eventually, after repeated protests, including a large one at the agency's headquarters in 1988, the FDA established accelerated approval processes for some drugs and established expanded access to drugs that were currently being tested. An example of this was the drug SAQUINAVIR, the first of the PROTEASE INHIBITORS (PIs), which was approved in a record three months, the fastest AIDS drug approval ever.

The FDA, along with many government agencies in the early 1980s, was slow to respond to the HIV epidemic. When it first became clear that blood and blood products, particularly clotting factors used in treating hemophilia, were probably transmitting the virus that was causing AIDS, the government agencies initially did nothing. It was more than two years before the government would issue requirements that clotting factors and blood donations be screened for HIV. The development of a test to detect HIV was the point when the FDA finally acted. Until then, even though the virus was known to be carried by blood, the government and blood industry groups refused to act to stop the use of potentially infected blood. The delays at the FDA in approving potential treatments, drug trials for HIV, and trials for drugs treating the OPPORTUNISTIC INFECTIONS (OIs) that occur led many early HIV patients to seek experimental treatments in other countries, as well as to try illegally importing any number of experimental drugs that were available in places such as Mexico. The early accounts of HIV patients revealed that many people were willing to go to great lengths to receive some potential relief where the FDA would give none and refused to provide guidance on potential treatments or imaginary cures that were being marketed to the HIV community. A particular example of this was the film star Rock Hudson, who traveled to France in 1985 for experimental treatment, as none was available in the United States at the time of his illness.

The FDA reviews and approves all HIV antiretroviral and treatment medications that are tested in various drug trials. It is responsible for the safety of all drugs on the market and reviews ongoing trials for any long-term issues after medications have entered the market It is the FDA that instructs manufacturers to issue warnings on medications, both prescription and nonprescription, if problems arise once they are being sold. The FDA is also responsible for withdrawing medications from the market if the need arises, as in the case of rofecoxib, an anti-inflammatory medication that was pulled from the market in 2004 after studies showed an increased risk of heart attacks and strokes among people who took the medicine on a regular basis. The FDA also is responsible for testing the effectiveness of condoms that are sold in the United States. All varieties of latex and polyurethane condoms, dental dams, female condoms, and barrier gloves used in hospitals and doctors' offices are studied and approved. The FDA also is in charge of the nation's blood supply, monitoring the blood banks, inspecting blood and plasma donation centers, and creating rules regarding products used in all the processes involved in blood and blood product donation.

Shilts, Randy. *And the Band Played On.* New York: St. Martin's Press, 1987.
United States Food and Drug Administration. "HIV and AIDS Activities." FDA.gov. Available online. URL: http://www.fda.gov/ForConsumers/ByAudience/ForPatientAdvocates/HIVandAIDSActivities/default.htm. Accessed July 24, 2011.

fosamprenavir   Fosamprenavir, one of the PRO-TEASE INHIBITORS (PIs), was approved by the U.S. FOOD AND DRUG ADMINISTRATION (FDA) in 2003. It is a prodrug of the PI AMPRENAVIR. A prodrug is an inactive drug that is changed by the body into an active drug that is useful for a particular treatment. Fosamprenavir is easier to use and less difficult to take than its predecessor amprenavir. It is available in both a liquid and a pill formulation and can be used by both adults and children older than two. Fosamprenavir is prescribed for use in conjunction with at least two other antiretrovirals in the treatment of HIV.

The drug is sold under the name Lexiva in the United States and under the name Telzir in other countries. The common abbreviation for the drug is FPV. It is manufactured by GlaxoSmithKline.

Dosage

Fosamprenavir is made in 700 mg tablets. The standard dose is 1,400 mg as either one 700 mg tablet twice a day or two tablets once a day. It is often prescribed in combination with ritonavir. This involves taking one 100 mg capsule of ritonavir with the 700 mg fosamprenavir schedule of twice-daily dosage or two 100 mg capsules with the 1,400 mg once-daily dosing. Dosage of the liquid formulation is generally only for CHILDREN and is based on their weight. As with the pill form, the liquid formulation can be taken either in conjunction with liquid ritonavir or without ritonavir. It is not recommended for children less than two years of age. Fosamprenavir can be taken with or without food.

Drug Interactions

Fosamprenavir is boosted when taking ritonavir and is often prescribed together with it. It may be taken with or without food but should not be taken with high-fat meals, which can reduce the absorption of the drug. Many other PIs interact with fosamprenavir, and the dosage of fosamprenavir or other PIs may be adjusted if prescribed at the same time as part of a multidrug HIGHLY ACTIVE ANTIRETROVIRAL THERAPY (HAART) regimen against HIV.

Herbal supplements should be discussed with a doctor. St. John's wort is known to cause a decrease in the bioavailability of PIs in the body. Other supplements that may cause decreased bioavailability of fosamprenavir include milk thistle and garlic supplements, which have been less studied than St. John's wort. Increased levels of fluticasone, an inhaled steroidal allergy or asthma treatment, may occur while taking fosamprenavir. Patients should be monitored for any changes due to this interaction.

Methadone levels in the body decrease substantially while taking fosamprenavir. People who are taking methadone for the treatment of opiate addiction should have dosages adjusted and monitored by a doctor.

Fosamprenavir interacts with a number of other medications, including the cholesterol-lowering drugs simvastatin and lovastatin, antibiotics used to treat infections such as TUBERCULOSIS, antidepressant or antipsychotic medications, and calcium channel blockers used in the treatment of heart ailments. It is important that a doctor know and understand all the medications and supplements a patient is taking when prescribing fosamprenavir.

Fosamprenavir also increases the amount of the drugs sildenafil (Viagra), vardenafil (Levitra), and tadalafil (Cialis)—all erectile dysfunction medications—in the blood and can therefore cause serious side effects. Lowering the dosage of these medications is recommended to prevent potential complications. The effectiveness of birth control pills may be decreased during fosamprenavir use. Heterosexual couples may want to consider the use of condoms or other barrier methods to prevent pregnancy if one or both partners are taking this medication.

Side Effects

Protease inhibitors, as a class of drug, often increase the cholesterol and triglyceride levels of patients, as does fosamprenavir. High lipid levels have been recorded in many patients. This side effect can be managed with appropriate cholesterol-lowering medications. It has also been associated with regimens that can cause LIPODYSTROPHY, or the redistribution of fat within the body. Symptoms are increased fat around the neck area, facial wasting, breast enlargement, and peripheral wasting. Some of these changes disappear when the drug is stopped. In late 2009, the FDA added a warning to fosamprenavir prescriptions notifying patients and doctors regarding the association of the drug with increased cholesterol and triglyceride levels and an increased risk of heart attacks among patients taking the antiretroviral.

Other side effects include diarrhea, nausea, malaise (discomfort or fatigue), and headache. About 20 percent of people who take fosamprenavir develop a skin rash initially. This can generally be managed, as it is mild or moderate in nature. There have been some severe skin reactions or allergies to the drug, which should be monitored by a doctor.

Fosamprenavir is a sulfa drug. People who have allergies to any sulfa drug should not take fosamprenavir.

AIDS InfoNet. "Fosamprenavir (Telzir, Lexiva)." AIDS InfoNet.org. Available online. URL: http://www.aidsinfonet.org/fact_sheets/view/448. Accessed March 11, 2011.

AIDSmeds. "Lexiva (Fosamprenavir)." AIDSmeds.com. Available online. URL: http://www.aidsmeds.com/archive/Lexiva_1560.shtml. Accessed March 11, 2011.

————. "Special Issues for Children with HIV." AIDSmeds.com. Available online. URL: http://www.aidsmeds.com/articles/Children_7566.shtml. Accessed March 11, 2011.

The Body. "Lexiva (Fosamprenavir, Telzir)." TheBody.com. Available online. URL: http://www.thebody.com/index/treat/908.html. Accessed March 11, 2011.

United States Department of Health and Human Services. "Fosamprenavir." Available online. URL: http://www.aidsinfo.nih.gov/DrugsNew/DrugDetailNT.aspx?int_id=337. Accessed March 16, 2011.

Global Fund to Fight AIDS, Tuberculosis, and Malaria (Global Fund)   The Global Fund is a partnership of governments around the world, private organizations, and citizens. It works with existing international and national organizations, nongovernmental organizations (NGOs), and local communities to provide additional funding to help combat the HIV epidemic. Unlike the Joint United Nations Programme on HIV/AIDS (UNAIDS), the Global Fund does not provide personnel for programs but simply funds existing or new programs.

The Global Fund was created in 2002 by the Group of Eight (G8), a forum of the leaders of eight Northern Hemisphere countries that control a large share of the world's economy. Members are Canada, France, Germany, Italy, Japan, Russia, the United Kingdom, and the United States. The group was strongly encouraged by the then–United Nations (UN) chief Kofi Annan to add funding to the fight against the HIV epidemic, as well as other world health problems. The funding model was devised by the Harvard academics Amir Attaran and Jeffrey Sachs in an article they wrote for the journal *Lancet*.

One of the strong arguments that the Attaran/Sachs article made for such a fund was that the countries and areas most affected should draw up their own design for programs that they felt they needed, as opposed to the model then used and often still used by the President's Emergency Plan for AIDS Relief (PEPFAR) and UNAIDS, which draws up programs and implements them for a country or region, often based on what the political leaders of the funders want. The Global Fund uses a panel of experts to select the best proposals according to criteria preselected to evaluate the proposals.

The Global Fund has been very successful in receiving donations and pledges for its work. The Bill and Melinda Gates Foundation has given more than $500 million to the fund. The pop singer Bono created a charity that gives proceeds to the foundation, thereby involving private citizens in the Global Fund effort. The United States has been the largest country donor to the Global Fund, but it still reserves most of its HIV funding for the PEPFAR program, which allows the U.S. government to control the way the money is allocated and spent. In addition to HIV, the Global Fund works on programs that target TUBERCULOSIS and MALARIA, three of the deadliest diseases in terms of deaths caused around the world. All three diseases saw broad medical advances for control and treatment in the late 1990s, which were part of the push behind the creation of the Global Fund.

The Global Fund is headquartered in Geneva, Switzerland. The current head of the fund is Michel Kazatchkine, who assumed that role in April 2007. Dr. Kazatchkine has been an HIV physician and researcher since 1983 in Paris. He was involved with the Global Fund from the beginning, as chair of the Technical Review Committee that reviews the merits of programs and awards grants to applicants. In 2009, the Global Fund began managing its own administrative tasks, which had been handled until then by the WORLD HEALTH ORGANIZATION (WHO). So far, the Global Fund has committed more than $15.6 billion to more than 570 programs in 140 countries. It is responsible for 75 percent of all funding to fight malaria, two-thirds of funding spent on tuberculosis prevention and treatment, and 25 percent of funding spent on HIV prevention and treatment. The Global Fund has given away 88 million bed nets to prevent malaria and 74 million malaria drug treatments. An estimated 5 million more people were treated for tuberculosis than would have been treated had the Global Fund not provided money. With Global Fund resources, an additional 2.3 million people are receiving HIV antiretrovirals who would have received no treatment otherwise. Where PEPFAR supports antiretroviral treatment in 15 countries, the Global Fund supports people in many more countries, including a majority of the countries in ASIA, where PEPFAR treats only people in Vietnam.

In early 2011, news reports by the Associated Press (AP) about fraud in the Global Fund caused some countries—in particular, Germany, the third-largest donor country—to announce shortly thereafter that they were suspending their donations to the fund until investigations into the alleged fund misuse were completed. Further investigation by other news and science organizations clarified that the fraud the AP referred to was already listed on the Global Fund's own Web site, and that the Global Fund had suspended grants to Mali, Mauritania, and Cameroon and had arranged for funds to Zambia to be handled by the UN rather than Zambian officials. The funds in question represented 0.3 percent of the total US$13 billion the Global Fund has given out since its creation. Although most articles that appeared on the story were measured and applauded the Global Fund for its transparency in announcing the frauds and working to stop misuse of the money, politicians in some countries have used the AP story to drum up support for cancelling aid to the Global Fund in a time of budget cutting. In March 2011, the Global Fund announced that it had appointed an independent review and audit panel to assure that funds are spent correctly. The panel will be headed by Michael Leavitt, former secretary of the U.S. Health and Human Services, and former president of Botswana Festus Mogae.

Agence France-Presse. "Africa Has 'Extraordinary Success' in AIDS Fight: Global Fund." Google. com. (23 July 2009). Available online. URL: http://www.google.com/hostednews/afp/article/ALeqM5ha3sXJjfWDahvBiNHgdDp_c-VSsA. Accessed March 16, 2011.

AllAfrica.com. "Africa: Global Fund Gets Tough on Corruption." AllAfrica.com. Available online. URL: http://allafrica.com/stories/201103160964.html. Accessed March 25, 2011.

Attaran, Amir, and Jeffrey Sachs. "Defining and Refining International Donor Support for Combating the AIDS Pandemic." *Lancet* 357 (6 January 2001): 57–61.

Cohen, Jon. "Media Rehash of Corruption Plagues Global Fund." Sciencemag.com. Available online. URL: http://news.sciencemag.org/scienceinsider/2011/01/media-rehash-of-corruption-plagues.html. Accessed March 25, 2011.

Gerson, Michael. "Putting Fraud in Global Health Spending in Context." *Washington Post*. Available online. URL: http://www.washingtonpost.com/wp-dyn/content/article/2011/02/03/AR2011020305176.html. Accessed March 16, 2011.

Global Fund. "The Global Fund to Fight AIDS, Tuberculosis and Malaria." GlobalFund.org. Available online. URL: http://www.theglobalfund.org/en/. Accessed March 16, 2011.

TreatASIA. "An Interview with Dr. Michel Kazatchkine—AIDS in Asia: The View from the Global Fund." AMFAR.org. Available online. URL: http://www.amfar.org/world/treatasia/article.aspx?id=7535. Accessed March 16, 2011.

University of Toronto. "G8 Information Centre." Utoronto.ca. Available online. URL: http://www.g8.utoronto.ca/. Accessed March 16, 2011.

H

hemophilia and HIV Hemophilia is a hereditary bleeding disorder caused by a deficiency or lack of one or more of several proteins involved in the process of blood coagulation. Because a person lacks or has a deficiency of a particular protein, the blood fails to clot and bleeding or hemorrhage can occur. Hemophilia is inherited from the X chromosome of one or both parents and predominantly occurs in men. It is extremely rare in WOMEN. There are different types of hemophilia, caused by a deficiency in a particular protein, or clotting factor. There are 20 factors that are required to allow blood to clot properly. The most common deficiency is in factor VIII; it is called hemophilia A, or classic hemophilia. It occurs in approximately one in every 5,000 births. Hemophilia B is caused by a deficiency in factor IX and occurs in approximately one in every 25,000 births.

Deficiencies in eight other numbered factors are extremely rare but are recorded in medical literature. They can occur in both men and women equally, unlike hemophilia A or B. In addition, von Willebrand disease is an inherited disorder found in 1 to 2 percent of the world's population that is caused by a deficiency in the von Willebrand factor, a protein essential to the initial stage of clotting. It is named after a Finnish doctor who discovered the factor while researching bleeding disorders. There are several types of von Willebrand disease, the differences based on the severity of the bleeding. Symptoms of hemophilia include bleeding excessively and bruising easily. External bleeding can occur easily with minor cuts, inside the mouth from biting, nosebleeds, or cuts that cannot stop bleeding even after pressure has been placed on the cut.

Internal bleeding can occur in joints or muscles as well as in the brain and be the result of minor bumps or falls. CHILDREN who have moderate to severe hemophilia often are bruised and bleed while learning to walk. Internal bleeding can occur at times from no known injury.

It was not until the 1930s that doctors found that plasma could be used to treat hemophilia patients. Whole blood transfusions or plasma were then used until the mid-1960s as the main treatment. In the mid-1960s, the clotting factors were identified and eventually isolated from plasma, thereby allowing the particular factor needed for the two main types of hemophilia to be given to patients to increase the amount of the deficient factor, allowing them to control their own clotting. Prior to this point, people who had hemophilia often died by the time they had reached their early 30s as a result of severe bleeding. By the 1970s, people were able to treat themselves at home with freeze-dried clotting factor that they could mix with water to inject themselves with as needed. These clotting factors made life longer and easier for hemophiliacs.

The commercial clotting factors that were created in the 1960s were chemically extracted from blood products donated by large numbers of people, numbering in the hundreds or thousands, that were mixed together to obtain enough of the needed factor. This created a situation in which hemophiliacs were exposed to the blood of thousands of different people each time they used a new batch of clotting factor. This led hemophiliacs to be exposed to a variety of HEPATITIS viruses and eventually, from the late 1970s, to HIV. By the time there was a test for

HIV to screen blood in 1985, more than half of the hemophiliacs in the United States were HIV positive. These sorts of numbers were repeated in many Western countries where clotting factors had become common in the treatment of hemophilia. Hemophiliacs were among the first people to be identified with HIV, and many became sick and died as a result.

In 1985, heat-treated factor concentrates became widely available, and the spread of HIV through clotting factors was reduced. Other viruses, including hepatitis C, continued to be a problem until 1989, when a new purified clotting factor using monoclonal antibodies was approved by the U.S. FOOD AND DRUG ADMINISTRATION (FDA). A second kind of high-purity clotting factor created through recombinant technology was introduced in 1992. These high-purity clotting factors have proven extremely safe in preventing most viruses from being transmitted to hemophiliacs, though hepatitis A, which can be prevented with a vaccine, can still be acquired in this manner. The higher-purity products have also proven to be extremely expensive, often running $100,000 a year for someone who has severe hemophilia.

Since 1985, the risk of being exposed to HIV through clotting factors has been reduced to nil. Another reason for this has been the screening of all donated blood for numerous viruses. Hemophiliacs still make up 1–2 percent of all HIV and AIDS cases in the United States; these people are long-term survivors exposed to HIV sometime between 1978 and 1985.

In 1998, the U.S. Congress recognized that people who had hemophilia had been especially vulnerable to HIV from the blood and blood products supply that was being monitored by government agencies during this time. They passed the Ricky Ray Hemophilia Relief Fund Act, which provided payment to people who had contracted HIV through contaminated blood products. Payments of $100,000 were made to individuals who had hemophilia who received HIV-contaminated clotting factor products between July 1, 1982, and December 31, 1987.

Spouses and children who contracted HIV from these individuals, as well as specified family survivors, were also eligible for payments. The program has made payments totaling in excess of $559 million to more than 7,000 people. The act was named for Ricky Ray, an Arcadia, Florida, hemophiliac child, who received national attention when it became known he had HIV. People in the community, who were afraid of the illness, set the Ray home on fire. Ricky Ray died of HIV complications in 1992 when he was 15.

National Hemophilia Foundation. "Guardian of the Nation's Blood Supply." hemophilia.org. Available online. URL: http://www.hemophilia.org/NHFWeb/MainPgs/MainNHF.aspx?menuid=3&contentid=37&rptname=bloodsafety. Accessed March 16, 2011.
———. "History of Bleeding Disorders." hemophilia.org. Available online. URL: http://www.hemophilia.org/NHFWeb/MainPgs/MainNHF.aspx?menuid=178&contentid=6&rptname=bleeding. Accessed March 16, 2011.
———. "Ricky Ray Program Office Set to Close." hemophilia.org. Available online. URL: http://www.hemophilia.org/NHFWeb/MainPgs/MainNHF.aspx?menuid=117&contentid=360. Accessed March 16, 2011.
———. "Welcome to the National Hemophilia Foundation." hemophilia.org. Available online. URL: http://www.hemophilia.org/NHFWeb/MainPgs/MainNHF.aspx?menuid=0&contentid=1. Accessed March 16, 2011.
United States Department of Health and Human Services, National Heart, Lung, and Blood Institute. "Hemophilia Signs and Symptoms, Bleeding, Bruising." NIH.gov. Available online. URL: http://www.nhlbi.nih.gov/health/dci/Diseases/hemophilia/hemophilia_signs.html. Accessed March 16, 2011.
———. "What Is Hemophilia, Hemophilia A, and Hemophilia B?" NIH.gov. Available online. URL: http://www.nhlbi.nih.gov/health/dci/Diseases/hemophilia/hemophilia_what.html. Accessed March 16, 2011.

hepatitis B   The term *hepatitis* means "inflammation of the liver." It has a number of causes, including viruses, medications, chemicals, alcohol, and bacteria. Hepatitis caused by a virus is sometimes called viral hepatitis. Hepatitis B (HBV) is the name for a particular virus that causes inflammation of the liver. It is one of several viruses commonly known as hepatitis. They are labeled by letters A through G to differentiate their specific actions and relations to each other. Although all are named for the symptoms of inflammation and irritation to the liver, the hepatitis viruses are not all related to each other, nor do they act in the same manner on the liver or body.

Hepatitis can cause scarring of the liver, including conditions referred to as fibrosis and cirrhosis. When this occurs, the liver cannot function properly as the filter for the body. The liver breaks down all types of chemicals in the body, either making them useful to the body or allowing them to be excreted out of the body. The liver processes fat in food, regulates the clotting of the blood, processes nutrients from food, and breaks down alcohol and other chemicals, including most medications. The liver also filters the blood, clearing chemicals, alcohol, and bacteria from the body. Fibrosis and cirrhosis interfere with the liver's ability to function and cause chemicals and nutrients to build up in the body.

Hepatitis B is spread the same ways that HIV is spread, through bodily fluids, particularly blood. Hepatitis B is much easier to spread than HIV and can live outside the body for up to a week. Shared use of needles, unprotected sexual intercourse, contact with an infected person's blood, and living with a person who has chronic HBV are the most common ways that it is spread. HBV is found around the world and is particularly common in AFRICA and parts of ASIA. In developed countries, it is less common than it used to be because of the availability of a vaccine and protection of the donated blood supply. In the United States, there were 46,000 new cases of hepatitis B in 2006, down from approximately 200,000 new cases a year diagnosed during the 1980s.

Symptoms and Diagnostic Path

There are two types of hepatitis symptoms: acute, meaning short-term hepatitis that can last from two weeks to six months, and chronic, which last a much longer, often for the remainder of a person's life. Both acute and chronic hepatitis can be very severe, and the terms are used to differentiate the actions of the illness rather than the type of virus.

The majority of people who become infected with hepatitis B will not show any symptoms upon infection and will only be diagnosed through blood tests. Some people will, however, develop acute hepatitis B symptoms. These can include jaundice, the yellowing of the skin and whites of the eyes; tiredness; stomach pain; nausea; vomiting; and aching joints and muscles. Acute symptoms can last for a few weeks and can cause severe health problems, including liver failure in some cases. Hepatitis B reproduces quite readily in the body, and the immune system often takes several weeks to begin mounting a response to the virus. Once the HUMAN IMMUNE SYSTEM begins mounting a response to the virus, it is generally cleared from the body, and someone who has cleared the active virus will develop antibodies and become immune to reinfection from hepatitis B.

Some people who become infected with hepatitis B have chronic hepatitis, meaning that inflammation will be long-lasting. Their immune system has not been able to clear the virus and they will have active virus in their body for an extended time. Studies show that 90 percent of babies who become infected from their mother during birth will have chronic hepatitis B throughout their lifetime. Chronic infection also means a person is capable of spreading the virus to others. In the United States, estimates are that 800,000 to 1.4 million people suffer from chronic hepatitis B. Globally, 350 million people are believed to have chronic hepatitis B. Anywhere from 15 to 25 percent of people who have chronic hepatitis B will develop severe liver problems at some point in their future.

Diagnosis for hepatitis B is through blood testing. Several tests are done to determine the type and severity of hepatitis B infection. The hepatitis B surface antigen (HBsAg) test measures a protein that is part of the HBV. A positive test result indicates the person is infectious and can spread the virus to others. The body produces antibodies to the protein as part of the immune system protecting the body. These antibodies are used to produce the vaccine against the HBV. A negative result means the person does not currently have active HBV. Most people will clear the HBsAg from their blood within 15 weeks of clearing the viral infection.

The hepatitis B surface antibody test (anti-HBs) is used to determine whether a person is immune to the virus. A positive test result means a person has some immunity that has developed either through clearing the virus during a previous infection or through receiving the immunization sometime in the past. A negative test finding indicates that there is no immunity or that the person has never had hepatitis B.

Total hepatitis B core antibody (anti-HBc) is used to determine whether a person has had a previous infection with hepatitis B. This blood marker appears at the start of a hepatitis B infection and remains with the person for life. This test simply indicates whether a person has ever been infected with hepatitis B, not whether the virus is currently active. A positive test result means a person has been infected at some point with hepatitis. A negative result indicates the person has not been infected before.

The immunoglobulin M antibody to hepatitis B core antigen (IgM anti-HBc) is a test that is used to determine whether a person is currently having an acute hepatitis B infection. A positive result indicates acute infection; a negative result indicates no acute infection.

These four tests are used to determine a person's hepatitis B status and whether the person is currently infectious, a chronic carrier of HBV, or has recovered and developed immunity. Doctors will interpret the results by looking at all of the results from these blood tests together. For instance, a positive HBsAg test result and a positive anti-HBc test result combined with a negative anti-HBs test result and negative IgM anti-HBc test result generally

means a person suffers from chronic hepatitis B. This is an example of the combinations of test results that need to be interpreted to determine hepatitis B infection and its severity and should be discussed with a doctor to receive an expert opinion.

A person who is determined to be in an acute or chronic infection stage will also undergo an HBV deoxyribonucleic acid (DNA) test, which can measure the amount of viral activity in the body. In addition, a hepatitis B e antigen (HBeAg) test and the hepatitis B e antibody (anti-HBe) test can be used to determine continued chronic infection in the body.

Other tests that may be conducted include a liver biopsy. For people who have had a hepatitis B infection or are tested as having chronic hepatitis B, a liver biopsy can determine the amount of damage the virus has done to the liver. A large needle is used to extract a small sample of liver tissue, which is tested for viral activity as well as fibrosis and cirrhosis. The biopsy, when combined with the viral load count of the HBV DNA test, can be used to decide a course of treatment, or whether a person may be in need of a liver transplant if the liver is shown to be severely damaged. Liver biopsies have a risk of complications such as excess bleeding and damage to the peritoneum, the lining of the abdomen, due to bile that escapes from the liver during the biopsy. Bile is the greenish fluid produced by the liver that helps to break down and use fats in the body. These complications, though rare, can cause problems, and monitoring any pain or physical changes in a patient after a liver biopsy is important.

People who are coinfected with HIV and HBV have an increased risk of liver damage because of chronic infection. They also have a higher risk of sustaining a chronic HBV infection than the general population. Because chronic inflammation of the liver can lead to other problems such as liver cancers, HIV-positive people also have a higher risk of liver cancer than a person infected only with HBV. Because both chronic HBV and liver cancer carry few outward signs initially, it is important for HIV-positive people to be tested for HBV as soon as possible after an HIV-positive diagnosis.

Symptoms and diagnosis of a person can be complicated with the addition of hepatitis D. Hepatitis D is a virus that is spread in the same manner as hepatitis B. It is a virus that must be in contact with hepatitis B in order to reproduce properly. Having the two viruses together is a serious concern, as the incidence of cirrhosis and liver cancer greatly increases with the presence of these two hepatitis viruses. There is currently no vaccine or treatment recommended for hepatitis D. Hepatitis D is not seen regularly in developed countries and is predominantly seen in INJECTION DRUG USE(R)S when it occurs. It is more predominant in sub-Saharan Africa, Southeast Asia, the MIDDLE EAST, and Mediterranean regions of the world.

Treatment Options and Outlook

In the past two decades, treatment for hepatitis B has greatly improved. Several medications have been approved for use in the fight against hepatitis B. These medications have been shown to reduce the viral load of HBV in chronic HBV carriers and can encourage the body's immune system to fight the HBV. Moreover, a chronic HBV carrier can seroconvert—that is, develop antibodies in the blood as a result of exposure to a virus or an immunization—to an inactive HBV carrier in some instances. This was once nearly impossible after a person had reached the chronic infection stage for HBV.

Acute hepatitis B is not generally treated. Most physicians recommend rest, plenty of sleep, and lots of fluids. HIV-positive people or people who have a serious acute hepatitis B infection may be started on antiretroviral medication of some variety that can stop the virus from reproducing and, ideally, protect the functioning of the liver.

The first medication approved for the treatment of hepatitis B was interferon alfa. It is given as a series of intramuscular injections over the course of several months. One dosing regimen involves a daily injection. Another involves a slightly larger amount of interferon alfa three times a week. Interferon alfa is a naturally occurring protein that is part of the immune system's own response to a ribonucleic acid (RNA) virus infection. Side effects of interferon alpha treatment are flulike symptoms that include nausea, sore muscles, body aches, fever, and depression. A slightly altered form of interferon alfa, known as pegylated interferon, which is only injected once a week, is also now available. It has the same side effects as interferon alfa. Although these treatments are approved for use in HIV-negative patients, they are not officially approved for use in HIV-positive people. Some physicians may opt to use the pegylated interferon medication anyway, as some studies have shown use by HIV-positive patients to be successful. Approximately 30–40 percent of patients who have the interferon treatments will seroconvert to HBeAG-negative status.

Other medications are varieties of antivirals. Some are the same medications already used to treat HIV, so these medications are more easily adjusted to or may fit in well with the HIGHLY ACTIVE ANTIRETROVIRAL THERAPY (HAART) that a person is already taking. LAMIVUDINE is one of the NUCLEOSIDE REVERSE TRANSCRIPTASE INHIBITORS (NRTIs). It was first approved for the treatment of HIV in 1995 and as a once-daily tablet in 2002. It was approved for the treatment of HBV in 1998. It should always be used in a combination therapy when treating someone who is also HIV positive. Lamivudine (also known as 3TC) is given in 150 mg tablets twice a day for HBV and HIV. HBeAg seroconversions are low in HIV-positive persons taking HAART and lamivudine for HBV, but the drug is good at suppressing the viral activity. The drug will stop working after a period of one to three years as the virus mutates to allow itself to reproduce.

Adefovir dipivoxil, or adefovir, is an NRTI that was approved for HBV treatment in 2002. It slows the viral replication in a similar manner to lamivudine but does not allow the virus to build resistance as easily as it does against lamivudine.

Adefivor does not show good seroconversion rates for people who have chronic HBV and HIV.

Entecavir was approved for HBV treatment in 2005. It is more effective than lamivudine is suppressing the HBV virus quickly, but, as is true with lamivudine, it should not be used as a monotherapy for people who are HIV and HBV positive, as it will confer drug resistance to the HIV virus. Entecavir is effective against lamivudine-resistant HBV. Recent studies conducted in Taiwan and released in the journal *Hepatology* demonstrated that extended use of entacavir reduced fibrosis among chronic hepatitis B patients. This is the first time a drug has been shown to reduce damage already done to the liver by hepatitis.

Telbivudine was approved for use in the United States in 2006. It is well tolerated, but over time, resistance by HBV is common. It is not effective against lamivudine-resistant HBV.

TENOFOVIR DISOPROXIL FUMARATE was approved for use against HBV in the United States in 2008. It has been shown to be more effective over time in suppressing HBV activity than adefovir. Some seroconversion of people on tenofovir has been recorded in studies.

All HBV treatments can be dangerous if stopped suddenly without a doctor's observing the patient for signs of hepatitis reactivation. Approximately 15 percent of people who stop these drugs show signs of a flare-up in their disease when stopping the medications. If treatment is stopped and a flare-up occurs, the recommendation is to resume treatment, as the reactivation of the virus may be life threatening.

An unknown number of chronic HBV carriers will spontaneously clear the viral infection over time. HBV clearance has also been shown to increase under some of the antiviral drugs used for suppression of HBV, though those numbers vary widely in studies and in effectiveness of each drug. Some people for reasons not completely understood will clear the virus after many years of being chronic HBV carriers. Once this occurs, the likelihood of the virus's becoming active again is very low, though this has

been shown to occur, particularly in immune-suppressed people. Once an HIV-positive person person has had HBV, monitoring of liver functioning through blood tests will occur to ensure that the virus remains dormant.

It has become more common for HIV-positive patients to find themselves on ORGAN TRANSPLANTATION lists just as any other person might who is suffering liver failure and is in need of a transplant. The well-known AIDS activist and author Larry Kramer received a liver transplant in 2001, and, more recently, transplants between HIV-positive people have been done in South Africa, further expanding the opportunities for HIV-positive people needing liver transplantation because of HBV. People who are good candidates for liver transplants are generally given the same consideration for placement on waiting lists as HIV-negative people. Regional hospitals in the United States have also become receptive to HIV patients in need of transplants.

Risk Factors and Preventive Measures
Hepatitis B is spread in the same manner in which HIV is spread—injection drug use and unprotected sex. People who are IDUs and those involved in unprotected sexual encounters are at highest risk for acquiring hepatitis B. Preventing exposure is important, so SAFER SEX, especially the use of condoms during sex, is the best method of preventing the virus from entering the body. Condoms and dental dams can prevent the exchange of bodily fluids and reduce the risk of the spread of hepatitis B. As hepatitis B is present at much higher levels in body fluids than HIV, it is actually easier to pass the virus to other people through the same means of transmission. Other risk factors affect health workers who have contact with blood on a regular basis or work with people and needles. IDUs are at risk because they often share needles. Cleaning needles with bleach and water or not reusing needles can prevent exposure to HBV.

People who live with HBV-positive people are not generally at risk if simple rules are followed in the household: Do not share common household items such as toothbrushes, razors, or sharp instruments; do not have contact with a household member's blood or sores; if you are a mother with a small baby, do not prechew your child's food; and do not share chewing gum with a child. HBV is present in greater quantities in the saliva than HIV and may be passed in that manner.

If a person believes he or she has been exposed to HBV, it is recommended that the person receive what is known as a hepatitis B immune globulin treatment. This is an intramuscular injection of a product derived from blood plasma that can help the body begin fighting the HBV before it starts reproducing. When used in conjunction with the HBV vaccination, it can prevent HBV from becoming active in the body in nearly 90 percent of cases studied. It conveys short-term immunity to the virus, while the vaccination can convey long-term immunity.

The vaccine for HBV is a series of three or four shots given over a period of six months. It is standard practice in developed countries to give the HBV vaccine beginning at birth to all children. After the vaccine became available in 1989, many school systems and states required VACCINATIONS of CHILDREN and young adults to try to prevent the spread of the virus any further. Although many people born after 1989 have received the vaccine, many adults and some children may not have received it. It has become standard practice for many professions to require the HBV vaccine of their employees. Health care workers, teachers, and employees of child care facilities are often required to be vaccinated for employment.

The HBV vaccine is effective in 90 percent of HIV-negative people receiving it. If a person is HIV positive, the effectiveness of the vaccine may depend on the health of the immune system. The vaccine has been shown to be less effective in people whose immune system is suppressed. Receiving the vaccine when an immune system has a CD4 T cell count greater than 350 has been shown to increase the chance of the vaccine's working effectively. Studies also tend to indicate that doubling the dosage amount of the vaccine in HIV-positive people increases the likelihood that the vaccine will provide immunity to HBV. It is recommended that if an HIV-positive person has not received the HBV vaccine, he or she should do so, as the combination of the two viruses makes treatment of both more difficult. Revaccination with the HBV vaccine series is recommended if the first series of injections does not take effect in an HIV-positive person. Having the vaccine more than once does not harm a person and may confer immunity to HBV on subsequent attempts. The vaccine does not help a person who has already become positive for HBV or someone who is a chronic carrier of HBV.

Babies born to mothers who are HBV positive will receive both the hepatitis B immune globulin injection as well as the series of HBV vaccinations. This method has been shown to be at least 95 percent effective in preventing the transmission of the virus to the infant.

Centers for Disease Control and Prevention. "Hepatitis B FAQs for the Public." CDC.gov. Available online. URL: http://www.cdc.gov/hepatitis/B/bFAQ.htm. Accessed March 16, 2011.

———. "Interpretation of Hepatitis B Serologic Test Results." CDC.gov. Available online. URL: http://www.cdc.gov/hepatitis/HBV/PDFs/Serologic Chartv8.pdf. Accessed March 20, 2011.

———. "Testing and Public Health Management of Persons with Chronic Hepatitis B Virus Infection." Available online. URL: http://www.cdc.gov/hepatitis/HBV/TestingChronic.htm. Accessed March 16, 2011.

Cutler, Nicole. "Outlook Brightens for Chronic Hepatitis B." Hepatitis-Central.com. Available online. URL: http://www.hepatitis-central.com/mt/archives/2010/09/outlook_brighte.html. Accessed March 25, 2011.

Hepatitis B Foundation. "Approved Drugs for Adults." HepB.org. Available online. URL: http://www.hepb.org/patients/hepatitis_b_treatment.htm. Accessed March 16, 2011.

HIVandHepatitis.com "Hepatitis B News Articles." HIVandHepatitis.com. Available online. URL: http://www.hivandhepatitis.com/hep_b.html. Accessed March 20, 2011.

McKenna, Phil. "Hepatitis B Drug Boosts HIV-Drug Resistance." NewScientist.com. Available online. URL: http://www.newscientist.com/article/dn11277 -hepatitis-b-drug-boosts-hivdrug-resistance.html. Accessed March 20, 2011.

NAM Aidsmap. "Hepatitis B." AIDSmap.com. Available online. URL: http://www.aidsmap.com/ Hepatitis-B/cat/1510/. Accessed March 16, 2011.

RxList. "HyperHep B (Hepatitis B Immune Globulin)." RxList.com. Available online. URL: http://www. rxlist.com/hyperhep-b-drug.htm. Accessed March 20, 2011.

World Health Organization. "Hepatitis." WHO.int. Available online. URL: http://www.who.int/topics/ hepatitis/en/. Accessed March 20, 2011.

hepatitis C   The term *hepatitis* means "inflammation of the liver." It has several potential causes including viruses, medications, chemicals, alcohol, and bacteria. Hepatitis caused by a virus is sometimes called viral hepatitis. Hepatitis C (HCV) is the name of a particular virus that causes inflammation of the liver. It is one of several viruses commonly known as hepatitis, which are labeled by letters *A* through *G*, to differentiate their specific actions and relations to each other. Although all cause symptoms of inflammation and irritation to the liver, the hepatitis viruses are not all related to each other, nor do they act in the same manner on the liver or body. HCV is a member of the *Flaviviridae* family of viruses. Research and drug discovery continue within that virus family, which includes the West Nile virus, yellow fever, and dengue fever.

HCV can cause scarring of the liver, including conditions referred to as fibrosis and cirrhosis. When this occurs, the liver cannot function properly as the filter for the body. The liver breaks down all types of chemicals in the body, either making them useful to the body or allowing them to be excreted out of the body. The liver processes fat in food, regulates the clotting of the blood, processes nutrients from food, and breaks down alcohol and other chemicals, including most medications. Fibrosis and cirrhosis interfere with the liver's ability to function and cause chemicals and nutrients to build up in the body.

HCV is a blood-borne virus, meaning it is carried in the blood and spread through contact with the blood of someone who is infected. It is common among INJECTION DRUG USE(R)S (IDUs), who have the majority of HCV infections in the United States. It is also common among people who have hemophilia and people who received blood transfusions prior to 1992, when testing for the virus in blood supplies became standard in the United States. Approximately 4 million people in the United States have antibodies to the virus, meaning they have been infected at some point in their lives. The WORLD HEALTH ORGANIZATION (WHO) estimates that 130 million people worldwide are chronic HCV carriers. In Egypt alone, the rates of infection in the Nile delta range upward of 60 percent in adult males.

HCV is the leading cause of liver cancer, liver failure, and liver transplantation around the world. In 20 percent of people who are chronic HCV carriers, cirrhosis will develop within 20 years of contracting the virus. HCV viral activity is accelerated in people who are also HIV positive. Other factors that increase the chance of developing cirrhosis include older age at time of infection, male gender, alcohol use, and advanced immune system suppression (fewer than 200 CD4 T cells/µl).

Symptoms and Diagnostic Path

There are two types of hepatitis symptoms: acute, meaning short-term hepatitis, which can last from two weeks to six months, and chronic, which lasts much longer, often for the remainder of a person's life. Both acute and chronic hepatitis can be very serious, and the terms are used to differentiate the actions of the illness rather than the type of virus, which the letters that follow the term *hepatitis* indicate.

Both acute and chronic hepatitis C are symptomatic in only 20 percent of people. Acute symptoms include jaundice (yellowing of the skin or whites of the eyes), darkening of the urine, mild pain in the area of the liver (upper right side of the abdominal area), mild fever, nausea, and vomiting. Blood tests can give an indication of acute hepatitis C through elevated alanine aminotransferase (ALT) and aspartate aminotransferase (AST) levels. ALT and AST are liver enzymes whose levels increase when the liver is stressed. Starting treatment for hepatitis C while the infection is acute can lead to better results, so diagnosing it at an early stage is important.

Chronic hepatitis C is much more often a result of infection with HCV than chronic hepatitis B is of HBV. Approximately 75 percent of people exposed to HCV become chronically infected. Other symptoms can be similar to those of acute HCV but also include symptoms of cirrhosis such as high blood pressure, splenomegaly (swollen spleen), spider angiomata (visible veins radiating out from a central red spot), and accumulation of fluid in the abdomen.

Tests used to diagnose HCV begin with an antibody test to determine whether someone has been exposed to the virus and has developed antibodies to the virus. Although false negative results can occur, they are not common when using sensitive blood tests. If the person has tested positive for antibodies, then other tests will be given to determine the viral load of HCV. The HCV ribonucleic acid (RNA) will help determine what therapy might be effective in treating the virus. In addition, genotyping the HCV has proven to be helpful in determining treatment. There are several different genotypes, or varieties, of HCV, and some are more common in various parts of the world. Genotype 1 accounts for 75 percent of all U.S. HCV infections.

Other blood tests can determine liver functioning, including ALT and AST. Higher levels of these enzymes indicate a higher probability that the disease has progressed. The other way to determine the condition of the liver and how well it is functioning is through a liver biopsy. A large needle is used to extract a small sample of liver tissue, which is tested for viral activity as well as fibrosis and cirrhosis. The biopsy, when combined with the viral load count of the HCV deoxyribonucleic acid (DNA) test, can be used to decide a course of treatment or whether a person may be in need of a liver transplant if the liver is shown to be seriously damaged. Liver biopsies have a risk of complications such as excess bleeding and damage to the peritoneum, the lining of the abdomen, due to bile that escapes from the liver during the biopsy. Bile is the greenish fluid produced by the liver that helps to break down and use fats in the body. These complications, though rare, can cause problems, and monitoring any pain or physical changes in a patient after a liver biopsy is important.

Treatment Options and Outlook

Treatment options have changed recently with the approval of two new drugs in early 2011. Until 2011, the only approved treatment for hepatitis C in the United States was the use of pegylated interferon alfa in combination with oral ribavirin. There are two types of pegylated interferon, alfa 2a and alfa 2b. They work similarly but are produced by different pharmaceutical companies. Ribavirin is an antiviral drug that is used to treat several different viral infections.

Interferon is given as a series of intramuscular injections over the course of several months. Pegylated interferon is given in a once-weekly injection. Interferon alfa is a naturally occurring protein that is part of the immune system's own response to an RNA virus infection. Side effects of interferon alfa treatment are flulike symptoms that include nausea, sore muscles, body aches, fever, and depression. Pegylated interferon cannot be used by pregnant WOMEN or women who do not use birth control because the medicine has been shown to induce abortions in laboratory tests. Other people who may not benefit from interferon include those individuals who suffer from depression.

Treatment with interferon is intended to clear the active virus from the person's body. Success rates in studies vary from 40–80 percent in HIV-negative people to 15–75 percent in HIV-positive people, depending on the genotype of the HCV involved. The treatment with interferon lasts almost a year; a second year of treatment may be needed if the virus does not clear the person's system after initial treatment.

ORGAN TRANSPLANTATION may be the only course of treatment available for those who have liver failure. This will not clear the body of HCV but may allow the person to receive further treatment for the virus with a fully functioning liver. Recently, transplants involving liver donations from healthy HCV-positive people have had some success, and an increase in their availability may help extend the lives of HCV patients.

With the approval of two new PROTEASE INHIBITORS in 2011 by the U.S. FOOD AND DRUG ADMINISTRATION, treatment for hepatitis C has vastly improved. Telaprevir (trade name Incivek) from Vertex Pharmaceuticals and boceprevir (trade name Victrelis) from Merck have shown improved cure rates when used in conjunction with pegylated interferon and ribavirin. Both drugs improve cure rates of hepatitis C to over 70 percent of cases. Telaprevir has shown slightly higher cure rates and has an easier dosing schedule. Both drugs are in pill formulations and are used in combination with, not in place of, the pegylated interferon and ribavirin. Although there are risks of side effects to the new treatments, including anemia, both new drugs will greatly improve the possibility of maintaining healthy liver function and longer lives in those affected with hepatitis C.

Risk Factors and Preventive Measures

HCV is spread predominantly through blood-to-blood contact. IDUs are at high risk. Other risk groups include health care workers who are in danger of needlesticks, hemophiliacs, and people who received blood transfusions prior to 1992. In areas outside developed countries, blood supplies are still not monitored closely, and people who receive transfusions in those areas of the world may be in danger of contracting hepatitis C. Hepatitis is not generally spread through sexual contact, though it has occurred in cases in which blood is exposed through sexual activities. Heterosexual sex is generally not a means of spread, though sex that causes tissue injury of some type increases the probability of virus spread. Anal sex increases the opportunity for HCV spread but is again not the primary route of infection. MEN WHO HAVE SEX WITH MEN (MSM) are not generally at high risk for spreading HCV through sexual activity. Other methods of potential spread include piercing and tattoo parlors that do not use hygienic means of sterilizing their equipment between customers.

Pregnant mothers do not often spread the HCV to their newborns through BREAST-FEEDING or through blood from the birth canal. The risk for the spread of HCV to newborns increases when the mother is also HIV positive. The rate of vertical TRANSMISSION (from the mother to the child) is in the range of 3–5 percent annually.

The best means of preventing transmission for all people is through not using injection drugs and, among those who do use injection drugs, not sharing injection drug needles.

There is no current vaccination for hepatitis C. Some positive vaccination study findings raised hope of developing an active vaccine in the near-future; studies continue at this time. One roadblock has been the highly changeable nature of HCV and its ability to evade control through mutation.

AIDS Treatment Data Network. "Viral Hepatitis Treatments and Resources." ATDN.org. Available online. URL: http://www.atdn.org/hepatitis.html. Accessed March 20, 2011.

Centers for Disease Control and Prevention. "Hepatitis C FAQs for the Public." CDC.gov. Available online. URL: http://www.cdc.gov/hepatitis/C/cFAQ.htm. Accessed March 20, 2011.

eMedicineHealth. "Hepatitis C." eMedicineHealth.com. Available online. URL: http://www.emedicinehealth.com/hepatitis_c/article_em.htm. Accessed March 20, 2011.

Gryta, Thomas. "Hepatitis C Drug Approved." Online. wsj.com. Available online. URL: http://online.wsj.com/article/SB10001424052702304520804576341360310326064.html. Accessed July 24, 2011.

HIVandHepatitis.com. "FDA Committee Sets Review Dates for HCV Drugs Boceprevir and Telaprevir." HIVandHepatitis.com. Available online. URL: http://www.hivandhepatitis.com/hep_c/news/2011/0318_2011_a.html. Accessed March 20, 2011.

———. "HCV Protease Inhibitor Boceprevir Accepted for Priority Review in U.S. and Europe." Hivand Hepatitis.com. Available online. URL: http://www.hivandhepatitis.com/hep_c/news/2011/0114_2010_a.html. Accessed March 25, 2011.

KGO-TV San Francisco. "Hepatitis C Vaccine Looks Promising." ABClocal.go.com. Available online. URL: http://abclocal.go.com/kgo/story?section=news/health&id=4278043. Accessed March 20, 2011.

Mayo Clinic Staff. "Hepatitis C." MayoClinic.com. Available online. URL: http://www.mayoclinic.com/health/hepatitis-c/DS00097. Accessed March 20, 2011.

National Institute of Allergy and Infectious Diseases. "Hepatitis C." NIAID.NIH.gov. Available online. URL: http://www.niaid.nih.gov/topics/hepatitis/hepatitisc/Pages/Default.aspx. Accessed March 20, 2011.

Pollack, Andrew. "Hepatitis C Drug Raises Cure Rate in Late Trial." *New York Times.* Available online. URL: http://www.nytimes.com/2010/05/26/health/research/26drug.html. Accessed March 20, 2011.

Vertex. "Telaprevir Clinical Development Plan." vrtx.com. Available online. URL: http://www.vrtx.com/current-projects/drug-candidates/telaprevir-VX-950.html. Accessed March 25, 2011.

World Health Organization. "Initiative for Vaccine Research: Viral Cancers." WHO.int. Available online. URL: http://www.who.int/vaccine_research/diseases/viral_cancers/en/index2.html#vaccine%20development. Accessed March 20, 2011.

herpes simplex virus Herpes simplex virus (HSV) is a group of viruses that cause painful ulcers and skin eruptions. Herpes simplex virus-1 (HSV-1) is the virus that generally causes what are known as cold sores or fever blisters in and around the mouth. It has in the past been called oral herpes, or "good" herpes. In reality, the virus simply settles into the trigeminal ganglion, a grouping of nerves found around the ears, where it enters remission or latency between outbreaks. Herpes simplex virus-2 (HSV-2) is the virus that causes what has generally been called "bad" herpes, or genital herpes. This virus has been shown to prefer to settle and remain latent in the sacral ganglion, a grouping of nerves found near the base of the spine, and cause eruptions and sores in and around that area of the body. Both HSV-1 and HSV-2 can occasionally be found in the opposite regions of the body, HSV-2 around the face and HSV-1 in the genital area.

HSV-1 is found in approximately two-thirds of Americans. It is most often acquired as a child or teenager and is generally passed from one person to another through kissing or close contact with the sore of a person infected with HSV-1. HSV-2 is found in 22 percent of Americans. It too is passed from one person to another when he or she has contact with the sore. Because this form of herpes is generally found in the genital region, it is not generally acquired until a person begins having sex in the late teens or adulthood. Having HSV-1 is strongly correlated to HSV-2's being asymptomatic in people who have both types of the virus. This means that if someone has HSV-1 at some point in one's life and then becomes infected with HSV-2 later on, he or she is more likely not to show visible signs of the infection, though it is still in the body and can be passed on to other people. Having HSV-1 orally is believed to protect a person from contracting HSV-1 genitally.

Symptoms and Diagnostic Path

The most common sign of herpes is a watery sore or eruption around the face or genital region. The blister appears on or near the mucous membranes in the regions HSV affects. The lesions in either area will generally last seven to 10 days and can recur several times a year. Lesions occur most frequently shortly after infection and decrease in intensity and occurrence through the years a person has the virus. These sores are often painful or itchy. Many people can be infected with either variety of HSV and never have any symptoms.

HSV can also cause infection in other areas of the body but generally only on rare occasions;

these conditions include HSV keratitis (red eye, with swollen painful lesion of the cornea), HSV hepatitis, HSV encephalitis, and a condition known as herpetic whitlow, in which the finger or thumb of an individual becomes the site of a herpes infection. This latter condition is most often identified in children, who spread herpes infections from their mouth to the thumb or fingers through sucking them, or in adults who work closely with the mouth such as dentists, dental hygienists, or even respiratory therapists. Use of proper protective medical equipment such as latex gloves can prevent most cases of this type of herpes.

In HIV-positive people, HSV can cause more frequent and more disruptive breakouts of sores or lesions that last for a longer period than is normally seen in herpes outbreaks. This effect can occur in other immune-compromised people, too, such as burn victims or transplant recipients. Also, HIV is affected by HSV in that HIV reproduces more rapidly in patients during HSV outbreaks. Another effect of HSV outbreaks in HIV-positive people is that the virus is much more easily spread to others with the open sores that HSV causes. Contact with herpes sores readily transmits both HSV and HIV in these cases. HSV infection is more prevalent among people who have multiple sexual partners.

BLOOD WORK/BLOOD TESTS that can identify HSV antigen, as well as viral load of the HSV, will be done on most HIV-positive patients. The type of HSV will also be determined at that point so that the patient and the physician know what variety of herpes virus the person has contracted. Most HIV-positive individuals have some type of HSV infection.

Treatment Options and Outlook

Treatment can be done on a daily basis or at the time of an outbreak of the virus. Control of the virus can be important in that HIV does become more active at times of HSV activity. Treatment of facial sores for an outbreak involves taking oral valacyclovir, famciclovir, or acyclovir for a period of a week to 10 days. A longer term of treatment is required for genital sores. In cases of serious sores, either large sores or sores spread over a large area, an initial course of intravenous (IV) acyclovir will probably be prescribed, followed by oral medication until the sores begin to heal.

People who take daily medication to suppress the severity or frequency of outbreaks will be treated with oral medications. Twice-daily regimens of valacyclovir, acyclovir, or famciclovir are the standard choices for this suppressive therapy. Suppressive treatment has been shown to reduce the viral load and number of lesions in a person. It is not known whether the infectiousness of the virus is also reduced by daily therapy. Treatment of recurrences as they happen does not influence the course of the illness nor reduce the number of times the virus will affect an individual.

On occasion, HSV can become resistant to acyclovir. If a person being treated for HSV does not see resolution of the sores after a week to 10 days of treatment, testing of the virus may determine that drug resistance exists. In that case, other medications may be used to treat the infection, such as IV foscarnet. Topical medications such as trifluridine, cidofovir, foscarnet, or imiquimod can also be used to treat the blisters, though this will generally require a longer period than oral or IV medications.

Risk Factors and Preventive Measures

Use of condoms during sex will help prevent the transmission of genital herpes. HIV-positive people who do not have HSV should avoid sexual contact with a partner when that person has clear signs of active herpes. Condoms will also help prevent the transmission if HIV. Other prophylaxis such as a dental dam can also help decrease the spread of oral herpes to the genital region.

Taking acyclovir during pregnancy is considered safe, including during the last trimester to prevent outbreaks and reduce the opportunity to pass the virus to the child, which generally occurs during natural birth. Many physicians still prefer to order a cesarean delivery for an HSV-positive mother, as the virus is shed from the body even during an asymptomatic outbreak.

Baeten, Jared M., M.D., and Connie Celum, M.D. "Herpes Simplex Virus and HIV-1." HIVInSite.ucsf. edu. Available online. URL: http://hivinsite.ucsf. edu/InSite?page=kb-05-03-02. Accessed March 20, 2011.

The Body. "Herpes Simplex (Cold Sores and Genital Herpes)." TheBody.com. Available online. URL: http://www.thebody.com/content/treat/art6052. html. Accessed March 20, 2011.

HerpesOnline. "Defining the Differences in Types of HSV." HerpesOnline.org. Available online. URL: http://www.herpesonline.org/hsv1vs2.html. Accessed March 20, 2011.

NAM aidsmap. "Herpes." AIDSmap.com. Available online. URL: http://www.aidsmap.com/Herpes/ page/1044860/. Accessed March 20, 2011.

Pinninti, Swetha G. "Pediatric Herpes Simplex Virus Infection." eMedicine.medscape.com. Available online. URL: http://emedicine.medscape.com/article/ 964866-overview. Accessed March 20, 2011.

USA Today. "Study Debunks Herpes-HIV link." USA Today. Available online. URL: http://www.usa today.com/news/health/2008-06-19-hiv-herpes_N.htm. Accessed March 20, 2011.

WebMD. "Genital Herpes and HIV." WebMD.com. Available online. URL: http://www.webmd.com/ genital-herpes/guide/risk-hiv. Accessed March 20, 2011.

Xu, Fujie, Julia A. Schillinger, Maya R. Sternberg, Robert E. Johnson, Francis K. Lee, Andre J. Nahmias, and Lauri E. Markowitz. "Seroprevalence and Coinfection with Herpes Simplex Virus Type 1 and Type 2 in the United States, 1988–1994." *Journal of Infectious Diseases* 185 (15 April 2002): 1019–1024.

highly active antiretroviral therapy (HAART)

Antiretroviral medications (ARVs) are used in the treatment of retrovirus infections. HUMAN IMMUNODEFICIENCY VIRUS (HIV) is a retrovirus, and when three or four ARVs are prescribed for the treatment of HIV infection, the combination of the drugs is generally called HAART. It is also common to see the phrase *antiretroviral therapy* (ART) used when referring to treatment with these medications. Use of four or more medications at the same time can also be known as mega-HAART.

There are several different types of ARVs that are used to make up a person's HAART. They include NUCLEOSIDE REVERSE TRANSCRIPTASE INHIBITORS (NRTIs), NUCLEOTIDE REVERSE TRANSCRIPTASE INHIBITORS (NtRTIs), NON-NUCLEOSIDE REVERSE TRANSCRIPTASE INHIBITORS (NNRTIs), PROTEASE INHIBITORS (PIs), fusion inhibitors, INTEGRASE INHIBITORS, ENTRY INHIBITORS, and combination drugs. There are also ARVs in development that fit into other categories, which are based on the method through which the retrovirus replication is stopped.

HAART first emerged as the standard of treatment for HIV in 1996. Within a short period, OPPORTUNISTIC INFECTIONS (OIs) had dropped 80 percent in most areas of the country. People who had been very ill suddenly were healthy again. People who were on disability leave for their illness returned to work. HAART is effective because the different types of ARVs work to stop the virus from replicating in different stages of its life cycle. When only one ARV is taken alone, the virus usually can find a way around this drug. The virus continues to disrupt the HUMAN IMMUNE SYSTEM in this situation. When three or more of the ARVs are used together in HAART, the virus has an extremely difficult time avoiding all of the different ways the medications stop the virus from replicating itself.

HAART produces both a reduction in the viral load (the amount of virus in a person's body) and an increase in the person's CD4 T cells. These two measures, determined through regular BLOOD WORK/BLOOD TESTS, help to determine whether a particular combination of ARVs is working well for a person. Other factors that will be used to determine a particular HAART regimen include a person's general health, risk factors for other illnesses, and the number and frequency of pills that must be taken to obtain the effect. HAART medications initially involved large numbers of pills during the day, some taken with food, others taken without food, and some taken two or three times during the day. Today, HAART is often a combination of pills taken only once a day. One ARV used in HAART is a subcutaneous injection drug (ENFUVIRTIDE). This means it is injected under the upper layers of skin, not into a vein or muscle.

It is important for a person who is on a HAART regimen to take the medication as directed. Maintaining the proper amount of the drug in the body is vital to preventing HIV from replicating. Studies have shown that patients who take their medications on time on a regular schedule do much better in the long term than people who miss doses or forget to take their medications on a regular schedule. Small amounts of the virus remain in the body even with optimal dosing of the ARVs and optimal adherence to the HAART schedule. New mathematical models are now being used to demonstrate the best HAART combination within the confines of what drugs a patient can take. New drug research is also developing different classes of ARVs that will increase the variety of HAART options for people with HIV. In addition, new drugs have been developed to draw out virus present in the body so that those virus particles can then be attacked by the HAART drugs.

Food and Drug Administration. "HIV and AIDS—Medicines to Help You." U.S. Department of Health and Human Services. Available online. URL: http://www.fda.gov/ForConsumers/ByAudience/ForWomen/ucm118597.htm. Accessed April 5, 2011.

HHMI News. "You've Gotta Have HAART." Howard Hughes Medical Institute. Available online. URL: http://www.hhmi.org/news/siliciano20080615.html. Accessed April 5, 2011.

Science Daily. "Waking Up Dormant HIV." Science Daily.com. Available online. URL: http://www.sciencedaily.com/releases/2009/03/090316120848.htm. Accessed April 5, 2011.

Wongvipat, Nancy. "HAART Works!" TheBody.com. Available online. URL: http://www.thebody.com/content/art4826.html. Accessed April 5, 2011.

histoplasmosis   *Histoplasma capsulatum* var. *capsulatum* is a fungus primarily found in the temperate regions of the world and is the most common fungus in the United States. It is endemic in the Ohio, Missouri, and Mississippi river valleys, where up to 90 percent of people in some of these regions have been exposed to the fungus. It lives in moist soils, particularly where bird and bat droppings accumulate. Infection is caused when the spore of the fungus is breathed into the lungs from soil and dirt that are disturbed and spores are spread into the air. People in certain professions such as farmers, construction workers, spelunkers, landscapers, and people who live within areas where those activities occur are more likely to be exposed, as the spores can carry for several miles in the wind. *H. capsulatum* var. *capsulatum* is also found occasionally in LATIN AMERICA, the CARIBBEAN, and Europe, though with less frequency than in the United States.

A second variety of the fungus, *H. capsulatum* var. *duboisii,* is seen only in western and central sub-Saharan AFRICA. Although it is less studied than the more common variety, it causes illness in those parts of Africa among immunocompromised people. Histoplasmosis is not as common there as it is in the Americas. This variety has not been studied well, and transmission through the pulmonary route has not been established. It is believed transmission occurs more through the skin and it is thought to be more often disseminated in the body. It is not known whether the fungus is misdiagnosed by local physicians or whether illness from other OPPORTUNISTIC INFECTIONS (OIs) kills before African histoplasmosis develops, or even whether *Histoplasma* var. *duboisii* is more virulent than *Histoplasma* var. *capsulatum.*

After the spores have been inhaled into the lungs, the immune system reacts and carries the fungus, which transforms from spore state to the yeast state in the body, to the lymph system. The macrophages of the immune system surround the fungus and quickly control the infection in people who have a healthy immune system. In HIV-positive people with weak immune systems, the fungus is quickly disseminated throughout the body because of impaired macrophage function. The granulomas that develop as macrophages kill the fungus can remain active for some time after initial infection, even in healthy people. Reactivation of granulomas can occur in HIV-positive people not currently traveling in or residing in areas of endemic infection who have been exposed to the fungus but did not initially develop any illness.

Symptoms and Diagnostic Path

Histoplasmosis is a disseminated infection in the body. Symptoms are general and may appear in different locations. Infection does not generally occur until the person's CD4 T lymphocyte count is below 150 cells/µL, and studies show an average count below 50 T cells/µL in histoplasmosis-infected patients.

General tiredness, fever, weight loss, and respiratory symptoms are most often named as complaints. More specific symptoms include swollen spleen, swollen liver, and generalized swollen lymph glands. Coughing, chest pain, and difficulty breathing can be signs of pulmonary infection. Skin infections also occur in some cases with flat lesions in groupings. Skin complications occur more often in cases from South America than in the United States. Infections in the eye and central nervous system are also possible. Signs of possible eye infection are swelling of the retina and spots in a person's vision. Central nervous system (CNS) infection can also cause meningitis, confusion, and possible seizures. CNS involvement indicates a severe form of histoplasmosis.

African histoplasmosis more often involves skin lesions and osteolytic lesions of the bones in the vertebrae, skull, and ribs. An osteolytic lesion is an area of weak bone, often destroyed or filled with holes by a particular bacteria or fungus.

Diagnosis can be done through urine or blood tests for antigen to *Histoplasma*, but this method is not reliable for testing for a pulmonary infection by the fungus. Biopsies can test for fungus growth, but these tests can take up to several weeks to grow, and treatment cannot be delayed in the case of disseminated infection. A diagnosis based on visible symptoms may be assumed if other causes can be eliminated.

Treatment Options and Outlook

Treatment for disseminated histoplasmosis is a lengthy process. Initially, an intravenous (IV) formula of lipid amphotericin B is given for a period of two weeks. The U.S. federal treatment guidelines recommend 200 mg of itraconazole three times a day for three days, then a year of 200 mg two times a day for 12 months. A lipid preparation of a drug means that the drug's molecules have been mixed with fatty molecules of some variety either to improve the body's ability to use the drug or to lower the toxicity of the drug. Standard amphotericin B can be toxic to the kidneys in some people. Blood tests will determine whether the amphotericin B is working properly and will measure the functioning of the kidneys so that any negative reaction to the medication is detected quickly. Some people will have initial adverse reactions to the amphotericin B and will be treated with other medications.

Other drugs that have been successfully used in patients for whom amphotericin B treatment fails or who cannot tolerate the drug are posaconazole and voriconazole.

For patients with less severe symptoms or histoplasmosis that is not disseminated, oral itraconazole is the treatment of choice in the United States. For patients who have confirmed CNS involvement, liposomal amphotericin B is given for a lengthier initial period followed by a year of oral itraconazole.

Risk Factors and Preventive Measures

As it is extremely difficult to avoid contamination if a person lives in certain areas where the fungus is endemic, he or she can try to avoid certain activities. HIV-positive people who have CD4 T cell counts below 150 cells/µL can avoid high-risk activities such as cleaning chicken coops, exploring caves, working with surface soil, or working on remodeling or cleaning old buildings. These activities can disturb the soil and send the fungus into the air, where it is readily breathed into the lungs.

Recurrence of the illness is possible if it is not eliminated through treatment. HIV-positive people who have disseminated infection should be on maintenance therapy for at least a year or until the CD4 T cell count has returned to greater than 150 cells/μL. Successful treatment with HAART for six months is another measure of whether to end suppressive therapy. The preferred treatment for maintenance is 200 mg of itraconazole daily. Other drugs that have been used successfully include fluconazole, voriconazole, and posaconazole. If CD4 T cell counts fall below 200, this therapy may be restarted as a precaution to prevent reinfection.

Gupta, Amita, M.D., and Karen Wendel, M.D. "HIV Guide: Histoplasmosis." Hopkins-HIVGuide.org. Available online. URL: http://www.hopkins-hivguide.org/diagnosis/opportunistic_infections/fungal/histoplasmosis. html. Accessed March 20, 2011.
Loulergue, Pierre et al. "Literature Reviews and Case Histories of *Histoplasma capsulatum* var. *duboisii* Infections in HIV-Infected Patients." *Emerging Infectious Diseases* 13, no. 11 (November 2007). Available online. URL: http://www.cdc.gov/EID/content/13/11/1647.htm. Accessed March 20, 2011.
Mayo Clinic Staff. "Histoplasmosis." MayoClinic.com. Available online. URL: http://www.mayoclinic.com/health/histoplasmosis/DS00517. Accessed March 20, 2011.
United States National Eye Institute. "Facts about Histoplasmosis." NIH.gov. Available online. URL: http://www.nei.nih.gov/health/histoplasmosis/histoplasmosis.asp. Accessed March 20, 2011.
Young, Erika M., and Mitchell Goldman, M.D. "Histoplasmosis and HIV Infection." HIVInSite.ucsf.edu. Available online. URL: http://hivinsite.ucsf.edu/InSite?page=kb-05-02-06. Accessed March 20, 2011.

HIV encephalopathy   HIV encephalopathy is the general term for the effect of HIV on the brain and nervous system. There are several components of the nervous system that can be affected by HIV. There are also several different terms that may be used by doctors or others in the medical field to describe the various effects HIV has on the brain. These include HIV-related dementia, AIDS-related dementia, HIV-associated progressive encephalopathy (HPE), and AIDS dementia complex (ADC).

It is known that HIV infects the brain early in the course of the disease, particularly during the initial seroconversion, when a person first becomes HIV positive. The word *encephalopathy* means "disease of the brain." This phase of infection is known to researchers as HIV encephalopathy. It is still unclear how exactly HIV reaches the brain, as most blood-borne diseases do not enter the brain. There is a separation of the cerebrospinal fluid, found in the spine and central nervous system, and blood, which circulates throughout a human body. The so-called blood-brain barrier is not an actual blockage, but a system of cells and body structures that keep bacteria and larger molecules out of the cerebrospinal fluid while allowing hormones, oxygen, immune cells, and carbons to pass between the two systems. Recent studies have led scientists to believe that part of the immune system, the monocytes, are the cells that transport HIV to the brain.

Symptoms and Diagnostic Path

Research has shown that HIV-positive people have high levels of lipopolysaccharides, which are generally only found in the lining of the intestine. They are a part of the structure of bacteria that generally can be found in the human intestine. HIV infection can cause a breakdown of the intestinal walls of some people early in the infection, causing these lipopolysaccharides to enter the blood and infect the monocytes that travel to the brain. Monocytes are white blood cells, part of the HUMAN IMMUNE SYSTEM, found in the blood. They are formed in the blood and then move into various body tissues to do their work protecting the body against bacteria and other foreign substances. Monocytes are referred to as undifferentiated white blood cells when in the blood. Once in the tissue, they change into specific white blood cells, such as macrophages or dendritic cells. Some research suggests that the monocytes, when combined with the lipopolysaccharides, seem to make the transition through the blood-brain barrier easy for the virus. These studies suggest that what is commonly termed a leaky gut may influence the way HIV enters the brain. The leaky gut theory has not received complete acceptance as a cause of the virus's crossing the blood-brain barrier but is presently the focus of more study as a potential cause. Another potential cause that has been suggested is that infected monocytes from the bone marrow may be entering the cerebrospinal fluid in some manner, thereby reaching the brain.

CHILDREN who are HIV positive tend to have a higher viral load than adults at initial infection and on a continuing basis if they are not receiving treatment. HPE is the term used to describe brain disease in HIV-positive children. Untreated HIV causes HPE in approximately 50 percent of children, far higher than the rate of HPE seen in adults with the illness. HIV encephalopathy in HIV-positive adults occurs in approximately 30 percent of adults diagnosed with AIDS.

The monocytes, once in the brain, become differentiated, meaning they change into different immune system cells, in particular, macrophages and their equivalent in the brain, microglial cells, which are believed to cause the most damage. It is believed that the cytokines, a type of protein, that are released in infection can alter the neurons of the brain, affecting the way that information is processed in the brain. Damage to neurons may also be caused by proteins in HIV itself, as it is released from dead immune cells or in the reproduction of the virus. Another theory is that particular subtypes of HIV may act differently in the brain and may account for why some HIV-positive people have more problems with brain involvement than other HIV-positive people. Another potential problem is that HIV releases the *tat* gene, which is used in the virus's reproduction. This gene

then circulates in the brain, causing toxicity to nerve cells.

HIV encephalopathy is a progressive illness. It is not one of the OPPORTUNISTIC INFECTIONS (OIs) but a direct result of the virus's acting on the brain. Symptoms can begin slowly and progress throughout the illness. It is seen much more frequently in people who have AIDS or who are untreated with antiretrovirals. Correlations between a high viral load and low CD4 T cell counts and the symptoms of HIV encephalopathy have been drawn in both children and adults. It is far more common in people with extremely weak immune systems than in those who are infected but being treated with antiretrovirals and are maintaining good control of the virus.

It is part of the virus activity that can begin slowly and not be noticeable initially, and may not be diagnosed by a doctor when it first begins to affect a person. Some of the early symptoms include poor concentration, difficulty learning new tasks, reduced productivity at work, lowered libido, forgetfulness, apathy, confusion, depression, and slow withdrawal from friends or family. Both doctors and patients can often interpret these symptoms as other issues. Some of them may initially seem to be side effects of HIGHLY ACTIVE ANTIRETROVIRAL THERAPY (HAART) medications, or the symptoms may be ignored on the assumption that they will end.

As time passes, symptoms will worsen. Walking and coordination will deteriorate, muscles will feel weaker, there may be vision problems, speech can become slurred, and there can be loss of bladder or bowel control. In some severe cases, psychosis can be evident, as well as seizures and sleep disturbances.

A neurologist or psychologist can give a test called a mental status examination. This will measure cognitive abilities and possibly pinpoint problems in a person's mental capabilities. It may be administered at different times to determine changes in a person's status. A mental status examination involves several different questions and tasks. It can involve questions about appearance, mood, anxiety levels, and even delusions.

It will also measure hand-to-eye coordination; memory; orientation to day, time, and place; and problem solving.

Computed axial tomography scans (CAT or CT scans), magnetic resonance imaging (MRI) scans, or single-photon emission computed tomography (SPECT) scans may also be used to detect HIV encephalopathy. CT scans can show signs of atrophy, or shrinking, of brain tissue. It should be noted that this alone does not necessarily correlate with mental impairment in a person. An MRI scan may be used for similar reasons if the CT scan result is inconclusive. MRIs can also detect white matter disease in the brain. White matter is the connective tissue of the brain, connecting neurons in different areas to each other. Some illnesses cause the white matter to atrophy, deteriorate, or interfere with the signals that are sent through these connective neurons that make up the white matter. SPECT scans use a radioactive material to measure blood flow in the brain's arteries. They can determine whether an area of the brain is no longer receiving proper blood flow, and are particularly useful at determining areas of the brain affected by seizures. SPECT scans are generally available only in larger medical centers. These scans can also help to eliminate other potential problems that may be causing neurological problems in an HIV patient such as TOXOPLASMOSIS, cryptococcal infections (see CRYPTOCOCCOSIS), PROGRESSIVE MULTIFOCAL LEUKOENCEPHALOPATHY, or lymphomas (see HIV-RELATED LYMPHOMAS). Diagnosis of HIV encephalopathy can often involve eliminating other possible problems before drawing a definitive conclusion.

A sample of cerebrospinal fluid may also be taken to test for high white blood cell count. Again, this does not necessarily mean a person has HIV encephalopathy, but the cerebrospinal fluid can be tested for other potential infections that may be causing the same symptoms. This fluid is collected by what is called a spinal tap or lumbar puncture. A long needle is inserted into the lower spine and some fluid removed for testing. The area is numbed during this procedure so patients will not feel pain, though a headache may occur afterward.

Treatment Options and Outlook

As knowledge about HIV has increased since the start of the epidemic, so has the understanding of HIV encephalopathy. When HAART first became available for treatment of HIV, remarkable turnarounds in people's HIV encephalopathy symptoms often occurred. The best treatment for HIV encephalopathy has proven to be controlling the HIV. Drops in viral load have been shown to correlate with an improvement in mental functioning in people who have HIV encephalopathy. Some antiretrovirals are better at crossing the blood-brain barrier to reach HIV in the brain. The following antiretrovirals are known to have better access in this area: LAMIVUDINE, STAVUDINE, ZIDOVUDINE, EFAVIRENZ, NEVIRAPINE, and INDINAVIR.

Symptoms such as depression may be treated with a variety of antidepressants. Antipsychotic medications may be used to treat people who have delusional thinking or hallucinations. Doctors may need to adjust the dosage of HAART medications in these cases, as many antidepressant and antipsychotic medications can interfere with the body's ability to take in many antiretrovirals.

Although HAART has proven to help those with HIV encephalopathy when the viral load drops, any return or rise in viral load may lead to the symptoms' returning. If HIV encephalopathy returns during treatment with HAART, a doctor will change medications or add to the regimen to try to bring about a positive change in symptoms. HIV encephalopathy is different from Alzheimer's disease. It affects different parts of the brain. HIV encephalopathy patients generally remain well aware of their day-to-day activities, unlike Alzheimer's disease patients. It is more closely related to the neurological illness seen in Parkinson's disease. Any sudden changes in a person who has HIV encephalopathy that involve deterioration or loss of daily orientation may reflect an OI of some kind, a reaction to medications, or significant liver or kidney problems.

For those people who are unable to take HAART medications or cannot take them as prescribed, the deterioration in brain functioning will be a slow, steady downward spiral in their health. They will become unable to handle day-to-day activities and personal care. Prior to HAART, when HIV encephalopathy was diagnosed, the average time a person lived was six months after diagnosis. A person will eventually be unable to communicate and be bedridden.

Risk Factors and Preventive Measures

People at greatest risk for HIV encephalopathy are those who have untreated HIV who have low CD4 T cell counts and high viral loads. There is no significant difference in race, ethnicity, or gender in those who get HIV encephalopathy in the general HIV population, so no one is more susceptible for those reasons. There is a significant rise in HIV encephalopathy cases with aging.

People who use cocaine and methamphetamine are believed to be at higher risk of HIV encephalopathy because these substances amplify the neurotoxic effects of the *tat* gene that is released by HIV in the brain.

The best preventive measure at this point is to maintain a low viral load count consistently on antiretroviral medications. Also, eating a well-balanced, nutritious diet that maintains, as much as possible, the health of the intestinal tract may be helpful in preventing ADC.

TheBody. "Dementia and HIV/AIDS." TheBody.com. Available online. URL: http://www.thebody.com/index/treat/neuro_dementia.html. Accessed March 20, 2011.

Doctor's Guide. "Leaky Gut Linked to HIV in Brain, Dementia." Pslgroup.com. Available online. URL: http://www.pslgroup.com/dg/229742.htm. Accessed March 20, 2011.

Project Inform. "AIDS Dementia Complex." TheBody.com. Available online. URL: http://www.thebody.com/content/treat/art4986.html. Accessed March 20, 2011.

Singh, Niranjan N., M.D. "HIV-1 Encephalopathy and AIDS Dementia Complex." eMedicine.Medscape.com. Available online. URL: http://emedicine.medscape.com/article/1166894-overview. Accessed March 20, 2011.

Thomas, Florian P., M.D. "Dementia Due to HIV Infection." eMedicineHealth.com. Available online. URL: http://www.emedicinehealth.com/dementia_due_to_hiv_infection/article_em.htm. Accessed March 20, 2011.

University of North Carolina School of Medicine. "AIDS Dementia Complex." UNC.edu. Available online. URL: http://www.med.unc.edu/medicine/web/AIDSDementia.pdf. Accessed March 20, 2011.

HIV-related lymphomas   Lymphomas are cancers of the lymph system. The lymph system is a network of vessels much like veins, which branch throughout the body carrying lymph fluid. This fluid is clear, colorless, and filled with white blood cells called lymphocytes. Along these branches are clusters of small knobs called lymph nodes that store immune system cells ready to fight infection in the body. The lymph system connects to the blood system in the area of the heart. Other organs that are part of the lymph system include the tonsils, spleen, appendix, and thymus. The spleen filters the lymph system. Because the lymph system runs throughout the body, a lymphoma can easily spread to other parts of the body, including the brain. As in all cancers, certain cells begin to reproduce rapidly, causing unnatural growth that can appear as a tumor and spread in tissue, blood, or lymph systems.

There are several varieties of lymphomas, and there are a few that occur in HIV-positive people with greater frequency than others. The main divisions of lymphomas are Hodgkin's lymphoma and non-Hodgkin's lymphomas. This is a visual division done under a microscope. Non-Hodgkin's lymphomas fall into several categories and are labeled most often by the speed of their spread; low-grade spreads slowly, and intermediate-grade and high-grade lymphomas spread much more quickly. Most lymphomas in HIV patients are B-cell lymphomas. The B cells start in the bone marrow and then migrate to the lymph system; the stage of development of the B cell determines the type of lymphoma. If an activated B cell, one that has been readied to fight an illness in the body, is malignant, it is called a diffuse large B-cell lymphoma. Central nervous system (CNS) lymphoma is an example of a large B-cell lymphoma. An immature B cell that becomes lymphoma is called a small noncleaved lymphoma. An example is Burkitt's lymphoma, a disease seen mainly in HIV-positive patients in AFRICA. Primary effusion lymphoma is another lymphoma associated with HIV illness.

Symptoms and Diagnostic Path

General symptoms are similar for most diffuse lymphomas and may not immediately differentiate lymphoma from other illnesses. Lymph nodes will be swollen but not necessarily sore or tender. Fever, tiredness, night sweats, unintentional weight loss, an unexplained feeling of fullness in the abdomen, and itchy skin are other common symptoms. Patients who have some or all of these symptoms for a period of two weeks or longer should consult a physician.

Systemic lymphoma generally occurs in HIV-positive people when their immune system is weakened, as with all OPPORTUNISTIC INFECTIONS (OIs). Median CD4 T cell counts between 100 and 200 have been reported in studies. The gastrointestinal (GI) tract is the predominant site where these lymphomas have been located, the stomach most often but also the large and small intestine, esophagus, and rectum. Other locations such as the bone marrow and the liver can also be affected as the malignant B cells spread rapidly through the lymph system. Tests for diagnosis include a complete blood count (CBC) (see BLOOD WORK/BLOOD TESTS) to determine the numbers of white and red blood cells, which can change from normal counts with lymphoma. A biopsy of the suspected lymph nodes can detect abnormalities. A test for the Epstein-Barr virus (EBV) will be done, as HIV-related lymphomas are predominantly associated with EBV reacti-

vation. EBV, also known as human herpes virus 4, causes mononucleosis, a common childhood illness. Bone marrow testing for lymphoma may be done to determine the spread of the lymphoma.

Primary CNS lymphomas will have different symptoms because the cancer is generally limited strictly to the brain in HIV-positive people. Confusion, headache, tiredness, memory loss, seizures, and paralysis can also occur. Magnetic resonance imaging (MRI) results of a brain scan resemble TOXOPLASMOSIS imaging results, with diffuse lesions throughout the brain in many cases. A thallium SPECT scan may be used, as studies have shown that lymphomas can be detected during such a scan, whereas toxoplasmosis lesions cannot. EBV deoxyribonucleic acid (DNA) assays of spinal fluid are performed to test for viral activity.

Burkitt's lymphoma is a high-grade, fast-spreading cancer of the B cells. There are two forms, the first seen predominantly in Africa in CHILDREN. It causes B cells to reproduce rapidly, often causing large watery tumors of the mouth or nasal area. This type of Burkitt's lymphoma is associated with EBV. The other type, found more often in the United States, often starts in the abdominal area and then spreads rapidly. It is the same type of high-grade small cleaved-cell cancer but is not associated with EBV according to research on the cancer. Burkitt's lymphoma is found in HIV-positive people who have very weakened immune systems.

Treatment Options and Outlook

There are several different forms of treatment for cancer in general and for lymphoma.

Chemotherapy Chemotherapy is a drug therapy for cancer that attempts to stop the growth of cancer cells, either by killing the cells or by stopping them from reproducing. Chemotherapy is generally oral or intravenous. When taken those ways, the medicine enters the bloodstream (or the muscle if given intramuscularly) and can spread through the whole body, fighting the systemic cancer, which may have spread to many locations in the body. In other types of chemotherapy, drugs are placed directly at the site of the main malignancy. Intraperitoneal chemotheraphy targets the intestines and other organs by infusion into the abdomen. Intrathecal chemotherapy can be administered directly into the spinal column, or, in the case of CNS lymphoma, a channel in the skull to reach into the brain directly.

Radiation therapy Radiation therapy is a form of X-ray or other type of radiation that is aimed by a machine toward the cancer. Sometimes it is done externally, using just the radiation machine, and at times a radioactive substance is placed in the body at the site of the cancer to focus the radiation to work more intensely on the cancer, destroy the cells, and prevent them from reproducing.

Chemotherapy with stem cell transplant Prior to beginning therapy, a patient may have the stem cells, which are immature blood cells, removed from the bone marrow and frozen. These cells later will be reintroduced to their body. Stem cells from a donor may also be used. With this type of therapy, a person then receives what is called high-dose chemotherapy that will attempt to kill all bone marrow and immune system cells as well as cancer cells. After the treatment, a person's stem cells or donated stem cells are reintroduced into the body, to allow them to produce new blood cells and restore the immune system.

The type of cancer treatment used will depend on the relative health of a person's immune system as well as the severity of the cancer. Most lymphomas in HIV-positive people occur when the immune system is already seriously weakened and make treatment of the lymphoma difficult. Newer types of treatment are being studied in clinical trials. Lymphoma in HIV-positive patients is difficult to treat and long-term success is not good. Most of the lymphomas seen in HIV-positive patients are high-grade, meaning they spread quickly and extensively. In some cases, particularly CNS lymphomas, there is not much that can be done currently to cure the disease. Life expectancy for a person who has HIV-related lymphomas and a weakened immune system is not long, generally less than six months. HIGHLY ACTIVE ANTIRETROVIRAL THERAPY (HAART) has been instrumental in restoring and maintaining immune system health, and, since the introduction of HAART, the incidence of CNS and Burkitt's HIV-related lymphomas has decreased significantly.

Risk Factors and Preventive Measures
The complete picture of how lymphomas begin in HIV-positive as well as HIV-negative people is not fully understood. It is clear that EBV activity can be detected in some varieties of lymphomas but not all of the different types. As more than 90 percent of the world's population has been exposed to EBV by the time they reach adulthood, it is nearly impossible to avoid exposure. In those lymphomas not associated with EBV, it is not clear how the B cells become proliferative, but research to understand all the potential causes continues.

Cleveland Clinic. "Diseases and Conditions: AIDS-Related Lymphoma." ClevelandClinic.org. Available online. URL: http://my.clevelandclinic.org/disorders/aids_and_hiv/hic_aids-related_lymphoma.aspx. Accessed March 20, 2011.

Lymphoma Information Network. "AIDS Related Lymphoma." LymphomaInfo.net. Available online. URL: http://www.lymphomainfo.net/nhl/types/aidsrelated.html. Accessed March 20, 2011.

Lymphomation.org. "B-Cell-Life-Cycle." Lymphomation.org. Available online. URL: http://www.lymphomation.org/images/b-cell-life-cycle.jpg. Accessed March 20, 2011.

———. "Lymphoma: A Detailed Description." Available online. URL: http://www.lymphomation.org/about-details.htm. Accessed March 20, 2011.

National Cancer Institute. "AIDS-Related Cancers." Cancer.gov. Available online. URL: http://www.cancer.gov/cancertopics/types/AIDS. Accessed March 20, 2011.

Ng, Valerie L., and Michael S. McGrath. "Pathogenesis of HIV-Associated Lymphomas." HIVInSite.ucsf.edu. Available online. URL: http://hivinsite.ucsf.edu/InSite?page=kb-00&doc=kb-06-03-01. Accessed March 20, 2011.

Remedy Health Media. "AIDS-Related Lymphoma Overview." OncologyChannel.com. Available online. URL: http://www.oncologychannel.com/AIDS/cancer/index.shtml. Accessed March 20, 2011.

Singh, Niranjan N. "eMedicine—HIV-1 Associated Opportunistic Neoplasms: CNS Lymphoma." eMedicine. medscape.com. Available online. URL: http://www.emedicine.com/neuro/topic454.htm. Accessed March 20, 2011.

UCSF Medical Center. "AIDS-Related Lymphoma." UCSFHealth.org. Available online. URL: http://www.ucsfhealth.org/conditions/aids-related_lymphoma/index.html. Accessed March 20, 2011.

HIV tests HIV testing is the basis for treatment and education programs around the world. There are a number of ways that people can be tested for HIV today; the most important aspect of testing is that it allows individuals to know whether they are HIV positive in order to seek the proper treatment and to prevent further spread of the virus through knowledge of transmission routes.

When the HIV epidemic started, it was an unknown disease. People were not sure what was causing the illnesses and deaths that had begun to appear in different locations around the world. Once the cause was discovered to be a virus and it was known that the virus was probably passed to people through sexual activity or blood products, then testing was developed to determine whether a person had the virus. In March 1985, the U.S. National Cancer Institute presented the first blood assay that tested for antibodies to the virus. The Pasteur Institute in Paris, France, also was eventually granted royalty rights to the test after suing the U.S. government. In 1983, Luc Montagnier, a French scientist at the Pasteur Institute, discovered a virus he believed caused AIDS, and he published a paper on the virus, which he called lymphadenopathy-associated virus (LAV). Pasteur sent a sample of the virus to the U.S. labs at the National Cancer Institute. In 1984, Robert Gallo, a researcher at the National Cancer Institute, was announced as the individual who had

discovered the "AIDS" virus by the U.S. Department of Health and Human Services secretary, Margaret Heckler. Gallo named his virus find *human T-lymphotropic virus III* (HTLV-III). Gallo applied for a patent, as had Montagnier. For several years, the two labs, as well as the two governments, argued in the press and in courts over who discovered the virus and the ability to test for it. Eventually, both scientists and both countries were given credit and royalty rights to the first test for HIV.

Antibody Tests

This first test that was developed is called the ELISA test, the enzyme-linked immunosorbent assay. This is generally the first test that is given when a person requests an HIV test at a doctor's office, hospital, or clinic. A sample of the person's blood is taken. The ELISA measures whether there are antibodies to HIV in the sample. An antibody is part of the HUMAN IMMUNE SYSTEM's response to a foreign substance, called an antigen. It is the job of antibodies to attack or isolate the antigen, thereby protecting the body. The ELISA involves placing the sample of the blood in contact with HIV antigens and looking through microscopes to determine whether the blood is reacting to the antigen.

The second test, which was developed shortly after the ELISA, for HIV is the Western blot test. This test looks for specific protein bands that are only found in HIV, and is also used to test for protein bands for many other illnesses. Therefore, it can detect whether a person's blood has the proteins, the antibodies, which are a response to the HIV antigen.

All standard HIV blood tests use the ELISA first; then, if the sample tests positive for HIV, the Western blot is used to check the sample again. If both tests yield positive findings for HIV, the person is notified that he or she has tested positive for the virus. The ELISA is considered a very sensitive test, meaning it is sensitive to the virus antibodies, and usually finds HIV antibodies if they are in the sample about 99.5 percent of the time. These are good tests to screen for a disease because they have a high degree of accuracy. The Western blot is considered a specific test. If it determines the antibody proteins for HIV are in a person's blood, then, in most cases, they are.

No matter how sensitive and specific the tests are, there will always be some people who test positive when they are negative or test negative when they are actually positive. The U.S. Centers for Disease Control and Prevention (CDC) state that the two tests in combination, the ELISA and the Western blot, provide an accuracy greater than 99 percent. If a person has a positive test result, the next step is to run the test again, to make sure that a different sample of the person's blood tests the same way. In this way, a person can be sure that he or she is indeed HIV positive.

The other possible result that a person may get from the standard HIV blood test is an indeterminate result. This means that the tests could not determine the results either negatively or positively for some reason. Often, this happens if the blood being tested is drawn during the time when a person is converting from HIV negative to HIV positive. A second blood test is definitely needed in these cases to determine the correct results.

In most people, developing antibodies to HIV requires anywhere from three weeks to three months. In some people, developing antibodies may take up to six months. During this time, the virus is replicating itself, and a person may have large amounts of the virus in the blood, breast milk, or sexual fluids. However, as there are yet no antibodies, the standard HIV antibody tests may not be able to detect the presence of the virus. This is called the window period. Most people who become infected have a window during which these tests will not work. It is also why doctors and testing centers strongly recommend testing again at least three months after the first test, particularly if there is a specific event or incident that causes a person to be tested for HIV. If two HIV tests over the course of six months, after a needle-sharing incident

or unprotected sexual encounter, are negative both times, then in all likelihood a person is HIV negative if he or she has not engaged in any other behavior that would be considered risky.

In recent years, the rapid test has been developed. Most blood tests require a waiting period of a few days to two weeks for results. The rapid test can produce an initial result in a matter of 20–40 minutes, making testing at community events, bars, and other outreach sites much easier. The most common rapid test uses a swab of cotton to collect mucus from the mouth, which is then tested for HIV antibodies. Antibodies for viruses, including HIV, can be found in saliva, but this does not indicate that HIV can be found in saliva. HIV is *not* spread through kissing, sharing utensils, spitting, or sharing drinking glasses. The oral rapid test is very accurate, but anyone who tests positive through an oral swab test will receive a confirmatory test using traditional blood tests. There are also several rapid tests that can use blood from a finger prick to determine whether a person is HIV positive.

Other tests for HIV antibodies that have been approved include a urine test, which allows people to be tested in clinics without having to draw blood. A urine sample can be taken and sent to a lab for antibody tests similar to those for blood samples. The same time frame of a few days to two weeks is needed for results. A U.S. Food and Drug Administration (FDA)–approved home HIV test is also sold in some pharmacies and online. This test allows a person to obtain blood by pricking the finger and placing a few drops on a specially treated card. This card is then mailed to a lab for analysis. A person can receive the results by calling a telephone number and requesting the results identified through a specific number assigned to each card. There is only one FDA-approved home test kit sold in the United States, and it is marketed under the name HomeAccess. Several other online products claim to give HIV test results, but they are not licensed to do so, and some have been prosecuted for their illegal activities.

All tests described in this section test for HIV antibodies, and the same window period exists for these tests, whether blood, oral mucus, or urine samples are used. It can take time to develop antibodies to HIV. Many people are anxious to know whether or not they are HIV positive, particularly if a certain event or activity has placed them at some risk for HIV. However, with these methods it is not possible to know, with absolute certainty until at least six months after an event whether a person has acquired HIV.

Other Tests

A test that is occasionally used in testing for HIV is the p24 antigen test. This blood test looks for the presence of the p24 protein, which is found in HIV. This protein is part of the capsid, or shell, of the virus and becomes visible shortly after infection with HIV. It remains detectable in the blood until antibodies are developed several weeks after infection. The protein disappears after the initial infection because the antibodies adhere to the protein and make it invisible to this test. It is generally only detectable after this initial period, as HIV continues to replicate in the body and the amount of virus in the blood overwhelms the immune system to the extent that there are not enough antibodies to fight the virus. It can still be used inexpensively in this manner to chart progression of the illness.

The p24 test is useful for people who believe they have been recently infected. It can detect infection earlier than an antibody test because it looks for the virus, not the body's response to the virus. It was used extensively early in the epidemic by blood product companies as a way to test for HIV early in the infection cycle. It is still used in resource-poor countries in detecting the virus in blood and blood products and is used as an inexpensive way to measure viral activity, but it is not used often in the United States or Europe any longer since the development of ribonucleic acid (RNA) and deoxyribonucleic acid (DNA) testing.

There are also tests that look for the RNA or DNA of the virus itself. These tests can be expensive and are not used often even in resource-rich countries for widespread HIV testing. They are used, however, in testing blood and blood products in many countries, as they are the most sensitive tests in detecting HIV.

The tests that look for RNA and DNA are called polymerase chain reaction (PCR) tests. The PCR test is also referred to as a nucleic acid amplification test, or NAT. The PCR test looks for the virus by amplifying the genetic code that is specific to HIV and identifying it in a sample of blood. Other tissue samples can be used if there is virus in the sample, such as semen. The PCR DNA test is most generally used as an initial test when screening newborn babies for HIV. Babies receive their initial immune system from their mother and will carry their mother's antibodies to HIV if the mother is HIV positive. These antibodies will remain in the baby for at least six months, often longer, so using the HIV antibody tests will only tell a doctor what is already known. The DNA PCR will allow the doctor to see whether there is virus in the newborn's immune system.

The RNA PCR test is the one run most usually by blood and blood product companies to test for HIV. This is the quickest test that exists for HIV. It can determine whether a person is HIV positive about 14 days after exposure to the virus. The DNA PCR test can detect the virus at about 20 days after exposure. If either of these tests is done for general HIV testing, the results will be confirmed by antibody tests when appropriate because there are more false positive results produced by the PCR tests.

The PCR tests are also referred to as viral load tests when they are used to measure the amount of the virus in the body. These tests have become standard ways to measure the function of the immune system. The more virus that is found in the blood, the less healthy a person is, and the more contagious he or she is. HIV viral load is highest at the first sign of infection as well as when the body can no longer fight the virus. PCR tests are used sometimes if a person believes he or she has been infected recently. This can allow a person to know the results quickly and make him or her aware of being infectious at that step of the infection process.

Testing Policy and Law

The CDC reports that each year about 20 million people are tested for HIV and that in the latest known statistics about 40 percent of all adults in the United States had been tested for HIV. However, the CDC also believes that more than 250,000 people in the United States are HIV positive and do not know that they have the virus. This means that the potential for spread of HIV continues, as these people are unaware that they can infect others.

Laws in the United States require the reporting of all HIV cases to the federal government. Initially, some states only reported AIDS cases, as defined by the CDC guidelines. Federal public health officials only know the number and location of cases and do not track names of individuals. This allows the government to track the spread of the virus in the population more accurately. There are 85 illnesses that the federal government tracks in a similar manner.

The name of a person who tests positive in a state or U.S. territory, however, is reported to the local and state public health officials if that person was tested in a setting that does not have anonymous testing. Anonymous testing does not record the name of the person being tested or the test results in any way. Some people are hesitant to have their name reported to government officials for any reason, under any circumstances. However, if individuals do test positive and then later seek treatment, it is still policy in all 50 states and six U.S. territories to report the name to public health officials. Several states have recently changed to reporting names for HIV cases at the urging of federal officials after many years of not collecting names. Most states offer anonymous testing at certain clinics, doctors' offices, and private health care settings. This allows people to be tested without any fear of reporting of names. Alabama, Idaho, Iowa, Mississippi, Nevada,

North Carolina, North Dakota, South Carolina, South Dakota, Tennessee, and the U.S. Virgin Islands do not have anonymous testing in any form, so the results of those tests will always involve name reporting. A person who has anonymous testing receives a code number that is associated with the blood sample and uses that code number when calling for test results. The other type of available testing is confidential. Confidential testing is not the same as anonymous testing. Confidential testing results in a person's name being associated with the fact that he or she has taken the test and with any results that are returned. Although theoretically the results are limited to the person being tested and to the doctor, some states require reporting of names to public health authorities in the event of a positive result. Insurance companies can see that an individual was tested for HIV, though they may not always see the results of the test.

Many states have adopted what is known as opt-in or opt-out testing for pregnant WOMEN. When a woman seeks medical care in 22 states, she is required to sign paperwork acknowledging that her blood will be automatically tested for HIV antibodies. If a woman does not want to be tested for HIV, she can sign a waiver declining the testing. This is known as opt-out testing. A person must opt out of the procedure, or it will be done automatically. In 28 states, the District of Columbia, and Puerto Rico, opt-in testing is done for pregnant women. A woman must declare she wishes to be tested for HIV; the test will not automatically be done. As the CDC now encourages opt-out testing, many states may be changing their laws regarding this procedure in the future. Currently, 10 states require HIV testing for newborn babies if the mother's HIV status is unknown. All infants born to mothers who are HIV positive will generally be tested as soon as possible after birth.

Public health data reporting is considered protected information. People in other forms of government, employers, and, in some cases, insurance companies do not have access to the information by a person's name or by illness. So even though reporting of HIV infection or AIDS takes place, it is considered to be very safe and secure information. Some state and local health departments do have partner notification programs. This means that the health department will request the name and contact information of sexual partners for someone who tests positive, so that those individuals can be notified that they may want to be tested for HIV. Some states do not require this but will offer counseling for people who test positive so that they may do such notification themselves. It is similar to partner notification that exists for other sexually transmitted infections as well as TUBERCULOSIS in many states.

Other testing laws involve immigrants and military personnel. All immigrants or candidates for permanent residency in the United States must undergo HIV testing. Until recently, all individuals who wanted to become permanent residents or citizens of the United States were required to be HIV negative. A person who tested HIV positive needed to apply for a waiver to this requirement. This requirement was rarely waived, and a person could be removed from the United States on the basis of HIV status. All U.S. military personnel are required to undergo regular HIV testing. Any active or reserve military personnel who test HIV positive are ineligible for deployment overseas. If a person in the U.S. military tests HIV positive while overseas, he or she will be returned to the U.S. mainland without delay. Certain types of military service are banned for people who are HIV positive.

The Joint United Nations Programme on HIV/AIDS (UNAIDS) and the WORLD HEALTH ORGANIZATION (WHO) support voluntary testing in all countries. However, UN statistics reveal that only 0.2 percent of people in resource-poor countries have been tested for HIV. There are several reasons for this low statistic; the chief among them include fear of stigma associated with testing, fear of reprisal for being HIV positive, and lack of medical care and/or treatment once a diagnosis is given. These reasons have led to the very high rates of HIV TRANSMISSION in many countries.

UNAIDS and WHO policy states that HIV testing involve what is called the three Cs: informed consent, counseling, and confidentiality. Guidelines also recommend that health providers make an opt-out style policy available for all. This was part of the agencies' hope for universal access to treatment and service by 2010. It is recognized that without proper funding and guidance in how to provide counseling and services, these goals will not be achievable. HIV testing for everyone who wants it is still lacking in many areas of the world.

AVERT: AVERTing HIV and AIDS. "History of AIDS up to 1986." AVERT.org. Available online. URL: http://www.avert.org/aids-history-86.htm. Accessed March 20, 2011.

———. "HIV Testing." AVERT.org. Available online. URL: http://www.avert.org/testing.htm. Accessed March 20, 2011.

Centers for Disease Control and Prevention. "Frequently Asked Questions." HIVTest.org. Available online. URL: http://www.hivtest.org/faq.aspx. Accessed March 20, 2011.

———. "HIV Testing." CDC.gov. Available online. URL: http://www.cdc.gov/hiv/topics/testing/index.htm. Accessed March 20, 2011.

Constantine, Niel. "HIV Viral Antigen Assays." HIV InSite.ucsf.edu. Available online. URL: http://hivinsite.ucsf.edu/InSite?page=kb-02-02-02-02. Accessed March 20, 2011.

Henry J. Kaiser Family Foundation. "HIV Name Reporting—Kaiser State Health Facts." statehealthfacts.org. Available online. URL: http://www.statehealthfacts.org/mcoparetable.jsp?cat=11&ind=559. Accessed March 20, 2011.

Kates, Jennifer, and the Henry J. Kaiser Family Foundation. "HIV Testing in the United States." KFF.org. Available online. URL: http://www.kff.org/hivaids/upload/6094-05.pdf. Accessed March 20, 2011.

MedPedia.com. "Sensitivity and Specificity." MedPedia.com. Available online. URL: http://wiki.medpedia.com/Sensitivity_and_Specificity. Accessed March 20, 2011.

San Francisco AIDS Foundation. "HIV Testing." The Body.com. Available online. URL: http://www.the

body.com/content/prev/art2497.html#sensitivity. Accessed March 20, 2011.

UNAIDS: Joint United Nations Programme on HIV/ AIDS. "Fast Facts about HIV Testing and Counseling." UNAIDS.org. Available online. URL: http:// www.unaids.org/en/media/unaids/contentassets/ dataimport/pub/factsheet/2008/20080527_fast- facts_testing_en.pdf. Accessed March 20, 2011.

HIV wasting syndrome   HIV wasting syndrome, also called AIDS wasting syndrome, is a major problem for HIV-positive people when their immune system is weakened. It is defined by the U.S. CENTERS FOR DISEASE CONTROL as "a weight loss of at least 10 percent in the presence of diarrhea or chronic weakness and documented fever for at least 30 days that is not attributable to a concurrent condition other than HIV infection itself." Wasting is linked to disease progression and death in HIV-positive people. Loss of just 5 percent of body weight can have the same negative effects.

Several studies have shown that wasting is highly correlated to disease progression in HIV-positive people and that preventing it can help prevent the disease from advancing to a stage in the illness when OPPORTUNISTIC INFECTIONS (OIs) can take hold and cause further damage. HIV and some opportunistic infections depress appetite or simply cause less interest in eating. In addition, some HIV medications must be taken on an empty stomach, others with particular types of food, and these disruptions in eating patterns can inadvertently cause a person to eat less than he or she would be eating on a regular schedule. Another cause of weight loss can be the HIGHLY ACTIVE ANTIRETROVIRAL THERAPY (HAART) medications that have side effects such as nausea, diarrhea, and tiredness.

Symptoms and Diagnostic Path
The chief symptoms is weight loss, both in fat and in muscle mass. Self-evident measures such as loss of appetite, weight loss that is unintentional, and loss of muscle in the arms can all

give a clear picture of wasting. Tests that may be done to measure wasting include body mass index (BMI), a measure of a person's height and weight that can give a doctor an idea whether a person is overweight or underweight according to healthy averages that have been determined through years of use and research into the measurement.

Another test that is commonly done in HIV-positive people is for testosterone levels. HIV-positive people in general have lower levels of testosterone in their body than HIV-negative people. This is true for WOMEN as well as men. It is unclear from studies that have been done in HIV-positive people whether the decreased testosterone is a result of medications that people are using, lack of food intake, or other possible causes. However, hormone levels of testosterone can be treated and people do seem to benefit in gaining lean muscle mass when receiving testosterone supplements.

Tests to determine whether intestinal illnesses are causing wasting usually involve taking several stool samples over a period of several days to look for various bacteria, helminths, viruses, or other potential causes of poor absorption of nutrients from food. A colonoscopy or biopsy of tissue can also allow closer examination of the intestinal tract for a clearer diagnosis.

Nutritional consultations may also be done with HIV-positive people to get a clear understanding of the food typically eaten by the patient. A balanced diet with steady levels of protein intake can help to minimize weight loss as well as ensure that the body has ample opportunity to absorb minerals and nutrients it needs for fighting illnesses.

Treatment Options and Outlook
Most treatment therapy for wasting involves lowering the viral load of HIV and raising the CD4 T cell count. HAART will allow the body to slow metabolism as the medications fight the virus and allow the immune system time to recover. Slower metabolism can allow a person to gain weight that'has been lost over time fight-

ing the virus. In addition, a person may have diagnostic tests to evaluate whether any intestinal illnesses or infections are present. Treatment for these illnesses will also involve drugs but will allow an increase in absorption of nutrients necessary to gain or maintain body weight.

There are also prescriptions that can help to improve digestion and food intake, and to add weight. Replacement testosterone is available as both intramuscular injections and adhesive patches that can be worn daily to allow the body to absorb the chemical through the skin. If an HIV-positive person shows regularly decreased levels of testosterone, this treatment may be a means to increase or stabilize weight.

Dronabinol is a synthetic tetrahydrocannabinol, the active ingredient in marijuana, which causes increased hunger in people. This may be prescribed to help with nausea or pain in HIV-positive people so that food intake can be increased and thereby weight loss minimized.

In states that allow medical prescriptions of marijuana, some HIV-positive people are prescribed the drug to counter nausea or pain to allow them to increase their food intake.

Risk Factors and Preventive Measures

Most HIV-positive people have fewer problems with wasting when they are on HAART. Antiviral medications can prevent the occurrence of OIs and, therefore, prevent potential problems with food intake and absorption. Good nutrition in general can prevent illness and maintain health. People who are HIV positive can request counseling in nutrition to improve their understanding of the nutritional needs of HIV-positive people.

AIDSmeds. "Wasting Syndrome." AIDSmeds.com. Available online. URL: http://www.aidsmeds.com/articles/Wasting_6934.shtml. Accessed March 20, 2011.

TheBody. "HIV Wasting Syndrome." TheBody.com. Available online. URL: http://www.thebody.com/content/living/art6604.html. Accessed March 20, 2011.

Hellerstein, Marc K., M.D. "Endocrine Manifestations of HIV." HIVInSite.ucsf.edu. Available online. URL: http://hivinsite.ucsf.edu/InSite?page=kb-04-01-07. Accessed March 20, 2011.

Mulligan, Kathleen, and Morris Schambelan, M.D. "HIV-Associated Wasting." HIVInSite.ucsf.edu. Available online. URL: http://hivinsite.ucsf.edu/InSite?page=kb-04-01-08. Accessed March 20, 2011.

Reiter, Gary S. "The HIV Wasting Syndrome." Available online. URL: http://aids-clinical-care.jwatch.org/cgi/content/full/1996/1101/1. Accessed March 20, 2011.

hospice Hospice is a type of care provided to people who are nearing death. At times, the term may be used to refer to a specific place where this type of care is provided, and at other times simply the type of care. It differs from palliative care in that hospice is geared specifically to the brief time before a person dies, whereas palliative care is designed to reduce pain, manage symptoms, and assist a person to manage his or her life. Although the two terms are often used together, people working in these fields see the two as very different areas of health care.

Hospice has played a large role in the care of HIV-positive people since the beginning of the epidemic in the United States. At that time, many hospitals and nursing homes would not admit people with AIDS or HIV. There was much that was not known about the illness, and fear existed about how the illness was spread. Even after knowledge became available that it was a virus and could not be spread through casual contact, there were many stories of people being turned away from small-town hospitals or other health facilities out of ignorance and fear. Hospice was a way for the community, particularly people in the gay community, to provide care for those who needed it.

Hospice grew out of the ideas of a physician, Cicely Saunders, in London, England, in the 1960s. She had studied dying patients and worked with them and their families to provide comfort care, and believed this care both was more supportive and provided better service to the patient and the family than the standard treatment provided in Western hospitals at the time. Her work at establishing the first modern hospice in the late 1960s led to an interest in the concept in U.S. nursing schools. Elisabeth Kübler-Ross, a psychiatrist in the United States, popularized and confirmed many of the hospice concepts in her famous book *On Death and Dying,* published in 1969. By the time the HIV epidemic began in the early 1980s, hospice as a concept and treatment method was beginning to take hold and replace the isolation of dying patients and the institutionalization of death.

These two different concerns, that of ending the isolation of a dying patient and the refusal to treat some patients, led to the establishment of hospice care and hospice facilities in cities where there were large populations of HIV-positive people. A very clear message was expressed by both the hospice community and the HIV patients, that dying with dignity was important. Both groups sought to end the early deaths of AIDS that had often been terrifying for patients, not knowing what was occurring and not having a place to feel safe when they were ill.

Palliative care works to reduce the pain and discomfort of a person and help with emotional, physical, and other needs during an illness. It is not focused on curing a patient. Some people who have HIV may be opposed to receiving advanced medical care because of spiritual beliefs or exhaustion from the illness. Other times, despite the advances of HIV health care, some people will not be helped with antiretrovirals or drugs to prevent OPPORTUNISTIC INFECTIONS (OIs). In these cases, palliative care may be considered the best available option for living. It is a plan of care that allows the patient to live as well as possible within the limits of the illness.

Hospice is the care that a person receives near the end of his or her life. It most often takes place in the patient's own home with familiar surroundings and people. Although there are residential hospices and some hospitals also maintain a hospice wing, many people choose to receive hospice care at their home. They usually have a person who is their primary caregiver, or

this may be a shared task of several friends or family members. All people involved are made aware of the choices the patient has made and the expectations for patient's care. A hospice in the home usually provides care from a nurse or a social worker; often a pastoral caregiver can be available if a person desires this. Pain medication and other necessary physical care can be arranged through the hospice workers or the person's primary doctor. Hospice plans vary from one location to the next, so a person needs to be informed of what the guidelines for care are and whether they fit his or her needs. Some may require a statement saying an individual does not want to be resuscitated; others may not allow tube feeding. These are choices an individual can make prior to entering a hospice-care setting.

Both hospice and palliative care remain quite important in the HIV community. There continue to be AIDS hospices across the United States and around the world that provide temporary ongoing care to ease pain and provide comfort for patients, in the physical hospice or in their own home. Medicare and Medicaid cover hospice services as they would cover other medical care. The patient's primary doctor must certify that a person has a six-months-to-live diagnosis. If a person makes a recovery during this time, hospice can be cancelled and a person may resume regular medical care. Some hospices can arrange respite care, if the primary caregiver must leave or needs a break from the duties of caregiving for a short time. It is most important that individuals work out their own plan for care at the end of their life so that the options that are chosen are in line with what they want. If they are not in the position to be capable of making decisions, it can be a relief to family and friends that these decisions are already made.

Center to Advance Palliative Care. "Palliative Care." GetPalliativeCare.org. Available online. URL: http://www.getpalliativecare.org/. Accessed March 20, 2011.

Chermack, John A. "Hospice and Supportive Care." TheBody.com. Available online. URL: http://www.thebody.com/content/art30590.html. Accessed March 20, 2011.

Hemphill, Mary Lynn. "Considering Hospice." The Body.com. Available online. URL: http://www.the body.com/content/living/art32488.html. Accessed March 20, 2011.

Hospice, Inc. "Hospice . . . for Patients and Families Facing Life-Threatening Illnesses." Hospicenet.org. Available online. URL: http://www.hospicenet. org/. Accessed March 20, 2011.

National Hospice and Palliative Care Organization. "History of Hospice Care." NHCPO.org. Available online. URL: http://www.nhpco.org/i4a/pages/index.cfm ?pageid=3285. Accessed March 20, 2011.

human herpes virus 6 and 7 (HHV-6 and HHV-7) HHV-6 and HHV-7 are herpes viruses that are not fully understood at this time. Both viruses are acquired early in life and are almost universal in nature, meaning close to 100 percent of all people have had these viruses at some point in life. Neither virus has as of yet been implicated in HIV illness or increased activity of HIV in a person's immune system. However, there have been several theorized possibilities about such connections.

HHV-6 is generally acquired within the first three years of life. More than 90 percent of CHILDREN show infection by one year of age and nearly 100 percent by age three. It is acquired most of the time from family members or caretakers, who shed the virus in their saliva from time to time as adults. It has recently been shown that HHV-6 can also, at times, become part of the human deoxyribonucleic acid (DNA). The reason that it integrates itself into the chromosomes of some people and is passed directly to children as part of their genetic makeup is not fully understood.

HHV-7 is also a childhood-acquired virus. More than 80 percent of adults show prior infection with this virus. It is also shed through saliva and can be detected there through testing.

Symptoms and Diagnostic Path

HHV-6 causes a childhood illness known as exanthem subitum, also called roseola. It often appears as a fever, with a rosy red rash that can cover portions of the child's skin when the fever breaks. It has been implicated in encephalitis and seizures during this infection. It is also known to cause problems in immunocompromised people, particularly those who have received ORGAN TRANSPLANTATION of some type and are using immunosuppressive medications. It has not been implicated in any HIV-associated OPPORTUNISTIC INFECTIONS (OIs).

HHV-7 has not been shown to cause any definitive illness in humans. There has been no implication of either HHV-6 or -7 in the viral activity or viral load of HIV-positive people.

HHV-6 and HHV-7 have both been associated with several illnesses. There has been no proof established yet that either virus causes anything other than infant fevers and roseola. Some writers and researchers believe that HHV-6 or -7 could be implicated in other illnesses such as muscular dystrophy, multiple sclerosis, autism, chronic fatigue syndrome, or any of a number of others. None of these hypotheses has been proven to be true as of this writing.

Treatment Options and Outlook

Ganciclovir and foscarnet have both been shown to reduce levels of HHV-6 in the blood. If any illness in an HIV-positive person could be shown to be HHV-6-related, these drugs would be recommended for use. HHV-7 causes no known illness, so treatment cannot be recommended.

Risk Factors and Preventive Measures

HHV-6 and HHV-7 are nearly universal, so avoidance is next to impossible. There is no current vaccine or vaccine trial for either of these herpes viruses.

Boutolleau, D., et al. "Detection of Human Herpesvirus 7 DNA in Peripheral Blood Reflects Mainly CD4+ Cell Count in Patients Infected with HIV." *Journal of Medical Virology* 76, no. 2 (June 2005): 223–228.

Campadelli-Fiume, Gabriella, Prisco Mirandola, and Laura Menotti. "Human Herpesvirus 6: An Emerging Pathogen." *Emerging Infectious Diseases* 5, no. 3 (May 1999). Available online. URL: http://www.cdc. gov/Ncidod/eid/vol5no3/campadelli.htm. Accessed March 12, 2011.

Centers for Disease Control and Prevention. "HHV-6 and HHV-7 Disease." HIVInSite.com. Available online. URL: http://hivinsite.ucsf.edu/InSite?page=md-agl-hhv. Accessed March 25, 2011.

NewsMedical. "Human Herpes Virus 6 Weaves Itself into the DNA Transferred from Parents to Babies." News-medical.net. Available online. URL: http://www.news-medical.net/?id=41120. Accessed March 20, 2011.

University of South Carolina School of Medicine. "Herpes Viruses." *Microbiology and Immunology On-line.* SC.edu. Available online. URL: http://pathmicro.med.sc.edu/virol/herpes.htm. Accessed March 20, 2011.

human herpes virus 8 (HHV-8, KSHV) HHV-8, also known as Kaposi's sarcoma–associated herpes virus (KSHV), is a member of the herpes virus family. It is found in 1–15 percent of the general population in the United States, and in greater prevalence in Mediterranean countries (10–20 percent of the population) as well as sub-Saharan Africa (30–80 percent of the population). It is also found at much higher rates of prevalence in MEN WHO HAVE SEX WITH MEN (MSM), among whom it is seen in 20–70 percent of the population in the United States, as measured in different studies.

HHV-8 is associated with several illnesses. All types of Kaposi's sarcoma (KS), including endemic and transplant-related KS, have been shown to be related to HHV-8 levels in the blood. Also, multicentric Castleman disease (MCD) and primary effusion lymphoma (PEL) have been shown to be associated with high levels of HHV-8 in the blood. MCD is a rare form of noncancerous tumor growth in multiple sites of the lymph system. PEL is a rare lymphoma of the B cells found predominantly in what are known as body cavities such as the pleural, pericardial, or peritoneal areas.

Symptoms and Diagnostic Path

People generally do not show a distinct pattern of symptoms for infection with HHV-8. There is some association with a syndrome of fever, rash, swollen lymph nodes, and bone marrow suppression, but studies have not positively confirmed this association. Diagnosis of infection with HHV-8 can be done through either antibody tests for an immune response to the virus of an individual or through analysis of blood samples for specific nucleic acids that make up the virus.

KS is generally diagnosed through observation. It is most often a nontender, purplish, and flat spot on the skin. It can often look like a bruise but when pushed does not change color as a bruise would. It can become patchy, with several spots, or lesions, growing together. Lesions can also become raised on the skin as they grow together. KS can spread in the mouth and esophagus and become disseminated, in some cases without any visible skin lesions. It can disseminate to the lungs, liver, intestines, and stomach, causing bleeding and therefore problems in eating and digestion. Weight loss can be common because of the pain involved in eating with disseminated internal KS. KS is a malignant overgrowth of the blood vessels at or just below the skin or mucous membrane, and most often occurs when a person's immune system has fewer than 200 CD4 T cells/µL of blood.

In the early years of the AIDS epidemic, KS was often the first visible sign of the illness. KS was one of the two illnesses that initially were discussed by the CENTERS FOR DISEASE CONTROL and Prevention (CDC) in the publication *Morbidity and Mortality Weekly Report* (*MMWR*), which began tracking several cases of KS that appeared one year in young men, as it was rare to find more than a few cases a year in all age populations.

MCD symptoms include high fever, anemia, weight loss, loss of appetite, swollen lymph glands, swollen spleen, and low white blood cell counts, due to overproduction of interleukin-6. It is a disease generally found in HIV-positive people, can occur at any level of immune system function, and can occur rarely in people who have received immunosuppressive drugs after ORGAN TRANSPLANTATION. In MCD, lymph nodes have noncancerous tumors in them. The term *multicentric* means that multiple lymph areas around the body are involved.

PEL also occurs most frequently at CD4 T lymphocyte levels below 200 cells/µL. Symptoms include shortness of breath and pain during breathing. PEL is a B-cell lymphoma. The cancerous cells are found in the buildup of fluid around the pleural cavities. There are no tumor masses involved, though the fluid does appear on X-rays of the lungs.

Treatment Options and Outlook

There is no specific treatment that is used against HHV-8. Some small studies have shown that KS lesions can be reduced or the spread of lesions stopped with the use of ganciclovir or foscarnet, two antiviral medications. The federal government has suggested further large-scale studies to decide whether these drugs help in the management of HHV-8 diseases. The best treatment for HHV-8 illness has been shown to be HIGHLY ACTIVE ANTIRETROVIRAL THERAPY (HAART). Once a person's immune system has begun to be restored through HAART, KS lesions often disappear, though disseminated disease does not generally disappear and will require additional chemotherapy.

KS can be treated with several methods. For patients who have disseminated KS, the most frequent treatment is chemotherapy. Doxorubicin, daunorubicin, and paclitaxel are three anticancer medications used for treating diffuse KS. For small or superficial KS lesions, freezing can often reduce and remove lesions. Lesions can also be surgically removed if they are not too numerous or deep in the tissue.

A PEL diagnosis is not a hopeful one for a patient, and recovery is not assured. Chemotherapy and HAART are the recommended forms of treatment. Intravenous ganciclovir or oral valganciclovir is recommended in conjunction with the HAART.

MCD can be treated with initiation of HAART. IV ganciclovir or oral valganciclovir is recommended in conjunction with HAART. The mono-

clonal antibody medication rituximab also can be helpful in MCD treatment

Risk Factors and Preventive Measures

Effective HAART has been shown to reduce and suppress KS lesions, as well as prevent any new lesions from forming. As both PEL and MCD do not appear except in HIV-positive people whose immune systems have fewer than 200 CD4 T lymphocytes/µL, it is also recommended that HAART be started in these instances.

IMMUNE RECONSTITUTION INFLAMMATORY SYNDROME (IRIS) has been reported in patients receiving HAART who have preexisting KS and MCD. However, as treatment with HAART to restore the immune system is the main focus of medication in HHV-8 diseases, it is recommended that HAART treatment be closely monitored for any signs of IRIS.

AIDSInfoNet.org. "Kaposi's Sarcoma (KS)." AIDSInfo Net.org. Available online. URL: http://www.aids infonet.org/fact_sheets/view/511. Accessed March 20, 2011.

Blankson, Joel N. "HIV Guide: HHV-8." Hopkins-HIV guide.org. Available online. URL: http://www. hopkins-hivguide.org/pathogen/viruses/hhv-8. html. Accessed March 20, 2011.

Casper, Corey, M.D. "Human Herpesvirus-8, Kaposi Sarcoma, and AIDS-Associated Neoplasms." Available online. URL: http://hivinsite.ucsf.edu/InSite ?page=kb-06-02-01. Accessed March 20, 2011.

Mayo Clinic Staff. "Castleman Disease." MayoClinic. com. Available online. URL: http://www.mayo clinic.com/health/castleman-disease/DS01000. Accessed March 20, 2011.

MedlinePlus. "Kaposi's Sarcoma." NIH.gov. Available online. URL: http://www.nlm.nih.gov/medlineplus/ ency/article/000661.htm. Accessed March 20, 2011.

MicrobiologyBytes. "Herpesviruses: HHV-8." Microb iologybytes.com. Available online. URL: http://www. microbiologybytes.com/virology/HHV8.html. Accessed March 20, 2011.

human immune system The human immune system is a complex, organized system of defense that the body has against substances such as antigens that can enter the body and cause illness. The network of cells, tissues, and organs that make up the immune system work together to maintain health and rid the body of any foreign matter.

The immune system is involved in five major activities in the body. It defends the body against foreign substances, such as viruses, bacteria, and fungi. It identifies and rids the body of abnormal cells to prevent their growth into tumors. It eliminates old and deteriorating cells and rejects cells from other organisms that might enter the body. It is sometimes involved in inappropriate responses to harmless substances, which lead to allergic reactions. These antigens are then called allergens. Finally, it at times can attack itself, resulting in an autoimmune disease, such as lupus and some types of arthritis.

The organs of the immune system are called lymphoid organs. These are the places where immune cells gather and communicate to fight off invaders to the body. These organs are connected to the lymph system, through small vessels similar to veins, where lymph fluid is carried. The lymphocytes, white blood cells, are carried through the lymph system in addition to the blood vessels. The lymphoid organs, located in different areas of the body, are the spleen, thymus, tonsils, adenoids, appendix, and Peyer's patches, the last located along the intestine. The spleen is the main filtering organ of the immune system. Blood is filtered there as well as lymph fluid. It is the organ that removes old blood cells, as well as the place where antibodies are generated. It is where B cells are activated in the body. The thymus, located in the center of the chest behind the breastbone, is the area where T cells migrate after leaving the bone marrow. They are filtered and gather information in the thymus before going out into the body. Lymph nodes, small bean-sized glands located in several spots in the body, filter the lymph fluid that flows throughout it. There are 600–700 lymph nodes in every human body, located mainly near the armpit, groin, and neck areas. The bone marrow also plays an important role in the lymph system,

as it is where lymphocytes are produced before they travel out to the rest of the body. Tonsils and adenoids are located in the mouth and sinus regions. They serve as a place for immune cells to gather and filter antigens as they enter the body. The appendix is located in the lower right portion of the abdomen. Although it is not completely clear what function the appendix serves, it is a lymphoid organ and does perform some function in filtering lymph. One theory is that the appendix serves as a place where good bacteria are stored for release into the intestine after a person has recovered from diarrhea or intestinal illness.

The immune system centers on the activity of the cells that recognize the self (the individual) and the non-self, the foreign cell or particle, known as the antigen. This is done through a unique set of markers on each cell of the body that the immune system recognizes as self. The ability of the immune system to recognize the difference between its own cells and those belonging to something else is called the major histocompatibility complex (MHC). A person's body recognizes these proteins that mark all cells. There are two types of MHC: MHC class I and MHC class II. MHC class II proteins are found only on certain immune cells such as dendritic cells, B lymphocytes, and macrophages. Most cells present MHC class I proteins, which allow the other immune cells to recognize the cells as self and ignore them, while finding cells or antigens that do not display these proteins, the non-self, and attacking them.

White blood cells, also called leukocytes, are created in the bone marrow. They are divided into two main types: phagocytes and lymphocytes. Phagocytes are responsible for "swallowing" pathogens and old or worn-out cells. Phagocytes are also divided into two types: monocytes/macrophages and granulocytes. Monocytes circulate in the blood; when they migrate into the body tissue, they become macrophages. Macrophages are responsible for moving and destroying foreign particles and diseased cells. They display pieces of a destroyed antigen on their surface, allowing lymphocytes to become activated and begin further immune system attacks on the foreign cells. There are different types of macrophages, which have individual names: Kupffer's cells in the liver, microglial cells in the brain and spinal cord, osteoclasts in the bone, histiocytes in connective tissue, epithelioid cells in granulomas, dust cells in the lungs, sinusoidal cells in the spleen, and mesangial cells in the kidneys.

There are three types of granulocytes: eosinophils, basophils, and neutrophils. They are known as granulocytes because they contain toxic granules that destroy invading pathogens. They travel in the blood and lymph. Eosinophils are involved in allergic responses and make up approximately 2 percent of leukocytes. Basophils comprise only about 1 percent of granulocytes and are involved in immediate response to antigens, as in asthma. Neutrophils are the predominant type of leukocytes, making up approximately 55–70 percent of granulocytes in the body. A related immune cell is the mast cell, which is found in tissue and near the interaction of antigens with the body, in mucosal linings such as those of the tongue, lips, and nasal passages.

Lymphocytes consist of several different types of cells. There are T lymphocytes, of which there are three types. Helper T cells inform the immune system of the presence of antigens and activate other cells in the immune system. They have a protein on their outer surface called CD4, so they are often called CD4 T cells. Inducer T cells also carry the CD4 protein. They recognize antigen on the surface of macrophages and secrete chemicals called cytokines that attract further intervention from phagocytes. Then there are cytotoxic T cells. These cells carry the protein CD8 and are often referred to as CD8 or T8 cells. These cells help eliminate infected cells by attaching themselves to the antigen cells and inducing cell death, or apoptosis. CD4 T cells are the prime cells that HIV attacks when it infects a person. CD4 memory cells are attacked during the acute phase of the infection, often killing many more than half of these cells during the first few weeks after exposure. Memory cells are the portion of the immune system that can recall previous infections and go into action immediately to protect a person against antigens in the body.

There are different types of cytokines. T and B cells release lymphokines. Macrophages and monocytes release chemokines called monokines. Other cytokines that are released from immune cells include interleukins, interferons, and growth factors. Cytokines serve as the communication system between cells. They "call" specific cells to an area for fighting, repairing, or protecting cells. Cytokines that call specific cells are referred to as chemokines.

Lymphocytes also include B cells, or B lymphocytes. B cells do not have the power to enter foreign cells or cells that have been infected by a virus or other parasite. They are sensitive to antigens and they produce antibodies known as immunoglobulins that are responsible for binding to an antigen and interfering with the antigen's role before encouraging phagocytes to enter the area. They prepare the antigen or cell for other immune cells such as the T cells that can penetrate or kill the invading antigen. There are a variety of different immunoglobulins (Ig). IgA is found predominantly in body fluids, guarding the body at the entrances such as the mucosa, nasal passages, and urethra. IgD is found in the stomach and the walls of the chest. The exact function of IgD antibodies is unclear; they seem to encourage other B-cell responses. IgE responds to parasitic infections and plays a role in allergies. People who have various allergies have high levels of IgE. IgG coats microbes and allows other immune cells to ingest the antigens and rid the body of them. IgG is produced primarily from memory cells that impart long-term immunity from previously recognized antigens. IgM is most effective at killing bacteria and the most numerous antibody in humans. It is an aggregate of other Ig antibodies and is found predominantly in the circulatory system.

Natural killer (NK) cells are another type of lymphocyte. NK cells recognize foreign cells of multiple antigen types. They are not informed of a specific antigen but may attack quickly by recognizing many types of foreign cells. Finally, there are dendritic cells. Dendritic cells are also antigen-presenting cells, as are macrophages. They take in an antigen and present the proteins for the antigen on the surface of the cell, allowing other immune system cells to recognize the invading cells to be killed or removed. It is believed that dendritic cells capture antigens and take them to lymphoid organs or lymph nodes where the cellular response is begun. Specialized dendritic cells called Langerhans cells are located in the skin.

Memory cells are T cells and B cells that are held in "storage" by the body to attack an antigen that has already entered. They recognize and recall the antigen and induce a quick response to it. There are also suppressor T cells, also known as regulatory T cells, which are used to shut off the immune system when the antigen has been eliminated from the body. Their role has only recently become more fully understood. Lack of regulatory T cells is known to play a role in autoimmune diseases, in which the immune system attacks the body.

There are different types of immunity to disease. Immunity is the ability to be resistant to or protected from a particular illness or disease—the capacity to respond to antigens, viruses, bacteria, fungi, and chemicals that are foreign to the body. Immunity is induced by exposure to the antigenic marker on an organism that invades the body or by administration of a vaccine that has the capability of stimulating production of specific antibodies (immunization). Immunity is also the response of the body and its tissues to a variety of antigens, including pollens, red cells, transplanted tissues, or the individual's own cells.

Acquired immunity is also called specific or adaptive immunity. This is a learned immunity. The body learns how to respond to certain antigens by being exposed to them; it develops the best way to respond to these antigens and remembers it. Acquired immunity can be divided into two parts: cell-mediated, resulting from activation of sensitized T lymphocytes that are created in the bone marrow but mature in the thymus; and humoral immunity, mediated by B lymphocytes that mature in the bone marrow and the spleen.

Acquired immunity is contrasted with natural, or innate, immunity, a more or less permanent immunity to disease with which an individual is born, the result of natural factors. Natural immunity may be due to the natural presence of immune bodies, but other factors such as diet, metabolism, temperature, or adaptive features of infectious organisms may be involved. Congenital immunity is natural immunity present at birth and may be natural or acquired; the latter results from antibodies received from the blood of the mother.

Some texts refer to active and passive immunity. Active immunity results from the development within the body of antibodies or sensitized T lymphocytes that neutralize or destroy the infectious agent. This mechanism results from the immune response to an invading antigen. It can also come about by a vaccine designed to spur an immune response. Passive immunity, on the other hand, is immunity acquired by the introduction of preformed antibodies into an unprotected individual. This can occur through injection of immune globulin, as when a person is inoculated against hepatitis A.

A last type of immunity is local immunity, which is immunity in a specific part of the body. HIV vaccine developers consider local immunity an important focus for vaccine research in HIV—for example, a focus on the mucous membranes. If immunity to HIV could be generated on the mucous membranes, then 90 percent of all cases could be prevented, since HIV mainly enters the body through the mucous membranes.

International AIDS Vaccine Initiative. "Understanding the Immune System and AIDS Vaccine Strategies." TheBody.com. Available online. URL: http://img.thebody.com/iavi/2009/understanding_the_immune_system.pdf. Accessed March 20, 2011.

———. "VAX Primers: The Science of AIDS Vaccines." IAVIreport.org. Available online. URL: http://www.iavireport.org/vax-primers/scienceofAIDSvaccines/Pages/TheScienceofAIDSVaccines.aspx. Accessed March 20, 2011

Linnemayer, Paul A. The Immune System—An Overview." TheBody.com. Available online. URL: http://www.thebody.com/content/art1788.html. Accessed March 20, 2011.

LymphNotes.com. "Understanding the Lymphatic System." LymphNotes.com. Available online. URL: http://www.lymphnotes.com/article.php/id/151/. Accessed March 20, 2011.

United States National Cancer Institute. "The Immune System." Cancer.gov. Available online. URL: http://www.cancer.gov/cancertopics/understandingcancer/immunesystem. Accessed March 20, 2011.

United States National Institute of Allergy and Infectious Diseases. "Immune System." NIH.gov. Available online. URL: http://www.niaid.nih.gov/topics/immunesystem/pages/default.aspx. Accessed March 12, 2011.

WebMD. "Immunoglobulins." WebMD.com. Available online. URL: http://www.webmd.com/a-to-z-guides/immunoglobulins. Accessed March 20, 2011.

human immunodeficiency virus (HIV) HIV is a virus that causes the depletion of the HUMAN IMMUNE SYSTEM. It interferes with the function of T cells that fight various infections in the body, causing the eventual death of these cells and allowing OPPORTUNISTIC INFECTIONS (OIs) by several unusual illnesses in the person whose T cells have been depleted. It causes the syndrome known as AIDS when the immune system becomes weakened enough for these opportunistic illnesses to affect a person. There is no known cure for HIV; however, antiretroviral medicine can control the virus reproduction in the body.

Symptoms and Diagnostic Path

The symptoms of exposure to HIV are initially a flulike illness that can affect people anywhere from 10 days to four weeks after initial infection. Although not everyone will have these flulike symptoms, they are the most common result of infection. The symptoms include nausea, diarrhea, fever, headache, rash, night sweats, sore throat, and swollen lymph nodes. This is known as acute or primary infection. About 70 percent of people who later test positive for HIV at some point report having these symptoms about the time that they believe they were exposed to the virus. During the acute illness, the virus is reproducing rapidly, and viral load can become quite high in some people. After this initial phase, the body's immune system reacts to the virus and begins to produce antibodies to try to control it. The flulike symptoms end a few days after they start.

These symptoms are the same as those of many other illnesses, from influenza to cold viruses. Simply having these symptoms does not indicate that a person is HIV positive. A person must take the HIV test that looks for viral load or antibodies to the virus to determine whether he or she is HIV positive. During the acute illness, the virus has moved from the site of infection to lymph nodes, where the virus begins reproducing. The body may take up to three months to react to the virus and begin producing antibodies. For this reason, the HIV enzyme-linked immunosorbent assay (ELISA) antibody test (see BLOOD WORK/BLOOD TESTS) is not considered accurate for at least three to six months after a person believes infection may have occurred. A viral load test can be performed to provide earlier indication that a person has been exposed to HIV. During this acute phase of the process, much of the body's immune system is being depleted of CD4 cells by the virus. A large portion of the CD4 memory cells are killed, leaving immature cells that do not recognize antigens from previous infections or illnesses, creating more opportunity for a person to become ill. A person who has acute HIV infection can readily pass on the virus to other people when he or she is unaware of being infected. The high viral load makes it much easier to pass along the virus through unsafe sexual behavior or any activities in which blood-to-blood contact is possible.

After the acute phase of the infection passes, a person's CD4 cells begin reproducing quickly to try to fight off the virus, and the viral load drops considerably from the high levels during this stage. If a person is unaware of being exposed to HIV or is not tested regularly, he or she may not notice symptoms of the virus until several years later. After the acute infection stage, the immune system begins a battle with the virus that continues all the time, inside the body. The body begins producing antibodies to the virus that hunt specific virally infected cells. The virus produces new viral particles that attempt to infect newly produced CD4 T cells. Although the virus behaves differently in different people, a general average of seven to 10 years may pass before a person becomes aware of being infected with HIV. During that time, the person's immune system is being weakened by the constant production of new virus and loss of immune system cells to fight infection. As this continues, a person may begin to notice being frequently tired, having difficulty fighting off colds or other common illnesses, having frequent night sweats and rashes, and having more frequent or constant fungal infections of the nails, mouth, and/or vaginal areas. Diarrhea, weight loss, and fevers also occur. This can happen gradually so that sometimes it is difficult for a person to be aware that anything different is happening. A person's CD4 T cells decrease over time and the viral load begins to increase as the body loses the fight against the virus.

As the human immune system weakens, a person becomes more susceptible to opportunistic infections. OIs take many forms, from common fungal infections such as thrush to rare and serious illnesses including Kaposi's sarcoma and PNEUMOCYSTIS PNEUMONIA (PCP). There are three major definitions used in assigning the diagnosis of AIDS in a patient. In the United States, the CENTERS FOR DISEASE CONTROL (CDC) Classification System for HIV Infection provides a case definition for AIDS and for statistical purposes allows the tracking of AIDS case numbers within the country. The WORLD HEALTH ORGA-

NIZATION (WHO) disease staging system for HIV infection and disease and the Bangui definition are used in other parts of the world to define and diagnose a person as having AIDS and for compiling statistics. Both the WHO and the CDC definitions rely on testing for HIV (see HIV TESTS) in the patient's blood. The Bangui definition is based on the systemic signs and the presence of one or more OIs and is generally used in regions where medical testing for HIV is not readily available. Both the WHO and the CDC have different guidelines for the definition and diagnosis of AIDS in children. When a person's CD4 T cell count falls below 200, the chance of becoming ill with an OI increases dramatically; when these T cells fall below 100, a person will probably become ill without preventive medicines to stop some of the OIs. Simply receiving a diagnosis of AIDS does not necessarily mean a person has an OI, but that their immune system is weak enough to offer that potential.

Treatment Options and Outlook

The first consideration for a person who learns he or she is HIV positive is to select a doctor who is familiar with the disease and how to treat it. Not all general practitioners have a detailed understanding of HIV. Research studies have shown that people who consult an HIV specialist in addition to their regular doctor have better survival rates than those who do not. Research has also shown that patients who talk with their doctor about treatment options and make decisions jointly with their doctor do better on HIV treatment than those who do not talk with their doctor. Both of these results demonstrate the importance of a knowledgeable doctor and a knowledgeable patient.

After testing positive, a person will then need to have their CD4 T cell counts and viral load tested to determine his or her current health. A full panel of different tests may be done to get a full picture. The articles on HIV TESTS and BLOOD WORK/BLOOD TESTS explain the many different tests doctors may order when patients are HIV positive. Currently, the CDC recommends treatment for HIV when a person's CD4 counts fall below 350. Research has repeatedly shown that the sooner a person begins HIV treatment, the longer and healthier his or her life will be. The virus is always at work reproducing itself in the body unless there is treatment. A little more than half of the experts on the CDC treatment panel recommend treatment for patients whose CD4 count is between 350 and 500. In the past, treatment was not started so early, but research continues to demonstrate that people treated early do better and live longer. At one time, it was thought that people could take what were termed drug holidays, during which they stopped antiretroviral medication for an extended period. It was thought that this might provide the same benefits, save patients money, and reduce some side effects of the medications. A large study known as the SMART (Strategies for Management of Anti-Retroviral Therapy) trial showed that patients who followed this treatment pattern had significantly more life-threatening events than patients who took their medication all the time without the drug holidays. So the recommendations are currently to treat early and treat well. Typically, a person who is known to be HIV positive requires regular blood tests to follow the HIV disease itself or the treatment they are using to make sure it is working. Most HIV-positive people have blood tested for viral load, CD4 count, and similar tests every two or three months.

There are several classes of antiretroviral medications today that can work together to stop HIV from reproducing in the body. These antiretrovirals are powerful drugs that have many side effects but can significantly extend the life of someone who is HIV positive. The combination of drugs that a person who has HIV takes is called HIGHLY ACTIVE ANTIRETROVIRAL THERAPY (HAART). Some people may also call it ART, for antiretroviral therapy. These combinations of drugs always involve at least three different pills, and at times four or five different drugs may be used. Some of the medications are combined into one pill, so that the amount of pills taken, the pill burden, is today relatively

low in comparison to that in the recent past, when treatment first became available. It was not unusual for patients to be required to take 15–20 pills a day at various times, with or without food, for optimal results.

There are currently five classes of drugs used to treat HIV. PROTEASE INHIBITORS (PIs), ENTRY INHIBITORS, NUCLEOSIDE REVERSE TRANSCRIPTASE INHIBITORS, NUCLEOTIDE REVERSE TRANSCRIPTASE INHIBITORS, NON-NUCLEOSIDE REVERSE TRANSCRIPTASE INHIBITORS, and INTEGRASE INHIBITORS each represent different areas of the viral reproduction cycle that can be stopped through the different classes of drugs. By combining different classes of drugs, the virus can be prevented from reproducing and ideally prevented from mutating to avoid all the actions of the drugs on its reproduction.

The outlook today for a person who is HIV positive and has access to treatment is significantly better than it has ever been. People are living much longer without suffering from OIs, and they are maintaining healthy, functioning immune systems as a result of treatment with HAART. Studies recently released show that HIV-positive people will on the whole have nearly the exact same life expectancy as people who are not HIV positive, as long as they begin taking medication before the CD4 cell count has fallen below 350 and maintain their medication schedules. Not everyone who receives treatment does well, but if the virus is stopped early enough, there is no reason a person cannot live a long, healthy life. Some people do not learn they are HIV positive until they become ill with an OI. This is a major reason to be tested for HIV on a regular basis if a person is sexually active with multiple partners, uses injection drugs with others, or has any reason to believe he or she may have been exposed to the virus in some manner. It is also important that people adhere to the instructions for taking the antiretroviral medications they are prescribed. If doses are missed regularly or taken at the wrong times, the virus can readily mutate to a form not affected by those drugs. Sometimes whole classes of drugs can be rendered useless because the virus has mutated and built RESISTANCE to them. Resistance can occur over time, or it can occur quickly, depending on different causes, but often the cause is that a person has not adhered to a regular schedule of taking the medications. If resistance develops, a person will be switched to a different combination of drugs that will work differently and, ideally, continue to prevent viral reproduction.

Risk Factors and Preventive Measures

Everyone is potentially at risk of exposure to HIV. The risk is higher among people who do not regularly use condoms or practice SAFER SEX during sexual encounters and higher in INJECTION DRUG USE(R)s who share needles. It is important to know one's HIV status. Testing can lead people to change their behaviors by practicing safer sex and not sharing needles. People who do use injection drugs need to remember not to share their needles or works with others, unless the equipment is thoroughly cleaned with soapy water and disinfected with bleach between uses. People who are not in mutually agreed upon monogamous relationships need to remember to practice safer sex including using condoms during intercourse, whether vaginal or anal. Unprotected intercourse is not a safer sex activity, and repeated unprotected sexual intercourse with different partners exposes a person to increased probability of HIV exposure. Smaller risks remain for people who received blood transfusions or blood clotting factor between 1978 and 1985. Although the majority of such cases have already been diagnosed, it is still possible for a person in this category to be HIV positive and not realize it if they have not been tested since that time.

In addition, recent studies show that a reduction in viral load correlates to a reduction in the spread of the virus. Studies conducted with sero-discordant partners—specifically, heterosexual couples, one of whom is positive and the other negative—have shown that when a person is taking antiretroviral medications and the virus

is under control, the rate of spread of the virus is very low. The study involved more than 3,000 couples. All were given counseling and condoms prior to the study. The couples with one person on HAART during the study showed a significantly lower rate of TRANSMISSION than those couples whose HIV-positive person was not on HAART. All people in the study were above the recommended cutoff for starting HAART. The transmission rate decreased from 2.23 percent in the non-HAART-using couples to 0.39 percent in the HAART-using couples. There was only one case of transmission recorded among the HAART-receiving couples. It has long been believed that HAART by itself may make transmitting the virus very difficult. Further studies, including some with gay males, are planned to test the advantage of using HAART for prevention of transmission. The rate of transmission among couples with one person on HAART was lower than that found in previous studies in which only condoms had been used.

HIV has been a devastating disease across the world. Several million people have died since it first was recognized in the early 1980s. Many millions more are currently infected and must take antiretroviral medications for the rest of their lives. Science continues to gain a better understanding of the virus and how the immune system works. Some promising genetic and other treatments are being explored. Trials of VACCINES AGAINST HIV/AIDS continue to prevent people from becoming infected. Although the virus has devastated several countries, there is more hope now than at any point in the nearly 30 years the virus has been seriously affecting the world.

Retroviruses

HIV is a RETROVIRUS. A retrovirus is a virus that enters a human cell, or other animal host cell, in some cases, and causes the cell to change the way it normally functions. It uses an enzyme called reverse transcriptase to produce deoxyribonucleic acid (DNA) from its own ribonucleic acid (RNA). The viral DNA is then made part of the host cell's DNA using another enzyme called integrase, and thereafter, when the cell reproduces, so does the virus. The ability of the RNA virus to change itself into DNA is called reverse transcription, because it is the reverse of what normally occurs within cells. There are several varieties of retroviruses. HEPATITIS B is a retrovirus also. HIV is part of the lentivirus subfamily of retroviruses. Lentiviruses are known as slow viruses. A slow virus takes a slow, progressive course that over months or years causes severe illness and, eventually, death. Other familiar lentiviruses besides HIV are feline immunodeficiency virus and the visna virus in sheep. Very little was known regarding retroviruses or lentiviruses until the epidemic of HIV that started in the 1980s. Lentiviruses have recently been found in the genetic makeup of small primates known as grey mouse lemurs on the island of Madagascar. This isolated group of primates has lentivirus built into their DNA, yet seem to have no ill effects from the virus. This shows that lentiviruses have been around for millions of years, as the island of Madagascar separated from Africa many millions of years ago, isolating these primates on the island. Study of these lemurs may lead to a better understanding of how they developed immunity to lentiviruses and aid HIV research. There are two major species of HIV, HIV-1 and HIV-2. HIV-1 is the more widespread of the two species, found across the world from southern AFRICA to NORTH AMERICA, South America, Europe, Australia, and ASIA. It is highly transmissible in specific instances and more deadly than HIV-2. HIV-2 is not as easily transmissible as HIV-1, and is predominantly found in West Africa. HIV-2 causes fewer deaths and has a much slower progression than HIV-1.

Subtypes and Groups

HIV-1 has been traced to an introduction of the simian immunodeficiency virus (SIV) to humans. The reason that the SIV created four different types of HIV-1 in humans is that the virus reproduces itself in the cells of the host, and each different introduction from animals to humans has led to a different form of the virus. Scientists have genetically traced the four different groups and can estimate at about what period the virus moved into the human population and where. The four groups are labeled group M, N, O, and P. In the case of groups M, N, and O, the transfer can be traced to SIV found in chimpanzees (Pan troglodytes troglodytes) in West Central Africa. Group M is also known as the main group and is the variety that has spread around the globe. Group O, for outlying group, is predominantly found in West Central Africa and accounts for about 2 percent of cases in that region. Group N, found in 1998, is rare and has only been found among a few people in Cameroon. In addition, in 2009, group P was discovered in a woman originally from Cameroon, living in Paris. Group P has been traced to SIV found in Western gorillas (Gorilla gorilla), meaning that this particular strain of SIV passed to humans and became the first known transfer of the virus to humans from that primate. More than 90 percent of all HIV-1 infections are from group M. There are at least nine subtypes, also known as clades, of group M. These subtypes are named by letters of the alphabet: A, B, C, D, F, G, H, J, and K. Type A is predominantly found in Africa, though it has also been seen increasingly in Russia and former Soviet countries. Type B is the major variety that predominates in North and South America, Australia, Europe, and Japan. Type C is the variety found in East and Southern Africa, India, LATIN AMERICA, and Nepal. It has been the most lethal variety of HIV, responsible for half of all HIV deaths. Type D is found in North and Central Africa and the Middle East. Type F has been found in Central Africa, Eastern Europe (see EASTERN EUROPE AND CENTRAL ASIA), and South America. Type G is found in Africa and Central Europe. Type H is found only in Central Africa. Type J is found in the CARIBBEAN and West and Central Africa. Type K is found only in Africa. It is possible to become infected with more than one subtype of HIV-1. Types that have combined in humans are known as circulating recombinant forms (CRFs), so that sometimes there are references to type A/G or type A/E. This is the result of two or more strains' forming a new and different strain of virus within humans. There are a variety of recombinant forms, and they account for approximately 18 percent of the HIV-1 cases in the world today. The epidemic in China is predominantly a recombinant form, as in the epidemic in South and Southeast Asia, excluding India. The recombinant forms account for only 0.7 percent of cases in North America but 89 percent of cases in Southeast Asia. Across the globe, type C accounts for 50 percent of cases; type A, 12 percent; type B, 10 percent; type G, 6 percent; type D, 2½ percent and types F, H, J, and K, just less than 1 percent of worldwide cases. CRF type A/G and type A/E account for 5 percent each of cases worldwide. The variety of CRF types show that it is possible to be exposed to more than one subtype of HIV-1, as this is how these varieties were first passed on to others.

In HIV-2, the virus was most closely related to SIV from the sooty mangabey (Cercocebus atys), a monkey found in West Africa. By studying genetic variations and the changes in the virus from the original SIV found in sooty mangabeys, scientists can determine that the virus passed to humans sometime in the 1930s in the area of Guinea-Bissau, a former Portuguese colony. The first cases of HIV-2 to appear outside Africa were in Portuguese soldiers returning from fighting in the civil war in Guinea-Bissau during the 1970s. HIV-2 is limited primarily to West Africa and is the predominant form of HIV found there. There have been only 79 cases of HIV-2 found in the United States according to the CENTERS FOR DISEASE CONTROL and Prevention (CDC). The majority of these cases have been in men who emigrated from West African countries. HIV-2 is considered endemic, meaning more than 1 percent of the people in the country test positive, in Cape Verde, Côte d'Ivoire, Gambia, Guinea-Bissau, Mali, Mauritania, Nigeria, and Sierra Leone. Significant numbers of cases have also been reported in Benin, Burkina Faso, Ghana, Guinea, Liberia, Niger, São Tomé, Senegal, and Togo. Angola and Mozambique, two other former Portuguese colonies in southern Africa, have also reported cases of HIV-2.

HIV-1 transferred to humans from the chimpanzee around 1890–1920 in south-central Cameroon, or in what is known today as the Democratic Republic of the Congo. Because the two different HIV viruses have subclasses, this transfer from ape to human occurred on several occasions, at least twice in the case of HIV-2 and four times for HIV-1. Spread from the original humans was accomplished in much the same way it is always spread, through the use of needles, sexual TRANSMISSION, or blood-to-blood contact. It is hypothesized that the virus traveled from Africa to the Americas via Haitian workers employed in Africa in the 1960s, and from Haiti on to the United States and elsewhere. Prior to the 1980s epidemic, there were several instances when the virus spread but did not cause an epidemic. A teenager in St. Louis died in 1969 of disseminated Kaposi's sarcoma (see HUMAN HERPES VIRUS 8), and his tissue was tested many years later and found to be positive for HIV. A Canadian woman died in 1981 after spending time doing social work with SEX WORKERS in Haiti, and a Danish surgeon died in 1977 after returning home from many years in Zaire. In the 1970s, at least five men in New York and a dozen in Europe died of symptoms that in the 1980s became recognized as AIDS. More than 50 deaths in Zaire from the 1970s have now been proven to have been caused by AIDS, showing that the virus existed before the epidemic struck. All of these early cases show that the virus was spreading undetected to many areas of the world long before it became recognized as an epidemic.

How HIV Works

HIV can enter the blood in several ways: through sharing of needles by INJECTION DRUG USE(R)s; through accidental cuts and bleeds, such as among medical personnel treating a person who is HIV positive; through blood transfusions or blood products that have not been tested prior to use; and through unprotected sexual encounters with someone who is already HIV positive. Once HIV is in the blood, it moves toward cells that it can infect—immune system cells—generally in the lymph nodes of the body. Once it locates CD4 T lymphocyte cells, HIV matches up to the cell receptors and binds to the cell, allowing the passage of viral RNA into the cell. HIV does this by matching proteins to the cell. There are two different proteins that must match up between HIV and the cell in order for HIV to pass on information that will cause the human cell to begin making more copies of the virus. The first is glycoprotein 120 (gp120), which is displayed on the surface of the virus after it has entered the body. The gp120 seeks out receptors on cells; in particular, there are receptors for gp120 on CD4 cells as well as on some macrophages. Once the gp120 has allowed the virus to bind to the cell, the virus then uses another small protein, gp41, to insert another binding key and allow the virus RNA to be emptied into the CD4 cell.

The surface of the CD4 cell contains a type of protein known as CCR5 (chemokine receptor type 5). This is a genetically encoded protein in humans. Most HIV, when it enters the body, seeks out this CCR5 protein on the surface of cells. This is the preferred entry coreceptor that HIV needs, but not the only one that it can use. Another coreceptor is known as CXCR4 (also called fusin in some articles). The virus that uses CXCR4 can act differently than the virus that uses CCR5, but the end result is generally the same—a weakened immune system over the long term if the virus is not stopped. About 10 percent of people of European descent have a genetically altered CCR5 gene, and HIV is unable to bind to the CD4 cells, effectively making the individual immune to most natural HIV infections. People who have two copies of this genetic difference make up the 10 percent; individuals who have one copy of this CCR5-delta 32 genetic mutation seem to have a delayed response to the virus and can maintain their immune system for an extended period. They are commonly known as long-term nonprogressors. It is not known how this mutation evolved, but it is thought that

it may have been the result of building immunity to the bubonic plague in the Middle Ages.

Once the connection between the virus and the cell has been established, the virus passes its RNA into the cell. The RNA is copied into the DNA of the cell using the viral enzyme reverse transcriptase, which creates DNA of the virus out of the RNA. This new DNA is carried into the cell's DNA through the viral protein integrase. This DNA is then known as a provirus, as it can now create viral proteins after infection. The DNA then creates messenger RNA, which can carry the instructions for creating new viral RNA out of the cell nucleus to the edge of the cell. Once at the edge of the cell, the proteins there use the enzyme protease to cut the polypeptides, the long chains of viral proteins created by the cell nucleus, into smaller pieces ready to infect other cells. The cell membrane allows the virus particles to slip out, taking a piece of the cell membrane to use as a new coat, without destroying the cell, allowing the production of new viral particles to continue indefinitely. The newly released viral cell then goes about looking for other CD4 cells or macrophages to infect to continue the process.

The drugs created through research have predominantly focused on the various enzymes of the virus to cause certain steps in the process to be halted. PROTEASE INHIBITORS try to stop the protease from cutting and creating new viral particles ready to leave the cell. Reverse transcriptase inhibitors (see NON-NUCLEOSIDE REVERSE TRANSCRIPTASE INHIBITORS) try to stop the enzyme reverse transcriptase from copying the viral RNA into DNA. INTEGRASE INHIBITORS try to stop the enzyme integrase from allowing the new viral DNA to be integrated into the cell's DNA. Unless these drugs are successful in stopping viral reproduction, it continues indefinitely. This eventually leads to the person's immune cells' slowly dwindling until there are no cells left to fight infection, allowing the potential for a number of diseases.

AVERT: AVERTing HIV and AIDS. "The Origin of HIV and the First Cases of AIDS." AVERT.org. Available online. URL: http://www.avert.org/origin-aids-hiv.htm. Accessed March 20, 2011.

BBC News. "Colonial Clue to the Rise of HIV." BBC. Available online. URL: http://news.bbc.co.uk/2/hi/health/7646255.stm. Accessed March 12, 2011.

Beaumont, Peter. "Primate Offers Missing Link to Ancestor of the AIDS Virus." *Guardian.* Available online. URL: http://www.guardian.co.uk/science/2008/dec/18/lemur-clue-for-aids-research. Accessed March 12, 2011.

Bowdler, Neil. "Key HIV Strain 'Came from Haiti.'" BBC. Available online. URL: http://news.bbc.co.uk/2/hi/health/7068574.stm. Accessed March 20, 2011.

Brown, David. "Researchers Say Antiretroviral (ART) Drugs May Prevent HIV Infection." *Washington Post.* Available online. URL: http://www.washingtonpost.com/wp-dyn/content/article/2010/02/19/AR2010021905215.html. Accessed March 20, 2011.

Buonaguro, L., M. L. Tornesello, and F. M. Buonaguro. "HIV-1 Subtype Distribution in the Worldwide Epidemic: Pathogenetic and Therapeutic Implications." *Journal of Virology* 81, no. 19 (18 October 2007): 10209–10219.

Chitnis, Amit, Diana Rawls, and Jim Moore. "Short Communication: Origin of HIV Type 1 in Colonial French Equatorial Africa?" UCSD.edu. Available online. URL: http://dss.ucsd.edu/~jmoore/publications/ChitnisEtAlHIVAIDSRes2000.pdf. Accessed March 20, 2011.

Hemelaar, Joris, Eleanor Gouws, Peter D. Ghys, and Saladin Osmanov. "Global and Regional Distribution of HIV-1 Genetic Subtypes and Recombinants in 2004." *AIDS* 20, no. 16 (24 October 2006): W13–W23.

Mayo Clinic Staff. "HIV/AIDS: Symptoms." MayoClinic.com. Available online. URL: http://www.mayoclinic.com/health/hiv-aids/DS00005/DSECTION=symptoms. Accessed March 20, 2011.

San Francisco AIDS Foundation. "The Stages of HIV Disease: HIV Is a Continuum." SFAF.org. Available online. URL: http://www.sfaf.org/aids101/hiv_disease.html. Accessed March 20, 2011.

Schmid, Randolph E. "New HIV Strain Discovered in Woman from Cameroon." ABC News. Available online. URL: http://abcnews.go.com/Health/wireStory?id=8233721. Accessed March 20, 2011.

Susman, Ed. "Antiretroviral Therapy Can Reduce Risk of HIV Transmission to Uninfected Sexual Partners." Pslgroup.com. Available online. URL: http://www.pslgroup.com/news/content.nsf/medicalnews/852576140048867C852576CF006E6E3E?OpenDocument&id=&count=10. Accessed March 20, 2011.

United States Department of Health and Human Services. "Adult and Adolescent Guidelines." aidsinfo.nih.gov. Available online. URL: http://aidsinfo.nih.gov/Guidelines/GuidelineHTML.aspx?GuidelineID=7&docID=1. Accessed March 20, 2011.

———. "HIV and Its Treatment: What You Should Know." aidsinfo.nih.gov. Available online. URL: http://aidsinfo.nih.gov/contentfiles/HIVandItsTreatment_cbrochure_en.pdf. Accessed March 20, 2011.

———, Agency for Healthcare Research and Quality. "Outcomes/Effectiveness Research: Patients with HIV Who Share Treatment Decisions with Their Doctor Have Better Outcomes." AHRQ.gov. Available online. URL: http://www.ahrq.gov/research/dec07/1207RA24.htm. Accessed March 20, 2011.

United States National Institute of Allergy and Infectious Diseases. "International HIV/AIDS Trial Finds Continuous Antiretroviral Therapy Superior to Episodic Therapy." NIH.gov. Available online. URL: http://www.nih.gov/news/pr/jan2006/niaid-18.htm. Accessed March 20, 2011.

———. "NIAID-Supported Scientists Discover Origin of HIV-1." NIH.gov. Available online. URL: http://www.niaid.nih.gov/news/newsreleases/1999/pages/hivorigin.aspx. Accessed March 20, 2011.

human papillomavirus (HPV) The human papillomavirus is a collection of more than 100 closely related viruses that cause warts in humans. All warts are caused by some variety of HPV. HPV types 1, 2, and 4 cause plantar warts or common warts on the feet and hands. HPV is spread through direct skin contact with another person or through virus particles that are shed from the wart. Common warts can be acquired easily through use of a towel or simply walking barefoot across a gym floor or in a shared shower. Scratching of the wart can increase the chance of spreading the virus. Nearly every human has been exposed to some variety of HPV. Warts are not as common in older people as they are in children, an indication that people build immunity to the virus as they age.

Certain HPV varieties cause warts in genital areas, such as the vagina, vulva, penis, cervix, or anus. Approximately 90 percent of genital warts, or warts acquired through sexual contact, are caused by HPV types 6 and 11. Sexually transmitted warts are also known as genital warts, venereal warts, or by their scientific name, condyloma acuminata. Genital warts are spread in the same manner as other HPV, through skin-to-skin contact, so touching the genital areas of someone who is infected with HPV can be all it takes to become infected. Condoms can prevent the spread of HPV but only in the areas that are covered by the condom, so if one's hand has contact with the virus, it can spread to his or her own genital area without difficulty.

HPV is the most common sexually transmitted infection (STI) and is found in more than 50 percent of sexually active people at some time in their life. It is more predominant in young adults and teenagers because they are at the age when people first begin having sex and have the opportunity to be exposed to the virus.

Symptoms and Diagnostic Path

Genital warts are generally painless, though they can cause some itching. Often they are small and difficult to see or feel. They can initially appear as small pink or reddish bumps. Sometimes they can cluster in groups, creating larger growths. They can be located in any or all areas that can be involved in sexual activities: penis, testicles, anus, urethra, vagina, vulva, cervix, and even the mouth and throat. It is also possible to have no outward sign of infection, no warts at all, yet still pass on the virus to other people. After exposure, a person will generally develop warts within a one- to six-month time frame, though it has been shown to be possible for warts to develop up to three years after exposure.

Diagnosis is made by a doctor, usually with a visual check of the area involved. For women who have an annual Papanicolaou test (also known as a Pap smear or Pap test), the check for HPV is part of the test. It has become more common for men to have a Pap smear during regular physical examinations because of the links between HPV and other conditions. A Pap test is a simple process in which the doctor uses a cotton swab or similar device to wipe a sample of tissue from an area, usually the cervix or the anus. This swab is then examined for any irregularities in the cells. It is called a Pap smear because it was named for the physician who invented the test, Georgios Papanicolaou. A blood sample can also be used to diagnose whether a person has been infected with HPV. In the last several years, it has been discovered that some varieties of HPV are linked to the development of precancerous lesions or cancer in certain areas of the body. HPV varieties 16, 18, 31, 33, 35, 39, 45, 51, 52, 56, 58, 59, 66, 68, and 73 have been linked to a number of cancers in men and women, including cervical cancer, anal cancer, vaginal and vulval cancers, penile cancer, and some oropharyngeal cancers. These types of HPV are not as common as the majority of HPV genital wart types but can be contracted in the same manner. HPV can cause changes in the skin in the areas mentioned. These types of changes are called dysplasia. *Dysplasia* is also a word that can be used to mean precancerous, meaning it is more likely to become a cancer than normal skin or mucous membrane. The types of dysplasia caused by HPV also have more specific terms. Anal intraepithelial neoplasia (AIN) and cervical intraepithelial neoplasia (CIN) are conditions in which a person has some abnormal tissue in those specific areas of the body, and those areas must be watched more closely for cancerous development. That is why people who have had HPV are advised to have an annual Pap smear during their regular physical examinations.

Treatment Options and Outlook

Treatment for genital warts is similar to the treatment for a wart on other parts of the body. Warts can be removed through freezing them with liquid nitrogen, chemically "burning" them off the area involved, or surgically removing that portion of the skin involved. The size or location of the genital warts can determine which method is used. On occasion, a cream or ointment that can slowly remove the warts will be prescribed. Removal of the warts does not remove the virus from a person's body. Warts can also disappear on their own or may return in the same or different locations.

CIN and AIN are treated differently because some dysplasias can develop into a cancer if not treated properly. There are different levels of dysplasia, usually numbered, such as CIN 1, CIN 2, or CIN 3. The higher the number, the more severe the dysplasia. This numbering is also used for other dysplasias such as AIN, vulvar intraepithelial neoplasia (VIN), or vaginal intraepithelial neoplasia (VAIN). There are most often no symptoms for any of the intraepithelial neoplasias. On occasion, there may be bleeding in more serious cases or a visible mass that may also be felt. A colposcope, a small microscope that can be inserted into the vaginal or anal opening, may be used for visual diagnosis of dysplasias. Biopsies of the lesions or mass may also indicate the severity of the condition and assist the physician in determining a specific treatment.

Treatment for CIN usually involves the removal of the dysplasia. This can be done in several ways, including laser treatment, freezing, burning the tissue, or surgical cutting away of the dysplasia. Frequent exams after such treatment will assure that the dysplasia was completely removed and has not returned. If dysplasias return, more significant surgical removal of the tissue may be required. For dysplasias that have developed into cervical cancer, the treatment is much more serious, involving radiation therapy or a radical hysterectomy and lymph node removal in the area. Similar treatments for vaginal and vulvar dysplasias will be followed. For cancer of the vulva or vagina, the surgical removal of the area can have serious consequences. Treatment for AIN is also similar; the least invasive method is chosen to restrict potential problems from developing with normal body excretory functions. Lesions may be treated with freezing or burning techniques, and there are topical ointments that can also be used

to treat lesions in or around the anus. Recent treatment with infrared light has also been shown to be effective in many cases. Radiation therapy for advanced dysplasias in the anal area is not part of standard treatment and is only used in cases involving anal cancers. Any of these cancers is usually treated by a specialist in that area of medicine.

Other cancers that are associated with HPV are cancer of the penis and oropharyngeal squamous cell cancers, which are cancers of the throat and neck areas. Treatment of these cancers does not differ for HIV-positive people and HIV-negative people. Cancers of the oropharyngeal areas caused by HPV have much higher rates of treatment success than those caused by other means.

People who are HIV positive have much higher rates of all of these conditions caused by HPV than do people who are HIV negative. It is known from studies that treatment of HIV with HAART does not seem to alter the course of the dysplasias or cancers associated with HPV. It does not slow the progression, improve the outlook, or cause further development, and it does not seem to affect whether or not a person develops warts at all. Recommendations from the government on the treatment of HPV-related conditions all call for regular screening and testing for dysplasias and cancers in patients who have HIV.

Risk Factors and Preventive Measures
HPV can be acquired through sexual activity, and, therefore, those who have more frequent sexual activity with a greater number of people increase their risk of acquiring the virus. As noted earlier, the incidence rate for HPV in the United States is higher than 50 percent of sexually active people. Young people who are just becoming sexually active are at greatest risk for acquiring the virus. Condoms can protect only areas of the body that are covered so are not effective at preventing all TRANSMISSION of the virus. People who are HIV positive are at greater risk of developing cancers associated with HPV and, therefore, need to be more vigilant in treating and following up treatment of genital warts.

There are now vaccines available to prevent certain strains of HPV. Gardasil is the brand name for one such vaccine, which prevents HPV strains 6, 11, 16, and 18. Strains 16 and 18 are responsible for more than 70 percent of all cervical cancer cases in the United States. Strains 6 and 11 are responsible for more than 90 percent of all genital warts. Currently, Gardasil is given to girls and women ages nine to 23 who have not previously been exposed to HPV. Gardasil is a series of three shots given over the course of six months. Patients need all three shots to build complete immunity to the virus. The vaccine is not effective in people who have already been exposed to HPV or have had genital warts. Recently, Gardasil has also been shown effective in young men in the prevention of HPV but is not yet approved for that use nor widely used among men at this time.

The other available HPV vaccine, Cervarix, is available only in Europe and Australia but has not yet been approved for use in the United States. Cervarix protects only against HPV types 16 and 18, the predominant cancer-causing strains of the virus.

AIDSmeds. "Hetero Men Also at Risk for Anal HPV." AIDSmap.com. Available online. URL: http://www. aidsmeds.com/articles/hiv_hpv_anal_1667_14406. shtml. Accessed on March 20, 2011.

Bloomberg News. "Merck Cancer Shot Cuts Genital Warts and Lesions in Men (Update 2)." Bloomberg. com. Available online. URL: http://www.bloomberg. com/apps/news?pid=20601202&sid=aajzweDaXZh0&refer=healthcare. Accessed March 20, 2011.

Carter, Michael. "Infrared Treatment for Pre-Cancerous Anal Lesions in HIV-Positive Patients Safe and Has Good Outcomes." AIDSmap.com. Available online. URL: http://www.aidsmap.org/en/news/9D28C5CC-3B04-42B7-A7FF-5DCB6788D642. asp. Accessed March 20, 2011

Centers for Disease Control and Prevention. "Frequently Asked Questions about HPV Vaccine Safety." CDC.gov. Available online. URL: http://www. cdc.gov/vaccinesafety/Vaccines/HPV/hpv_faqs. html. Accessed March 20, 2011.

———. "STD Facts—Human Papillomavirus (HPV)." CDC.gov. Available online. URL: http://www.cdc.

gov/STD/HPV/STDFact-HPV.htm. Accessed March 20, 2011.

Hill-Kayser, Christine. "Anal Cancer: The Basics." Oncolink.com. Available online. URL: http://www. oncolink.com/types/article.cfm?c=5&s=10&ss=776&id=9497. Accessed March 20, 2011.

Immunization Action Coalition. "HPV Vaccine: What You Need to Know." Immunize.org. Available online. URL: http://www.immunize.org/vis/hpv. pdf. Accessed March 20, 2011.

National Cancer Institute. "Human Papillomaviruses (HPV) and Cancer." Cancer.gov. Available online. URL: http://www.cancer.gov/cancertopics/factsheet/risk/HPV. Accessed March 20, 2011.

———. "Human Papillomavirus: The Basics." The Body.com. Available online. URL: http://www.the body.com/content/art5109.html. Accessed March 20, 2011.

Palefsky, Joel. "Biology of HPV in HIV Infection." *Advances in Dental Research* 19, no. 1 (April 2006): 99–105.

Pereira, A., et al. "Prevalence and Factors Associated with Anal Lesions Mediated by Human Papillomavirus in Men with HIV/AIDS." *International Journal of STD & AIDS* 19, no. 3 (2008): 192–196. Available online. URL: http://ijsa.rsmjournals.com/cgi/content/abstract/19/3/192. Accessed March 20, 2011.

Project Inform. "HPV and HIV." TheBody.com. Available online. URL: http://www.thebody.com/content/art5108.html. Accessed March 20, 2011.

Shenefelt, Phillip D. "Nongenital Warts." eMedicine. com. Available online. URL: http://www.emedicine. com/derm/topic457.htm. Accessed March 20, 2011.

United States National Institute of Allergy and Infectious Diseases. "Human Papillomavirus and Genital Warts." NIH.gov. Available online. URL: http://www3.niaid.nih.gov/topics/genitalWarts/. Accessed March 20, 2011.

hydroxyurea Hydroxyurea is an antineoplastic drug that has been used in conjunction with antiretroviral medications in the treatment of HIV. An antineoplastic drug is one that is effective at stopping neoplasms, the abnormal growth of cells. It is used predominantly for blood cancers and blood disorders, such as sickle-cell disease. It stops the reproduction of cells in the bone marrow, thereby lessening the reproduction of blood cell disorders. It is never prescribed alone in the treatment of HIV, as it does not affect HIV at all, but it has been used as part of combination therapy because it increases the effectiveness of some NUCLEOSIDE REVERSE TRANSCRIPTASE INHIBITORS (NRTIs). It has been used in the past in conjunction with DIDANOSINE and STAVUDINE. It is not approved by the U.S. FOOD AND DRUG ADMINISTRATION (FDA) for use in the treatment of HIV, but nevertheless has been prescribed for that purpose and may continue to be used in that manner.

Hydroxyurea is the common name used for the drug, but it is also known by a variety of trade names (Hydrea, Droxia), as well as the official common name hydroxycarbamide. It is manufactured by Bristol-Myers Squibb.

Dosage

In studies that were conducted for the treatment of HIV, one 500 mg pill twice a day was the given dosage. Some studies have used lesser doses, which did not seem to lessen the effect of the drug. There is no set dosage for treatment of HIV in CHILDREN, as no studies have advanced to the point of treating children with the medication.

Drug Interactions

Hydroxyurea was studied because of its interactions with other drugs. It interferes with the enzymes needed to build cells. Because it blocks these enzymes, cells that multiply rapidly such as neoplasms are forcibly slowed. It works well with NRTIs because these drugs imitate some of these same building blocks. HIV chooses the false building blocks to try to reproduce, but cannot because they do not contain the proper enzymes. Hydroxyurea slows the normal cells from reproducing, thereby increasing the opportunity for HIV to choose the wrong building blocks and further complicating the reproductive process of HIV. In particular, hydroxyurea has performed well with didanosine and stavudine in studies.

Hydroxyurea should not be taken in conjunction with ZIDOVUDINE because both drugs can interfere with bone marrow production, potentially causing problems for patients.

Side Effects

Side effects of hydroxyurea were problematic in the research studies. Because hydroxyurea slows cell production, HIV-positive patients in the studies did not see large gains in their CD4 cells. These cells were slowed in their production as well as other cells. Although viral load reduction was good, cell growth was not, and for people in need of repairing their immune system cells with healthy cells, this approach was viewed as counterproductive.

Hydroxyurea also intensified the side effects of didanosine and stavudine, namely, peripheral NEUROPATHY incidents, which increased during the studies. It also increased the risk for pancreatitis, a potentially life-threatening inflammation of the pancreas. Hydroxyurea also causes bone marrow suppression, leading to lowered red blood cell counts (anemia) and lowered white blood cell counts (neutropenia or leukopenia). It also can cause lowered platelet counts (thrombocytopenia), which can lead to excessive bleeding. People who already have low CD4 counts, especially below 200, or previous bone marrow suppression problems should not use hydroxyurea.

The drug is known to have potential to cause birth defects. Pregnant women or women who may become pregnant should not use hydroxyurea.

Side effects of high doses of hydroxyurea during cancer treatment include nausea, headache, vomiting, hair loss, weight gain, and changes in skin color. The problems with hydroxyurea have caused research into its use as a potential drug in the fight against HIV to be stopped. It has not been approved for use for HIV but is available for use in cancer treatment, as well as in other illnesses. Some HIV-positive people may still be taking it as part of some form of antiretroviral treatment. A doctor should closely monitor blood counts and monitor the patient for signs of pancreatitis.

AIDSInfoNet. "Hydroxyurea (Hydrea)." AIDSInfoNet. org. Available online. URL: http://www.aidsinfo net.org/fact_sheets/view/427. Accessed March 20, 2011.

AIDSmeds. "Droxia." AIDSmeds.com. Available online. URL: http://www.aidsmeds.com/archive/Droxia_ 1901.shtml. Accessed March 20, 2011.

AIDS Treatment Data Network. "Simple Fact Sheets: Hydroxyurea (Hydrea)." AEGIS.com. Available online. URL: http://www.aegis.com/factshts/net work/simple/hydr.html. Accessed March 20, 2011.

MedLinePlus. "Hydroxyurea: MedlinePlus Drug Infor- mation." NIH.gov. Available online. URL: http:// www.nlm.nih.gov/medlineplus/druginfo/meds/ a682004.html. Accessed March 20, 2011.

I

immigration and travel Immigration is the act of moving to live in a country other than the country of one's birth. Usually this is done as a means of seeking employment, an increase in opportunity for a person or a family, or, in some instances, as an escape from an ongoing civil conflict or other threat to one's self. With the spread of HIV during the past 30 years, countries all over the world have set up barriers against people with HIV or AIDS to protect their own citizens or to protect the stability of their health care system. In response, the WORLD HEALTH ORGANIZATION (WHO) has offered admonitions that HIV-positive people are not a threat to countries or their health systems in most instances.

The WHO has stated on different occasions that there is no solid reason for restrictions on travel, entry, or immigration from a public health viewpoint. HIV is not communicable through casual contact, as are TUBERCULOSIS and severe acute respiratory syndrome (SARS). WHO also refers to restrictions on travel and immigration as discriminatory and potentially harmful to the country and people affected by the regulations. The restrictions can foster an attitude of discrimination and stigma for people affected by HIV and cause fear or hate of foreign travelers or of people who have HIV. A belief that citizens of a country must be protected against foreigners is not uncommon in countries with such restrictions. Such regulations also imply that the HIV-positive person cannot or will not act responsibly in their relations and will spread the virus willingly or maliciously. Regulations against HIV-positive travelers can lead to problems discussing HIV in general, fostering a belief

that the virus has been kept out of the country and is not a concern within the country because of the regulations. Travel and immigration regulations create a sense of fear among HIV-positive travelers or migrants that can lead them to lie to enter a country, hide their medications and HIV status, and thereby create a culture of fear and silence. This can cause more problems for the country and the individual in the long run, as misconceptions may prevent the country from providing education or the individual from seeking proper treatment.

Some countries have all-purpose bans on HIV-positive people. Questions on visa forms, or entry forms, ask whether a person is HIV positive. If the answer is yes, that country can refuse entry to an individual for that reason alone. Border agencies often examine luggage and refuse entry to people who have antiretroviral medications. As of early 2011, there were 11 countries that banned even short-term stays of HIV positive people outright in their country or required a disclosure of HIV infection for even a short stay: Brunei, Equatorial Guinea, Iraq, Jordan, Papua New Guinea, Qatar, Singapore, Solomon Islands, Sudan, United Arab Emirates, and Yemen. China had been on this list but lifted the restrictions prior to the 2008 Beijing Olympics under pressure from many sources. Suriname has recently passed regulations requiring people from specific resource-poor countries to disclose their HIV status, and now requires papers detailing the existence of health insurance for travelers from those regions. Although visitors have the option to lie on required forms regarding their HIV status, border agencies and employees are often given wide-ranging leeway in enforcement of laws to bar entry to people suspected of being HIV positive or to bar people carrying antiretroviral medications. Stories of refusal of entry, immediate deportation, and jail time in some instances have been recorded in nations listed as banning immigration and travel because of HIV.

The United States, despite internal opposition from activists as well as external opposition from the WHO and several governments, maintained restrictive policies toward most HIV-positive travelers and immigrants until the ban was lifted on January 4, 2010. Restrictions were initially written by the U.S. Public Health Service (PHS) in 1987 when the PHS added HIV and AIDS to the list of reasons for excluding someone from applying for immigration to the United States. It became one of 33 different reasons, including "contagious" diseases, that excluded someone applying for citizenship. The Immigration and Naturalization Service (INS) began testing applicants for HIV as part of their immigration application. The Immigration Act of 1990 completely revised the grounds for exclusion. It also permitted for the first time a waiver of exclusion on health-related grounds for permanent resident and visa applications. Early in 1993, then-president Clinton indicated that he would remove HIV as one of the reasons for exclusion. The PHS drafted regulations to match the Clinton decision. In reaction to these moves, the opposition party–controlled U.S. Congress passed the National Institutes of Health Revitalization Act of 1993, which specifically codified HIV infection as a grounds for exclusion for visas and resident applications. This created a statutory ban on the admission of people with HIV to this country. In 2008, the U.S. Senate, under continuing pressure, passed the reauthorization bill for the President's Emergency Plan for AIDS Relief (PEPFAR), which President George W. Bush had requested. Attached to this bill was the change in the law activists had long sought. Although technically the law requiring that visitors to the United States be only HIV negative has been changed, the Department of Health and Human Services (HHS) has not yet written the rules that will implement the law. President Bush's HHS staff simply ignored the rule, leaving the task of writing the new rules to the Obama administration. Once the Obama administration was in place, one of their first acts was to draft rules that removed HIV as a reason to block admission or immigration to the United States. South Korea also recently removed the HIV restriction as a block to travel there.

Before the recent change, it had been illegal to immigrate to this country or work in the United States for an extended time if one were HIV positive. People had to apply for a waiver to this rule under several different circumstances; these included being the spouse, unmarried son, unmarried daughter, or unmarried adopted child of a U.S. citizen or legal permanent resident; the parent of a son or daughter who was a U.S. citizen or legal permanent resident; or a refugee or asylum seeker who fell under a "humanitarian" exception to the HIV ban. There are other instances, also, but these were the most commonly filed reasons for waivers. There are specific classes of people who, even though they may normally be eligible for immigration or extended visa stays, are not allowed under the ban on HIV-infected people. These include people eligible for extended work visas, visa lottery picks, brothers and sisters of citizens of permanent residents, and adult children of permanent residents or citizens. There have been cases of HIV-positive people filing for asylum status in the United States because of the threat to them by their government or people in their native country. These cases are not generally publicized, but the people are on record as having gained asylum based on their HIV status.

The ban on travel created a great many problems for HIV-positive travelers in the United States and these other countries. Travelers were known to mail or ship medications to themselves or friends and relatives ahead of time to avoid carrying their medications with them. They were known to take a "holiday" from their antiretroviral medications, thereby putting themselves at higher risk for illness because the virus was not under control while they were not taking their medications. This could also allow RESISTANCE to the medications, as a physician was not monitoring their drug holiday.

There are currently 6.7 billion people in the world. Each year nearly one in every seven people—approximately 900 million—travel internationally, leaving their home to go to another country. There are 191 million people employed in a place other than the country of their citizenship. There are nearly 21 million refugees who have fled their native country. It is estimated that 40 million people are living with HIV world-wide. Given these numbers, it is not difficult to see the scope of the prolems both in trying to stop HIV-positive people from traveling or migrating for work and in preventing them from entering specific countries. Yet, despite these numbers, and United Nations attempts to change the thinking of these governments, nations continue to attempt to ban HIV-positive people from traveling, living, and working in them.

In addition to the 11 countries mentioned earlier, the following countries deport HIV-positive people if their status is found out either during a visit or during the time they are applying for worker status or have already been working and living in the country: Armenia, Bahrain, Bangladesh, Bulgaria, China, Hungary, North Korea, Kuwait, Malaysia, Moldova, Mongolia, Russia, Saudi Arabia, Singapore, Syria, Tajikistan, Taiwan, and Uzbekistan. In addition, there are 32 nations that have special restrictions regarding HIV-positive people. There are also 33 countries that have vague, randomly enforced, or unstated and contradictory regulations regarding HIV-positive people.

Deutsche AIDS-Hilfe. "HIVTravel." HIVTravel.org. Available online. URL: http://www.hivtravel.org/. Accessed March 20, 2011.

Human Rights Watch. "Discrimination, Denial, and Deportation." HRW.org. Available online. URL: http://www.hrw.org/en/reports/2009/06/18/discrimina tion-denial-and-deportation. Accessed March 20, 2011.

Immigration Equality. "HIV Ban Is History." ImmigrationEquality.org. Available online. URL: http://www.immigrationequality.org/template.php?page id=5. Accessed March 20, 2011.

International AIDS Society. "Denying Entry, Stay and Residence Due to HIV Status." TheBody.com. Available online. URL: http://img.thebody.com/ias/2009/travel_restrictions_English_WEB.pdf. Accessed March 20, 2011.

McNeil, Donald G., Jr. "Discrimination in Visa Laws Poses Risk to Those with AIDS, Rights Group Says." *New York Times*. Available online. URL: http://www.nytimes.com/2009/06/23/health/23glob.html?_r=2&emc=eta1. Accessed March 20, 2011.

Neilson, Victoria. "HIV-Based Persecution in Asylum and Immigration Decisions." *Human Rights Magazine* (Fall 2004). Available online. URL: http://www.abanet.org/irr/hr/fall04/persecution.htm. Accessed March 20, 2011.

UNAIDS: Joint United Nations Programme on HIV/AIDS. "HIV-Related Travel Restrictions." UNAIDS.org. Available online. URL: http://www.unaids.org/en/KnowledgeCentre/Resources/FeatureStories/archive/2008/20080304_HIVrelated_travel_restrictions.asp. Accessed March 20, 2011.

immune reconstitution inflammatory syndrome (IRIS)   IRIS is a collection of symptoms that began appearing in HIV patients after HIGHLY ACTIVE ANTIRETROVIRAL THERAPY (HAART) was initiated in the mid-1990s. It is also called immune reconstitution syndrome (IRS) or immune reconstitution disease (IRD). IRIS is not an illness in and of itself, but a reaction to a particular illness and the body's sudden ability to recognize and fight an illness that was already active.

Symptoms and Diagnostic Path

Most people respond well when they start HIV treatment with antiretroviral medications, with rises in their CD4 T cell count and a corresponding drop in their viral load. However, there are some people who respond to HAART with a surprising relapse into an illness that was previously treated or thought cured, or a response to a previously unknown illness that had not been treated. IRIS can appear anywhere from a few weeks to a few months after initiation of HAART. The most common time frame is between two and six weeks after beginning the treatment. It has not been extensively studied, but appears to occur in people whose immune system was very weak when they started antiretroviral treatment, most often those who had CD4 T cell counts lower than 100. Inflammation is the swelling, redness, or soreness associated with a part of the body that is involved in an injury or illness. The body requires immune cells to fight off illnesses, and so numerous cells are sent to an area of the body where there is an injury. This results in the common swelling, aches, and pains of an injury's healing. When a person has HIV and the immune system has been very weak, it is believed that the body has not been able to respond properly to different illnesses that have been present in the body for a while. Once the immune system begins regeneration with the assistance of HAART, it suddenly detects an illness that it had been unable to respond to previously and goes into overdrive, so to speak, to respond to it, sending an array of HUMAN IMMUNE SYSTEM cells to the region to fight the illness.

When IRIS occurs, it does so most often in people who have mycobacterial infections. Studies reveal about two in every five cases of IRIS involve either TUBERCULOSIS (TB) or *MYCOBACTE-RIUM AVIUM* COMPLEX (MAC). Other illnesses that have been known to initiate an IRIS event are CYTOMEGALOVIRUS (CMV), HEPATITIS B and HEPA-TITIS C, herpes, HUMAN PAPILLOMAVIRUS (HPV), Kaposi's sarcoma, PROGRESSIVE MULTIFOCAL LEU-KOENCEPHALOPATHY (PML), and *PNEUMOCYSTIS PNEUMONIA* (PCP).

Treatment Options and Outlook

There is no standard treatment for IRIS, as the illnesses that activate the immune response differ. Diagnosis and treatment of the instigating illness are the best way to control the symptoms of IRIS. If IRIS symptoms are detected, a doctor may suggest anti-inflammatory medications

such as aspirin, ibuprofen, and naproxen. These are available at most drugstores. Corticosteroids may also be used in more severe cases to decrease the inflammation.

Some cases of IRIS can be life threatening. The body produces such a powerful immune response that the swelling, inflammation, and associated fever can cause more problems than the illness itself. Some studies have shown that treatment with leukotriene inhibitors, such as those used to treat asthma attacks, may have a beneficial effect in cases of IRIS.

On the other side of the coin, although these symptoms in most cases can be bothersome and not life threatening, they also are a good sign that the body is strengthening its immune system. Some studies have suggested that people who show an IRIS response after initializing treatment do better in the long run in returning to good general health with their HIV under control.

Risk Factors and Preventive Measures

People at most risk for developing IRIS are those who have extremely weakened immune systems when they start antiretroviral treatment. Other potential risk factors are starting treatment during an infection with a particular illness, especially those mentioned earlier. A shorter interval between beginning antiretroviral treatment and receiving diagnosis and treatment for an illness makes IRIS likelier to occur. Another risk is to those people who have the greatest drop in viral load due to HAART treatment, drops of 2.5 logarithmic units (logs) or more. A log is a way of measuring viral load. It refers to the number 10 to a specific power, or exponent. A two-log drop in viral load is written 10^2 and indicates 100 times. So, if a viral load is measured at 1,000,000 copies of virus and has a two-log drop, the viral load is then at 10,000 copies of virus. It is also possible to have IRIS symptoms if a person has been off HAART medication for a while and restarts treatment with antiretrovirals.

Prevention of IRIS is often not considered a reason for delaying initiation of HAART, particularly because most people benefit from HAART.

It may become an issue if proper tests have been run and it is determined there is a triggering illness that needs to be treated first before HAART is started. TB and MAC are such examples. Some doctors have begun to treat these illnesses first in HIV-positive people, before starting HAART, to lower the risk development of IRIS.

AIDS Education and Training Centers. "Immune Reconstitution Syndrome." AIDSetc.org. Available online. URL: http://www.aidsetc.org/aidsetc?page=cm-304_immune. Accessed March 20, 2011.

Cheonis, Nicholas. "Immune Reconstitution Syndrome." TheBody.com. Available online. URL: http://www.thebody.com/content/treat/art2525.html. Accessed March 20, 2011.

Jacobson, Mark A. "Clinical Implications of Immune Reconstitution in AIDS." Available online. URL: HIVInSite.ucsf.edu. http://www.hivinsite.org/InSite?page=kb-03-04-03. Accessed March 20, 2011.

Murdoch, David M., Willem D. F. Venter, Annelies Van Rie, and Charles Feldman. "Immune Reconstitution Inflammatory Syndrome (IRIS): Review of Common Infectious Manifestations and Treatment Options." *AIDS Research and Therapy* 4, no. 9 (2007). Available online. URL: http://www.aidsrestherapy.com/content/4/1/9. Accessed March 20, 2011.

Project Inform. "IRIS: A Concern for People Starting HIV Therapy." ProjectInform.org. Available online. URL: http://www.projectinform.org/info/iris/index.shtml. Accessed March 20, 2011.

indinavir Indinavir was first approved for use in the United States in 1996. It was one of the first PROTEASE INHIBITORS (PIs) approved for use in the treatment of HIV in combinations with other drugs. It is manufactured by Merck and Company and sold under the trade name Crixivan. Its three-letter abbreviation is IDV. It may also be called indinavir sulfate in some research materials. There is no formulation of the drug for CHILDREN, and it is approved only for adults and teenagers who have HIV.

Dosage

Indinavir is approved by the U.S. FOOD AND DRUG ADMINISTRATION (FDA), to be taken as two 400 mg capsules three times a day (every eight hours). Indinavir should be taken on an empty stomach, meaning a person should not eat for two hours prior to taking a dose of indinavir or for one hour afterward. This was the dosage specified by the FDA in 1996.

A second method of dosage is used more frequently. This involves two doses of indinavir taken with ritonavir each day. Different doctors use several different combinations of ritonavir and indinavir: 400 mg of indinavir plus 400 mg of ritonavir, 800 mg of indinavir plus 100 mg of ritonavir, or 800 mg of indinavir plus 200 mg of ritonavir. All of these doses are taken twice a day. These have not been officially approved by the FDA.

Indinavir is not one of the recommended medications for initial treatment of HIV. People who have not taken medication before are advised to choose one of several other options. However, it is a recommended medication when combined with ritonavir for people for whom a PI-based drug regimen has failed in the past.

Drug Interactions

Indinavir interacts with many HIV medications. It is not recommended that indinavir and ATAZANAVIR SULFATE be taken at the same time, as both can cause hyperbilirubinemia, a rise in the bilirubin levels in the blood, causing a yellowing of the eyes and nails. The multidrug pill KALETRA increases the amount of indinavir in the body. If they are prescribed together, the recommended dosage of indinavir is 600 mg twice a day with Kaletra. Indinavir increases the amount of SAQUINAVIR in the body. NELFINAVIR increases the amount of indinavir, and indinavir increases the amount of nelfinavir in the body.

Indinavir also interacts with NON-NUCLEOSIDE REVERSE TRANSCRIPTASE INHIBITORS (NNRTIs), another type of anti-HIV medication. EFAVIRENZ and NEVIRAPINE both decrease the amount of indinavir in the body. Indinavir doses should be increased to 1,000 mg for each dose if it is prescribed at the same time as either of these

NNRTIs. DELAVIRDINE increases the amount of indinavir available in the body and the quantity should be reduced to 600 mg of indinavir at each dose.

The drug interacts with a number of other medications including the cholesterol-lowering drugs simvastatin and lovastatin, antibiotics used to treat infections such as TUBERCULOSIS, antidepressant or antipsychotic medications, and medications to fight some fungal infections. It should not be taken with any drugs containing ergot, which is used in many migraine medications. It is important that a doctor know and understand all the medications and supplements a person is using when prescribing indinavir.

Indinavir also increases the amount of the drugs sildenafil (Viagra), vardenafil (Levitra), and tadalafil (Cialis)—all erectile dysfunction medications—in the blood and therefore can cause serious side effects. Lowering the dosage of these medications is recommended to prevent potential complications.

Indinavir increases the amount of estrogen-based birth control pill medication in the body. There is usually no recommended dosage change in the oral contraceptive.

St. John's wort, an herbal supplement, should never be taken with a PI, as it has been shown to reduce the amount of PI in the body greatly. Other supplements that may affect the level of indinavir in the body include garlic pills and milk thistle supplements.

Side Effects

The major drawback to the use of indinavir is the potential to develop crystals in the urine. This can lead to kidney stones, in addition to kidney pain, back pain, and difficulties in urination. These events occur more frequently in younger people who use indinavir. People who use indinavir are strongly encouraged to drink at least six eight-ounce glasses of water each day to prevent the formation of urine crystals and kidney stones.

Protease inhibitors, as a class of drug, often increase the cholesterol and triglyceride levels of patients. High lipid levels have been recorded in some indinavir patients. This side effect can be managed with appropriate cholesterol-lowering medications. Indinavir has also been associated with treatment regimens that can cause LIPODYS-TROPHY, or the redistribution of fat within the body. Symptoms are increased fat around the neck and stomach area, facial wasting, breast enlargement, and peripheral wasting in the arms and legs. Some of these changes disappear when the drug is stopped.

Indinavir also has been linked to drier skin, brittle hair and nails, and dark patches on the skin called hyperpigmentation.

Other side effects include nausea, vomiting, headache, diarrhea, and loss of appetite. These side effects generally are of short duration and disappear after a person has used the medication awhile.

AIDS InfoNet. "Indinavir (Crixivan)." AIDSInfoNet.org. Available online. URL: http://www.aidsinfonet.org/fact_sheets/view/441. Accessed March 11, 2011.

AIDSmeds. "Crixivan (Indinavir)." AIDSmeds.com. Available online. URL: http://www.aidsmeds.com/archive/Crixivan_1557.shtml. Accessed March 11, 2011.

———. "Special Issues for Children with HIV." AIDS meds.com. Available online. URL: http://www.aids meds.com/articles/Children_7566.shtml. Accessed March 11, 2011.

The Body. "Crixivan (Indinavir)." TheBody.com. Available online. URL: http://www.thebody.com/index/treat/crixivan.html. Accessed March 11, 2011.

United States Department of Health and Human Services. "Indinavir." aidsinfo.nih.gov. Available online. URL: http://www.aidsinfo.nih.gov/DrugsNew/DrugDetailNT.aspx?int_id=233. Accessed March 11, 2011.

injection drug use(r) (IDU) An injection drug user (IDU) is a person who uses a hypodermic needle to inject drugs, legal or illegal. The term is used in most instances to refer to a person who is using illegal substances such as heroin, cocaine, steroids, or methamphetamines, but can also refer to someone who uses any injection medication such as insulin in the treatment of diabetes. Injection drug use in and of itself does not cause someone to contract HIV or AIDS. HIV is transmitted between IDUs when the needle is shared by different users without being sterilized or when the IDU cannot secure clean needles before using the drug.

Injection drug use is often a preferred way to administer a drug because the drug, whether legal or illegal, bypasses the filtering of the body and does what it was created to do directly. When a pill is swallowed, the stomach or the intestines break down the drug. The liver serves as the body's means of filtering the chemicals and lessening the impact of a substance on the body. Drugs introduced directly into the blood have a much stronger effect. IDUs generally use a hollow needle and a syringe, known in slang terms as the equipment or works, and inject the drugs intravenously, directly into a vein. Injection can also be done intramuscularly, into a muscle, or subcutaneously, just below the skin. Any of these methods bypasses the body's initial filtering systems. When it is done intravenously, the injector will generally pull back the plunger on the syringe to make sure it has entered a vein; when this is done, some blood will be drawn back into the syringe and the person will know it has entered the vein. When the drug is then injected, small amounts of blood are left in the syringe. This is why it is easy to for IDUs pass on viruses and other blood-borne illnesses to others. A second person who then uses the needle and syringe is injecting small amounts of another person's blood into his or her own, unless a thorough cleaning and sterilizing of the equipment are completed between uses.

There are an estimated 11.5 million IDUs worldwide. Injection drug use continues to become more popular in areas where it previously was not common. As drug cartels have expanded their reach in the world, the supply of heroin in a form that can be inhaled or smoked has decreased, and the processed injectable form has become more available and more acceptable for use. Injected heroin use continues to grow in Central and Southeast ASIA as well as Russia and

Eastern Europe. In other parts of the world, injection use of other substances is more common. In LATIN AMERICA, the primary injection drug used is cocaine; in parts of Europe, methamphetamines are the most common illegal injected substances.

Nonprescription injection drug use is illegal in all countries of the world. As a result, a culture of drug users who hide from authorities has developed. Reaching IDUs in most countries is a difficult task. Public shaming of IDUs is common, and discrimination against IDUs is a given. Even in countries where drug treatment is available and possession of clean needles is allowable, there are many reports of police or governmental harassment of IDUs. Injection drug use also overlaps with other HIV TRANSMISSION routes. Some people use illegal drugs for recreational purposes. This can lead to a lowering of inhibitions among users and influence behavior. Recreational drug users of all substances report an increase in unsafe sexual activities during drug use. People forget SAFER SEX principles, are unconcerned about protection, or feel invulnerable at the time of the drug use and engage in behavior they might not normally practice with a friend or stranger. In addition, regular users of illegal drugs report higher rates of sex work, which is often used to pay for the drugs. SEX WORKERS report high rates of illegal and injection drug use. Some countries' epidemics have been traced to the IDU community and continue to be spread predominantly through interactions within the IDU community. Studies have shown that when the rate of HIV infection reaches 10 percent in the IDU community, it then has the potential to spread to nearly 50 percent within one to four years. This type of close interaction in IDU communities then can drive epidemics among sex workers and among non-IDU populations because of overlapping activities involved when using illegal drugs.

HIV-prevention strategies in reaching communities of IDUs have proven successful when HIV education is provided in conjunction with access to clean needles. Needle exchange programs have been successful in significantly reducing the spread of HIV and HEPATITIS B and HEPATITIS C, which are also readily spread through IDU. Needle exchange programs work to reduce the overall potential harm by allowing the exchange of old, used needles and syringes with new, clean ones. By reducing the potential harm that IDUs can do to themselves and friends by using dirty equipment or sharing equipment, needle exchange programs can reduce the TRANSMISSION of various viruses among people who cannot or will not stop the use of various injectable drugs. Drug treatment programs, as well as drug replacement programs, which substitute methadone for heroin, also significantly reduce the potential for HIV spread through reduction in both sexually risky activities and needle sharing. Despite the proven effectiveness of these programs in preventing the spread of HIV and other illnesses, such programs are often underfunded or nonexistent. Only 25 percent of IDUs are receiving treatment for addiction in the United States at any one time. In addition, needle exchange programs are illegal in many parts of the United States, because the harm-reduction strategy is seen as simply encouraging injection drug use.

IDU intervention cannot be stressed enough in the prevention of HIV. In some countries, IDU is the main means of the spread of the virus, and the largest driver of the epidemic in that part of the world. In Russia, 83 percent of HIV-positive people are infected via IDU. Other countries with similarly high rates include Kyrgyzstan, Kazakhstan, Ukraine, Malaysia, and Indonesia. In the United States, 36 percent of all AIDS cases are the result of IDU. Programs that provide clean syringes, drug treatment instead of imprisonment, and education about HIV and ways to stop its spread are rare. In many countries, including the United States, syringe exchange is illegal, and programs running such exchanges are not able to provide HIV education or condoms in addition to safe needles. Drug treatment programs are not generally able to provide clean needles in addition to treatment and withdrawal of the illegal drug. Harm-reduction methods that have proven successful need to receive a stronger look in governmental funding in order to have a greater impact on HIV spread through injection drug use.

In the United States each year, approximately 450,000 people above the age of 12 use illegal injection drugs. This is less than two-tenths of the U.S. population. Of those people, more than half have injected heroin, one-third have injected cocaine, and one-third have injected methamphetamines, indicating that some people use more than one injection drug over the course of a year. IDU is responsible for approximately 11 percent of all new cases of HIV in the United States. This is a decrease over time in the rate of new cases resulting from IDU and may be related to the education efforts of community agencies. It is unclear whether the rate has decreased because the availability of needles is greater or whether the individuals using injection drugs have stopped sharing needles. In the United States, more people of color use injection drugs in urban areas than whites. However, more rural white people use injection drugs than rural people of color. IDU accounts for more than 25 percent of all HIV infections among black people and more than 30 percent among Hispanics. The HIV infection rate among white IDUs is approximately 19 percent. IDU-related HIV is also a larger percentage of total cases among WOMEN and adolescents in the United States, as compared to men. IDU-related HIV or having sex with partners who inject drugs accounts for 57 percent of all HIV cases among women.

IDU is a problem in some communities of gay men in Western countries. There is a culture of drug use among some gay men and injection use of methamphetamines is often a part of that culture. People who use methamphetamines are referred to as tweakers, and "being tweaked" is the phrase used to describe being high on methamphetamines. *Tweaking* is a slang term derived from a person's constant fidgeting and tweaking of objects around him or her when high on methamphetamines. *Slamming* is the word used to describe injecting methamphetamines. People use methamphetamines because they believe the drugs will heighten their sexual pleasure or increase the time they can spend having sex because the drugs often causes a delay in the buildup of the sexual release. Use of methamphetamines has been linked to reduced use of condoms and other SAFER SEX practices among gay men. In addition to the increase in sexual encounters on methamphetamines, there is an increased risk of passing the virus through the injection process.

The terms *works* and *rig* refer to the IDU equipment that is required to prepare and use a drug that is injected. It generally includes a needle, syringe, some material to filter the drug prior to injection, a spoon or other item to hold the drug while it is being heated, and something to use as a tourniquet to make the vein more readily accessible for injection. Sharing of needles or syringes is the most common way for HIV to spread among IDUs. It is often done as a cost-saving measure because needles can be expensive and difficult to locate. Studies have shown that HIV can live inside a syringe for a significantly longer period than if it is simply exposed to air, where it dies within seconds. This is why it is vital for an IDU to clean the needle and syringe with soap and water, and then disinfect them with undiluted household bleach prior to and between uses with anyone. Cleaning substances must also be thrown out and not reused for multiple cleanings. Thorough rinsing and drying of the syringe is also important so a user does not inject the cleaning substance into the body. Disinfection, however, only reduces the amount of virus on a surface and is not guaranteed to kill all virus particles. The process does not sterilize the syringe and should not be considered as safe as using a new, sterile syringe. Though using injection street drugs such as methamphetamine or heroin is never completely safe, through such simple steps a person can protect himself or herself to some degree from many viruses and other blood-borne microbes that can produce an infection in people who are sharing or reusing needles and syringes.

Treatment of heroin addiction often involves the use of a methadone substitution program. Methadone is an opiate drug that has shown some benefit in allowing heroin users to stop using injection drugs while not suffering as many withdrawal symptoms. However, use of methadone can be complicated while administering antiretrovirals in the treatment of HIV. In order to prescribe the proper antiretroviral treatment, a physician will need to be aware of any drug treatment program that an HIV-positive person is participating in.

AVERT: AVERTing HIV and AIDS. "Injecting Drugs, Drug Users, HIV and AIDS." AVERT.org. Available online. URL: http://www.avert.org/injecting.htm. Accessed March 20, 2011.

The Body. "Injection Drug Use and HIV/AIDS." The Body.com. Available online. URL: http://www.thebody.com/index/whatis/druguse_overview.html. Accessed March 20, 2011.

Centers for Disease Control and Prevention. "Fact Sheet: Drug-Associated HIV Transmission Continues in the United States." CDC.gov. Available online. URL: http://www.cdc.gov/hiv/resources/Factsheets/idu.htm. Accessed March 20, 2011.

DeCarlo, Pamela, and David R. Gibson. "Center for AIDS Prevention Studies Fact Sheet: What Are Injection Drug Users' (IDU) HIV Prevention Needs?" UCSF.edu. Available online. URL: http://caps.ucsf.edu/uploads/pubs/FS/pdf/IDUFS.pdf. Accessed March 20, 2011.

Hall, H. Irene, et al. "Estimation of HIV Incidence in the United States." *JAMA: The Journal of the American Medical Association* 300, no. 5 (6 August 2008): 500–529.

San Francisco AIDS Foundation. "Reducing the Risk of Getting HIV from Injection Drug Use." TheBody.com. Available online. URL: http://www.sfaf.org/aids101/injection.html. Accessed March 20, 2011.

———. "Welcome to Tweaker.org." Tweaker.org. Available online. URL: http://www.tweaker.org/home.html. Accessed March 20, 2011.

Strathdee, Steffanie A., and Francisco Inacio Bastos. "Injection Drug Use and HIV Infection: Encyclopedia of Public Health." enotes.com. Available online. URL: http://www.enotes.com/public-health-encyclopedia/injection-drug-use-hiv-infection. Accessed March 20, 2011.

United States Department of Health and Human Services, Substance Abuse and Mental Health Services Administration. "Injection Drug Use and Related Risk Behaviors." SAMHSA.gov. Available online. URL: http://www.oas.samhsa.gov/2k9/139/139IDU.cfm. Accessed March 20, 2011.

integrase inhibitors Integrase is an enzyme necessary for the reproduction of HIV in a person's body. Once the HIV has entered a cell, a reaction takes place that is used by HIV to change its ribonucleic acid (RNA) to deoxyribonucleic acid (DNA). The HIV DNA must insert itself into the cell's DNA in order to ensure that as the cell reproduces it also reproduces more HIV DNA. The enzyme used to insert itself into the cell's DNA is called integrase. The integrase inhibitor, as the name implies, blocks the integration of the viral DNA to the cell's DNA.

There are three steps believed to occur when HIV integrates its DNA into the cell's DNA. First, the integrase binds itself to the cell's DNA. Second, the viral DNA is processed for integration. The final step is the insertion of the viral DNA into the cell's DNA. Several attempts to create integrase inhibitors that worked on either of the first two steps of the integration process were not successful. The drugs that have been developed for use in stopping the third step in the process have been much more successful.

Integrase inhibitors are a new class of anti-HIV medication. The first drug in this class, RALTEGRAVIR, was approved by the U.S. FOOD AND DRUG ADMINISTRATION in 2007. There is at least one other integrase inhibitor currently in drug trials around the country. Integrase inhibitors will provide a different manner of stopping the virus that has not been available. Many people cannot use the other classes of drugs because of their side effects or because they have been unable to achieve a viral load low enough to prevent the virus from mutating into a new form that makes the HIGHLY ACTIVE ANTIRETROVIRAL THERAPY (HAART) inactive. Drug trial results for integrase inhibitors have been very good, showing large decreases of viral activity, particularly when used in combination with other medications. It is unclear what the long-term side effects of integrase inhibitors might be, if any. Two other integrase inhibitors are currently under development. One, ELVITEGRAVIR (GS-9137), is from Gilead Sciences; the other, dolutegravir (GSK-572), is from ViiV Healthcare.

AIDSmeds. "Integrase Inhibitors." AIDSmeds.com. Available online. URL: http://www.aidsmeds.com/archive/Integrase_1687.shtml. Accessed March 20, 2011.

The Body. "Comparing Two Integrase Inhibitors." The Body.com. Available online. URL: http://www.the body.com/content/art48990.html. Accessed March 20, 2011.

Havlir, Diane V. "HIV Integrase Inhibitors—Out of the Pipeline and into the Clinic." *New England Journal of Medicine* 359, no. 4 (24 July 22008): 416–418. Available online. URL: http://www.nejm.org/doi/full/10.1056/NEJMe0804289. Accessed March 20, 2011.

isosporiasis Isosporiasis, also known as cystoisosporiasis, is a human intestinal illness caused by the protazoon *Isospora belli* (also called *Cystoisospora belli*). This protazoon is found predominantly in tropical regions of the world and is endemic in Australia, southeast ASIA, AFRICA, LATIN AMERICA, and the CARIBBEAN. It is not a common infection in the United States. It is only found in humans, and there are no known animal carriers of this protozoan. The life cycle of the protozoon requires that the oocysts (eggs) be exposed to the air before it becomes an adult. A human excretes the oocysts of the protozoon in feces. The oocysts then develop over the course of at least 24 hours into adult forms, which are then taken back into the body when someone else has contact with them, probably through contaminated water or food. The protozoon can live for many months in the adult stage of the human. It is in the same family of protazoon as *Cryptosporidium,* the protazoon that causes CRYPTOSPORIDIOSIS. Isosporiasis is generally a time-limited illness in people who are HIV negative and have healthy immune systems. In HIV-positive people, it can cause a chronic diarrhea that leads to severe dehydration, weight loss, and exhaustion.

Symptoms and Diagnostic Path

Isosporiasis is an intestinal illness marked by copious watery diarrhea. Other symptoms may include bloating, severe cramping, low-grade fever, vomiting, and noxious gas; because of the malabsorption of food and nutrients, it leads to weight loss and tiredness. Infection outside the intestinal tract has been seen in the liver, spleen, bile ducts, and lymph nodes of patients who have been studied in autopsies.

Fecal samples are the most common means of identifying the oocysts of the protozoan. Several samples may be needed, as the oocysts are shed only intermittently and not in great quantities. If this method does not work, a colonoscopy may be required to perform a biopsy on tissue from the intestines.

Treatment Options and Outlook

The main treatment is the use of trimethoprim/ sulfamethoxazole (TMP-SMX). This has been effective in studies in Africa and in Haiti, where isosporiasis is one of the major AIDS-related illnesses. Other medications can be used if a patient is allergic to sulfa medications. One such treatment course is a combination of pyrimethamine and leucovorin. Side effects of TMP-SMX are common and include fever, rash, and a decrease in white blood cell counts.

A patient will also be given plenty of fluids to replace the lost nutrients and liquid lost through diarrhea. Because the illness is so severe in HIV-positive people, it can lead to wasting and death if the proper diagnosis is not made.

Risk Factors and Preventive Measure

For people in the United States, the risk of acquiring *I. belli* is low. Travelers to areas of endemic infection may be given a prophylaxis of TMP-SMX before a trip to protect them against various "traveler's diarrheas." Studies have shown that the introduction of HIGHLY ACTIVE ANTIRETROVIRAL THERAPY (HAART) has led to a decrease in the cases of isosporiasis except among immune-suppressed people with CD4 T lymphocyte counts below 50.

Once isosporiasis has been diagnosed and treatment has been successful, patients who have T cell counts less than 200 may be placed on a maintenance dosage of TMP-SMX to prevent recurrence. In studies, recurrence occurred in about 50 percent of patients not given a maintenance prophylaxis.

AIDSmeds. "Isosporiasis: What Is It?" AIDSmeds.com. Available online. URL: http://www.aidsmeds.com/articles/Isosporiasis_6874.shtml. Accessed March 20, 2011.

Centers for Disease Control and Prevention. "DPDx—Cystoisosporiasis." CDC.gov. Available online. URL: http://www.dpd.cdc.gov/dpdx/HTML/Cystoisosporiasis.htm. Accessed March 20, 2011.

Minnaganti, Venkat R., M.D. "Isosporiasis." eMedicine.com. Available online. URL: http://www.emedicine.com/med/topic1194.htm. Accessed March 20, 2011.

Kaletra Kaletra is the trade name for a combination protease inhibitor (PI) drug manufactured by Abbott Laboratories. The U.S. FOOD AND DRUG ADMINISTRATION (FDA) approved it for use in 2000. It is the first, and still only, combination pill created that combines the required booster PI ritonavir with another drug, in this case, the PI lopinavir. The abbreviation for Kaletra is LPV/r or LPV/RTV. It may also be called lopinavir/ritonavir in research articles. It is sold under the trade name Aluvia in some other countries. The single pill combines 200 mg of lopinavir and 50 mg of ritonavir. There are also low-dose tablets containing 100 mg of lopinavir and 25 mg of ritonavir for CHILDREN and a liquid formulation for infants. Kaletra is always used in combination with at least one other drug as part of a multidrug treatment regimen against HIV.

Dosage

The dosage for a person who is treatment experienced, someone who has taken anti-HIV medications before, is two Kaletra twice a day, or 5 mL of the liquid Kaletra twice a day. Dosage for someone who is treatment naïve, a person who has not had anti-HIV medication previously, is two Kaletra twice a day or four Kaletra once a day. It is not important whether Kaletra tablets are taken with or without food, but the liquid form of Kaletra should be consumed with some food for better absorption in the body.

The liquid formulation of Kaletra can be used by children as young as two weeks of age. Dosages should be based on weight. The liquid formulation does contain alcohol, and care should be considered when prescribing this.

Drug Interactions

Kaletra is metabolized (broken down in the body) by the liver, as are many of the PROTEASE INHIBITORS (PIs). This can affect the ways the various anti-HIV medications interact when used together. Because of the way Kaletra is broken down by the liver, it has the potential to reduce the amount of ZIDOVUDINE and ABACAVIR in the body if either drug is taken with Kaletra. It is unknown exactly how much reduction is involved, and dosing suggestions are not available currently. Kaletra increases the amount of the anti-HIV drugs FOSAMPRENAVIR and TENOFOVIR DISOPROXIL FUMARATE available in the body. Both drugs, if used in combination with Kaletra, can cause an increase in adverse reactions that can be dangerous if not monitored. It is unclear what dosage recommendations should be made for these two drugs when used with Kaletra.

Herbal supplements should be discussed with one's doctor. St. John's wort is known to cause a decrease in the bioavailability of PIs in the body. Other supplements that may cause decreased bioavailability of Kaletra include milk thistle and garlic supplements; these substances have not been studied as extensively as St. John's wort.

Antifungal medications such as ketoconazole, itraconazole, and voriconazole are affected by Kaletra. Amounts of ketoconazole and itraconazole are increased in the blood, while the quantity of voriconazole is decreased. Care needs to be used in prescribing azole antifungals so that the proper dosage to treat the fungal infection while not causing harm to the person taking Kaletra is determined.

Increased levels of fluticasone, an inhaled steroidal allergy and asthma treatment, may occur while using Kaletra. Patients should be monitored for any changes due to this interaction.

Methadone levels in the body decrease substantially while taking Kaletra. People taking methadone for the treatment of opiate addiction should have dosages adjusted and monitored by a doctor.

Kaletra interacts with a number of other medications including the cholesterol-lowering drugs simvastatin and lovastatin, antibiotics used to treat infections such as TUBERCULOSIS, antidepressant or antipsychotic medications, and antiarrhythmics and calcium channel blockers used in the treatment of heart ailments. It is important that a doctor know and understand all the medications and supplements a patient uses when prescribing Kaletra.

Kaletra also increases the amount of the drugs sildenafil (Viagra), vardenafil (Levitra), and tadalafil (Cialis)—all erectile dysfunction medications—in the blood, with the potential to cause serious side effects. Lowering the dosage of these medications is recommended to prevent potential complications. The effectiveness of birth control pills may be decreased during Kaletra use. Heterosexual couples may want to consider the use of condoms or other barrier methods to prevent pregnancy if taking this medication. Kaletra liquid contains alcohol in the formulation. It should not be prescribed to people who are taking either disulfiram, for the treatment of alcohol dependence, or metronidazole, used to treat parasitic infections. These medications can make people who drink alcohol or take medications with any alcohol in them very sick.

Side Effects

Diarrhea, nausea, vomiting, and headache are the most common initial reactions. Skin rashes have occurred also. These reactions are generally mild and will pass given time. Elevated liver enzyme levels can also occur, particularly in people who have chronic HEPATITIS.

Protease inhibitors, as a class of drug, generally increase the cholesterol and triglyceride levels of patients. Very high lipid levels have been recorded in some Kaletra patients. This side effect can be managed with appropriate cholesterol-lowering medications. Kaletra has also been associated with treatment regimens that can cause LIPODYSTROPHY, or the redistribution of fat within the body. Symptoms are increased fat around the neck and stomach area, facial wasting, breast enlargement, and peripheral wasting in the arms and legs. Some of these changes disappear when the drug is stopped.

Pancreatitis has been observed in patients who use Kaletra. Those who have had previous cases of pancreatitis should be monitored for further reactions. Some of these cases have been life threatening.

Kaletra has also been implicated in several varieties of heart dysrythymias. Care should be given to prescribing Kaletra for people who have specific types of heart dysrythymias such as long QT syndrome.

Kaletra may also increase the risk of worsening a person's diabetes or causing diabetes in people who were not previously diabetic. Blood sugar levels should be monitored in people susceptible to diabetes.

AIDS InfoNet. "Lopinavir + Ritonavir (Kaletra)." AIDS InfoNet.org. Available online. URL: http://www.aidsinfonet.org/fact_sheets/view/446. Accessed March 11, 2011.

AIDSmeds. "Kaletra (Lopinavir + Ritonavir)." AIDSmeds.com. Available online. URL: http://www.aidsmeds.com/archive/Kaletra_1559.shtml. Accessed March 11, 2011.

———. "Special Issues for Children with HIV." AIDSmeds.com. Available online. URL: http://www.aidsmeds.com/articles/Children_7566.shtml. Accessed March 11, 2011.

The Body. "Kaletra (Lopinavir/Ritonavir)." TheBody.com. Available online. URL: http://www.thebody.com/index/treat/kaletra.html. Accessed March 11, 2011.

United States Department of Health and Human Services. "Lopinavir/Ritonavir." aidsinfo.nih.gov. Available online. URL: http://www.aidsinfo.nih.gov/Drugs New/DrugDetailNT.aspx?int_id=316. Accessed March 11, 2011.

KP-1461 KP-1461, a new form of the NUCLEO-SIDE REVERSE TRANSCRIPTASE INHIBITORS (NRTIs), which causes a constant mutation in the virus. It has also been referred to as a mutagen or as a viral decay accelerator. This would be a new type of NRTI that has not been used before against HIV. Unlike other antiretrovirals that work to prevent HIV from mutating and to prevent the reproduction of the virus, KP-1461 encourages mutation in the viral deoxyribonucleic acid (DNA). Eventually, this unrestrained mutation causes the virus to weaken significantly, and, in laboratory experiments, this has caused the eventual death of the virus because the mutations created were not able to reproduce the virus. It has also shown in vitro activity against drug-resistant strains of the virus. Some people using the drug had large reductions in viral load, while others in the phase IIa study had lesser reductions. It is unclear whether the mutation rates were the same or whether the amount of time on the drug needed to be adjusted for some individuals. Further research may answer these questions. It is an exciting possibility that taking one drug for a predetermined amount of time could potentially force the virus to reproduce itself out of existence.

Dosage
In phase II studies, 1,600 mg doses were given twice a day. It is unknown as of yet whether this is the optimal dosage for this drug. Further studies are being planned and will probably determine the optimal dosing for KP-1461. KP-1461 is taken orally.

Drug Interactions
Drug interactions were not measured in the limited studies so far. In the small human trials that have been done, the drug was taken as a single drug, not in combination with other medications.

Side Effects
No known side effects have been seen so far in studies. It generally was well tolerated in early human studies. However, given that the purpose of the drug is to cause mutations in viral DNA, there is some concern among researchers, and the U.S. FOOD AND DRUG ADMINISTRATION (FDA), that the drug might cause mutations in DNA that does not need to be mutated. These mutations might over the long term cause other problems for somebody who uses the medication. Researchers at Koronis Pharmaceuticals and at the University of Washington believe that so far the drug has not been shown to cause such other mutations in animal models. Longer-term studies in humans are needed before approval by the FDA is likely.

Bland, Eric. "HIV Mutates to Death with New Drug." Discovery.com. Available online. URL: http://dsc.discovery.com/news/2009/02/09/hiv-mutation.html. Accessed March 20, 2011.

Evans, David. "KP-1461: A Novel Anti-HIV Drug in Limbo?" SFAF.org. Available online. URL: http://www.sfaf.org/hiv-info/hot-topics/beta/beta_2010_winspr_drugwatch.pdf. Accessed March 20, 2011.

HivandHepatitis.com. "New Analysis Shows Novel Nucleoside Analog KP-1461 Demonstrates Clinical Activity against HIV." HIVandhepatitis.com. Available online. URL: http://www.hivandhepatitis.com/recent/2009/052209_d.html. Accessed March 20, 2011.

Koronis Pharmaceuticals. "Koronis: KP-1461 for HIV." Koronispharma.com. Available online. URL: http://www.koronispharma.com/KP1461forHIV.html. Accessed March 20, 2011.

United States Department of Health and Human Services. "KP-1461." aidsinfo.nih.gov Available online. URL: http://www.aidsinfo.nih.gov/DrugsNew/DrugDetailT.aspx?int_id=416. Accessed March 20, 2011.

United States National Institutes of Health. "Safety and Efficacy Study of KP-1461 to Treat ART-Experienced HIV+ Patients." ClinicalTrials.gov. Available online. URL: http://clinicaltrials.gov/ct2/show/NCT00504452. Accessed March 20, 2011.

L

lactic acidosis Lactic acidosis is a life-threatening condition caused when lactate builds up in the blood. Human cells contain structures called mitochondria that use oxygen in the blood to change sugars from the food people eat into energy. If the blood does not contain enough oxygen or the mitochondria are damaged in some way, cells will make energy in other ways that produce lactic acid as a by-product. As the lactic acid remains in the blood, it in turn changes into lactate. This by-product causes the blood to become more acidic. The liver breaks down lactate and removes it from the body. If there is too much lactate, the liver will be strained to keep removing the lactate from the body. In addition to lactic acidosis, a lesser condition of a similar nature is called hyperlactatemia, in which the amount of lactate in the blood is consistently above normal but not high enough to cause life-threatening conditions. As the liver begins to fail to remove the lactate, it can shut down, causing further stress on other organs and potentially death.

Symptoms and Diagnostic Path

Lactic acidosis is a condition that builds over time, usually a period of several weeks to a few months; however, it is known to develop quickly at times. Symptoms are sometimes difficult to recognize and are not always distinguishable from those of other illnesses or general complaints. They include nausea, general tiredness, weakness of muscles, vomiting, generalized abdominal pain, rapid breathing, rapid heartbeat, weight loss, and swollen or painful liver.

Liver abnormalities are common in lactic acidosis. Swollen liver (hepatomegaly), fatty liver (steatosis), and raised liver transaminase levels that can be measured through BLOOD WORK/BLOOD TESTS are also common. The normal range for lactate in the blood is 0.5–1.0 millimoles per liter. In people who have persistent hyperlactatemia, a range of 1.5–3.5 millimoles per liter is common. Many HIV-positive people who receive a HIGHLY ACTIVE ANTIRETROVIRAL THERAPY (HAART) regimen containing NUCLEOSIDE REVERSE TRANSCRIPTASE INHIBITORS (NRTIs) have persistent hyperlactatemia. It is important that lactate levels be measured regularly to determine any unusual increases in blood lactate levels. At levels greater than 5 millimoles per liter, doctors generally switch a person's HAART regimen. Levels of 10 millimoles per liter are extremely serious and require immediate medical attention.

Lactic acidosis is relatively rare and occurs in approximately 1–2 percent of HIV-positive people who are taking HAART. Hyperlactatemia is believed to occur in up to 25 percent of HIV-positive people on HAART regimens that contain an NRTI. In particular, the NRTI STAVUDINE has been implicated in close to half of all lactic acidosis cases. DIDANOSINE has also been implicated as presenting a higher risk for lactic acidosis than other NRTIs. When it does occur, lactic acidosis has been fatal in approximately 70 percent of cases.

Treatment Options and Outlook

There is no treatment for lactic acidosis other than to stop HAART treatment. Some doctors may offer various vitamins and antioxidants that may help prevent hyperlactatemia from developing into lactic acidosis, but there are no studies that support this approach. Once a person has lactic acidosis, breathing assistance as well as hemodialysis may be required to assist recovery. Outlook is poor for individuals who have lactic acidosis that has reached that point, and recovery is not guaranteed.

Risk Factors and Preventive Measures

Lactic acidosis occurs when either the liver is not working properly and cannot clear the lactate from the blood or the mitochondria are damaged in some way and cannot produce cell energy in the usual manner. Lactic acidosis occurs in HIV patients most often when they are taking a HAART regimen with an NRTI. HIV-positive WOMEN, in particular pregnant women, are at higher risk for lactic acidosis than HIV-positive men. Although several NRTI drugs have been implicated in lactic acidosis cases, it is a rare occurrence. The probability of experiencing lactic acidosis is increased among people who are being treated for HEPATITIS C with the drug ribavirin, which increases lactate in blood during treatment.

The Body. "Lactic Acidosis." TheBody.com. Available online. URL: http://www.thebody.com/content/art12779.html. Accessed March 20, 2011.

Chow, Dominic C., M.D., Larry J. Day, M.D., Scott A. Souza, M.D., and Cecilia M. Shikuma, M.D. "Metabolic Complications of HIV Therapy." HIVInSite. ucsf.edu. Available online. URL: http://hivinsite.ucsf.edu/InSite?page=kb-03-02-10#S5X. Accessed March 20, 2011.

Goldman, Bonnie. "This Month in HIV: 2009 Update on Body Shape Changes and HIV/AIDS." TheBody.com. Available online. URL: http://www.thebody.com/content/treat/art51106.html?getPage=1. Accessed March 20, 2011.

John, Mina, et al. "Chronic Hyperlactatemia in HIV-Infected Patients Taking Antiretroviral Therapy." AIDS 15, no. 6 (April 2001): 717–723.

NAM AIDSmap. "Lactic Acidosis." AIDSmap.com. Available online. URL: http://www.aidsmap.com/cms1045058.aspx. Accessed March 21, 2011.

lamivudine   Lamivudine was approved by the U.S. FOOD AND DRUG ADMINISTRATION (FDA) in 1995 for use in combination therapy against HIV. It was first developed in 1989 in Canada and licensed to GlaxoSmithKline by the discovering company. It is one of the NUCLEOSIDE REVERSE TRANSCRIPTASE INHIBITORS (NRTIs). It is commonly referred to as 3TC, which is an abbreviation derived from the chemical structure name 2',3'-dideoxy,3'-thiacytidine. It is closely related to the drug ZALCITABINE, whose chemical structure name is 2',3'-dideoxycytidine. The trade name is Epivir.

Dosage

Lamivudine is marketed as two different pills, 150 mg and 300 mg, for the treatment of HIV. The 150 mg pill is taken twice a day, the 300 mg pill just once a day. Lamivudine is always used as part of a combination of antiretroviral medications and not by itself. For CHILDREN above the age of four, the 150 mg tablet can be broken to provide two smaller 75 mg doses. One of these can be taken twice a day. For children below the age of four, a liquid formulation is available.

It is also approved for use in the treatment of HEPATITIS B (HBV) in a smaller dose (100 mg) than that needed for HIV. If a person is coinfected with HBV and HIV, then the higher HIV dosage should be used.

Lamivudine has an interesting resistance mutation that can develop quite quickly, even if the drug is taken properly. This mutation actually causes HIV not to reproduce properly, thereby allowing lamivudine to continue working even though the virus has mutated against it. This is one HIV mutation that doctors do not worry about much, and lamivudine can still be part of many people's HIGHLY ACTIVE ANTIRETROVIRAL THERAPY (HAART) regimen despite the mutation.

Drug Interactions

Lamivudine is one of the easiest drugs to take for HIV. It is used in many of the antiretroviral combinations and can be taken with most other antiretrovirals. Lamivudine should not be taken at the same time as any other medication containing lamivudine. This includes the combination pills EPZICOM, TRIOMUNE, COMBIVIR, and TRIZIVIR. Lamivudine is also very close in structure to the antiretroviral drug EMTRICITABINE, and they act in the same manner against HIV. It is recommended that the two medications not be prescribed together, as doing so may not confer any added benefit to treatment. Emtricitabine is also found in the combination pills TRUVADA and ATRIPLA. If a person has developed drug resistance to emtricitabine, then lamivudine will not be one of the drugs chosen for another regimen, as the two drugs generally have the same resistance patterns.

Lamivudine can increase in concentration in the body when taken with trimethoprim/sulfamethoxazole (TMP-SMX), a common antibiotic used to treat PNEUMOCYSTIS PNEUMONIA. Dosages do not generally need to be adjusted, though a doctor may withhold lamivudine if there is a concern about this interaction.

The drug is also approved by the FDA for the treatment of chronic hepatitis B. If a doctor needs to change a patient's HAART medications and lamivudine is one of those drugs, the doctor may monitor the patient for any changes in liver function. Anytime that hepatitis B treatment is stopped, there remains a chance that the hepatitis B will flare up, causing potential damage to the liver.

Side Effects

Lamivudine is generally well tolerated. On occasion, side effects such as nausea, headache, diarrhea, and gas have been reported.

Lamivudine is an NRTI; several potential serious side effects are associated with drugs of this type. NRTI use has been linked to LIPODYSTROPHY, the loss of fat from some areas of the body and the accumulation of fat in others. NRTI use can also cause a rise in cholesterol and triglyceride levels. Although lamivudine has not been directly linked to these conditions, it is part of the class of drugs that have been associated with these side effects.

LACTIC ACIDOSIS has also been linked to NRTIs. It is a rare condition but can occur with greater frequency in WOMEN and obese individuals. Lactic acidosis is very dangerous and should be monitored closely. Hyperlactatemia, higher than normal levels of lactate in the blood, can be an indication that someone might be at risk for the more serious lactic acidosis. If symptoms of nausea, stomach pain, shortness of breath, irregular heartbeat, vomiting, weakness, and tiredness occur while taking lamivudine, a patient should consult a doctor immediately. Although other NRTIs are more often associated with lactic acidosis, the potential for lamivudine to be the cause of this illness exists.

AIDS InfoNet. "Lamivudine (Epivir)." AIDSInfoNet. org. Available online. URL: http://www.aidsinfo net.org/fact_sheets/view/415. Accessed March 11, 2011.

AIDSmeds. "Epivir (Lamivudine, 3TC)." AIDSmeds. com. Available online. URL: http://www.aidsmeds. com/archive/Epivir_1579.shtml. Accessed March 11, 2011.

———. "Special Issues for Children with HIV." AIDS meds.com. Available online. URL: http://www.aids meds.com/articles/Children_7566.shtml. Accessed March 11, 2011.

The Body. "Epivir (3TC, Lamivudine)." TheBody.com. Available online. URL: http://www.thebody.com/ index/treat/3tc.html. Accessed March 11, 2011.

United States Department of Health and Human Services. "Atazanavir." aidsinfo.nih.gov. Available online. URL: http://www.aidsinfo.nih.gov/DrugsNew/Drug DetailNT.aspx?int_id=126. Accessed March 11, 2011.

Latin America Latin America consists of the countries south of the U.S. border with Mexico, other than Belize, Guyana, French Guiana, and Suriname, which are considered part of the CARIBBEAN culturally. There are 1.6 million people in Latin America living with HIV/AIDS according to the United Nations (UN). More than 730,000 of these people live in Brazil. Other countries with large populations of people living with HIV/AIDS are Mexico, with 220,000;

Colombia, 160,000; Argentina, 110,000; and Peru, 75,000. More than 600,000 people have died since the beginning of the epidemic in this region. Statistics in this article are drawn from the latest UN reports available for the countries discussed.

Estimated prevalence rates for countries in Latin America generally show higher rates in Central America and lower rates in Mexico and some of the Andean countries. Panama has the highest rate of prevalence at 1 percent. Other countries' prevalence rates are Panama, 0.9 percent; El Salvador, Honduras, and Guatemala, 0.8 percent; Venezuela, 0.7 percent; Brazil, Colombia, and Argentina, 0.5 percent; Chile, Ecuador, and Peru, 0.4 percent; Costa Rica, Paraguay, and Mexico, 0.3 percent; and Bolivia and Nicaragua, 0.2 percent. Increases in prevalence have been seen in Argentina, Chile, Costa Rica, and Uruguay since 2001. A decrease was seen in Panama and Honduras during the same period, according to the UN statistical estimates.

The spread of HIV in Latin America is predominantly via sexual activity of MEN WHO HAVE SEX WITH MEN (MSM). Although not all statistics gathered by some governments reveal this as the main cause, the history of discrimination against MSM, as well as the stigmatizing of such activity, is believed to keep the numbers artificially low. The culture of many Latin American men is one of machismo, the chauvinistic man in charge. Because MSM are perceived by some as not conforming to this cultural norm, their sexual practices are often ignored, in this case at the peril of the health of the country. MSM in Latin countries do not think of themselves as gay in the sense that many gay men in other Western countries do. It is not unusual for MSM in Latin countries also to be having sex with wives or other women to affirm their machismo. Guatemala is one country that has not spent money on education among MSM; nor do statistics reflect MSM sexual activity as a main cause of the spread of the virus. However, local activists indicate that the problem of MSM unsafe sex is present, and testing among MSM revealed an

HIV rate of 10 percent in 2005, with a higher rate of 18 percent in the capital, Guatemala City. Other countries such as Peru and Mexico clearly acknowledge that spread of HIV has taken place mainly in and from the MSM communities. Education programs as well as medical services to MSM populations have been important in preventing further spread of the virus in those countries.

Brazil initially saw HIV/AIDS cases in the early 1980s. The majority of these cases were in MSM populations in the large cities of São Paulo and Rio de Janeiro. By 1986, blood donations were being screened in the larger cities and then throughout the country by 1988, halting spread of HIV through those routes. In the late 1990s, after HIGHLY ACTIVE ANTIRETROVIRAL THERAPY (HAART) had proven effective in arresting the virus, Brazil's government began supplying medications to all who needed them. Doing so was seen as a requirement of the constitution, which guarantees medical care for everybody in the country. Brazil began manufacturing its own generic versions of antiretrovirals shortly thereafter to minimize costs. This measure also immediately caused a drop in mother-to-child TRANSMISSION from 16 percent nationwide to 4 percent. Brazil has also shown the cost benefits of its large distribution of medicines through the decrease in hospitalization costs and other medical expenses, all owing to the availability of HAART for those who need it. Studies in Brazil have also shown that risk-reduction education can reduce the spread among and from the INJECTION DRUG USE(R) (IDU) population. HIV spread through this population has actually been reduced in recent years in Brazil, through outreach to IDUs as well as harm-reduction programs such as needle exchanges. Unprotected sex among MSM remains the number-one way that HIV is spread in Brazil. Spread of HIV is also high in populations of PRISONS, where 6 percent of men and 14 percent of women tested positive in recent studies.

In Argentina, the majority of HIV-positive people live in urban Buenos Aires and surrounding suburban areas. Four of five new cases in

Argentina were attributed to unprotected sex, mainly heterosexual, during 2005. MSM test at a rate of 14 percent positive in Buenos Aires. Injection drug use in general has decreased in the country as a result of HIV education as well as the availability of smokable alternatives to injectable drugs, of which cocaine is one example. Only 5 percent of IDUs said that they currently injected in 2003 as compared to 44 percent in 1998. The other country with a mainly heterosexually based HIV epidemic is Uruguay. Two-thirds of new cases in 2005 were attributed to unprotected heterosexual activity. As in Argentina, the epidemic is concentrated around the capital—in Uruguay, the region of Montevideo—which lies nearly directly across the Rio de la Plata from Buenos Aires. MSM prevalence rates in the capital were found to be near 22 percent in recent studies. IDUs account for 18 percent of new HIV cases, and IDUs tested in the capital show a prevalence rate of 19 percent. Argentina claims to provide antiretrovirals to anyone who needs them, but UN statistics report that approximately 70 percent of those who need the medications actually receive them. Uruguay also provides antiretroviral medication to approximately 70 percent of those who need the medication.

In Paraguay, the HIV epidemic is centered around the capital but also through the major trade routes along the border with Brazil and Argentina, indicating the spread through commercial SEX WORKERS who are available in trade centers there. Male sex workers show a much higher rate of HIV infection in Paraguay, at 11 percent, than female sex workers, at 2 percent. However, rates of other sexually transmitted infections are relatively equal, indicating that the opportunities for HIV spread are present for both populations. Currently, 70 percent of HIV-positive people in Paraguay are male, indicating an MSM-spread epidemic for the most part. IDUs in the country also test positive at a high rate, 13 percent, so the opportunity for spread in that community also is strong.

In Peru, studies have shown the virus predominantly affects the MSM population. Rates of HIV prevalence range from 18 to 22 percent among the MSM population and have been steady in different studies conducted by the government over the last 15 years. It is believed that condom use is increasing as rates of all sexually transmitted infections have been dropping among the MSM population. Those same studies show, however, that MSM who also have sex with women have not increased condom use, and an increasing number of women are becoming infected in Peru. Prevalence rates among female sex workers remain relatively low, below 2 percent. The most recent national studies also show a high rate of infection among indigenous peoples of the Amazon, among whom condom availability is low, and sex between men seems relatively common according to studies. An HIV rate of more than 7 percent was detected among the Chayahuita people.

Chile, Bolivia, and Ecuador all show similar epidemics: higher proportions of men who are HIV positive, low prevalence among female sex workers, and an increasing number of heterosexual women who are becoming infected by their male sex partners who also engage in MSM activities. In Bolivia, education programs have typically focused on the female sex workers, and education directed at the MSM population has been absent. In Chile, more than 90 percent of female sex workers report condom use on a regular basis, but the MSM population reports far lower adherence to regular condom use.

Colombia and Venezuela both have large numbers of HIV-positive people. Both countries border the Caribbean and are near the Guyanas, where HIV prevalence rates are significantly higher than on the rest of the continent. Travel between the Caribbean and these two nations may drive the prevalence rates higher without significant education available to the public. Female sex workers in cities along the Colombian coast show higher rates of HIV than female sex workers in the capital or other interior cities. Prevalence rates among the MSM populations are in the 10–18 percent range in both countries.

In Central America, a concerted effort to track HIV statistics has not been implemented. Up-to-date reports are difficult to obtain. Travel in and among the countries is fairly high, and the opportunity for spread is great. The Caribbean coastal regions of these nations all reflect higher HIV rates than interior or Pacific coastal regions. HIV prevalence rates among MSM are significantly higher than in the general population. Rates in Nicaragua among MSM are 38 percent higher than in the general population, in Honduras 7 percent higher. Other countries fall between these two. SAFER SEX is infrequent among some MSM populations, reflecting poor educational programs, particularly in Guatemala and Nicaragua. Other regional studies cited by the UN show that a large percentage of MSM populations also regularly have sex with women: Between one-quarter and one-third do so in all Central American countries except Panama. This could lead to new HIV infections in many women in these countries if educational efforts do not reach out to this population group.

Mexico's epidemic is largely concentrated among MSM, IDUs, and commercial sex workers. Rates of infection among the MSM population in the capital are around 10 percent. Among male sex workers, the rate of infection is double that. Similar numbers can be found among male sex workers in resort and U.S. border regions. Rates among female sex workers are lower, just 5 percent along border cities. IDUs in that area test HIV-positive at rates of 2–4 percent. Higher rates among IDUs involved in sex work have also been detected. Mexico was able to secure its blood supply early in the epidemic, and no case of spread through these means has been seen in several years. There are concerns among HIV experts that the indigenous populations of the country may be at higher risk than the general population. Language is a barrier in some areas of the country, as Spanish is not spoken in the home and educational materials are not being provided in regional languages. The same concerns also have been voiced in Guatemala, where the Maya are believed to be

at higher risk than other people because of low socioeconomic status and the unavailability of educational materials. Mexico's government maintains that all people who need HAART treatments are receiving them; however, statistics gathered by the UN suggest that the rate of people who are receiving medications is closer to three-quarters of the total who need them. Machismo is a cultural standard that threatens Mexico's female population in this epidemic. It is difficult for women to initiate condom use, and general surveys indicate that more than 15 percent of Mexican men have had sex with someone other than their wife or cohabiting partner in the past year. Of that number of men, fewer than 10 percent used a condom in any of their sexual activities.

The epidemic in Latin America has been stabilized in some of the countries with large populations, but continues to spread in areas where it had been until recently a small epidemic. Ignorance and unsafe sexual practices may cause a further expansion of the epidemic if education and governmental awareness do not keep up with the virus.

AVERT: AVERTing HIV and AIDS. "HIV and AIDS in Brazil." AVERT.org. Available online. URL: http://www.avert.org/aids-brazil.htm. Accessed March 20, 2011.

———. "HIV & AIDS in Latin America." AVERT.org. Available online. URL: http://www.avert.org/aids latinamerica.htm. Accessed March 20, 2011.

Cohen, Jon. "Special Online Collection: HIV/AIDS—Latin America and Caribbean." Sciencemag.org. Available online. URL: http://www.sciencemag.org/sciext/aidsamericas/. Accessed March 20, 2011.

UNAIDS: Joint United Nations Programme on HIV/AIDS. "Latin America." UNAIDS.org. Available online. URL: http://www.unaids.org/en/Country esponses/Regions/LatinAmerica.asp. Accessed March 20, 2011.

———. "UNAIDS Report on the Global AIDS Epidemic, 2010." Available online. URL: http://www.unaids.org/globalreport/. Accessed March 20, 2011.

United States Agency for International Development. "HIV/AIDS Health Profile Latin America and the Caribbean." Available online. URL: http://www.

usaid.gov/our_work/global_health/aids/Countries/
lac/hiv_summary_lac.pdf.
———. "HIV/AIDS Health Profile: Mexico." USAID.gov.
Available online. URL: http://www.usaid.gov/our_
work/global_health/aids/Countries/lac/mexico
_profile.pdf. Accessed March 20, 2011.
World Bank. "HIV/AIDS—HIV/AIDS in Latin America
and the Caribbean Brief." Worldbank.org. Available
online. URL: http://web.worldbank.org/WBSITE/
EXTERNAL/COUNTRIES/LACEXT/EXTLACREGTO
PHEANUTPOP/EXTLACREGTOPHIVAIDS/0,,content
MDK:20560003~menuPK:841626~pagePK:34004
173~piPK:34003707~theSitePK:841609,00.html.
Accessed March 20, 2011.

Latino/a Americans   *Latino* is a term used to group together people of a wide variety of ethnic backgrounds on the basis of their cultural similarities. Another term often used by the U.S. government is *Hispanic,* which traditionally meant someone who is or speaks Spanish. Both terms are umbrella terms used to define people whose ethnic background is one in which Spanish is or was at one time the primary language in the home. It is not a racial category, but an ethnicity. *Latino* can be more narrowly defined as someone from Latin America, where the term originated. Because of the large ethnic diversity of Latin America, these categories can and do include people of Asian, indigenous, African, European, and other racial or cultural backgrounds. The term *Hispanic* does not include Brazilians or people who speak languages other than Spanish, whereas the term *Latino* often includes people from countries where English, Portuguese, or other languages are spoken, as these individuals feel an affinity for this ethnic description and choose to consider themselves Latino.

Latinas/os make up approximately 15 percent of the U.S. population, the largest ethnic group in the United States after non-Hispanic Europeans. By far the largest number of Latinos in the United States are of Mexican descent: approximately 64 percent. People of Puerto Rican descent make up 9 percent of Latinos;

Cuban descent, 3.5 percent; Salvadoran (from El Salvador) descent, 3.2 percent; and Dominican (from the Dominican Republic), 2.7 percent. Smaller percentages of Latinos are from other countries of Latin America. Approximately 7 percent of U.S. Latinos simply use that term to describe themselves, indicating no other cultural background or descent in governmental surveys.

Although Latinos/as make up 15 percent of the U.S. population, they make up approximately 20 percent of the people who are HIV positive. Latino males are three times more likely than non-Latino white males to be HIV positive. Latina WOMEN are five times more likely to be HIV positive than non-Latina white women. Both Latino men and women are nearly three times more likely to become sick and die of HIV illnesses than their non-Latino white counterparts. Latinos are more likely than non-Latino whites to have been infected with HIV through heterosexual sex or through injection drug use (IDU) (see INJECTION DRUG USE(R)) and less likely to be infected through MEN WHO HAVE SEX WITH MEN (MSM) sexual encounters. Within the Latino community, people of Puerto Rican birth or descent are more likely than other Latinos to become HIV positive through IDU, while Latinos of Mexican birth or descent are more likely to become HIV positive through MSM sexual activity.

The difference in infection rates between Latinos in the United States and non-Latino whites in the United States is related to socioeconomic issues. More Latinos are in poverty than their non-Latino white counterparts. More Latino CHILDREN are raised in poverty than non-Latino white children. Educational levels are lower for Latinos, particularly for people of Mexican birth or descent, than for other groups of Latinos in the United States. Latinos are less likely to have health care benefits from their jobs than non-Latino whites. Latinos are more likely to be unemployed than non-Latino whites in the United States. In addition to these difficulties, language can play a role in whether or not a person receives good medical care, can communicate well with a medical provider, or can receive proper HIV prevention if the only available prevention materials are in English rather than in Spanish. Latinos repeatedly report discrimination in many areas of life in the United States, particularly in jobs and in schools. In recent years, some states have implemented bans against dual language instruction, allowing only instruction in English, which has an inherent bias against children who speak a language other than English when they enter schools.

Latinas in the United States face multiple stigmas in relation to HIV. In traditional Latin American cultures, a woman's role is predominantly in the home and less in the community or as part of the main workforce, the norm in the United States. Women who arrive in the United States do not have the same levels of freedom as Latina women born in the United States. They are less likely to speak English than men in the community. Medical care is less assessible than for their Latino partners, as the language barrier can create struggles in receiving proper or regular care. As in other male-dominated cultures around the world, women report not being aware of their male partner's activities, so men who participate in IDU or engage in MSM activity do not always make these activities known to their female partners. Fear of testing among Latinas is high because of language barriers as well as the perceived risk among some of being sent back to their country of origin if they are in the country as temporary or illegal workers. Because of this lack of information and lack of medical care, Latinas often find out they have an HIV infection late in the course of the illness, leading to an earlier death from HIV than among women in other cultural or racial groups.

MSM from Latino families report high levels of discrimination and harassment within the Latino community. This level of discrimination is higher among those who speak Spanish in the home, according to studies. Seventy percent of Latino MSM in the United States report hiding their sexual activities because of the high levels of disapproval of family and community.

MSM who do not identify as gay or bisexual are recognized as one of the main reasons for the higher rate of HIV infection among Latinas than among non-Latina white women. Men who are engaging in MSM activity as well as sexual relations with women are referred to as men "on the down low," or as *bugarrones,* in some Spanish dialects. Although studies do show a decrease in the level of disapproval among Latinos who were born in the United States, this attitude remains rooted in the religious and cultural upbringing of many Latinos.

Education, available in Spanish as well as English, remains the best way to reach Latinos and prevent the further spread of HIV. *Rechazo,* "rejection" in English, is the word used by many HIV-positive people to refer to the stigma that surrounds the topics of HIV and MSM sexuality among Latinos. Because more than one-third of the Latino population of the United States is below the age of 18, it is vitally important that discussion of sexuality and HIV be undertaken to prevent the spread among young people. Rising levels of HIV in Latino MSM and Latinas indicate that current education is not reaching some of this population. The numbers of new Latino/a immigrants are highest in the American South. Large numbers of Latinos/as have moved to states such as North Carolina, Arkansas, and Alabama in recent years. This area of the country typically has less access to medical care that is available in Spanish, and rates of sexually transmitted infections (STIs) are higher here than in the rest of the United States. These two factors could make for a poor combination of factors in the near future for some U.S. Latinos/as. Recognition of the differences between Latinos/as and non-Latino/a populations is a must in reaching and educating people about HIV. Working within the strength of the family and the church is a requirement for effective communication of information to the community. Open and honest discussion of sexuality and STI prevention is a necessity to prevent any further spread within the growing community of Latinos/as in the United States.

Centers for Disease Control and Prevention. "HIV/AIDS among Hispanics/Latinos." CDC.gov. Available online. URL: http://www.cdc.gov/hiv/hispanics/index.htm. Accessed March 20, 2011.

Diaz, Rafael M., and George Ayala. "Social Discrimination and Health: The Case of Latino Gay Men and HIV Risk." TheTaskForce.org. Available online. URL: http://www.thetaskforce.org/downloads/reports/reports/SocialDiscriminationAndHealth.pdf. Accessed March 20, 2011.

Greico, Elizabeth M. "Race and Hispanic Origin of the Foreign-Born Population in the United States 2007: American Community Survey Reports." Census.gov. Available online. URL: http://www.census.gov/prod/2010pubs/acs-11.pdf. Accessed March 20, 2011.

Latino Commission on AIDS. "Shaping the New Response: HIV/AIDS and AIDS in the Deep South." TheBody.org. Available online. URL: http://img.thebody.com/press/2008/DeepSouthReportWeb.pdf. Accessed March 20, 2011.

National Latino AIDS Awareness Day. "A National Perspective of the HIV/AIDS Epidemic on Hispanics/Latinos in the U.S." LatinoAIDS.org. Available online. URL: http://www.latinoaids.org/docs/hiv_on_latinos_us.pdf.

United States Bureau of the Census. "Hispanics in the United States." Available online. URL: http://www.census.gov/population/www/socdemo/hispanic/files/Internet_Hispanic_in_US_2006.pdf. Accessed March 20, 2011.

United States Department of Health and Human Services, Office of Minority Health. "HIV/AIDS and Hispanic Americans." Available online. URL: http://minorityhealth.hhs.gov/templates/content.aspx?ID=3327. Accessed March 20, 2011.

leishmaniasis Leishmaniasis is an illness caused by flagellate protozoa that belong to the genus *Leishmania* spp. It is spread predominantly through the female sandfly, which feeds on blood. There are more than 30 varieties of the sandfly genus *Phlebotomus* or *Lutzomyia* that carry the more than 20 varieties of *Leishmania* species among dogs, rats, opossums, humans, and other mammals. One variety of the illness, visceral leishmaniasis, is becoming endemic in parts of the world where it had not been seen previously because of coinfection with HIV.

There are four forms of leishmaniasis that occur in humans. Depending on the individual person and the species of *Leishmania,* this could be local cutaneous, diffuse cutaneous, mucosal, or visceral leishmaniasis. Disseminated visceral leishmaniasis, also known as kala-azar or black fever, is a severe form of the disease that is nearly 100 percent fatal if untreated. Typically, 90 percent of visceral leishmaniasis cases have been found in six countries: India, Bangladesh, Nepal, Sudan, Ethiopia, and Brazil. Since the HIV epidemic began, visceral leishmaniasis has become more prevalent in areas where previously it had not been widespread.

About 1.5–2 million new cases of leishmaniasis are identified each year. It is endemic in 88 countries, across all continents except Australia. Visceral leishmaniasis has been identified in 28 countries. Leishmaniasis among HIV-positive people has been reported all around the Mediterranean region, including Italy, Spain, Portugal, and France, as well as India and Brazil.

Leishmaniasis is spread through the sandfly of the genus *Phlebotomus* in ASIA, AFRICA, and the Pacific (see OCEANIA) and the *Lutzomyia* genus in NORTH AMERICA and South America. *Leishmania* are tiny creatures, 3–6 micrometers long by 1.5–3 micrometers in diameter. They are absorbed into the sandfly's intestine from an infected mammal when the female sandfly bites it to secure blood needed for breeding her eggs. Sandflies live and breed in warm, moist organic matter, so garbage, deteriorating walls, and decaying plant matter can be inviting homes for them to produce larvae. As with mosquitoes, the male sandflies do not bite and cannot spread leishmaniasis. When the sandfly bites a mammal infected with *Leishmania* sp., the protozoon is ingested along with the blood. At this point, the protozoon is in the smaller of its two forms, called an amastigote, which is round, unable to move freely, and very small.

Taken into the stomach of the sandfly, the amastigotes quickly transform into a second *Leishmania* form, called the promastigote. This form is larger than the amastigote and has a flagellum, a taillike structure that allows self-movement. As the sandfly bites the next mammal, the promastigotes are delivered into the bite site. When the promastigotes penetrate the skin, the human immune response is to send macrophages to attack the antigens by swallowing them. Once inside the macrophage, they transform back into the smaller amastigote form. After reproduction reaches a certain stage, the protozoa leave the macrophage, either passing through the membrane of the macrophage or simply killing the cell through bursting the membrane, and then traveling through the blood or lymph system. In visceral leishmaniasis, the protozoa travel throughout the body, locating new macrophage hosts to breed inside repeatedly.

Symptoms and Diagnostic Path

Cutaneous leishmaniasis produces skin ulcers at the site of the sandfly bite from a few days to weeks after the event. Ulcers appear singly or in groups. The ulcers generally heal themselves in a few months in immunocompetent people but leave scarring. Diffuse cutaneous leishmaniasis also generally heals spontaneously after several months, but the scarring from the ulcers or skin nodules can be extensive. Historically not found in the United States, cutaneous leishmaniasis has recently been seen in patients in Texas and Oklahoma. Causes for this are thought to be the recent spread of either the sandfly or other animal vectors such as the armadillo or rat.

In mucosal leishmaniasis, the infected person has large ulcers in and around the mouth, nose, pharynx, and larynx, areas with the largest mucosal coverage. Ninety percent of mucosal leishmaniasis cases occur in Bolivia, Brazil, and Peru. The disease leaves extensive and disfiguring scarring. Leishmaniasis is also known in South America as *espundia*. Infection of the mucosal tissue can occur months to years after the initial bite of the sandfly and rarely is self-healing.

Visceral leishmaniasis is a systemic disease that occurs months or years after initial infection by the protozoan. Symptoms include fevers, weakness, loss of appetite, enlarged lymph nodes, swollen spleen, swollen liver, and pancytopenia (reduction of the numbers of red and white blood cells as well as platelets). In India, visceral leishmaniasis is also known as *kala-azar,* a Hindi term that translates as "black fever." The name refers to the darkened skin around the head, abdomen, and extremities that was often associated with the disease in India. In addition, a syndrome known as post–kala-azar dermal leishmaniasis (PKDL) can affect people after they have received treatment for and been cured of visceral leishmaniasis, particularly those coinfected with HIV. It causes diffuse nodules of swelling under the skin of the affected individual and can resemble symptoms of Hansen's disease (leprosy), making the diagnosis difficult. It has been seen predominantly in India and Sudan.

Visceral leishmaniasis is diagnosed when possible with biopsies of the affected areas. Scrapings of the ulcers usually allow for enough pathogen to provide a diagnosis in cutaneous or mucosal disease. In visceral leishmaniasis, diagnosis can be achieved through bone marrow testing, spleen biopsy, or cultures from the blood. A negative serum test finding for leishmaniasis in HIV-coinfected people is not uncommon because of a lack of any immune response. In poorer regions of the world, diagnosis is often done simply through visual means, and therefore unknown cases of *Leishmania* that may exist in a person will activate once treatment for HIV begins triggering the body suddenly to produce antibodies and a defense against the protozoa.

Treatment Options and Outlook

Pentavalent antimony drugs, sodium stibogluconate and meglumine antimoniate, have been used as the first line of treatment for more than 70 years in many areas of the world, including the United States. Both drugs are given in injections or intravenously. There are no oral compounds of these drugs. Duration of treatment on the antimonials can be from three to four weeks. Antimonials reduce the amount of the parasite in the body but do not kill it completely, and relapses can occur, particularly in people with compromised immune systems. CENTERS FOR DISEASE CONTROL and Prevention (CDC) recommendations for treatment include the addition of a granulocyte-macrophage colony-stimulating factor (GM-CSF) to enhance the effectiveness of the antimonials in individuals who have neutropenia. Antimonials frequently can be toxic, particularly in people who have underlying issues of malnutrition or those in advanced disease states. Side effects can include cardiac dysrhythmias and acute pancreatitis. Monitoring of the patient's condition is necessary when using these medications.

Some areas of India have seen leishmanias that are resistant to the antimonial drugs, so amphotericin B has become the standard of treatment. Although there are oral forms of amphotericin B available in Europe and other parts of the world, intravenous forms of the drug are recommended for use in the treatment of leishmaniasis because the oral forms are not effective outside the gastrointestinal tract. Again, severe side effects are common with this drug. Kidney toxicity and renal failure, often reversible, are the most common side effects of the drug. Monitoring for kidney and liver toxicity, electrolyte changes, and infusion area allergic reactions is necessary. In particular, hypokalemia, or low blood potassium levels—which can lead to cardiac arrest—need to be monitored in people receiving amphotericin B. Some of these side effects can be prevented with corticosteroids or acetaminophen and the consumption of plenty of fluids. Intravenous fluids are generally used prior to administration of amphotericin B to increase hydration and decrease the risk of kidney toxicity. Tylenol and Benadryl as well as corticosteroids can also be given prior to amphotericin B administration to reduce the possible allergic side effects to the drug, which include chills, fever, and headache. Pentamadine isethionate is also used as another line of treatment in the case of unresponsiveness to pentavalent antimonial drugs. The high cost of amphotericin B has caused problems in treatment in many areas of the world where patients or governments cannot afford to pay for this medicine. Lipid-based formulations of amphotericin B are considered safer and have become the standard of treatment in the United States. They are also more expensive than non-lipid-based amphotericin B. Since 2008, manufacturers of amphotericin B have lowered the price of the drug significantly for overseas markets where it is most needed.

Some countries (Germany, India, and Colombia) have approved the use of miltefosine in the treatment of leishmaniasis. It is an oral, as well as an intravenous, treatment that has been shown to be as effective as sodium stiboglutinate in clinical trials. A daily dose of 2.5 mg is the general amount prescribed. Miltefosine has been shown to be teratogenic (causing birth defects) and therefore should not be prescribed to women who are pregnant or considering pregnancy. The cost of this course of treatment is significantly lower than that of other drugs, at a range of $125–$200 per course of treatment versus $3,000–$5,000 per treatment course for amphotericin B. Side effects are relatively minimal; gastrointestinal distress and elevated blood levels of creatinine and alanine are the most common. Strict adherence to the treatment regimen is required, as resistance to the drug has been shown to occur in vitro.

Paromomycin is an antibiotic that has received orphan drug status through the U.S. and European Union authorities. It has been approved for treatment of leishmaniasis in India. In the United States, it is approved for the treatment of intestinal amebiasis in a different form than the one used to treat leishmaniasis. It has been shown to provide strong antileishmanial activity in drug and clinical trials. Side effects were minimal, including reversible hearing loss and elevated transaminase levels in less than 2 percent of patients. It is a daily oral drug that has an extremely low cost of $5–$10 per treatment regimen. Delivery of the drug is difficult in the United States, as the primary supplier has discontinued its manufacture here as of early 2008. It continues to be manufactured in India.

Treatment of HIV-positive individuals with HIGHLY ACTIVE ANTIRETROVIRAL THERAPY (HAART) prior to treatment with antileishmanial drugs has been shown to increase the effectiveness of the body's response to the parasite as well as the drug against the parasite. Relapse has been seen in HIV-positive individuals at a higher rate than in the general public, leading to cases of PKDL.

Risk Factors and Preventive Measures

Leishmaniasis is endemic in many countries around the world. Sandflies that can transmit the protozoan live in warm moist areas, so rotting garbage or plant material as well as any place that collects moisture can serve as a breeding ground. The other mammals that can host the protozoan include dogs, which constitute the main carrier in many countries. Elimination of infected animals has been shown to decrease infection rates of humans, but this type of program is unlikely to eliminate the other host animals completely. In India, studies have shown that the use of lime (calcium carbonate) in the mixture of mud used to build most houses there can reduce the infestation of sandflies in homes by 90 percent, thereby reducing the opportunities to be bitten by the bug. Sandflies are susceptible to the same pesticide-spraying campaigns that exist against mosquitoes. However, any stoppage of spraying campaigns only allows the sandfly to return. The pesticides have their own toxicity issues, which are not addressed here. Application of bug sprays can prevent many types of insects from biting humans. In addition, use of bed netting can reduce the transmission of many insect-spread illnesses, such as leishmaniasis and malaria. Travelers to areas of endemic leishmaniasis should include bug spray or sleeping nets as part of their travel supplies.

Centers for Disease Control and Prevention. "Treating Opportunistic Infections among HIV-Infected Adults and Adolescents." *MMWR* 53, no. RR15 (17 December 2004): 1–122. Available online. URL: http://www.cdc.gov/mmwr/preview/mmwrhtml/rr5315a1.htm. Accessed March 20, 2011.

Chappuis, Francois, Shyam Sundar, Asrat Hailu, Hashim Ghalib, Suman Rijal, Rosanna W. Peeling, Jorge Alvar, and Marleen Boelaert. "Visceral Leishmaniasis: What Are the Needs for Diagnosis, Treatment, and Control?" *Nature Reviews Microbiology* 5, no. 11 (November 2007): 873–882.

Davis, Antony J., and Lukasz Kedzierski. "Recent Advances in Antileishmanial Drug Development." *Current Opinion in Investigational Drugs* 6, no. 2 (February 2005): 163–169.

Institute for OneWorld Health. "Drug Program." OneWorldHealth.org. Available online. URL: http://www.oneworldhealth.org/drug_program. Accessed March 20, 2011.

Medical News Today. "Dermatologists Identify North Texas Leishmaniasis Outbreak." MedicalNewsToday.com. Available online. URL: http://www.medicalnewstoday.com/articles/82576.php. Accessed March 20, 2011.

Sundar, Shyam, T. K. Jha, Chandreshwar P. Thakur, Prabhat K. Sinha, and Sujit K. Bhattacharya. "Injectable Paromomycin for Visceral Leishmaniasis in India." *New England Journal of Medicine* 356, no. 25 (21 June 2007): 2571–2581.

Sundar, Shyam, et al. "Amphotericin B Treatment for Indian Visceral Leishmaniasis: Conventional versus Lipid Formulations." *Clinical Infectious Diseases* 38, no. 3 (2004): 377–383. Available online. URL: http://cid.oxfordjournals.org/content/38/3/377.full. Accessed March 25, 2011.

lipodystrophy   Lipodystrophy is the redistribution of body fat that occurs in up to 50 percent of people who take antiretroviral medications for HIV infection. Lipodystrophy may also be referred to as body-fat abnormalities. The word is derived from two Greek words: *lipo*, meaning "fat," and *dystrophy*, meaning "abnormal condition." It is a general term used by many people to refer to several conditions that can affect people with HIV who use antiretroviral drugs. These different conditions include lipoatrophy, the loss of subcutaneous fat from face and limbs; lipohypertrophy, the accumulation of fat in the central areas of the body, breast, stomach, and shoulders; lipomas, the accumulation of fat in small deposits just below the skin; and METABOLIC SYNDROME, which is a term used to describe a combination of medical problems, including increased cholesterol, increased fasting blood sugar levels, increased triglycerides level, high blood pressure, and obesity in the waist area.

Symptoms and Diagnostic Path

Symptoms can vary, depending on the type of syndrome involved. Lipoatrophy is the loss of fat in the extremities, the buttocks, and the face. Fat is lost from just below the skin and can cause a person to look different, feel bad about his or her appearance, and appear ill to others. Cheeks can look sunken; legs and arms can appear quite skinny with veins showing easily, and a person's pants will appear saggy, as the buttocks can lose the majority of fat from them. Lipoatrophy can be measured in various ways by taking measures of the arms and legs prior to beginning treatment, taking photographs of the person prior to treatment, or recording various fat measurements. Loose skin can be observed by the patient or by the doctor.

Lipohypertrophy, the accumulation of fat, can appear around the stomach. It was first noticed among people who took the drug INDINAVIR, marketed under the name Crixivan. People have referred to the fat accumulated in the stomach as crix-belly. Fat can also accumulate on the lower neck or shoulders; the term *buffalo hump* refers to this symptom. Women also have reported increased breast size. In many cases, this too can be observed after the start of treatment with antiretrovirals. Buffalo hump is an observable change in body structure, as are larger breasts in women.

Lipomas are accumulations of fat that form small benign tumors, which can vary in size from about the size of a pea to the size of a glass marble. These generally form on the trunk—chest, stomach, and buttocks—but can also appear on the arms, face, and pubic areas. The lumps of fat are often noticeable and can be annoying or painful when they are located in a spot on the body that has regular contact with objects. Lipo-

mas can be a genetic condition in some people. If there is no previous history of the development of lipomas, then the sudden occurrence of one or more lipomas may be related to antiretroviral fat redistribution.

Treatment Options and Outlook

Lipoatrophy is not seen currently as much as it was in the few years after antiretrovirals became available for patients. In particular, lipoatrophy has been closely related to two antiretrovirals taken either individually by some people when treatments were first begun or as part of a combination therapy, as is recommended at this time. The two drugs implicated in lipoatrophy are ZIDOVUDINE and STAVUDINE, both NUCLEOSIDE REVERSE TRANSCRIPTASE INHIBITORS (NRTIs). Stavudine is no longer considered for initial treatment for most people in the United States or Europe, though it is part of the combination pill TRIOMUNE, which is available throughout much of the developing world. Zidovudine is still used frequently, but doctors are aware of the potential body changes that can occur over the long term with the use of the drug. Replacing the two antiretrovirals as part of HIV treatment can stop the further changes, and over time body changes will reverse themselves when patients use other medications.

Loss of facial fat can cause great problems for some people, as it is strongly associated with self-image and by others as a sign of illness. Sunken cheeks, visible bone structure, creases in facial skin, and loose facial skin are all signs of lipoatrophy of the face. Regaining the fatty tissue in the face is the slowest part of fat recovery in patients who stop the drugs that have been linked to lipoatrophy. The U.S. FOOD AND DRUG ADMINISTRATION (FDA) has approved a treatment called poly-L-lactic acid, sold under the name Sculptra in the United States and New-Fill in other countries. It is an injectable substance used to fill the spaces below the skin where fat has been lost. It is considered plastic surgery and is covered by some medical insurance plans, particularly if the need for the surgery is shown to be the result of treatment with anti-retroviral medications. Although some people have undergone other types of plastic surgery, including implants, to regain facial structure, the advantage of poly-L-lactic acid is that it is a biologically inert substance that over the course of two to three years is absorbed and taken out of the body through normal body metabolism. Poly-L-lactic acid is administered over the course of multiple treatments and does not cause allergic reactions. It encourages the body to produce more collagen, which will replace some of the lost fat in the areas injected.

Lipohypertrophy can occur in up to 30 percent of people taking some HIV antiretrovirals. It was first noticed in people who were using PROTEASE INHIBITORS (PIs) shortly after they became available in the late 1990s. Although some studies have indicated that there is no difference between fat gain in HIV-positive and HIV-negative people of the same age groups, it is difficult to ignore the problem among some people who are taking these antiretroviral medications. The European AIDS Clinical Society guidelines for treatment of HIV call for clear discussions with the patient regarding diet and exercise. The organization recommends plenty of exercise and a low-fat diet that would be recommended to most people who wanted to maintain weight or lose excess weight. Although PIs may be linked with the additional fat gain, it is also thought that the process of clearing the virus and increased health in patients may be the root cause of the sudden fat gain. There is no FDA-approved treatment for such weight gain. Some patients have had fat-removal treatment, particularly when it involves the fat accumulated around the neck and shoulders (buffalo hump). Not all patients react the same way to all medications, and those patients who have had the greatest problems with fat accumulation also have the greatest loss in the fat over time after stopping certain medications.

Lipomas have not been linked with any particular antiretroviral medication or treatment regimen. However, they are clearly associated with some aspect of antiretroviral treatment, as the number of patients suddenly developing lipomas can be seen in any HIV treatment setting. It is believed by some researchers to be related to the PI class of drugs. A dermatologist or surgeon can remove the lipomas easily. Patients report that stopping particular drugs or drug treatment combinations ends the formation of lipomas.

Risk Factors and Preventive Measures

Doctors and researchers believe that people who are at higher risk genetically for fat gain and body weight problems may have a higher disposition for lipodystrophy complications when taking antiretrovirals. Prevention of weight gain is becoming part of discussions between doctors and patients when antiretroviral treatment is started. Antiretrovirals such as stavudine and zidovudine are recognized as causing some problems with lipoatrophy over time. Medications can be switched to replace these drugs if problems arise. Similarly, if PIs are causing large fat gains in some people, different combination therapies can be tried to remedy the situation.

Lipodystrophy is a side effect of antiretroviral treatment that was not expected to occur. When HIV treatment began to be available, concern focused on saving the life of the patient and not drug side effects. As the drugs have proven so successful and people live longer, complications with the medicines have become better understood. Once a person has adjusted to the idea that he or she is going to survive, these often major changes in body appearance can be startling to patients and those around them. Lipodystrophy is a cause for concern for both doctor and patient and can be addressed from the start of treatment so that potential body changes can be addressed before such changes are detrimental to the patient.

AIDS Education & Training Centers. "Abnormalities of Body-Fat Distribution." AIDS-ed.org. Available online.

URL: http://www.aids-ed.org/aidsetc?page=cm-308_fat. Accessed March 20, 2011.

AIDSInfoNet. "Body Shape Changes (Lipodystrophy)" AIDSInfoNet.org. Available online. URL: http://www.aidsinfonet.org/fact_sheets/view/553. Accessed March 20, 2011.

AIDSmeds. "Lipodystrophy: What Is Lipodystrophy?" AIDSmeds.com. Available online. URL: http://www.aidsmeds.com/articles/Lipodystrophy 10726.shtml. Accessed March 20, 2011.

Chow, Dominic C., M.D., Larry J. Day, M.D., Scott A. Souza, M.D., and Cecilia M. Shikuma, M.D. "Metabolic Complications of HIV Therapy." HIVInSite. ucsf.edu. Available online. URL: http://hivinsite.ucsf.edu/InSite.jsp?page=kb-03-02-10. Accessed March 20, 2011.

European AIDS Clinical Society. "EACS—Euro Guidelines 2009." EuropeanAIDSClinicalSociety.org. Available online. URL: http://www.european aidsclinicalsociety.org/guidelinespdf/EACS-Euro Guidelines2009FullVersi on.pdf. Accessed March 20, 2011.

Frascino, Bob, M.D. "The Lipoatrophy Resource Center—Doctor Views: Dr. Bob Frascino." TheBody.com. Avail-able online. URL: http://www.thebody.com/content/art47314.html. Accessed March 20, 2011.

Goldman, Bonnie. "This Month in HIV: 2009 Update on Body Shape Changes and HIV/AIDS." TheBody.com. Available online. URL: http://www.thebody.com/content/treat/art51106.html?getPage=1. Accessed March 20, 2011.

Lichtenstein, Kenneth, Ashok Balasubramanyam, Rajagopal Sekhar, and Eric Freedland. "HIV-Associated Adipose Redistribution Syndrome (HARS): Definition, Epidemiology and Clinical Impact." *AIDS Research and Therapy* 4, no. 16 (16 July 2007). Available online. URL: http://www.aidsrestherapy.com/content/4/1/16. Accessed March 20, 2011.

Manfredi, R. "Lipomatosis and HIV Disease during Antiretroviral Therapy." European Society of Clinical Microbiology and Infectious Diseases. BlackwellPublishing.com. Available online. URL: http://www.blackwellpublishing.com/eccmid14/abstract.asp?id=14304. Accessed March 20, 2011.

Sharp, Matt. "Metabolic Complications Associated with HIV Disease." TheBody.com. Available online. URL: http://www.thebody.com/content/art1110.html. Accessed March 20, 2011.

M

malaria Malaria is a tropical disease caused by a parasite that is transmitted through the bite of the *Anopheles* mosquito. There are several species of the parasite *Plasmodium*, each limited to a certain geographic area. *Plasmodium vivax* is the most common of the family of parasites and is found in LATIN AMERICA, ASIA, and parts of AFRICA. *P. ovale* is endemic in West Africa, the Philippines, eastern Indonesia, and Papua New Guinea. *P. knowlesi* is limited in range to Southeast Asia and predominantly the island of Borneo and the country of Malaysia. *P. malariae*, like *P. vivax*, is found worldwide but is not considered as serious as other varieties. By far, the most dangerous variety is *P. falciparum*, which can be found worldwide and is the predominant variety in sub-Saharan Africa. It also accounts for 80 percent of severe malaria infections and 90 percent of malaria deaths worldwide.

Symptoms and Diagnostic Path

Malaria was eradicated from mosquitoes within the United States in the 1940s through insecticide spraying and other control measures. There are approximately 1,500 cases of malaria a year in the United States, most of them in travelers from countries where malaria is an endemic disease or seasonal problem. There have been several outbreaks of mosquito-borne malaria in the United States from mosquitoes biting travelers who have returned with the illness, so it is conceivable that malaria could return to the country at a future time if the illness is not discovered and the insects eliminated. It is also possible to acquire malaria parasites through blood transfusions, though this method is rare, and blood is screened in most developed countries to prevent the occurrence.

People who live in areas where malaria is endemic develop immunity to the illness over time through repeated activation of their immune system to fight the parasite. Immunity for malaria consists of the ability to fight the amount of parasite in the body, but does not prevent repeated reinfection. Some genetic ability to fight malaria also exists in people who have the sickle-cell trait. This blood cell marker prevents the severe illness and death that can occur from falciparum malaria.

Malaria and HIV interact with each other to create different courses of each disease. HIV illness prevents the acquired immunity to malaria seen in endemic areas. Because HIV weakens the HUMAN IMMUNE SYSTEM gradually, malaria becomes increasingly more dangerous in HIV-positive individuals in these endemic areas. HIV-positive people show greater amounts of parasite in their blood and more frequent incidence of illness than HIV-negative people in those regions. Malaria, as with other OPPORTUNISTIC INFECTIONS (OIs), allows the HIV to increase its reproduction, leading to higher HIV viral loads in people. This can lead to a greater risk of TRANSMISSION of HIV, it is believed.

Malaria symptoms can be wide ranging and depend on the variety of *Plasmodium* species that infects a person. Typical symptoms in nonimmune people are fever, chills, sweats, muscle aches, headache, diarrhea, vomiting, and other general signs. These signs can be mistaken in nonendemic areas of the world for flu or other illness, and misdiagnosis is common. Falciparum malaria often presents more serious symptoms, including swollen spleen, severe anemia, breathing problems, coma, mental confusion, and other neurologic complications. It is often referred to as cerebral malaria.

Malaria can cause special concerns during pregnancy. WOMEN who do not have acquired immunity to malaria face more complications than people who are not pregnant if they become infected with malaria. In addition to increasing the chance of anemia, it can lead to serious birth defects in the child, low birth weight, or abortion of the fetus. This is particularly true of HIV-positive pregnant women. In women who have some acquired immunity to malaria, this acquired immunity lessens during pregnancy, leading to similar results.

Malaria is known for classic recurring symptoms that start quickly and return every 48 hours in *P. vivax* and *P. ovale.* Symptoms in *P. malariae* cycle every 72 hours. Symptoms in *P. fulciparum* do not often follow strong cycles. This presentation of symptoms can be variable for people and may not occur in all cases. Because of the nature of the parasite's life cycle, it is possible for malaria to recur in people who have recovered from the illness many years after initial illness. The liver is the location in the body where *Plasmodium* lives and can reproduce until it returns to the blood.

Tests that can detect malaria include examining the patient's blood under a microscope for the parasite, and antigen tests to detect reaction to malarial parasites. In people who are not immune, often symptoms of illness begin before parasites are measurable in the blood, so repeated tests may be needed.

Treatment Options and Outlook

Treatment for malaria is the same for HIV-negative and -positive people. There are several medications that can be used. Treatment for falciparum malaria is generally administered on an inpatient basis because of the seriousness of the illness. Treatment for other varieties is done on an outpatient basis. *P. falciparum* can cause severe illness and death in as little 12–24 hours once symptoms start, and it is vital that a person suspected or known to have this variety of malaria receive treatment immediately.

Treatment of falciparum malaria employs intravenous medication and fluids. Chloroquine, sulfadoxine-pyrimethamine, mefloquine, atovaquone-proguanil, quinine, doxycycline, and artemisin derivatives (which are not available in the United States but often used in other countries) are all possible drugs that can be used to treat an active malaria infection. The drug used will depend on allergies or reactions to those drugs, other health issues, other medications the person is taking, and the type of malaria and location where it was acquired. For instance, falciparum malaria acquired in Costa Rica is not generally resistant to chloroquine at this time, so treatment would be with that medication; however, if falciparum malaria were acquired in Africa, treatment would use other medications, as resistance to chloroquine is relatively high in African falciparum malaria.

If it is treated promptly, death rates from falciparum malaria are lessened considerably. Treatment of the other varieties of malaria can completely clear the parasite if begun early in the infection. Some treatments may require more than one drug, as the parasite can hide in the liver for extended times and must be cleared from that area of the body; otherwise, relapse can occur months or years later.

Risk Factors and Preventive Measures

Because people who have HIV are more likely to have severe illness when infected with *P. falciparum,* travel to areas where malaria is endemic should be avoided by people who have low CD4 T cell counts. If travel is required, prophylactic treatment is also required. Other means of preventing malaria are using insecticide-treated bed netting when sleeping. Use of these nets has been shown to reduce TRANSMISSION of malaria, particularly in CHILDREN, in several endemic areas. Insect repellent also is a requirement for people traveling to malaria endemic areas.

People who grew up or lived in areas where acquired immunity to malaria exists will lose this immunity in a short time frame after living away from the endemic area. Returning to that area places this person at the same risk for developing or redeveloping malaria as someone who has never suffered the illness. Prophylactic treatment will be the same in these individuals.

Three different drugs are primarily used for malaria prevention. The prescriptions are the same whether the person is HIV positive or HIV negative. Atovaquone-proguanil, mefloquine, or doxycycline will be prescribed for travelers to malaria endemic areas depending on which is best for the individual, and the possible resistance to these drugs in the area being visited. For instance, mefloquine resistance has become more common in Southeast Asia, and this drug would probably not be prescribed for prophylaxis if traveling to this region. All of the drugs have some side effects, and some should not be mixed with certain other medications; therefore, individuals will receive different drugs depending on which is best for them. Antimalarial prophylaxis is generally very effective if taken according to prescription directions. Medicines should be started prior to a trip to endemic areas and generally continue for a month after the trip is completed.

Atovaqone-proguanil is taken orally once a day. It is used in areas where *P. falciparum* has developed resistance to other antimalarial drugs. Side effects can include nausea and headache; they are uncommon in most people. Mefloquine is taken orally once a week. Side effects include vivid dreams, nightmares, sleeplessness, anxiety, headache, and nausea. Side effects are more common in people who are taking dosages to treat malaria rather than prevent it, in which case dosage is lower. It is eliminated slowly from the body, and side effects may continue for some time after the drug is stopped. People who have a history of depression or psychotic episodes should not be prescribed mefloquine. Doxycycline is taken orally once a day. It should be taken with food, and may cause side effects such as nausea and sun sensitivity. People allergic to tetracycline should not take doxycycline.

Two other medications may also be used in the prevention of malaria, but are prescribed less frequently. Chloroquine can be used to prevent malaria in some but not all regions of Central and South America, and not in Asia or Africa, as the *Plasmodium* spp. has developed immunity to the drug. It is taken once weekly. Primaquine is primarily used in the prevention of *Plasmodium vivax* and not other varieties of *Plasmodium*. Primaquine is taken daily but cannot be taken by pregnant or nursing women, and people must be tested to determine whether they have a glucose-6-phosphate dehydrogenase (G6PD) deficiency. G6PD deficiency can lead to an abnormal breakdown of red blood cells both in the blood and elsewhere in the body. Primaquine can cause a severe reaction in people who have G6PD deficiency.

Centers for Disease Control and Prevention. "Malaria Facts." CDC.gov. Available online. URL: http://www.cdc.gov/malaria/facts.htm. Accessed April 1, 2011.

Cox-Singh, Janet, et al. "*Plasmodium knowlesi* Malaria in Humans Is Widely Distributed and Potentially Life Threatening." *Clinical Infectious Diseases* 46, no. 2 (15 January 2008): 165–171.

Huff, Bob. "Malaria and HIV." TheBody.com. Available online. URL: http://www.thebody.com/content/treat/art13512.html. Accessed April 1, 2011.

Kakkilaya, B. S. "Malaria Site: Clinical Features of Malaria." MalariaSite.com. Available online. URL: http://www.malariasite.com/malaria/Clinical Features.htm. Accessed April 1, 2011.

National Institute of Allergy and Infectious Diseases. "Understanding Malaria." NIH.gov. Available online. URL: http://www.niaid.nih.gov/topics/Malaria/understandingMalaria/Pages/default.aspx. Accessed April 1, 2011.

National Library of Medicine. "MedlinePlus: Malaria." MedlinePlus. Available online. URL: http://www.nlm.nih.gov/medlineplus/malaria.html. Accessed April 1, 2011.

Whitworth, James. "Malaria and HIV." HIV InSite. Available online. URL: http://hivinsite.ucsf.edu/InSite?page=kb-05-04-04. Accessed April 1, 2011.

World Health Organization. "Malaria." World Health Organization. Available online. URL: http://www.who.int/malaria/en/. Accessed April 1, 2011.

maraviroc Maraviroc is one of the ENTRY INHIBITORS, or fusion inhibitors; it received accelerated approval by the U.S. FOOD AND DRUG ADMINISTRATION (FDA) in 2007 and general approval in 2008. Another name for this type of drug is a CCR5 antagonist. It works specifically on HIV-1 that uses the CCR5 molecule to enter the cells. A person must be tested to determine whether he or she has the CCR5 tropic virus; if not, this drug will not have an effect on their virus. Some people who have HIV have a form of the virus that uses the CXCR4 receptor to enter human cells, and some people have a form of the virus that enters by using both types of receptors. Among treatment-experienced people, approximately 55 percent have the CCR5 tropic virus. The blood test that determines whether a person's virus is CCR5 tropic can only be performed on people who already have a measurable viral load. In addition, the test is expensive. This is currently a drawback to the use of the drug.

Pfizer Laboratories manufactures maraviroc. It is sold under the trade name Selzentry in the United States and as Celsentri elsewhere. It is abbreviated as MVC. Maraviroc is always prescribed as part of a multidrug combination of anti-HIV medications. In November 2009, it was approved for use in treatment-naïve people, but not for anyone below the age of 16; it has not been tested in pregnant or nursing women.

Dosage

Maraviroc is available in 150 mg and 300 mg tablets. Dosage varies, depending on what other medications the patient in taking. Use of maraviroc with drugs that can induce or inhibit liver metabolism affects the amount of maraviroc in the body. A doctor or pharmacist will discuss the correct dosage with the patient. It can be taken with or without food.

Drug Interactions

Maraviroc interacts with a number of drugs because it is metabolized by the cytoprotein 450 3A (CYP3A). Drugs that inhibit or induce the protein can cause a drop or rise in the amount of maraviroc in the body. Grapefruit juice is one common CYP3A inhibitor and should be avoided when taking maraviroc.

Medications that can inhibit the CYP3A include ketoconazole, KALETRA, ritonavir, SAQUINAVIR, and ATAZANAVIR SULFATE. Doses of maraviroc will be lowered with these medications. Dosage is likely to be one 150 mg pill twice a day.

EFAVIRENZ, rifampin (an antibiotic), and some other medications decrease maraviroc; in such cases the dosage of maraviroc will be increased. Dosage with these medications will probably be two 300 mg maraviroc pills twice a day.

TIPRANAVIR, NEVIRAPINE, ENFUVIRTIDE, and the antibiotic TMP-SMX require a dosage of one 300 mg twice a day. Since there are several potential interactions with commonly prescribed HIV medicines, the patient must ensure that the doctor and pharmacist know of all current medications.

Other than CYP3A metabolism, there do not seem to be any drug interactions that have been mentioned in the literature.

Side Effects

The most common side effects of short-term duration were cough, fever, colds, rash, muscle and joint pain, stomach pain, and dizziness.

An increase in heart attacks was seen in drug studies involving maraviroc. The manufacturer warns that the drug should be prescribed with caution for people who are at higher risk for cardiac problems.

There is some concern that there may be an increased risk of malignancies or liver problems with this medication, but studies and postapproval reports have not yet indicated this to be a problem. Some researchers have expressed concern that long-term blocking of the CCR5 receptor, which plays a role in immune system surveillance, may lead to an increase in other immune system misfunctions. However, preliminary ongoing studies of maraviroc have not found any increase in cancers or other immune system problems at this time.

AIDSmeds. "Selzentry or Celsentri (Maraviroc)." AIDS meds.com. Available online. URL: http://www.aids meds.com/archive/selzentry_1629.shtml. Accessed April 1, 2011.

———. "Special Issues for Children with HIV." AIDS meds.com. Available online. URL: http://www.aids meds.com/articles/Children_7566.shtml. Accessed March 11, 2011.

The Body. "Selzentry (Celsentri, Maraviroc)." The Body.com. Available online. URL: http://www.the body.com/content/art40488.html. Accessed April 1, 2011.

Highleyman, Liz. "Maraviroc (Selzentry) Not Associated with Elevated Cancer Risk in Clinical Development Program." HIVandHepatitis.com. Available online. URL: http://www.hivandhepatitis.com/2010_confer ence/AIDS2010/docs/0817c_2010.html. Accessed April 1, 2011.

United States Department of Health and Human Services. "Maraviroc." aidsinfo.nih.gov. Available online. URL: http://www.aidsinfo.nih.gov/DrugsNew/Drug DetailNT.aspx?int_id=408. Accessed April 1, 2011.

maturation inhibitors Maturation inhibitors prevent HIV from assembling the proper proteins in the coating of the virus particle. By stopping the final assembly of the virus, they prevent it from maturing into a form that would be dangerous to a person, hence the name of this class of drugs, maturation inhibitors. Currently, there is one maturation inhibitor drug under phase II testing, BEVIRIMAT; however, others are under development. Maturation inhibitors will be a new class of anti-HIV drugs if approved by the U.S. FOOD AND DRUG ADMINISTRATION (FDA). They would constitute a sixth class of medication available to treat HIV-infected individuals. Because HIV mutates regularly, sometimes medications lose effectiveness against the virus. Often, if the virus becomes resistant to one drug in one of the six classes of drugs, it can also be resistant to treatment by other drugs in the same class, rendering several drugs useless for that individual. Developing new classes of drugs, or drugs that work in slightly different ways, against the virus allows several different options for patients who may need those options the longer they take medications.

After the human cell has released new viral particles that HIV forces the cell to produce, the last step before these particles become infectious is called maturation. During this phase, the shell of the viral particle must change from one type of protein to another in order to become infectious to other human cells. Technically, these proteins are called p25 and p24; p25 is known as a precursor protein, while p24 is known as a capsid protein. The change from p25 to p24 is vital for the virus to become infectious. The *gag* (group-specific antigen) gene informs and codes the basic structure of the virus, and this is what maturation inhibitors prevent from occurring. By interfering with this *gag* gene, the maturation inhibitor can cause a variety of harmless mutations to occur, so that these particles cannot cause infection in human cells. Blocking this change in the capsid protein prevents full development of the virus.

Currently, testing of the one maturation inhibitor under phase II development has shown that people who have developed some specific resistance mutations to PROTEASE INHIBITORS (PIs) may also have a resistance to that particular maturation inhibitor. Other maturation inhibitors under development have not progressed as far in testing, so it is unclear whether or not they will work in a different type of maturation. There are several steps in the process of viral maturation, and therefore potentially several places where a drug could interfere as the virus tries to mature to become infectious.

DeJesus, Edwin, M.D. "HIV Antiretroviral Agents in Development." TheBody.com. Available online. URL: http://www.thebody.com/content/art1352.html #mi. Accessed April 1, 2011.

Hosein, Sean R. "A Maturation Inhibitor Reappears." AEGIS.com. Available online. URL: http://www.

aegis.com/pubs/catie/2009/CATIE173-01_EN.html. Accessed April 1, 2011.

Li, F., et al. "PA-457: A Potent HIV Inhibitor That Disrupts Core Condensation by Targeting a Late Step in Gag Processing." *PNAS: Proceedings of the National Academy of Sciences* 100, no. 23 (11 November 2003): 13,555–13,560.

Salzwedel, Karl, David E. Martin, and Michael Sakalian. "Maturation Inhibitors: A New Therapeutic Class Targets the Virus Structure." *AIDS Reviews* 9, no. 3 (July 2007). Available online. URL: http://www.aids reviews.com/resumen.asp?id=970&indice=200793. Accessed April 1, 2011.

men who have sex with men Men who have sex with men (MSM) include men who would consider themselves gay and those who consider themselves bisexual. It is a term used more predominantly in non-Western countries, where more familiar terms such as *gay, homosexual,* or *bisexual* are associated with culturally negative laws, emotions, and behaviors. There are many men around the world who do not feel that they are gay or bisexual but do have sex with other men. The phrase "men who have sex with men" is therefore used to encompass all men who engage in these activities regardless of other associations with other terms.

In the United States, people generally refer to themselves by one of several social categories based upon with whom they engage in sexual or committed relationships. Gay men are individuals who have sex or are in relationships with other men. Heterosexual, or straight, men are those who have committed relationships or sex with women. A person who says he or she is bisexual acknowledges having sexual relationships with both men and WOMEN. This is different among some people in American society. Some men do not acknowledge publicly, or to their spouses, that they are engaged in having sex with men, either regularly or on an irregular basis. In the United States, this has become known in the last few years as being on the down low, or simply DL. Being on the DL means a man is having sex with men as well as being in a committed relationship with a woman. The term can be used to describe any person who is engaged in sexual activity outside the committed relationship, whether with a woman or a man, but has come to be used by MSM who do not wish, for any number of reasons, to be identified with being gay or bisexual.

When the HIV epidemic began, the first populations of people affected outside the African continent were MSM in Western countries—the United States, Europe, and Australia. Men in large U.S. cities in particular were initially affected. New York City, Los Angeles, and San Francisco had large populations of HIV-infected gay men. Other cities with large populations of MSM soon followed: Atlanta, Miami, Washington, D.C., Houston, Dallas, and Chicago. Because many MSM at that time were not open about their sexual identity, it became clear during the initial HIV epidemic studies that many men led lives that were unknown to their friends and families. When it was falsely believed that gay people lived in cities and not rural areas, it became clearer as people became ill that MSM lived all over the United States, and these men were vulnerable to the virus at rates higher than others in the country in that initial epidemic.

A strong reaction from the affected community of gay men and women in the United States and the education programs they began lowered the TRANSMISSION rate for HIV significantly among MSM, particularly after federal funding for HIV education was begun in the late 1980s. The use of condoms was stressed, and negotiation between men prior to sexual encounters taught people that it was healthy to discuss status, condoms, and behavior prior to engaging in sexual behavior. Although rates of HIV increased in other populations of U.S. citizens, such as the INJECTION DRUG USE(R) (IDU) community and heterosexual individuals, rates of new infections among gay men fell steadily from the mid-1980s until the late 1990s, when they leveled off. Gay community organizations in all these regions, where sexual behavior is more liberalized than in many other parts of the world, continue to provide educational programs, support groups, and condom distribution in neighborhoods and bars. Unlike at the height of the epidemic in the United States, this is no longer supported through many government programs, as George W. Bush–era regulations forbade the use of federal funds in what they viewed as encouraging homosexual behavior.

MSM accounted for about 10 percent of all HIV cases worldwide as of 2009; however, in many Western countries, HIV has predominantly affected MSM. In the United States, Australia, New Zealand, Canada, and many countries of Western Europe, more people have become infected through MSM encounters than other activity. About 50 percent of all new HIV cases in the United States in 2009 were among MSM. The great majority of these men are between the ages of 15 and 35. Although it is unknown exactly how many men fall into the MSM category in the United States, it is estimated from statistics that do exist that approximately 20 percent of MSM in the United States are HIV positive. There has been a slight increase in the last few years in new HIV-positive test results among gay men in the United States, and a large number of these men are young and AFRICAN AMERICAN. Black MSM between the ages of 13 and 29 are twice as likely as their white or Latino counterparts of the same age group to be HIV positive. The 13–29 age group has the largest number of new HIV cases among black and LATINO AMERICAN MSM who are in the most recent year for which data are available (2009). The age group that has the highest level of new cases among white MSM is the 30–39 age group. In the United States, MSM are the only category of people who have an increasing number of new cases. Other groups measured show steady or slightly declining levels of new cases. Health care workers and community educators have different ideas about the cause for this rise. Some believe it is the result of poor government funding of sex education and sole focus on ABSTINENCE instead of on a full spectrum of sex education. Others think that a culture of unpro-

tected sex has arisen in the MSM community and that young men are not aware of the danger of HIV since the access to antiretroviral drugs has greatly lowered the death rates from HIV. In addition, people in both camps agree that men who do not discuss their sexual behavior openly are less likely to be reached through education programs aimed at particular communities. Some increase in cases among MSM in other Western countries has also been noted.

United Nations (UN) data from LATIN AMERICA show that HIV has been predominantly spread by MSM, with lesser epidemics among heterosexuals and IDUs. Data from Mexico show that 60 percent of HIV cases to date are the result of spread among MSM. Studies in Colombia by Mejia indicate a 10–25 percent HIV-positive rate among the groups of MSM in Colombian cities. Latin American countries highlight issues for public health educators as well as public policy realities. In Peru, for instance, approximately 10–18 percent of MSM are HIV positive according to Peruvian government studies cited by the UN. In addition, the studies showed that about 10 percent of all men, when asked, stated that they did have sex with other men regularly. Of those 10 percent, a full 90 percent said they also regularly had sex with women. This shows the potential for MSM spreading the virus to their female partners through heterosexual sex. Men in Latin America often state that though they have sex with other men, they consider themselves heterosexual and not gay. A culture of machismo exists in many Central and South American countries, in which men feel they are invulnerable and lead lives in which they are in charge at home. Decisions about not using condoms are often made because men from this sort of culture feel that they do not need them, they are healthy men, their women should not tell them to use a condom, and doing so is an unnecessary intrusion into their pleasure.

In AFRICA, the culture of MSM is kept hidden. Most men who participate in such activities are also married because of the negative cultural view that is expressed by the governments on the continent. Only South Africa guarantees equal protection under the law and allows couples of the same gender to marry, a right enshrined in their constitution. Most of the continent still has laws drafted by the colonial rulers of France, Britain, Belgium, Germany, and Portugal that are used to enforce very strict anti-sodomy laws. Recently, Uganda, which has had a large, predominantly heterosexual, HIV epidemic, tried to pass legislation that would have made the death sentence the norm for people found guilty of being gay. African leaders often say that the behavior of MSM is chosen and was imported from European colonists. Strict evangelical Christianity, which was introduced to Africa by the colonizers, also led to strong anti-MSM beliefs among some Africans. Despite such strict legal and moral control, MSM populations exist in Africa as they do in every country. Some studies that have been done on the populations in different countries have found results similar to those in other regions of the world. MSM are difficult to reach for education purposes, if education is available; men are viewed as the head of households and hold control over whether condoms are used at all; men from all stations in life participate in sexual activity with both men and women, though they do not view themselves as gay in the Western sense. The numbers of MSM in African countries are not known exactly; nor is it clear how MSM contribute to the spread of HIV in Africa, which has predominantly had a history of HIV spread through heterosexual activity. Condom use was reportedly higher among MSM than among heterosexuals in parts of Africa, but still very low in comparison to other parts of the world due to cost and limited availability of condoms.

In ASIA, some of the same cultural prohibitions against MSM exist that are common in Africa. Many men who have sex with other men are married. Many men involved in MSM activities do not view themselves as gay in the Western sense of the term. Research into MSM in Asia reveals a very active and often very visible culture, but one that is relegated to the shadows of what is seen as proper or approved activity. Many of the first cases of HIV in Asia were in MSM. Epidemics among MSM in some countries such as China, Cambodia, India, Thailand, and Vietnam stand to prove that MSM are present and that they are at risk of contracting HIV and spreading it to their wives and children. Recent court decisions in India and Nepal have repealed laws instituted during colonial times against MSM activities. Whether these changes will encourage other countries to address legalization of MSM activity and provide these men with easier access to education is unknown. In Thailand, MSM activity is frequent. A notably large sex tourism economy exists, and male SEX WORKERS are common in tourist areas. Condom use is high in Thailand among MSM in comparison with some other countries in Asia, thanks to a strong education program run by the government. Again, as in Africa, the lack of affordable condoms makes their use difficult for many people unless the government provides the condoms or encourages their use widely. China recently stepped up campaigns to educate MSM on the use of condoms and the prevalence of HIV in the MSM community. According to UN-cited studies, approximately 11 percent of all HIV cases in China are in MSM, but the number has been rising in relation to that of other groups of HIV-positive people in recent years. This is a sign that the government recognizes that MSM activity exists, something new for the government, which had previously denied that it was an area of concern.

MSM are a high-risk category for the spread of HIV predominantly because anal sex is a more effective way to spread the virus. The linings of the anus and colon are made of different tissue than the lining of the vagina. The blood passes easily through the tissues of the colon and the anus. Penetrative sex can cause small, unnoticeable tears in the anus, causing an opening that the virus can enter easily if an HIV-positive man ejaculates during anal sex with a woman or a man. An HIV-positive person who is receptive during anal sex can also pass on the virus to an

HIV-negative person who is "topping," or in the insertive role, during anal sex. Although the risk is lower for the insertive partner, HIV can be passed in this manner also. The urethral opening in the penis is muscosal tissue, as is the foreskin in uncircumcised men, and can allow the virus into the body if a receptive partner is bleeding during anal sex. A condom should be used to prevent passing the virus between either partner during anal sex. Oral sex is a significantly lower-risk activity that MSM can engage in, though this too can carry risks if a person has cuts inside the mouth or gums that bleed readily from infections. Any cut in the mouth or on the lips allows breaks in the mucous membrane, letting blood leave and other fluids enter the bloodstream, potentially causing infection. The best way for MSM to avoid exposing themselves to HIV is to know their HIV status. MSM remain uneducated about the virus, as shown in the statistics of young men who become HIV positive. By knowing their HIV status, people can take the proper safety measures when having sex with others, thereby protecting themselves. As long as MSM remain a persecuted minority and the public maintains a judgmental attitude toward funding education and outreach for this population, the virus will continue to spread.

AVERT: AVERTing HIV and AIDS. "HIV, AIDS and Men Who Have Sex with Men." AVERT.org. Available online. URL: http://www.avert.org/men-sex-men. htm. Accessed April 1, 2011.

———. "Latin America HIV/AIDS Statistics." AVERT. org. Available online. URL: http://www.avert.org/ southamerica.htm. Accessed April 1, 2011.

The Body. "Marking World AIDS Day, the NYC Health Department Reports That HIV Infections Continue to Rise among Young Men Who Have Sex with Men: New Studies Confirm Risky Behaviors." The Body.com. Available online. URL: http://www.the body.com/content/news/art54667.html. Accessed April 1, 2011.

Bowen, Anne. "Rural MSM and HIV Prevention." Effec-tiveInterventions.org. Available online. URL: http:// www.effectiveinterventions.org/files/Rural_MSM _HIVPrev.pdf. Accessed April 1, 2011.

Centers for Disease Control and Prevention. "CDC Fact Sheet: HIV and AIDS among Gay and Bisex-ual Men." CDC.gov. Available online. URL: http:// www.cdc.gov/NCHHSTP/newsroom/docs/Fast Facts-MSM-FINAL508COMP.pdf. Accessed April 1, 2011.

The Global Forum on MSM and HIV. "MSMGF: The Global Forum on MSM and HIV." msmgf.org. Available online. URL: http://www.msmgf.org/. Accessed April 1, 2011.

Housing Works. "Where Are the Black Gay Men?" The Body.com. Available online. URL: http://www.the body.com/content/whatis/art50605.html. Accessed April 1, 2011.

IRIN (Integrated Regional Information Networks), UN Office for the Coordination of Humanitarian Affairs. "NEPAL: HIV Awareness amongst MSM Still Low." IRINNews.org. Available online. URL: http:// www.irinnews.org/Report.aspx?ReportId=71738. Accessed April 1, 2011.

Kincaid, Timothy. "The Prevalence of HIV in the Gay Com-munity." BoxTurtleBulletin.com. Available online. URL: http://www.boxturtlebulletin.com/the-preva lence-of-hiv-in-the-gay-community. Accessed April 1, 2011.

Londish, Gregory J., et al. "Minimal Impact of Circum-cision on HIV Acquisition in Men Who Have Sex with Men." *Sexual Health* 7, no. 4 (November 2010): 463–470. Available online. URL: http://www.pub lish.csiro.au/view/journals/dsp_journal_fulltext.cfm ?nid=164&f=SH09 080. Accessed April 1, 2011.

Mejia, A., et al. "HIV Seroprevalence and Associated Risk Factors in Men Who Have Sex with Men in the Villavicencia City, Colombia, 2005." *AIDS 2006: XVI International AIDS Conference.* IASociety. org. Available online. URL: http://www.iasociety. org/Default.aspx?pageId=11&abstractId=2196286. Accessed July 24, 2011.

Ottosson, Daniel. "State-Sponsored Homophobia 2009: A World Survey of Laws Prohibiting Same Sex Activity between Consenting Adults." ILGA. org. Available online. URL: http://ilga.org/historic/ Statehomophobia/ILGA_State_Sponsored_Homo phobia_2009.pdf. Accessed April 1, 2011.

Thomas, Monifa. "Illinois: 17 Percent of Gay Men Here HIV-Positive, New Stats Confirm." AEGIS.com. Avail-able online. URL: http://www.aegis.com/news/ads/ 2009/AD091336.html. Accessed April 1, 2011.

UNAIDS: Joint United Nations Programme on HIV/ AIDS. "China to Tackle HIV Incidence amongst MSM."

UNAIDS.org. Available online. URL: http://www. unaids.org/en/KnowledgeCentre/Resources/Feature Stories/archive/2009/20090116_MSMAsia.asp. Accessed April 1, 2011.

———. "Strengthening Work with MSM in Africa." UNAIDS.org. Available online. URL: http://www.unaids. org/en/KnowledgeCentre/Resources/FeatureStories/ archive/2008/20080523_strengthening_work_msm_ africa.asp. Accessed April 1, 2011.

Verghese, Abraham. *My Own Country: A Doctor's Story.* New York: Vintage Press, 1995.

metabolic syndrome Metabolic syndrome is a collection of symptoms and conditions that can lead to an increased chance of heart attack, stroke, and diabetes. It can affect anyone, though it occurs more frequently as people age and with increased weight. Symptoms of metabolic syndrome include insulin resistance, higher levels of low-density lipoprotein (LDL) in the blood (higher "bad" cholesterol), high levels of triglycerides (another blood fat), high blood pressure, and weight gain around the middle of the body. Metabolic changes have also been associated with the treatment of HUMAN IMMUNODEFICIENCY VIRUS (HIV) with antiretroviral medications, though definitive correlation has not been sufficiently drawn to satisfy all researchers or doctors. However, most doctors would agree that there are body changes that result from use of antiretrovirals, HIV illness itself, or a combination of the two processes.

Symptoms and Diagnostic Path

BLOOD WORK/BLOOD TESTS can be performed to measure LDL, triglyceride, blood sugar, and insulin levels. These tests generally require a person to fast (eat no food for a specific period), before the blood can be drawn and sent to a lab. Blood pressure can be measured in a doctor's office or clinic. Weight gain can be measured using a scale or visually; weight gain around the middle of the body can be seen through photographs.

Coronary heart disease (CHD) is a serious concern at any age, but in many HIV-positive people it has become a worse problem at an earlier age. Studies have shown a double the normal risk of CHD for HIV-positive men 25–35 and a rate six times the HIV-negative rate for men 18–25 years of age. Studies have shown this increased risk in HIV-positive men did not vary according to whether or not they were taking particular antiretrovirals. Other studies have suggested that there are certain PROTEASE INHIBITORS (PIs) that do increase cholesterol and triglyceride levels making these a strong factor in potential CHD.

Studies have presented conflicting reasons for these metabolic changes. One large study done by Kaiser Permanente showed an increased risk based on the number of years taking HIGHLY ACTIVE ANTIRETROVIRAL THERAPY (HAART) and no increased risk depending on whether the treatment regimen was based on protease inhibitors or on NUCLEOSIDE REVERSE TRANSCRIPTASE INHIBITORS (NRTIs). Other studies have shown a correlation with the number of years spent on PI-specific treatment regimens. What this means is that there may be certain antiretroviral medications that can lead to metabolic changes in HIV-infected people. It is not clear at this time which medications may cause these metabolic effects.

Another metabolic change that has been observed among HIV-positive people on antiretrovirals is a decrease in bone density. Instances of osteoporosis, osteopenia, or osteonecrosis have been cited. Each of these terms refers to specific deterioration of the bone and increased chance for the bone to deteriorate to the point that it breaks or crumbles when a particular action happens. Physicians have reported the need for hip replacement among HIV-positive people at young ages, bone density loss prior to menopause in women and in men of varying ages, and bone breaks resulting from everyday bumps and actions. A large study known by the acronym SMART involving HIV-positive people showed that bone density loss can be correlated with particular medications and can be seen most frequently the longer a person is taking antiretrovirals.

Insulin resistance occurs in people when they cannot process insulin properly in their body and the body produces more insulin to try to take the converted sugars and fats from the food we eat into the cells. Eventually, blood sugars build up and insulin produced by the body is no longer sufficient to process the blood sugars. The liver also begins to accumulate more fats, which can cause further problems. Prior to antiretroviral treatment, there was no record of HIV-positive people having insulin resistance issues at higher rates than the general population. Studies have shown that 15–25 percent of people who use HAART may have some form of insulin resistance.

Treatment Options and Outlook

Treatment for metabolic changes involves the same options available to HIV-negative individuals. High triglyceride and cholesterol levels can be treated with lipid drugs that lower blood cholesterol and triglyceride levels. In addition, changes in personal habits are also necessary. Eating a diet that is lower in saturated fats, quitting smoking, and regularly exercising are all extremely important in lowering cholesterol and triglyceride levels. Statin drugs are the recommended medication for lowering lipid levels; in particular, atorvastatin and pravastatin have been shown to interact less with antiretroviral medications than other statins. Fenofibrate can be used to lower triglyceride levels if this is required. Studies have shown that these drugs are less successful when a person is taking a protease inhibitor regimen of antiretrovirals.

Bone density issues do not have a particular standard of care in HIV and AIDS. There have not been studies to test particular treatments among HIV-positive people with osteonecrosis or osteoporosis. If problems are suspected or if pain occurs in and around bones, then magnetic resonance imaging (MRI) scans can be useful in determining whether bone density deterioration has occurred. Patients who have suspected osteoporosis can benefit from calcium and vitamin D supplements, in addition to regular exercise, weight loss, and quitting smoking. Osteonecrosis can be treated with standard pain

medications, and bone replacement surgery has been done in HIV-positive people with no difference in efficacy from that for HIV-negative patients of the age group. Biophosphonates have been shown to be useful in treating osteoporosis and osteopenia in HIV-positive individuals, and a larger study is currently measuring the success of these medications.

Insulin resistance can be treated by dietary changes and exercise as an initial option. Weight loss is also important in the treatment of HIV-positive patients who have insulin resistance. Switching HAART regimens to eliminate INDINAVIR, and using the PI ATAZANAVIR SULFATE, have been shown to cause fewer incidents of insulin resistance. Replacing PIs with NON-NUCLEOSIDE REVERSE TRANSCRIPTASE INHIBITORS (NNRTIs) also has been used to eliminate the potential for insulin problems in HIV-positive patients already at risk for insulin resistance.

Risk Factors and Preventive Measures

Some risk factors that accompany metabolic changes are hereditary. Some people are born with a higher risk of osteoporosis, diabetes, and a higher cholesterol level. If an HIV-positive person has a family history of these conditions, it is possible that antiretroviral treatment may enhance this tendency and lead to various metabolic changes in that individual. A close monitoring by the doctor of each patient prior to starting antiretroviral therapy can allow a quicker response to changes in a person's metabolic status. By knowing the risks and starting point prior to HAART, an individual can receive better overall care from a physician.

The antiretroviral indinavir has been associated with glucose metabolism impairment. Other PIs also have been discussed as potentially increasing insulin resistance but are less clearly associated than indinavir. Atazanavir sulfate is a PI that has *not* been shown to be related to insulin resistance.

On the other hand, atazanavir sulfate has, in some studies, been shown to be associated with bone density issues during antiretroviral treatment. As is always the case with metabolic change studies, another large study found no relation between atazanavir sulfate and bone density, but did find such a correlation with the NRTI drugs STAVUDINE and ZIDOVUDINE.

Many doctors and researchers will make changes in the antiretroviral medications if there is any reason to believe that the current combination has led to a metabolic problem. Others may take a wait-and-see approach as long as the patient is monitored and the antiretroviral combination is working well. Periodic monitoring of all of the blood work can show any changes in cholesterol, triglyceride, blood sugar, and insulin levels. Bone density scans or other means of determining bone strength can help to determine the person's bone health and the potential harm that may be occurring at that level. Given that there is as yet no clear understanding of the full effect of HIV on metabolic syndrome or the full effect of HAART in the known increase of metabolic syndrome events in HIV-positive patients, further studies are planned and being conducted currently.

AIDSInfoNet. "Body Shape Changes (Lipodystrophy)." AIDSInfoNet.org. Available online. URL: http://www.aidsinfonet.org/fact_sheets/view/553. Accessed April 1, 2011.

Chow, Dominic C., M.D., Larry J. Day, M.D., Scott A. Souza, M.D., and Cecilia M. Shikuma, M.D. "Metabolic Complications of HIV Therapy." HIVInSite.org. Available online. URL: http://hivinsite.ucsf.edu/InSite.jsp?page=kb-03-02-10. Accessed April 1, 2011.

European AIDS Clinical Society. "EACS—European-Guidelines 2009." European AIDS Clinical Society.org. Available online. URL: http://www.europeanaidsclinicalsociety.org/guidelinespdf/EACS-EuroGuidelines2009FullVersion.pdf. Accessed April 1, 2011.

Fichtenbaum, Carol J., M.D. "Coronary Heart Disease Risk, Dyslipidemia, and Management in HIV-Infected Persons." Thomasland.com. Available online. URL: http://thomasland.metapress.com/content/p07mhnt8l08g5tku/fulltext.pdf. Accessed April 1, 2011.

Goldman, Bonnie. "2009 Update on Body Shape Changes and HIV/AIDS." TheBody.com. Available online. URL: http://www.thebody.com/content/treat/art51106.html?getPage=1. Accessed April 1, 2011.

Hakeem, Lukman, Ian W. Campbell, and Diptendu Nath Bhattacharyya. "HIV-Associated Lipodystrophy—A New Metabolic Syndrome: Abstract and Introduction." Medscape.com. Available online. URL: http://www.medscape.com/viewarticle/576642. Accessed April 1, 2011.

Highleyman, Liz. "Insulin Resistance and Diabetes." TheBody.com. Available online. URL: http://www.thebody.com/content/art2534.html. Accessed April 1, 2011.

Klein, Daniel, Stephen Sydney, Charles P. Quesenberry, Jr., and Leo B. Hurley. "Do Protease Inhibitors Increase the Risk for Coronary Heart Disease in Patients with HIV-1 Infection?" *JAIDS: Journal of Acquired Immune Deficiency Syndromes* 30, no. 5 (15 August 2002):471–477. Available online. URL: http://journals.lww.com/jaids/pages/articleviewer.aspx?year=2002&issue=08150&article=00002&type=abstract. Accessed April 1, 2011.

Lichtenstein, Kenneth, Ashok Balasubramanyam, Rajagopal Sekhar, and Eric Freedland. "HIV-Associated Adipose Redistribution Syndrome (HARS): Definition, Epidemiology and Clinical Impact." *AIDS Research and Therapy* 4, no. 16 (16 July 2007). Available online. URL: http://www.aidsrestherapy.com/content/4/1/16. Accessed April 1, 2011.

Mascolini, Mark. "Bone Loss in SMART Study." i-base.info. Available online. URL: http://i-base.info/htb/305. Accessed April 1, 2011.

Sharp, Matt. "Metabolic Complications Associated with HIV Disease." TheBody.com. Available online. URL: http://www.thebody.com/content/art1110.html. Accessed April 1, 2011.

microbicides A microbicide is a substance or an agent that kills microbes (bacteria, viruses, or other pathogens). From the time that HIV was discovered to be the cause of the epidemic, researchers have looked for ways to develop a microbicide to kill the virus that causes AIDS prior to its entering the body. Scientists have attempted to use any number of substances or create new ones that would kill the virus before it could enter a person's body and cause illness. The benefit to having a microbicide available to people is that it could be used prior to or during sexual activity to reduce or prevent infection with HIV or other sexually transmitted infections (STIs). Microbicides are seen as potentially helpful in the fight against HIV because they would allow WOMEN and men the opportunity to protect themselves reasonably easily prior to sexual intercourse. It is at times difficult for individuals to use a condom, particularly women, and SEX WORKERS in general. Around the world, it is often difficult for women to use condoms or other birth control and disease prevention devices. Their partners often refuse to allow the use of a condom, and attempting to use one can place a woman at risk of physical harm. Commercial sex workers also report difficulties using these items with demanding or abusive clients. A safe, effective, and for the most part undetectable intervention that can be controlled by women has long been sought to prevent the spread of STIs as well as HIV.

One of the first attempts at such a substance was the use of nonoxynol-9, also known as N-9, as a general microbicide. Nonoxynol-9 was used as a spermicide initially for its ability to kill sperm and prevent pregnancy, and it is often found as an ingredient in gels used by women who use contraceptive sponges or diaphragms for birth control. During the late 1980s and the 1990s, it was included in many sexual lubricants available in pharmacies, as well as in lubricants preapplied to most condoms manufactured in developed countries. However, a study conducted by van Damme et al. and reviewed ethically by the joint United Nations Programme on HIV/AIDS (UNAIDS) and the CENTERS FOR DISEASE CONTROL and Prevention (CDC) in AFRICA among commercial sex workers, published in 2002, found that the women who used nonoxynol-9 were 50 percent more likely to contract HIV than those women who used a lubricant with no microbicide in the gel provided by the study. Further study of nonoxynol-9 found that the substance serves as an irritant to both vaginal and rectal cell tissue and increases the opportunities for HIV spread, thereby providing no benefit and

some harm to those using products containing nonoxynol-9.

The International Partnership for Microbicides (IPM) was formed in 2002 as a way to focus efforts at finding an effective microbicide that women could use safely to protect themselves from HIV transmission as well as other STIs. It was formed through activists, researchers, and funding organizations that desire to speed the process of microbicide development. IPM has offices in the United States as well as Europe and southern Africa. It is funded through donations from large investors such as the European Commission, U.S. Agency for International Development, Bill and Melinda Gates Foundation, and several other countries' development offices and foundations. Other groups such as the Global Campaign for Microbicides are also active in raising awareness, funding, and drug trials of various potential substances that might be used against HIV.

Several microbicide drug trials are under way around the world to test the efficacy of particular substances believed to be potentially helpful in the fight against HIV. The different products being tested have different ways of attempting to prevent the virus from entering the body. Some of the products currently in trials include a TENOFOVIR DISOPROXIL FUMARATE–based gel, products that balance the pH of the vagina to prevent HIV survival, gels of ENTRY INHIBITORS to block HIV entry into the cells, and absorption inhibitors to prevent the virus from associating with the necessary cells. One large multiyear trial of a microbicide was stopped in 2009 when it was shown that the microbicide did no better at protecting women from HIV than the placebo gel being used in the trial. The product in question, PRO-2000, had shown some effectiveness in a small earlier trial. Dapivirine vaginal rings are in a phase III trial as of 2011. Dapivirine, one of the NON-NUCLEOSIDE REVERSE TRANSCRIPTASE INHIBITORS (NNRTIs), is provided in a silicone ring and disperses itself throughout the vagina over the course of one month. The NRTI is not absorbed into the body, but remains in the vagina and is believed to prevent transmission or greatly reduce it. The trial of the dapivirine rings is being conducted in several clinic sites in eastern and southern Africa. In addition to vaginal microbicides, anal microbicides are being developed and tested.

The Economist. "Dashed Hopes." *Economist* (19 December 2009). Available online. URL: http://www.econ omist.com/node/15125189?story_id=E1_TVTN VTRJ. Accessed April 1, 2011.

Gayle, Helene D. "Study: Nonoxynol-9 Does Not Protect against HIV." TheBody.org. Available online. URL: http://www.thebody.com/content/art30552. html. Accessed April 1, 2011.

Global Campaign for Microbicides. "Global Campaign for Microbicides: About the Campaign." Global -Campaign.org. Available online. URL: http://www. global-campaign.org/about.htm. Accessed April 1, 2011.

International Partnership for Microbicides. "Dapivirine Microbicide Rings." IPMGlobal.org. Available online. URL: http://www.ipmglobal.org/node/532. Accessed April 1, 2011.

International Rectal Microbicide Advocates. "IRMA." RectalMicrobicides.org. Available online. URL: http:// www.rectalmicrobicides.org/. Accessed April 1, 2011.

Van Damme, L., et al. "Effectiveness of COL-1492, a Nonoxynol-9 Vaginal Gel, on HIV-1 Transmission in Female Sex Workers: A Randomised Controlled Trial." *Lancet* 360, no. 9338 (28 September 2002): 971–977.

microsporidiosis Microsporidiosis is the name for the illnesses caused by a number of protozoan parasites of the phylum Microsporidia. There are at least 14 known parasites in the family, among some 1,200 species, that can cause illness in humans. The following Microsporidia are known to cause various infections: *Brachiola algerae, B. connori, B. vesicularum; Encephalitozoon cuniculi, E. hellem, E. intestinalis; Enterocytozoon bieneusi; Microsporidium ceylonensis, M. africanum; Nosema ocularum; Pleistophora* sp.; *Trachipleistophora hominis, T. anthropophthera; Vittaforma corneae.*

The most common form of the parasites is *Enterocytozoon bieneusi,* which infects the lining of the small intestine and causes severe diarrhea. It has also been linked to sinusitis and cholangitis (inflammation of the biliary ducts leading to the liver). Other microsporidia can cause infections of the eye, lungs, kidney, and muscles as well as the sinus and intestines. The microsporidia are ingested in some manner by the human and attach themselves to the intestine lining or other cell specific to the species with a small, taillike appendage known as a polar tubule. The spore then transfers infective material into the cell, where it reproduces spores until the cell is filled and bursts, spreading further spores into the host animal. Prior to the HIV epidemic, microsporidiosis had only been reported in medical literature in 11 cases.

Symptoms and Diagnostic Path

The most general symptom with *Enterocytozoon bieneusi* is watery diarrhea, along with weight loss (wasting), gas, abdominal pain, and dehydration. Other microsporidia can bring about different symptoms. *E. cuniculi* is associated with hepatitis, encephalitis, and disseminated infection. *E. intestinalis* can cause keratoconjunctivitis (inflammation of the cornea and the clear area of the eye) and diarrhea. *E. hellem* can also cause keratconjunctivitis, as well as sinusitis, respiratory disease, infection of the prostate, and disseminated illness. *Brachiola algerae* causes muscle and skin infections. These are just a few of the various symptoms that can be seen with microsporidia infection.

Diagnosis must be done with an electron microscope because of the small size of the protozoa. Samples from stools, bowel biopsies, or fluid from the sinuses or eyes and biopsies of the muscle or skin can be used for this examination. Staining, the biochemical technique of adding dye to a sample to highlight particular features, is used first to identify whether the illness is microsporidia related, and then to determine the particular species of microsporidia. Many microsporidia cannot be cultivated in a laboratory, making this method preferred to attempting to cultivate a particular species in vitro.

Treatment Options and Outlook

Generally, treatment of an HIV-positive person with HIGHLY ACTIVE ANTIRETROVIRAL THERAPY (HAART) has proven the most effective at ridding the body of the various microsporidia. Most patients who have microsporidiosis have a CD4 T lymphocyte count of fewer than 100 cells/μL, so restoring the immune system to a functioning level will allow the patient's own immune system to rid the body of microsporidia on its own. People who have a CD4 T cell count of greater than 200 cells/μL for longer than six months will probably be taken off any medications specifically used to treat microsporidiosis.

In eye infections, treatment with fumagillin, a veterinary medicine often used to treat bee colonies for infections, has been shown to clear the eye of infection. It is available only as a topical medicine in the United States and therefore needs to be mixed with a saline (salt water) solution before use for such treatment. In order to clear microsporidiosis from the rest of the body, albendazole is recommended so the eye infection does not recur.

Albendazole is the recommended treatment for a number of microsporidia, though it is not specifically approved for treatment of the infection in the United States. It is not, however, effective against *E. bieneusi* or *V. corneae* because these microsporidia have amino acids that have been seen in albendazole resistance. Other antibiotics that have also shown some effectiveness against some microsporidia include itraconazole, nitazoxanide, metronidazole, and oral fumagillin. (The last is not available in the United States.)

Risk Factors and Preventive Measures

The only recommendation that the government provides for the prevention of microsporidiosis is to avoid drinking water from untreated sources. As the spread of microsporidia is mainly through human and animal excrement, it can be assumed that general hand washing and personal hygiene are also good recommendations. Unprotected sexual activity can also be a cause of the spread of some microsporidia.

For people who have been treated for ocular microsporidiosis, continuing treatment after restoration of the immune system has proven to be the best way to prevent recurrence of the infection, which has been shown to return if the medicine is stopped.

On the basis of recent data, it is now known that some domestic and wild animals may be naturally infected with the following microsporidian species: *E. cuniculi, E. intestinalis,* and *E. bieneusi.* Birds, especially parrots (parakeets, love birds, and budgies), are naturally infected with *E. hellem. E. bieneusi* and *V. corneae* have been identified in surface waters, and spores of *B. algerae* have been identified in ditch water. Avoidance of these sources may help to protect a person who has a weakened immune system from developing microsporidiosis.

AIDSmeds. "Microsporidiosis: How Is It Treated or Prevented?" AIDSmeds.com. Available online. URL: http://www.aidsmeds.com/articles/Micro_6882.shtml. Accessed April 1, 2011.

Centers for Disease Control and Prevention. "Microsporidiosis." CDC.gov. Available online. URL: http://www.dpd.cdc.gov/DPDX/HTML/Microsporidiosis.htm. Accessed April 1, 2011.

Molina, Jean-Michel, et al. "Fumagillin Treatment of Intestinal Microsporidiosis." *New England Journal of Medicine* 346, no. 25 (20 June 2002): 1963–1969. Available online. URL: http://www.nejm.org/doi/full/10.1056/NEJMoa012924. Accessed April 1, 2011.

NAM AIDSmap. "Microsporidiosis." AIDSmap.com. Available online. URL: http://www.aidsmap.com/cms1032607.asp. Accessed April 1, 2011.

Middle East and North Africa   There are more than 460,000 people living in this region who have HIV, according to United Nations (UN) statistical estimates at the end of 2009. That is lower than previous estimates, though growing in comparison to the number in the rest of the world. From 2003 to 2007, this region showed a 300 percent increase in HIV/AIDS cases, as opposed to a 20 percent increase in the Western world during the same period. Sexual activities appear to be the main route of TRANSMISSION, though increases in the number of injection drug users (IDU) (see INTRAVENOUS DRUG USE(R)) in the region who have tested positive have been recorded since 1999. The highest rates of known prevalence include Djibouti, 2.5 percent; Algeria, 0.1 percent; Israel, 0.2 percent; Sudan, 1.1 percent; Iran, 0.2 percent; and Morocco, 0.1 percent.

One of the more outrageous stories during the epidemic has been the Libyan government's jailing, trying, and convicting five Bulgarian nurses and one Palestinian medical intern of transmitting AIDS purposefully to more 400 children during the worst nosocomial (hospital-acquired) transmission of HIV recorded. Although originally arrested in 1999, the group was not sentenced to death until 2004, and the Libyan highest court approved the sentence in 2006. The French government intervened, and the group was released to the European Union, eventually being freed in Bulgaria in 2007. It later became clear the group had been tortured to confess to the crimes and that unsafe medical practices at Al-Fateh Hospital in Libya's second-largest city, Benghazi, had allowed the extensive transmission of HIV. A fund was set up by several countries to cover the cost of caring for the children, an act that helped to encourage the release of the medical workers. Elsewhere in Libya, transmission by IDUs is the largest known infection route, a problem compounded by the number of IDUs who pay for sex and the small numbers of men in Libyan studies who say they use condoms.

In Egypt, heterosexual transmission is the main route of infection; MEN WHO HAVE SEX WITH MEN (MSM) transmission routes also play an important role. MSM tested during an Egyptian Ministry of Health study in 2006 were 6 percent HIV positive, indicating an active epidemic in that community. A 2006 study in Sudan of MSM showed 9 percent of MSM were HIV positive. Both studies are cited in the 2007 Joint United Nations Programme on HIV/AIDS (UNAIDS) regional update. MSM sex is illegal and highly criminalized in all countries of this region except Israel. Injection drug users in Egypt as well as Syria, Iraq, and Jordan are a small but worrisome population, as in most parts of the world, as studies conducted on these populations show extensive use of commercial SEX WORKERS, thereby opening up other populations to HIV infection.

In Sudan, the epidemic is also largely heterosexually spread and is a great concern for a country that has been engaged in civil war for most of its independence. Rates of infection at pregnancy clinics in Sudan range from 0.8 percent to 3 percent across all regions of the country. More than half the Sudanese men in the previously mentioned MSM study said they engaged in commercial sex and rarely used a condom.

In Saudi Arabia, approximately 0.05 percent of the population has tested HIV positive, though, according to the UNAIDS Saudi report, 75 percent of these numbers are foreign nationals in the country. Most foreigners who do test positive are jailed, then deported. Citizens who test positive are provided care and necessary medications free, as is the policy of the government in all health care. The primary means of transmission is heterosexual sex, with lower rates of IDU and mother-to-child transmission. The report clearly states that sex work and MSM activities are illegal and consistently prosecuted and that it is nearly impossible to track incidence.

In general, this is a culturally conservative part of the world. Men hold positions of power in society and government. Discussion of sexual behavior is actively discouraged. Condom use is particularly frowned upon because condoms encourage men and women to practice sexual activity outside marriage. Men also have the right to be polygamous in several countries. In addition, substantial percentages of men have reported in studies that they either visit sex workers or engage in sexual activity outside marriage. This leads HIV/AIDS experts to be concerned about the potential for HIV spread, particularly among large extended polygamous families.

In Turkey, the epidemic is driven by heterosexual spread. IDU is minimal compared to that of both neighboring Central Asian and Eastern and Central European standards. There is an epidemic among commercial sex workers, who are predominantly from other countries, and in the MSM population.

Morocco has always had an active commercial sex industry that is not generally discussed because of conservative cultural mores. HIV infection is driven through sexual activity, predominantly heterosexual in nature. WOMEN comprise a higher portion of the infected than in most countries of this region, and large numbers of infected women there are married.

Education still has an opportunity to curb infection in an area that has always had a minimal HIV infection rate. Growing rates in several countries, including Algeria and Tunisia, do not bode well for the opportunity to educate, as it may have passed without the countries' taking advantage of the chance to stop an epidemic before it started.

The Body. "HIV/AIDS in Arab World Up 300 Percent." TheBody.com. Available online. URL: http://www.thebody.com/content/world/art40433.html. Accessed April 1, 2011.
Fattah, Hassan M. "Saudi Arabia Begins to Face Hidden AIDS Problem." NYTimes.com. Available online. URL: http://www.nytimes.com/2006/08/08/world/middleeast/08saudi.html. Accessed April 1, 2011.
International HIV/AIDS Alliance. "Morocco." AIDS Alliance.org. Available online. URL: http://www.aidsalliance.org/sw7218.asp. Accessed April 1, 2011.
Smith, Craig A. "Libya Sentences 6 to Die in H.I.V. Case." NYTimes.com. Available online. URL: http://www.nytimes.com/2006/12/20/world/middleeast/20libya.html?ex=1167454800&en=7c536420bc24c815&ei=5070. Accessed April 1, 2011.
UNAIDS: Joint United Nations Programme for HIV/AIDS. "Middle East and North Africa." UNAIDS.org. Available online. URL: http://www.unaids.org/en/regionscountries/regions/middleeastandnorthafrica/. Accessed April 1, 2011.
———. "Middle East and North Africa: AIDS Epidemic Update, Regional Summary, 07." Available online. URL: http://data.unaids.org/pub/Report/2008/jc1531_epibriefs_mena_en.pdf. Accessed July 24, 2011.
———. "UNGASS Country Progress Report: Saudi Arabia." UNAIDS.org. Available online. URL: http://www.unaids.org/en/dataanalysis/monitoringcountryprogress/2010progressreportssubmittedbycountries/saudiarabia_2010_country_progress_report_en.pdf. Accessed April 1, 2011.

molluscum contagiosum Molluscum contagiosum is a common viral infection of the skin that causes one or more small, firm bumps, which are generally painless but can cause itchiness. In most cases, the bumps recede within a year, even if no treatment is given. As the virus only affects the outer layer of skin and does not affect internal organs, it generally poses no problem to a healthy individual. Once the skin bump is gone, the virus has cleared the body. New bumps can form as older ones are scratched.

The molluscum contagiosum virus (MCV) is a member of the poxvirus family, which includes smallpox. The virus is common in CHILDREN and is readily spread person to person through touching or contact with personal or common items such as door handles, toys, or faucets touched by someone who has the virus. In adults, the virus is often spread through sexual contact.

In HIV-positive people, MCV can spread to large areas of the face or body when the HUMAN IMMUNE SYSTEM is weakened. Bumps can be large, gather in clusters, and be annoying in appearance and cause great itching and redness. This variety of molluscum is often referred to as giant molluscum. Most molluscum in children is produced by a different strain of the virus than the strain that affects HIV-positive people, but the bumps and the general course of the virus are the same.

Symptoms and Diagnostic Path

The bumps are generally small, less than two millimeters. Giant molluscum can be up to two centimeters in size. The bumps, large or small, are always rounded in appearance and have a slight depression in the middle. They can be single bumps or can be spread to create groups of bumps through scratching behavior in children. In HIV-positive people, the bumps can cover the whole trunk of a person, as well as large parts of the face, and gather in clusters of several bumps, particularly around the eyelids. HIV-positive people who have weakened immune systems have a higher risk of being affected by molluscum than HIV-positive people who have well-functioning immune systems.

Treatment Options and Outlook

With the initiation of HIGHLY ACTIVE ANTIRETROVIRAL THERAPY (HAART), molluscum cases have dropped dramatically. People have stronger immune systems because of the antiviral medications, and the virus does not have the opportunity to become active as a result. Once established in HIV-positive people, molluscum can spread to large areas quickly. Giant molluscum are difficult to treat and there are no specific antiviral medications at this time to treat the infection.

All treatments for molluscum involve the removal of the bumps in some manner. The bumps are not dangerous and cause no internal problems, but can be cosmetically displeasing as well as difficult to prevent from spreading unless removed. The standard treatments for removal involve surgically removing the bumps, freezing the bumps, using a laser to burn them off, or using medicinal creams with salicylic acid or another chemical to destroy the bumps while leaving the skin around them intact. Topical cidofovir and imiquimod are also used in some resistant cases of molluscum.

Risk Factors and Preventive Measures

The virus is fairly common and is readily spread. Children should be cautioned not to scratch the molluscum bumps so they do not spread to other parts of the skin. The same is true in adults. Prevention is the same as for all common cleanliness. Hands should be washed thoroughly and frequently so that germs from contaminated surfaces do not spread. Contact with another person's molluscum should be avoided, as it spreads easily.

American Academy of Dermatology. "Molluscum Contagiosum." AAD.org. Available online. URL: http://www.aad.org/skin-conditions/dermatology-a-to-z/molluscum-contagiosum. Accessed April 1, 2011.
Centers for Disease Control and Prevention. "Molluscum (Molluscum Contagiosum)." CDC.gov. Available online. URL: http://www.cdc.gov/ncidod/dvrd/molluscum/faq/everyone.htm. Accessed April 1, 2011.
Kauffman, Catharine Lisa. "Dermatologic Manifestations of Molluscum Contagiosum." Medscape.com. Available online. URL: http://emedicine.medscape.com/article/1132908-overview. Accessed April 1, 2011.
Martins, Ciro R., and David Kouba. "Molluscum Contagiosum." Hopkins-HIVGuide.org. Available online. URL: http://www.hopkins-hivguide.org/diagnosis/organ_system/dermatologic/molluscum_contagiosum.html. Accessed April 1, 2011.
Mayo Clinic Staff. "Molluscum Contagiosum." Mayo Clinic.com. Available online. URL: http://www.mayoclinic.com/health/molluscum-contagiosum/DS00672/DSECTION=prevention. Accessed April 1, 2011.

Mycobacterium avium complex *Mycobacterium avium* complex (MAC) is an infection caused by a group of related bacterial species of the genus *Mycobacterium*. Mycobacteria are common throughout the human environment. *M. avium* and *M. intracellulare* are the most common; however, other species that have not yet been classified can also cause infection. In people who have a healthy immune system, MAC rarely causes any illness. A subspecies of *Mycobacterium* *avium* has been implicated as a possible cause of Crohn's disease, but researchers are unsure of the connection between the bacteria and the supposed genetic links of Crohn's disease. However, in HIV-positive individuals, MAC can disseminate throughout the body, causing a very serious illness, almost always in people whose CD4 T lymphocyte count is less than 50 cells/μL.

MAC is probably transmitted through inhalation of the bacteria through the respiratory tract, though the possibility exists of its transmission through the intestinal tract via ingestion. It has been found in water and soil samples as well as in other common contaminants such as house dust, birds, farm animals, and tobacco. Understanding of the transmission process is as of yet incomplete. Initially, it was thought that a previous MAC infection could be reactivated after the immune system began failing, but studies demonstrating a lack of antibodies to the MAC infection show that infections are new to the body and not an older infection reactivated. The bacteria first inhabit the mucosal lining of the intestinal or respiratory tract and then infect the macrophages located there. Once this occurs, the macrophages carry the infection to the lymph or blood system, where dissemination occurs.

Prior to the introduction of HIGHLY ACTIVE ANTIRETROVIRAL THERAPY (HAART), 20–40 percent of all HIV patients developed disseminated MAC in some form. The incidence rate has dropped dramatically in the HAART era. People who have MAC most often have a disseminated illness that is found not only in the lungs and intestinal tract but also the liver, spleen, lymph system, adrenal glands, bone marrow, and kidneys. The body seems unable to respond to MAC after the immune system becomes weak, often allowing the infection to spread widely uncontrolled.

Symptoms and Diagnostic Path

Early symptoms of a disseminated MAC infection can include abdominal pain, fever, night sweats, weight loss, diarrhea, and fatigue. Localized MAC infections can occur in people who have begun HAART or have been on HAART for a short time. These can appear as lung infections predominantly and as lymphadenitis in children.

In a study conducted at San Francisco General Hospital (Chin et al., 1994), signs of a disseminated MAC infection were looked for among HIV-positive patients who self-reported various health issues. Clinical testing was done to evaluate the patients for MAC and for abnormalities in BLOOD WORK/BLOOD TESTS. The following three were found to have a strong correlation to a MAC infection: a history of fever for more than 30 days, a hematocrit (the proportion of blood volume occupied by red blood cells) of less than 30 percent, or a serum albumin (a plasma protein in the blood) level less than 3.0 grams/dL.

Blood tests for disseminated MAC infection are highly sensitive to the bacteria and can be very reliable. Biopsies of various tissues can also provide a diagnosis of MAC.

Treatment Options and Outlook

Treatment of MAC infection needs to use at least two antimycobacterial drugs to prevent or delay resistance to the treatment. Three-drug treatments are also common. The drug treatments should last a minimum of 12 months. Clarithromycin and azithromycin are the two most commonly used antimycobacterials. Rifabutin and ethambutol are the most common second or third drugs added to the combination. In some cases of severe immune deficiency, an injectable drug such as clarithromycin or amikacin can be added. People who are first diagnosed HIV positive at the time of their MAC diagnosis should not start HAART immediately, but should wait for the MAC to be treated for at least two weeks to prevent drug interactions as well as the occurrence of IMMUNE RECONSTITUTION INFLAMMATORY SYNDROME (IRIS).

MAC can become resistant to drug treatment if not carefully monitored and if the patient does not take the dosage daily. Second- and third-line treatments should use a combination of the drugs mentioned and possibly others, such as a quinolone drug (moxifloxacin, ciprofloxacin, or levofloxacin).

Risk Factors and Preventive Measures

There are no means to avoid infection with MAC, as it appears in most environments and the spread is poorly understood at this time. Adults and adolescents who have been diagnosed with disseminated MAC should continue to use MAC medications until their immune systems have recovered (CD4 T lymphocyte count greater than 100 cells/μL) for a minimum of 12 months. Those who continue to have infections should remain on the medications indefinitely to protect them against a recurrence of disseminated disease.

Preventive medications are the same medications used in the treatment of MAC. If a patient's CD4 T lymphocyte count is below 50 cells/μL, then a prophylaxis treatment should be started. Treatment with either azithromycin or clarithromycin is the norm. Treatment with both drugs for prevention is not necessary. Rifabutin can be given in conjunction with azithromycin, although the costs of the added drug, along with the added side effects and drug interactions for rifabutin, may not make it feasible.

AIDS Education and Training Centers. "*Mycobacterium avium* Complex." AIDSetc.org. Available online. URL: http://www.aidsetc.org/aidsetc?page=cm-522_mac. Accessed April 1, 2011.

Centers for Disease Control and Prevention. "*Mycobacterium avium* Complex." CDC.gov. Available online. URL: http://www.cdc.gov/ncidod/dbmd/disease info/mycobacteriumavium_t.htm. Accessed April 1, 2011.

Chin, D. P., et al. "*Mycobacterium avium* Complex in the Respiratory or Gastrointestinal Tract and the Risk of *M. avium* Complex Bacteremia in Patients with Human Immunodeficiency Virus." *Journal of Infectious Disease* 169, no. 2 (February 1994): 289–295. Available online. URL: http://www.ncbi.nlm.nih.gov/pubmed/7906290?dopt=Abstract. Accessed April 1, 2011.

Jacobson, Mark A., M.D., and Judith A. Aberg, M.D. "*Mycobacterium avium* Complex and Atypical Mycobacterial Infections in the Setting of HIV Infection." HIVInSite.ucsf.edu. Available online. URL: http://hiv insite.ucsf.edu/InSite?page=kb-05-01-05. Accessed April 1, 2011.

Koirala, Janak. "*Mycobacterium avium–Intracellulare*." Medscape.com. Available online. URL: http://emedicine.medscape.com/article/222664-over view. Accessed April 1, 2011.

NAMES Project AIDS Memorial Quilt (AIDS Memorial Quilt)   The AIDS quilt, or the AIDS Memorial Quilt, is the largest community art project in the world. It was begun in 1987 by the San Francisco activist Cleve Jones and several friends as a way to remember friends who had died during the AIDS epidemic.

Cleve Jones is an activist who had been involved in planning and leading a yearly memorial march to honor Harvey Milk, a San Francisco city council member, and George Moscone, mayor of San Francisco, who had been assassinated in 1978 by another city council member, Dan White. During the 1985 march, Jones put together a display of 1,000 placards that people in the march carried. Each placard contained the name of a person who had died in San Francisco of AIDS. The placards were then hung on the San Francisco Federal Building wall at the end of the march, and Jones says that he thought at the time that the wall looked like a large quilt. In 1986, Jones created the first panel of a patchwork quilt for his friend Harvey Feldman. He then teamed up with friends in 1987 officially to form the NAMES Project, which began collecting quilt panels from around the country as a memorial to people who had died.

In his book *Stitching a Revolution,* Jones recalls that the initial volunteers were mostly people who themselves were ill or family members of people who had died. They felt a need to document themselves or loved ones in some manner, afraid that society and history would ignore them. The decision to make the quilt panels three feet by six feet was made, as this was the standard size of a grave. There was a

definite attempt to tie the panels to the deaths of the people they represented. Because of the discrimination faced by people who had HIV and AIDS in those days, families often did not hold funerals for people who died of AIDS, and funeral homes were known to refuse to accept the bodies for services. There was a fear that the illness could be spread by touch or through the air, and families were shamed when a member died as a result of the illness.

The three-by-six panels were stitched together into twelve-by-twelve blocks that allowed people to move around the quilt, to touch the panels without having to crawl over the panels of other people. The display of the quilt was completed by running white fabric around and between the twelve-by-twelve blocks so that it appeared as one giant quilt laid out on the ground. The white sashing between the blocks could be used as the place for people to walk around each block and view the designs and see the names and words that were written on each block. Panels have been constructed or created out of almost any imaginable fabric and decorated by an enormous number of varied items. Some are simple fabric panels with the name and the birth and death dates of an individual. Others are highly stylized statements about the individual. They are constructed in burlap, cotton, nylon, leather, bubble wrap, and silk. They are festooned with buttons, Barbie dolls, coins, hair, records, compact disks, uniforms, ribbons, feather boas, school awards, love letters, shoes, wedding rings, car keys, silk flowers, rhinestones, T-shirts, jockstraps, and nearly anything else one can imagine as long as it can be securely sewn to the panel.

The first time the quilt was displayed in full to the public was in Washington, D.C., at the National Gay and Lesbian March on Washington in October 1987. Jones and his volunteers had collected more than 2,000 panels by that time from all around the country. Word had spread through news stories, speaking engagements, and simple word of mouth. Panels began showing up with stories attached about the people the panel represented. Nearly half a million people saw the quilt during the weekend that it went on display. The quilt then went on a tour of several cities around the country. It was used by the people who brought the quilt to their city as a fund-raising and educational tool as well as a memorial to the people who had died.

In October 1988, the quilt returned to Washington, D.C., for another display. By this time, there were more than 8,000 panels, and the quilt filled a much larger space on the National Mall. The quilt again toured several cities, raising funds for local AIDS service and education nonprofit agencies. The quilt was displayed again in 1992 and 1996 in Washington, D.C. Some panels were included in President William Clinton's inaugural parade in 1993. The last time that the full quilt was displayed anywhere was in 1996. It had simply outgrown the space available to display it on the National Mall. In 2004, the most recent 1,000 panels were on display in Washington, D.C., as part of the National HIV Testing Day educational efforts. The quilt continues to be used in educational and fund-raising events in many different locations around the country and the globe. Panels are requested and sent to locations for display in local areas.

In total, there are now more than 47,000 panels composing the quilt. There are more than 91,000 names on the quilt, as some panels represent more than one individual. The quilt covers approximately 1.3 million square feet of space (approximately 29 acres or 12 hectares) if it is spread out, and weighs more than 54 tons. It contains panels from every state in the United States plus Puerto Rico and Guam, as well as 35 countries, from Argentina to Zambia. The quilt has been credited with raising more than $4 million for various AIDS organizations around the country. It is believed that more than 91 million people have viewed the quilt since the first exhibit in Washington, D.C. Some well-known people who have panels in the quilt include Peter Allen, Arthur Ashe, Mel Boozer, Tina Chow, Roy Cohn, Easy E, Elizabeth Glaser, Keith Haring, Rock Hudson, Liberace, Freddy Mercury, Tim Richmond, Max Robinson, Sylvester, Ryan White, and Pedro Zamora.

In 1989, the quilt was nominated for the Nobel Peace Prize. It was the subject of the Academy Award-winning documentary *Common Threads: Stories from the Quilt.* The musical *Quilt: A Musical Celebration* was based on stories from the quilt. Several books have been written about the quilt or have used it as inspiration.

The AIDS Memorial Quilt and the NAMES Project are now based in Atlanta, Georgia. The quilt is stored in a special warehouse. Visitors can view specific panels at the warehouse if the panels are currently not on display around the country. The quilt has also been digitized, and each panel can be viewed online. The letters and stories that are associated with each panel have also been preserved and can be seen at the Atlanta location.

Jones, Cleve, and Jeff Dawson. *Stitching a Revolution: The Making of an Activist.* New York: HarperSanFrancisco, 2000.

NAMES Project Foundation. "The AIDS Memorial Quilt." AIDSquilt.org. Available online. URL: http://www.aidsquilt.org/index.htm. Accessed April 1, 2011.

The World Bank. "The Names Project AIDS Memorial Quilt." WorldBank.org. Available online. URL: http://web.worldbank.org/WBSITE/EXTERNAL/TOPICS/EXTHEALTHNUTRITIONANDPOPULATION/EXTHIVAIDS/0,,contentMDK:20728719~menuPK:376507~pagePK:64020865~piPK:149114~theSitePK:376471,00.html. Accessed April 1, 2011.

nelfinavir Nelfinavir, one of the PROTEASE INHIBITORS (PIs), is manufactured by Agouron Pharmaceuticals. The U.S. FOOD AND DRUG ADMINISTRATION (FDA) approved it in 1997. It is always prescribed as part of a multidrug regimen for the treatment of HIV. The drug is sold under the brand name Viracept and is abbreviated NFV. It is available in both pill form and a powder that can be mixed with water or juice for CHILDREN or people unable to swallow pills.

Nelfinavir was recalled from the European market in 2007 after the maker of the drug noted that high levels of a chemical used in the manufacture of the drug had been found to be in the medication. The chemical, ethyl methanesulfonate (EMS), is a known cancer-causing agent in humans. Studies of the drug in the United States found some EMS in the drug, and it was discontinued as a recommended drug for pregnant women and children. It has since been reclassified as acceptable for all HIV-positive people, after the company reviewed manufacturing and corrected the problem.

Nelfinavir has been used in sub-Saharan AFRICA and elsewhere as an effective drug for pregnant women at the onset of the delivery. A single dose of nefinivir has been given to the mother to prevent the passing of HIV to the newborn during the delivery process. Nelfinavir has also been used as part of a prophylactic regimen for health care workers who have been potentially exposed to HIV through needlesticks or other medical accidents.

Dosage

Nelfinavir has a high dose requirement that has made it a less popular treatment option as newer, easier-to-dose medications have become available to HIV-positive people. It is sold in either 250 mg tablets or 625 mg tablets. It is to be taken as 1250 mg, five 250 mg tablets, twice a day; two 625 mg tablets twice a day; or 750 mg, three 250 mg tablets, three times a day.

A scoop found in the container measures the powdered form. It measures 50 mg of medicine in each level scoop. Recommended dosage is 45–55 mg per kilogram of body weight for children above the age of two. Food is always to be taken with nelfinavir, whether it is in the powder or tablet form. It is absorbed into the body better on a full stomach. If swallowing tablets is difficult, the tablets can be crushed and mixed with water or food to aid ingestion.

Drug Interactions

Nelfinavir is one PI that is not helped by low-dose ritonavir. There is no benefit to prescribing the two drugs together. Other PIs in the body can affect concentrations of nelfinavir; however, no dosing changes are recommended for these drug level changes.

The drug interacts with a number of other medications, including the cholesterol-lowering drugs simvastatin and lovastatin, antibiotics used to treat infections such as TUBERCULOSIS, antidepressant or antipsychotic medications, and medications for some fungal infections. It should not be taken with any drugs containing ergot, which is used in many migraine medications. It is important that a doctor know and understand all the medications and supplements a person is using when prescribing nelfinavir.

Nelfinavir also increases the amount of the drugs sildenafil (Viagra), vardenafil (Levitra), and tadalafil (Cialis)—all erectile dysfunction medications—in the blood, causing severe side effects. Lowering the dosage of these medications is recommended to prevent potential complications.

Estrogen-based birth control methods are less effective when taking nelfinavir. WOMEN who are using these forms of birth control may seek to use a barrier protection method such as condoms while taking nelfinavir.

Methadone levels in the body decrease substantially while taking nelfinavir. People who use methadone for the treatment of opiate addiction should have dosages adjusted and monitored by a doctor.

St. John's wort, an herbal supplement, should never be taken with a PI, as it has been shown to reduce the amount of PI in the body significantly. Other supplements that may affect the level of nelfinavir in the body include garlic pills and milk thistle supplements.

Side Effects

The main side effect of nelfinavir use is diarrhea. Explosive diarrhea is experienced by 20–40 percent of the people taking the drug initially. It ceases in many people over time, but the remainder experience the diarrhea as long as they are taking the drug. Other side effects include nausea, vomiting, tiredness, and headache.

Protease inhibitors, as a class of drug, often increase the cholesterol and triglyceride levels of patients. High lipid levels have been recorded in some nelfinavir patients. This side effect can be managed with appropriate cholesterol-lowering medications. Nelfinavir has also been associated with treatment regimens that can cause LIPODYS-TROPHY, or the redistribution of fat within the body. Symptoms are increased fat around the neck and stomach area, facial wasting, breast enlargement, and peripheral wasting in the arms and legs. Some of these changes disappear when the drug is stopped.

Cases of increased blood sugar level, onset of diabetes, or worsening of existing diabetes when using nelfinavir have also been recorded.

AIDS InfoNet. "Nelfinavir (Viracept)." AIDSInfoNet. org. Available online. URL: http://www.aidsinfo net.org/fact_sheets/view/444. Accessed March 11, 2011.

AIDSmeds. "Special Issues for Children with HIV." AIDSmeds.com. Available online. URL: http://www. aidsmeds.com/articles/Children_7566.shtml. Accessed March 11, 2011.

————. "Viracept (Nelfinavir)." AIDSmeds.com. Available online. URL: http://www.aidsmeds.com/archive/ Viracept_1564.shtml. Accessed March 11, 2011.

The Body. "Viracept (Nelfinavir)." TheBody.com. Available online. URL: http://www.thebody.com/index/ treat/viracept.html. Accessed March 11, 2011.

United States Department of Health and Human Services. "Nelfinavir." aidsinfo.nih.gov. Available online. URL: http://www.aidsinfo.nih.gov/DrugsNew/Drug DetailNT.aspx?int_id=263. Accessed March 11, 2011.

neuropathy   Neuropathy, also referred to as peripheral neuropathy, is an abnormal degenerative or inflammatory condition of the peripheral nervous system. *Peripheral* refers to the nerves that are outside the central nervous system of the brain and spinal cord. Nerves are responsible for, among other functions, the movement of muscles and the sensation of touch, including the sensation of pain. Neuropathy is frequent in people who have diabetes and HIV and in people who consume excessive quantities of alcohol.

Symptoms and Diagnostic Path

In people who have HIV, the most frequent symptoms are painful feet and legs. Individuals experience numbness or tingling in the hands and/or feet; weakness in the muscles of the legs, feet, and hands; or a burning pain in the soles of the feet and the ends of the fingers and toes. Some describe the sensation as extreme pain that can interfere with walking or using the hands. In some people, the symptoms may simply be loss of feeling or sense in the extremities, more of an annoyance, while other people can find it to be very painful. In people who have severe conditions, even the lightest touch of the area affected can cause extreme pain. For instance, socks and shoes can be painful to wear, and sheets or other bed linens can cause a restless night of sleep by simply lying on top of the feet. Symptoms can wax and wane, not always affecting an individual the same way.

Testing for neuropathy involves checking the reflexes of the ankles or other affected areas. Occasionally, measuring electronically the nerve impulses may be done to check the level of functioning of the nerves. Otherwise, there is no special test that is generally done that could help with diagnosis other than a person's discussing the symptoms with a doctor. The main discussion will be in regard to other factors.

Neuropathy is more prevalent in older HIV patients and in those who have higher viral load counts. The condition is seen in approximately 30 percent of HIV patients as the disease progresses. It also is seen more frequently in people who have taken or currently take one of the "D drugs" as part of their highly active antiretroviral therapy (HAART) regimen. Stavudine (d4T), didanosine (ddI), and zalcitabine (ddC) are the D drugs, and neuropathy is a known side effect for some people. As these medications were all approved early in the HIV epidemic, many patients developed these side effects while on the drugs. As other medications have become available and doctors have learned more about side effects of the D drugs, management of peripheral neuropathy has improved, and more doctors are aware of the potential for its development in people who use these drugs.

Treatment Options and Outlook

The first option for a doctor would be to change a patient's HAART regimen if neuropathy were believed to be the result of the medications a person was currently taking. Removing the particular drug and replacing it with a different antiretroviral requires a doctor to know the best method of withdrawal from one antiretroviral and replacement with another so as not to allow any potential resistance to the medications to develop.

If a person is not using one of the medications that can cause neuropathy, a doctor will examine other potential causes such as diabetes or heavy alcohol use. HIV viral load levels will also be examined. Neuropathy in HIV patients is more prevalent with age and high viral load. Other medications used in the treatment of some opportunistic infections (OIs) may also cause neuropathy. An overabundance of vitamin B_6 is also known to cause these problems.

Treatment remains a matter of trying to end the pain, or the cause of the problem. By stopping the alcohol or the antiretroviral that causes nerve damage, neuropathy can sometimes be stopped, too. Many people regain the senses in the extremities and have reduced pain over a course of several weeks once the medication has been stopped.

If the neuropathy is the result of HIV disease, then pain medications will often be prescribed to make it easier for the individual to get through the day. Ibuprofen is often recommended for mild cases. Antidepressants such as amitriptyline or nortriptyline cause the brain to send more nerve signals and can decrease pain and increase sensation in some patients. Other pain medications such as lidocaine or capsaicin, which are available as rub-on ointments, have been used with some success.

In the event that pain is severe, then codeine or another opiate-based pain reliever can be prescribed. Some patients have found pain relief with medical marijuana. This may also be prescribed in areas where its use is allowed. The drug dronabinol, synthesized from tetrahydrocannabinol (the active chemical in marijuana), has also been used with some success in managing neuropathy pain.

Risk Factors and Preventive Measures

Age and alcohol use increase the chance of having neuropathy as part of HIV disease. The use of the D drugs, as noted, also can cause neuropathy. The fact that a person is HIV positive and that the disease is progressing will also cause neuropathy in some people. It is not an avoidable part of the illness for some patients. Removal of the causes of the neuropathy or management of the problem is the main focus of prevention and treatment.

AIDSInfoNet. "Peripheral Neuropathy." AIDSInfoNet. org. Available online. URL: http://www.aidsinfo net.org/fact_sheets/view/555. Accessed April 1, 2011.

AIDS Treatment Data Network. "Simple Facts: Peripheral Neuropathy." AEGIS.com. Available online. URL: http://www.aegis.com/factshts/network/simple /neurop.html. Accessed April 1, 2011.

Goldman, Bonnie, and Scott Evans. "Peripheral Neuropathy Still Common among HIV-Infected Patients on HAART: Risk May Increase with Age." TheBody.com. Available online. URL: http://www. thebody.com/content/confs/croi2009/art50885. html. Accessed April 1, 2011.

McGuire, Dawn, M.D. "Neurologic Manifestations of HIV." HIVInSite.org. Available online. URL: http://hiv insite.ucsf.edu/InSite?page=kb-04-01-02. Accessed April 1, 2011.

University of Chicago, Center for Peripheral Neuropathy. "Types of Peripheral Neuropathy." UChicago.edu. Available online. URL: http://millercenter.uchicago. edu/learnaboutpn/typesofpn/inflammatory/hiv _aids.shtml. Accessed April 1, 2011.

nevirapine Nevirapine was the first of the NON-NUCLEOSIDE REVERSE TRANSCRIPTASE INHIBITORS (NNRTIs) when the U.S. FOOD AND DRUG ADMINISTRATION (FDA) approved it in 1996. It is manufactured by Boehringer Ingelheim, a German pharmaceutical company, and sold under the trade name Viramune. It is prescribed as part of a multidrug combination in the treatment of HIV. It is also found as one of the ingredients in the combination pill TRIOMUNE (STAVUDINE/ LAMIVUDINE/NEVIRAPINE), which is available in areas outside the United States. Nevirapine is used extensively in AFRICA and other resource-poor countries to prevent the TRANSMISSION of HIV between mothers and their infants during childbirth. Nevirapine is also successful at passing the blood-brain barrier, allowing the drug to reach HIV that has entered the brain and that can cause various neurological complications in some cases.

Dosage
Nevirapine is available in 200 mg tablets and in a liquid formula for CHILDREN and infants. Starting nevirapine is a two-step process. For the first two weeks, a person takes one 200 mg tablet once a day. If, after this period, a person has no serious side effect symptoms, the dosage increases to one 200 mg tablet twice a day. Some doctors currently prescribe two 200 mg tablets once a day after the start-up period. It is believed that this will work in the same manner as the two separate doses, but the FDA has not yet approved this method of once-daily dosing.

Children and infants are prescribed dosages of liquid nevirapine based on their body surface area. There is also a start-up period for the liquid formula. It is recommended that people who are undergoing dialysis take a single 200 mg tablet after each dialysis treatment.

Single-dose treatment of pregnant WOMEN just prior to delivery has been shown to be very effective in the prevention of transmission of the virus to the newborn child. A newborn may also be given a brief three-day dosage to increase the chance the virus is not passed from the mother.

In March 2011, the FDA announced approval of a new once-daily dosage of an extended-release version of nevirapine; the drug will be sold under the name Viramune XR.

Drug Interactions
Nevirapine can interact with some PROTEASE INHIBITORS (PIs) and significantly reduce their effectiveness in treating HIV infection. These include ATAZANAVIR SULFATE, SAQUINAVIR, INDINAVIR, KALETRA, and AMPRENAVIR. It can increase the amount of ritonavir, DARUNAVIR, and NELFINAVIR in the blood. Prescribing nevirapine with saquinavir, indinavir, and Kaletra generally includes the addition of ritonavir to boost the amount of these drugs in the bloodstream. Atazanavir sulfate is generally *not* prescribed with nevirapine, as in addition to decreasing the amount of atazanavir sulfate, the combination increases the amount of nevirapine in the body, thereby increasing the potential for side effects.

The drug can interact with some antibiotics used to treat TUBERCULOSIS (TB) and *MYCOBACTERIUM AVIUM* COMPLEX (MAC), which are OPPORTUNISTIC INFECTIONS (OIs) that sometimes occur in HIV-positive people. These antibiotics can reduce the effectiveness of nevirapine. Some antifungal medications used in the treatment of CANDIDIASIS (thrush) and other fungal OIs can cause the levels of nevirapine to rise in the body, increasing the potential for dangerous side effects.

Nevirapine can decrease the effectiveness of oral birth control pills by lowering the amount of the active ingredient in the body. Women who wish to prevent pregnancy should consider the use of another method of birth control (condom or intrauterine device) while taking nevirapine.

People who are taking methadone may need to have their dosage of that drug adjusted, as nevirapine can reduce the amount of methadone in the blood, causing withdrawal symptoms in patients. The herbal supplement St. John's wort should not be taken while on nevirapine, as it reduces the amount of nevirapine in the body.

Antifungal drugs such as ketoconazole and antibiotics such as clarithromycin also interact with nevirapine, and a doctor will need to evaluate these types of drugs before prescribing them at the same time as nevirapine. Patients should check with a doctor for a full list of potential drug interactions when taking nevirapine. They should always provide a full list of medications and herbal supplements so that a doctor can fully understand and explain the potential risks of mixing different medications.

Side Effects

The most common potential side effects of taking nevirapine include headache, nausea, fever, rash, and vomiting. In children, granulocytopenia (a shortage of granulocytes, a type of white blood cell) is also seen. The 14-day start-up dosage can reduce the incidence of rash and possibly other initial side effects. If a rash develops and becomes more severe over time, a person will need to stop taking nevirapine. A potentially fatal drug reaction known as Stevens-Johnson syndrome can result from this rash. Symptoms of Stevens-Johnson syndrome include inflammation and redness of the eyes, blistering rashes, aching muscles and joints, prolonged fever, and general exhaustion.

Cases of hepatitis and liver toxicity have also occurred in people starting nevirapine. It can be associated with the previously mentioned reaction or be a side effect in itself. Women whose CD4 counts are greater than 250 and men whose CD4 counts are greater than 400 are at greatest risk of liver problems, but this reaction can potentially happen to anyone. Two-thirds of these liver events occur within the first 12 weeks of nevirapine treatment, though the FDA recommends monitoring thoroughly for at least the first 18 weeks of treatment, and notes that the hepatitis reaction can occur at any point during treatment. Those individuals who do experience a severe liver reaction will need to stop nevirapine treatment and never start it again. Some instances of hepatitis among nevirapine patients do not stop even after discontinuing the drug but continue to worsen afterward. People who start nevirapine will need to be monitored for any liver problems during the full course of treatment. Nevirapine should never be prescribed for individuals who are already suffering with any type of hepatitis because of these liver complications.

Despite the potential for serious side effects, nevirapine remains a beneficial drug because it works well in combination therapy. As with any NNRTI, when resistance to one NNRTI does develop, resistance to several of the NNRTI medications is likely. A drug resistance test will be given to determine which types of NNRTIs will be effective after resistance to nevirapine has occurred.

AIDS InfoNet. "Nevirapine (Viramune)." AIDSInfoNet. org. Available online. URL: http://www.aidsinfonet. org/fact_sheets/view/431. Accessed March 11, 2011.

AIDSmeds. "New Viramune Tablet Approved for Once-Daily Use." AIDSmeds.com. Available online. URL: http://www.aidsmeds.com/articles/hiv_viramune _xr_1667_20144.shtml. Accessed April 15, 2011.

———. "Special Issues for Children with HIV." AIDS meds.com. Available online. URL: http://www.aids meds.com/articles/Children_7566.shtml. Accessed March 11, 2011.

———. "Viramune (Nevirapine)." AIDSmeds.com. Available online. URL: http://www.aidsmeds.com/ archive/Viramune_1616.shtml. Accessed March 11, 2011.

The Body. "Viramune (Nevirapine)." TheBody.com. Available online. URL: http://www.thebody.com/ index/treat/viramune.html#basics. Accessed March 11, 2011.

United States Department of Health and Human Services. "Nevirapine." aidsinfo.nih.gov. Available online. URL: http://www.aidsinfo.nih.gov/DrugsNew/Drug DetailNT.aspx?int_id=116. Accessed March 11, 2011.

new research on HIV therapy The new generation of drugs and treatments against HIV use not only a pharmacological approach but also an effort based on the extensive knowledge scientists have accumulated over the years on the molecular biology and genetics of the virus and its interaction with host cells, offering the possibility of new treatments and potential cure in the next decade.

Despite research success in the battle against the HUMAN IMMUNODEFICIENCY VIRUS (HIV), it remains an incurable but manageable disease. The virus can be controlled and kept at bay for years, as shown with increasing lengths of survival time, but currently there is no means to eradicate it from the body, as it integrates within the genes, hiding in a person's deoxyribonucleic acid (DNA) and becoming part of the individual. Current treatments interfere with viral replication, with its process of assembly of the virus, and with its entry to cells; however, those treatments do nothing about the source of the new viruses, the integrated DNA. When treatment is stopped, viral load will increase again from the stored templates distributed around the body in each infected cell. Any therapy able to cure HIV will have to eliminate the viral DNA in the genome. A combination of traditional HIGHLY ACTIVE ANTIRETROVIRAL THERAPY (HAART), to clear the virus from blood, and this hypothetical new therapy, to wipe out viral DNA, would offer the possibility of a definitive cure for HIV.

There are several approaches to excise viral DNA from the genome. One of them is an artificial enzyme called *Tre* recombinase, a molecular scissors that is able to recognize DNA sequences specific to HIV, make cuts on the sides of the recognized fragment, excise it, and then rejoin the DNA. This cuts information necessary for the virus to replicate, so even if some viral DNA remains in the genome, it is not enough to allow the construction of new viruses. *Tre* recombinase was developed by using a natural enzyme, *Cre* recombinase, as model. *Cre* recombinase recognizes the *cre* sites on DNA and excises them. *Tre* recombinase is the result of a mutation process on *Cre* recombinase that continues until it is able to recognize DNA sequences specific to HIV instead of the original *cre* sequences. In cultured human cells, *Tre* recombinase is able to remove HIV's DNA from the cells completely in three months, confirming the feasibility of this approach. A drawback of *Tre* recombinase is that it is a protein—a big, complex, and sensitive molecule—and that it must act inside the cells, so the delivery mechanism will be the most difficult part of this idea. One possible way to do this is with stem cells that can be transplanted into a person, so that over time, these engineered stem cells will replace the infected resting T cells that replicate and cause the continuous reproduction of HIV in the body. Potential uses of this extremely promising theoretical way to remove HIV from DNA are being explored.

Even if DNA contains all the information needed to make an organism, that is not enough to make a functional organism, as not only is having the instructions important but also regulating and timing them. Some genes are used only in very specific tissue, or during development; therefore, it is important to regulate their expression. The cell does this with a series of chemical flags on DNA that enhance or prevent the transcription of genetic information, binding or unbinding regulatory molecules to the DNA strand. Among these processes, the methylation of DNA is very important, allowing the expression of a gene, or inhibiting that expression completely, or marking its activation. Methylation patterns are involved in keeping the HIV provirus, the genome of the virus that is integrated into the DNA, alive but inactive, ready to begin reproduction when a person stops taking antiretrovirals. Methylation offers the possibility of a therapeutic target to disrupt the infection cycle and cure the disease. In 2008, researchers at the Gladstone Institute of Virology, affiliated with the University of California in San Francisco, discovered that inhibiting the methylation of the viral DNA causes its reactivation. The study also discovered a human protein that binds exclusively to the methylated DNA and has a key role in perpetuating viral latency. The researchers tested a drug that inhibits HIV methylation, called aza-CdR, and causes the reactivation of the virus. There are at least two other molecules that cause the reactivation of the virus, rendering host cells vulnerable to therapy. One of the molecules, called HMBR, has toxic side effects; however, a similar chemical, suberoylanilide hydroxamic acid (SAHA), has already been approved by the FDA as a drug for leukemia, and the doses necessary to produce the activation effect were within the clinical levels, meaning that human trials could begin sooner, as the FDA approval process has already been completed. By reactivating the latent virus, theoretically the antiretroviral medications already being taken by an individual could then remove that virus from the infected person.

Despite its devastating effects on the immune system, HIV does not infect all the T cells in its initial stages and remains dormant on a special population of cells called memory T cells, from which it spreads to the rest of the immune system. A 2009 study found that the specific memory cells harboring the HIV could be identified and targeted with drugs that inhibit other processes that keep the provirus in the human genome.

A drastic approach to the problem of dormant HIV's hiding in the immune system is its complete replacement. This is a very radical method that has been suggested in the past but deemed too dangerous, cumbersome, and unfeasible, as the way to do it is by performing a bone marrow transplant. Finding bone marrow donors would be only one of many obstacles, as the process of bone marrow transplant is long and involves completely destroying immune system of the person receiving the transplant by using chemotherapy and radiation, and tiny amounts of remaining virus could still attack the newly grafted cells. However, in cases of HIV patients with leukemia, the transplant is necessary, so scientists have tried to study its effect on the disease. In 2006, a German HIV patient was diagnosed with leukemia. One of the available bone marrow donors had the CCR5-delta 32 muta-

tion: That is, the donor's T cells lacked the receptor used by HIV to enter the cell. The transplant was performed by using this particular bone marrow, and it was a success, not only for curing the leukemia, but also for eliminating the HIV. Results of HIV tests performed after the transplant were negative; the virus could not even be found using high-sensitivity genetic methods in biopsies of specific tissues that it usually invades. The patient had remained free of antiretroviral therapy for four years, as of 2010. Caution is needed here, as this is a one-case sample; however, it suggests that eradicating the virus from the immune system can end HIV infection.

Researchers have used this success to develop potential therapy that would similarly block or change the structure of the CD4 cell to block the CCR5 or CXCR4 coreceptors from allowing the virus to merge and become part of the immune system. Using what is called zinc-finger nuclease technology, developed by Sangamo BioSciences, researchers ran a phase I study to test the potential of this zinc-finger treatment. Patients had blood withdrawn from the body, which was then filtered to remove T cells and returned to the body. The T cells were then treated at a lab with the zinc-finger nuclease that was carried to the T cells by a genetically modified viral vector. The zinc-finger nuclease caused a break in the *CCR5* gene that deleted the receptor from the T cells. The T cells were then returned to the participants in the study through reinfusion. In all the patients in the study, their own newly modified T cells were accepted back into their body and began reproduction of new cells. All but one of the patients responded with jumps in CD4 counts as well as a normalization of CD4-to-CD8 cell ratio, which is disrupted in HIV-positive patients. The results were positive and proved to the researchers that what occurred in the Berlin patient may be replicated in others in the future, without the need for full bone marrow replacement.

Another research trial that is looking into HIV eradication from the body is the use of interleukin-7 (IL-7). IL-7 is a naturally produced cytokine. It helps the body produce T cells and stimulate certain immune functions such as causing CD4 cells to begin their functions in the body. Researchers for the pharmaceutical company Cytheris are testing the use of IL-7 along with two other antiretrovirals to stimulate the immune system, thereby flushing out resting CD4 cells, where HIV is "hiding" when a person's viral load is unmeasurable. Most people who have unmeasurable viral loads maintain what is known as a reservoir of resting HIV that remains quiet until a person stops taking the antiretrovirals or until the HIV mutates enough to cause the drugs to fail. These resting cells then start production of HIV again. This experimental treatment, now in a phase II trial, will attempt to show that HIV can be suppressed more significantly or perhaps even eliminated fully by using the new IL-7 along with several antiretrovirals to kill the latent HIV that has been reactivated.

In the future, it is likely that a combination of the methods discussed will be used successfully to end HIV infections with minimal side effects, and potentially offer protection against new infections, as new gene therapy techniques would allow transformation of immune system cells into cells lacking the CCR5 receptors and expressing *Tre* recombinase using a single injection. It is reasonable to expect that most of the patients currently undergoing HAART, as well as the newly infected, may soon survive to witness the end of HIV.

AIDSmeds. "New HIV Eradication Study in Progress." AIDSmeds.com. Available online. URL: http://www.aidsmeds.com/articles/hiv_cytheris_eradication_1667_19272.shtml. Accessed April 14, 2011.

Contreras, X., et al. "Suberoylanilide Hydroxamic Acid Reactivates HIV from Latently Infected Cells." *Journal of Biological Chemistry* 284, no. 11 (9 January 2009): 6782–6789. Available online. URL: http://www.natap.org/2010/HIV/091310_06.htm. Accessed April 1, 2011.

Goldman, Bonnie. "The First Man to Be Cured of AIDS: An Update on the Amazing Story." TheBody.com. Available online. URL: http://www.thebody.com/content/art53624.html?mvg. Accessed April 1, 2011.

Hofmann-Sieber, H., et al. "Excision of HIV-1 Proviral DNA Using *Tre*-recombinase: An eExperimental Update." [Abstract] AIDS2010update.org. Available online. URL: http://pag.aids2010.org/Abstracts.aspx?AID=12417. Accessed April 1, 2011.

Kauder, Steven E., et al. "Epigenetic Regulation of HIV-1 Latency by Cytosine Methylation." PubMed.gov. Available online. URL: http://www.ncbi.nlm.nih.gov/pmc/articles/PMC2695767/?tool=pubmed. Accessed April 1, 2011.

Krauss, Kate, Stephen LeBlanc, and John S. James. "AIDS Cure Research for Everyone." AIDSPolicyProject.org. Available online. URL: http://www.aidspolicyproject.org/documents/The%20Cure%20Final.pdf. Accessed April 1, 2011.

NAM AIDSmap. "Zinc Finger Gene Therapy Produces HIV-Resistant CD4 T-Cells." AIDSmap.com. Available online. URL: http://www.aidsmap.com/page/1681138/. Accessed April 1, 2011.

Nature Reviews. "DNA Methylation." Nature.com. Available online. URL: http://www.nature.com/reviews/focus/dnamethylation/index.html. Accessed April 1, 2011.

Savarino, Andrea, et al. "'Shock and Kill' Effects of Class I-Selective Histone Deacetylase Inhibitors in Combination with the Glutathione Synthesis Inhibitor Buthionine Sulfoximine in Cell Line Models for HIV-1 Quiescence." *Retrovirology* 6, no. 52 (June 2009). Available online. URL: http://www.retrovirology.com/content/6/1/52. Accessed April 1, 2011.

ScienceDaily. "Scientists Identify Key Factor That Controls HIV Latency." ScienceDaily.com. Available online. URL: http://www.sciencedaily.com/releases/2009/06/090625210423.htm. Accessed April 1, 2011.

———. "Waking Up Dormant HIV." ScienceDaily.com. Available online. URL: http://www.sciencedaily.com/releases/2009/03/090316120848.htm. Accessed April 1, 2011.

Trono, Didier, et al. "HIV Persistence and the Long-Term Drug-Free Remissions of HIV-Infected Individuals." *Science* 329, no. 5988 (9 July 2010): 174–180.

Vergel, Nelson. "Zinc Fingers and Gene Therapies for HIV: Mimicking the Cured Berlin Patient." The Body.com. Available online. URL: http://www.thebodypro.com/content/art60675.html. Accessed April 1, 2011.

non-nucleoside reverse transcriptase inhibitors (NNRTIs) A nucleoside is one of the building blocks of deoxyribonucleic acid (DNA), which is the basis through which genetic information is passed on in future generations of all living things. Reverse transcriptase is an enzyme, a substance that makes a chemical reaction take place, which is used by HIV to change its ribonucleic acid (RNA) to DNA once it is inside a person's cell. This change is required in order for HIV to infect the cell and to reproduce itself. NNRTIs are also known as non-nucleoside analogs or non-nukes in research and popular literature. In medical chemistry, an analog is an artificial replacement for a natural substance. Therefore, the name *NNRTI* describes what the medication does.

NNRTIs interfere with the reproduction of HIV during the reverse transcription phase. HIV requires an enzyme called reverse transcriptase to change the genetic information contained in its RNA into DNA in the infected person's cells. NNRTIs bind to the reverse transcriptase enzyme in a different manner than NUCLEOSIDE REVERSE TRANSCRIPTASE INHIBITORS (NRTIs), but both block the enzyme from working properly. The resulting bond that NNRTIs form on the reverse transcriptase prevents the change from viral RNA to DNA in the cell. The cell cannot be infected and forced to reproduce HIV in the presence of the NNRTI drug.

NNRTIs were the second type of antiretroviral medication that was developed for the treatment of HIV. They do not work well when taken individually and must be taken as part of a combination therapy. They work well when taken with NRTIs. NNRTIs on the market currently are ETRAVIRINE, DELAVIRDINE, EFAVIRENZ, and NEVIRAPINE.

AIDSmeds. "Non-Nucleoside Reverse Transcriptase Inhibitors (NNRTIs)." AIDSmeds.com. Available online. URL: http://www.aidsmeds.com/archive/NNRTIs_1612.shtml. Accessed April 1, 2011.

Lee, Jean. "The Non-Nukes." TheBody.com. Available online. URL: http://www.thebody.com/content/art878.html. Accessed April 1, 2011.

The Well Project. "HIV Drugs and the HIV Lifecycle." WellProject.org. Available online. URL: http://www.thewellproject.org/en_US/Treatment_and_Trials/Anti_HIV_Meds/Lifecycle_and_ARVs.jsp. Accessed April 1, 2011.

North America North America, as described in this article, consists of the United States of America (U.S.), Canada, and Greenland, an integral part of the European country of Denmark. For information on Mexico and Central America see the article on LATIN AMERICA. Across most of the United States and Canada, the HIV/AIDS epidemic resembles that of Western Europe. In the far north of Alaska; the Canadian territories of Northwest Territories, Nunavut, and Yukon; as well as Greenland, the epidemic is somewhat different, as the majority of the population in these areas is indigenous in origin, and the virus was late in arriving in some of these regions.

Prevalence rates for the countries as a whole are as follows: United States, 0.6 percent; Canada, 0.2 percent; and Greenland, 0.2 percent. Infection rates among some high-risk groups are higher, as in most other countries. The largest proportion of HIV-positive results in the United States are found among men, who made up close to 74 percent of all diagnoses in 2006. Of those newly diagnosed that year, 53 percent were MEN WHO HAVE SEX WITH MEN (MSM). Unprotected heterosexual activity resulted in 33 percent of new cases that year. The remainder were predominantly INJECTION DRUG USE(R) (IDU) TRANSMISSION cases. The largest percentage of females diagnosed in the United States in 2006 were exposed through heterosexual activities, at the rate of 80 percent. The United States does not track commercial SEX WORKERS nor conduct general surveys on such activity, as it is considered illegal in all but a few areas of the state of Nevada, and only in registered brothels in those areas. The HIV prevalence rates of commercial sex workers in the United States is unclear. The United States does measure HIV prevalence by ethnic and racial background.

The United States was one of the first countries to have AIDS cases appear in the very early 1980s. Like most governments at that time, the U.S. government was slow to address the virus, which was quickly spreading through several populations. In particular, MSM, IDUs, and recipients of blood products were becoming ill and dying. Political leaders were unwilling or unable to discuss the nature of the illness until several high-profile individuals had died. When a virus was discovered as the cause, the United States slowly began making changes in blood donation testing; eventually, few new diagnoses were among people who receive donated blood. Education programs sponsored by the affected communities began to have immediate impact and were initially adopted by federal and state governments to educate those at high risk. Wide-scale testing for the virus was begun and gained general acceptance after medications became available in the mid- to late 1990s. In the late 1990s and during the 2000s, more restrictive education and funding led to a drop in the availability of educational materials, which some believe has led to the more recent higher rates of infection seen among the MSM population. Restrictions on discussion of sexual behavior in educational materials and defunding of programs that discuss such behavior have been common.

In the United States in particular, the virus has gone from being one of predominantly gay white men to an illness of socioeconomic status. The numbers of infected went from nearly 80 percent gay men to more than 50 percent heterosexuals among new cases. Poor people have become much more likely to experience the epidemic than middle- or upper-class individuals. This prevalence may be due to several factors. As opposed to many developed countries, the United States does not fund general medical care for its citizens. This is a privatized function in U.S. society, although some changes to this may occur in the future, as the United States has adopted new health care regulations requiring all citizens to have health insurance by 2014. A majority of people in the United States receive medical insurance through their job. Therefore, people who do not hold jobs or people who may not receive benefits from their job are not likely to have health insurance, as private health insurance can be very expensive to purchase in the United States. It is estimated that 15 percent of people living in the United States had no health care coverage as of 2010 and therefore were not likely to have regular medical appointments, receive medications, or seek preventive health care. The United States also incarcerates a greater percentage of its population by far than any other country, and HIV has proven especially difficult to handle among populations of PRISONS. MSM and IDU activities often occur in greater concentration in prison populations than in the general population of a country. In addition, prison populations reflect a greater number of minority and underclass people. Therefore, in the United States, HIV has come to be seen as a minority and underclass illness, rather than an illness that can affect any person. This has made it far more difficult to educate and inform the population, as the government is slow to provide consistent public health funding and in general does not want to fund any type of program dealing with activities that are seen as illegal or immoral, such as MSM sexual activities or IDU. Prison populations do not receive education or prevention materials to the extent that would be available outside a prison setting. Education in SAFER SEX practices is unfunded, and only abstinence as a preventive measure has been funded for the past several years. Needle exchange or safe injectable equipment purchased over the counter is illegal in the United States. The U.S. government has also defunded some programs in the country in order to fund programs abroad, leading many in the United States to believe that the virus is more of a concern elsewhere than in the United States.

For those who do have medical and prescription medicine insurance, there is good access to HIV medications in the United States, though less in communities where prescription drug coverage is unavailable. Access to a wide range of highly active antiretroviral therapy (HAART) medications and options to switch medications that are unavailable in many countries have led to longer life for people who are HIV positive. Government programs to pay for most or all of the drug costs often have long waiting lists, however. All of these conditions have led the United States to have the highest rate of HIV prevalence of any developed nation.

Canada also has a diverse population and a varied HIV epidemic. Like the United States, Canada has seen an increase in the number of HIV-positive people in the country because of advances in medical care. The level of newly diagnosed cases has been relatively stable in Canada, at approximately 2,400 annually in the first decade of the 21st century. Also, like the U.S. epidemic, it is believed that one in four Canadians living with HIV is unaware of being infected. Approximately 51 percent of Canadians were infected through MSM activity. Women are increasingly becoming infected with HIV in Canada. In 2005, women comprised 27 percent of new diagnoses, up from just 12 percent in 1985 and 24 percent in 2002. Aboriginal women were disproportionately affected, as they make up 60 percent of infections among aboriginal peoples who live in Canada. A substantial number of new HIV infections are being diagnosed in people who were born in areas where the infection is considered endemic, the CARIBBEAN and sub-Saharan AFRICA. Their rate of infection is measured at 12 times higher than that of the general population in Canada. Prevalence rates of IDUs in Canada remain high—in the range of 20 percent as measured in studies cited by the United Nations (UN)—in the capital, Ottawa, and in Montreal.

Greenland has a smaller epidemic than either the United States or Canada; however, there are signs of concern, as the prevalence of other sexually transmitted infections, particularly gonorrhea and chlamydia, are relatively high in comparison to prevalence in other locations. The majority, 88 percent, of HIV-positive Greenlanders were infected through heterosexual contact.

IDU and MSM activities are considered rare in the small population of just above 50,000 on the large island.

AVERT: AVERTing HIV and AIDS. "HIV and AIDS in America." AVERT.org. Available online. URL: http://www.avert.org/america.htm. Accessed April 1, 2011.
———. "United States HIV and AIDS Statistics by Exposure Category." AVERT.org. Available online. URL: http://www.avert.org/usastatg.htm. Accessed April 1, 2011.
Canadian Broadcasting Corporation. "Understanding the Global AIDS Epidemic." CBC.ca. Available online. URL: http://www.cbc.ca/news/health/story/2009/11/24/f-aids-hiv-global-epidemic.html. Accessed April 1, 2011.
Centers for Disease Control and Prevention. "HIV Prevalence Estimates—United States, 2006." CDC.gov. Available online. URL: http://www.cdc.gov/mmwr/preview/mmwrhtml/mm5739a2.htm. Accessed April 1, 2011.
Harrison, Paige M., and Allen J. Beck. "Prisoners in 2005." USDOJ.gov. Available online. URL: http://bjs.ojp.usdoj.gov/content/pub/pdf/p05.pdf. Accessed April 1, 2011.
Henry J. Kaiser Family Foundation. "Health Reform Source." KFF.org. Available online. URL: http://healthreform.kff.org/. Accessed April 1, 2011.
King's College London. "Prison Briefs—Highest to Lowest Rates." KCL.ac.uk. Available online. URL: http://www.kcl.ac.uk/depsta/law/research/icps/worldbrief/wpb_stats.php. Accessed April 1, 2011.
Law, Dionne Gesink, Elizabeth Rink, Gert Mulvad, and Anders Koch. "Sexual Health and Sexually Transmitted Infections in the North American Arctic." *Emerging Infectious Diseases* 14, no. 1 (January 2008): 4–9.
Lohse, Nicolai, Karin Ladefoged, and Niels Obel. "Implementation and Effectiveness of Antiretroviral Therapy in Greenland." *Emerging Infectious Diseases* 14, no. 1 (January 2008). Available online. URL: http://www.ncbi.nlm.nih.gov/pmc/articles/PMC2600136/. Accessed April 1, 2011.
Moore, Solomon. "Prison Spending Outpaces All but Medicaid." NYTimes.com. Available online. URL: http://www.nytimes.com/2009/03/03/us/03prison.html. Accessed April 1, 2011.
Reuters. "Insured Losing Access to Healthcare: U.S. Study." Reuters.com. Available online. URL: http://

uk.reuters.com/article/healthNewsMolt/idUKN
2538627220080626. Accessed April 1, 2011.

UNAIDS: Joint United Nations Programme on HIV/
AIDS. "North America, Western and Central Europe."
UNAIDS.org. Available online. URL: http://www.
unaids.org/en/CountryResponses/Regions/NAmer
ica_WCEurope.asp. Accessed April 1, 2011.

**nucleoside reverse transcriptase inhibitors
(NRTIs)**   A nucleoside is one of the building
blocks of deoxyribonucleic acid (DNA), which
is the basis for genetic information to be passed
on in future generations of all living things.
Reverse transcriptase is an enzyme, a substance
that makes a chemical reaction take place, that
is used by HIV to change its ribonucleic acid
(RNA) to DNA once it is inside a person's cell.
This change is required in order for HIV to infect
the cell and to reproduce itself. NRTIs are also
known as nucleoside analogs or nukes in medical and popular literature. In medical chemistry, an analog is an artificial replacement for a
natural substance. Therefore, the name *NRTI*
describes what the medication does.

NRTIs interfere with the reproduction of HIV
during the reverse transcription phase. HIV
requires an enzyme called reverse transcriptase
to change the genetic information contained in
its RNA into DNA in the infected person's cells.
NRTIs contain faulty nucleosides in the form of
the drug, so the change from viral RNA to DNA
cannot be completed successfully in the virus.
The cell cannot be infected and forced to reproduce HIV in the presence of the drug. Studies
have shown that HIV is more likely to choose
the nucleosides from an NRTI to use in its replication than the natural ones it is supposed to
use.

NRTIs were the first class of medications
used to fight HIV infection. Drugs that fall into
this class are EMTRICITABINE, LAMIVUDINE, ZID-
OVUDINE, STAVUDINE, ABACAVIR, DIDANOSINE, and
ZALCITABINE. There are also several currently
unnamed drugs in this classification that are in
development for future use.

NRTIs generally make up at least one of the
medications in a patient's HIGHLY ACTIVE ANTI-
RETROVIRAL THERAPY (HAART) prescription. They
are considered prodrugs, drugs that must first
be processed by the body for use. The body
changes the nucleoside by adding phosphate to
the structure before it can be used to fight the
virus. There are known side effects of several of
the NRTIs that can cause mild to serious problems. These are detailed in the entries on the
individual drugs.

AIDSmeds. "Nucleoside/Nucleotide Reverse Transcriptase Inhibitors (NRTIs)." AIDSmeds.com. Available
online. URL: http://www.aidsmeds.com/archive/
NRTIs_1082.shtml. Accessed April 1, 2011.

Encyclopaedia Britannica Online. "Nucleoside." Britan-
nica.com. Available online. URL: http://www.britan
nica.com/EBchecked/topic/421972/nucleoside.
Accessed April 1, 2011.

Seattle Treatment Education Project. "Know Your
HIV Drugs: NRTIs (the Nukes)." The Body.com.
Available online. URL: http://aids.about.com/od/
glossary/g/nucs.htm. Accessed April 1, 2011.

Tibotec Pharmaceuticals. "HIV Treatment and Drug
Classes." Tibotec-HIV.com. Available online. URL:
http://www.tibotec-hiv.com/bgdisplay.jhtml?item
name=treatment_and_drug_classes. Accessed April
1, 2011.

**nucleotide reverse transcriptase inhibitors
(NtRTIs)**   A nucleotide is one of the building
blocks of deoxyribonucleic acid (DNA), which
is the basis for genetic information to be passed
on in future generations of all living things.
Reverse transcriptase is an enzyme, a substance
that makes a chemical reaction take place, that
is used by HIV to change its ribonucleic acid
(RNA) to DNA once it is inside a person's cell.
This change is required in order for HIV to infect
the cell and to reproduce itself. NtRTIs are also
known as nucleotide analogs or nukes in medical and popular literature. In medical chemistry, an analog is an artificial replacement for a
natural substance. Therefore, the name *NtRTI*
describes what the medication does.

NtRTIs interfere with the reproduction of HIV during the reverse transcription phase. HIV requires an enzyme called reverse transcriptase to change the genetic information contained in its RNA into DNA in the infected person's cells. NtRTIs contain faulty nucleotides in the form of the drug, so the change from viral RNA to DNA cannot be completed successfully. The cell cannot be infected and forced to reproduce HIV in the presence of the drug. Studies have shown that HIV is more likely to choose the nucleotides from an NtRTI to use in its replication than the ones it is supposed to use.

The difference between a nucleoside reverse transcriptase inhibitor (NRTI) and an NtRTI is that the NtRTI does not need to be processed by the body first in order to work against the virus. It essentially does the same thing that an NRTI does, but does not require the extra step. NtRTIs are sometimes described in the same drug class because they function in the same manner as NRTIs, but the initial action in the body is different. There is only one NtRTI on the market at this time for the treatment of HIV, TENOFOVIR DISOPROXIL FUMARATE. A second NtRTI initially tested for use against HIV is adefovir, which is prescribed for use against HEPATITIS B but was considered toxic at the much larger doses found necessary for its use against HIV.

AIDSmeds. "Nucleoside/Nucleotide Reverse Transcriptase Inhibitors (NRTIs)." AIDSmeds.com. Available online. URL: http://www.aidsmeds.com/archive/NRTIs_1082.shtml. Accessed April 1, 2011.

Encyclopaedia Britannica Online. "Nucleoside." Britannica.com. Available online. URL: http://www.britannica.com/EBchecked/topic/421972/nucleoside. Accessed April 1, 2011.

Seattle Treatment Education Project. "Know Your HIV Drugs: NRTIs (the Nukes)." The Body.com. Available online. URL: http://aids.about.com/od/glossary/g/nucs.htm. Accessed April 1, 2011.

Tibotec Pharmaceuticals. "HIV Treatment and Drug Classes." Tibotec-HIV.com. Available online. URL: http://www.tibotec-hiv.com/bgdisplay.jhtml?itemname=treatment_and_drug_classes. Accessed April 1, 2011.

Oceania Oceania comprises the island nations of the Pacific Ocean along with Australia, New Zealand, and Papua New Guinea. HIV infection in this region remains low in most countries. Some locales have not recorded any cases of HIV, though medical clinics and doctors are often few and far between on the islands, and it is difficult to estimate prevalence in such a widespread area.

After Australia and New Zealand began to see HIV infections in the early 1980s, they both began strong public education programs. Television advertisements as well as government collaborations with community organizations to provide education and condom distribution allowed both countries to reach affected populations quickly. Both countries saw a quick leveling off and decline in annual HIV infections until 2001. Since that time, there has been an increase in yearly diagnoses, particularly among MEN WHO HAVE SEX WITH MEN (MSM), who are the main population infected by HIV in both countries. In Australia, new MSM cases rose 30 percent between 2000 and 2006. An increase in unsafe sexual practices is believed to be the cause, and both countries have recently begun public education efforts again to reach younger males who were not of age when the epidemic first materialized. The number of men reporting not using condoms during anal intercourse increased from 13 percent in 1996 to 26 percent in 2006 in Sydney. Other large cities reported similar findings.

In Australia, indigenous peoples, particularly indigenous WOMEN, are at a higher risk for HIV TRANSMISSION than the general population or women in general in the country. Indigenous women are 18 times more likely to be HIV positive than women in the general population. The indigenous INJECTION DRUG USE(R) (IDU) population was also a greater concern because 18 percent of HIV-positive indigenous people are IDUs, whereas only 3 percent of HIV-positive nonindigenous people are IDUs in Australia.

New Zealand also shows a higher rate of HIV infection among indigenous women than women in the general population. Maori women comprise 23 percent of the heterosexually acquired HIV cases, but Maori constitute only 11 percent of the population. Heterosexually spread HIV is increasing in New Zealand; studies cited in the United Nations (UN) yearly reports show that many people acquire the virus overseas and take it into the country, thereby increasing the chance for spread among their regular sex partners in New Zealand.

The Pacific Island nations continue to report fewer than 300 cases in each of the countries. French Polynesia, Guam, Fiji, and New Caledonia, all territories of Western countries, show HIV prevalence rates of 0.1 percent. All other countries and territories show prevalence rates below 0.1 percent. The territories of Niue, Pitcairn, and Tokelau have never recorded a case of HIV. Many other Pacific Island nations still report fewer than 10 cases of HIV total for the whole of the epidemic. However, the high prevalence of other sexually transmitted infections is a cause for concern. Condoms generally are not used and often are unavailable on many islands. In addition, certain cultural traditions such as tattooing, penile piercing, and scarification may cause the spread of HIV among islanders. MSM sexual activity is not well studied among the Pacific Island peoples. But some islands, such as Samoa, where 22 percent of men said they had sex with other men, have the potential for spread through these communities.

According to the most recent United Nations statistics, by far the largest number of HIV cases and highest prevalence of HIV is in the country of Papua New Guinea. Since 2001, the number of HIV-positive people has increased from 14,000 to 34,000. This gives the country a prevalence rate of 0.9 percent, much higher than Australia's 0.2 percent, the next highest in the region. New infections are running at double the rate from a few years ago. More than 80 percent of infections are in the rural parts of the country, where 80 percent of citizens live. Papuans live in a time of profound changes for the country. High levels of urbanization, migrancy, crime, unemployment, and drug and alcohol use exist both in the capital, Port Moresby, and in the countryside. There are large gender inequalities, which are reflected in the physical violence and rape that often accompany sex in parts of the nation. The most recent United Nations reports show HIV prevalence among women 15–29 years of age is twice the rate among men of the same age. The main method of transmission in the country is heterosexual sex. Most people report having multiple partners, and in surveys many women report sexual violence and coercion. Surveys among working men report that 60 percent of soldiers and truck drivers and 30 percent of dock workers have paid for sex in the past year. Sex in exchange for gifts or services is also highly common. Community-based studies around the country found that 40 percent of the population is infected with some type of sexually transmitted infection (STI). This is bad news for future HIV spread, as HIV is easier to pass among people in the presence of other STIs. In STI clinics around the country, 13 percent of patients test positive for HIV. Sexual activity among men is also common. Of men surveyed, 12 percent report having sex with other men, and three-quarters of those report also having sex with women. A limited health care system, ineffective clinics, and low economic opportunities are not good national indicators that the epidemic in Papua New Guinea will be controlled soon. What medical system currently exists is often overburdened with HIV-related illnesses. Studies show that 70 percent of beds in the capital's hospital are already filled with HIV patients. It is unclear how the proximity to and the cultural similarities with neighboring island nations such as the Solomon Islands and New Caledonia may affect the HIV epidemic in those nations.

Buchanan-Aruwafu, Holly. "An Integrated Picture: HIV Risk and Vulnerability in the Pacific." HE.net. Available online. URL: http://ssltd.he.net/~piaf2/images/pdf_hiv_in_the_pacific_articles/hiv%20risk%20a nd% 20vulnerability%20in%20the%20pacific.pdf. Accessed April 1, 2011.

Huang, Julia. "Confronting the AIDS Epidemic in the Pacific." EpochTimes.com. Available online. URL: http://en.epochtimes.com/n2/australia/aids-epidemic-in-the-pacific-6711.html. Accessed April 1, 2011.

PIAF: Pacific Islands Aids Foundation. "HIV in the Pacific." HE. Net. Available online. URL: http://ssltd.he.net/~piaf2/index.php?option=com_content &task=view&id=77&Itemid=111. Accessed April 1, 2011.

UNAIDS: Joint United Nations Programme on HIV/AIDS. "Fact Sheet—Oceania." UNAIDS.org. Available online. URL: http://www.unaids.org/documents/20101123_FS_oceania_em_en.pdf. Accessed April 1, 2011.

———. "Oceania: AIDS Epidemic Update, Regional Summary 07." UNAIDS.org. Available online. URL: http://data.unaids.org/pub/Report/2008/jc1533_epi briefs_oceania_en.pdf. Accessed April 1, 2011.

———. "UNAIDS Report on the Global AIDS Epidemic, 2010." UNAIDS.org. Available online. URL: http://www.unaids.org/globalreport/. Accessed April 1, 2011.

opportunistic infections An opportunistic infection (OI) is an illness that arises when the HUMAN IMMUNE SYSTEM is suppressed or otherwise compromised. The effect of HIV is the gradual destruction of key immune system cells, particularly CD4 T lymphocytes, which causes the individual's immune system to struggle to fight illnesses that may normally be kept in check or not cause problems in many cases for an HIV-negative person. The infections take the opportunity provided by the weakened immune system to flourish unhindered in the body. Most people who die of HIV disease do not die of the virus but of an OI that is able to take advantage of the person's ineffective immune system. OIs can also occur in other people who have weakened immune systems for reasons other than infection with HIV. Chemotherapy for some cancers can cause a weakening of the immune system. People who have had ORGAN TRANSPLANTATION are often required to take immune-suppressing drugs to prevent the rejection of the donated organ. These individuals are also at risk of developing a wide range of opportunistic infections. People who are elderly also are at risk because of a gradual weakening of the immune system due to the aging process.

OIs result from all types of microbes that can infect humans. Viruses, bacteria, fungi, and protozoan parasites, as well as a variety of cancers, all fall into the category of OI. Many of the OIs are not new infections to the body. Illnesses such as TOXOPLASMOSIS are normally in the body, but a normal immune system can fight the infection and keep it controlled. Most people are exposed to toxoplasmosis when they are CHILDREN but do not develop any illness; however, the parasite remains in the body in a dormant or inactive state. When the immune system weakens, the toxoplasmosis can develop into a dangerous parasitic infection that can quickly kill a person if not controlled.

Viruses that are common in the population but do not cause serious problems include the JC virus, which causes PROGRESSIVE MULTIFOCAL LEUKOENCEPHALOPATHY, and CYTOMEGALOVIRUS. These viruses are seen in nearly all of the world's population but rarely cause serious illness. Viruses reproduce inside the cells of the host, or person, who is carrying the virus. The virus is able to reproduce using the cell itself to assemble new virus, often encoding itself into the person's deoxyribonucleic acid (DNA) or ribonucleic acid (RNA) so that each new cell the body creates is infected with the virus. A virus is too small to be seen with a standard microscope and can only be seen with electron microscopes. Viruses are 100 times smaller than bacteria.

Bacteria are one-celled animals that can be seen under a microscope. Bacteria can live in a range of places from hot, sulfuric water to cold, frozen land. Some bacteria eat hazardous materials, and others cause illness in plants, animals, and humans. Common bacterial infections that can cause problems in HIV-positive people include *MYCOBACTERIUM AVIUM* COMPLEX, TUBERCULOSIS, and shigella.

Protozoa, also sometimes called protozoan parasites, are small, one-celled creatures that range from algae to amoebas. Not all protozoa cause illness, but some do. LEISHMANIASIS and MALARIA are caused by protozoa; they are severe illnesses on their own, and when combined with HIV create very serious infections. Protozoa have different life stages that can allow them to be transmitted from their host to other vectors, or carriers. Protozoa can be seen under a standard microscope.

Fungi are primitive plantlike organisms. Fungal infections can occur on the skin or mucous membranes in all people but can become extremely dangerous in HIV-positive people with weakened immune systems. The fungus can spread to organs and the central nervous system, causing the body to stop functioning as the fungus grows rapidly. HISTOPLASMOSIS, CANDIDIASIS, and COCCIDIOIDOMYCOSIS are examples of fungal infections that can be seen in immune-compromised people.

Some OIs found in HIV patients are cancers. A cancer is an uncontrolled division of cells that spreads, often forming growths, tumors, which obstruct functions of the body. Cancers can spread via the blood or lymph system. Cancers that are discussed as OIs include Kaposi's sarcoma and several types of lymphoma, or cancer of the lymph system cells, lymphocytes. Burkitt's lymphoma is a severe OI found predominately in AFRICA.

Although a person who has a weakened immune system is susceptible to any number of OIs, it is unlikely that any one person will have all of the illnesses. The types of infections vary by the part of the world a person lives in or what the individual has been exposed to in life. Whenever possible, it is imperative to prevent OIs from having the opportunity to infect a person. HIGHLY ACTIVE ANTIRETROVIRAL THERAPY (HAART) has been responsible for restoring a person's immune system to a functioning state and has reduced the number and severity of OIs since its introduction to HIV treatment in the mid-1990s. HAART treatment has proven to be the most effective way to restore a person who has HIV infection to health and thereby prevent OIs from gaining a foothold in the person's body.

Primary prophylaxis is the term used by doctors for preventing the acquisition of a disease. An example of primary prophylaxis is taking mefloquine to prevent infection by the malaria protozoan, *Plasmodium*. This drug can prevent a person from becoming infected. Secondary prophylaxis is defined as taking a medication to prevent a recurrence of an illness after it has been treated or taking a medication to prevent an acute phase of such an infection from recurring. An example of secondary prophylaxis would be treating a person with trimethoprim/sulfamethoxazole (TMP-SMX) for PNEUMOCYSTIS PNEUMONIA to prevent it from reactivating when a person's immune system measurements indicate a weakened state.

AIDSmeds. "Opportunistic Infections (OIs)." AIDS meds.com. Available online. URL: http://www.aids meds.com/articles/OIs_4898.shtml. Accessed April 1, 2011.

AIDS.org. "Opportunistic Infections." AIDS.org. Available online. URL: http://www.aids.org/factSheets/500 -Opportunistic-Infections.html. Accessed April 1, 2011.

Centers for Disease Control and Prevention. "1993 Revised Classification System for HIV Infection and Expanded Surveillance Case Definition for AIDS among Adolescents and Adults." CDC.gov. Available online. URL: http://www.cdc.gov/mmwr/pre view/mmwrhtml/00018871.htm. Accessed April 1, 2011.

University of California Museum of Paleontology. "Introduction to the Bacteria." Berkeley.edu. Available online. URL: http://www.ucmp.berkeley.edu/ bacteria/bacteria.html. Accessed April 1, 2011.

———. "Introduction to the Viruses." Berkeley.edu. Available online. URL: http://www.ucmp.berkeley. edu/alllife/virus.html. Accessed April 1, 2011.

University of California, San Francisco, Center for HIV Information. "Opportunistic Infections and AIDS-Related Cancers." HIVInSite.ucsf.edu. Available online. URL: http://hivinsite.ucsf.edu/insite?page=pb-diag-04 -00. Accessed April 1, 2011.

oral hairy leukoplakia   Oral hairy leukoplakia (OHL) is a virally induced infection of the mouth found predominantly in HIV-positive people, though it is also seen in other immune-suppressed people. It can be found in the mouth of HIV-positive persons who have stable immune systems and reasonably high CD4 T lymphocyte counts above 500 but generally first appears if CD4 T cell counts have fallen below 200. It is caused by the Epstein-Barr virus (EBV).

EBV is one of the herpes viruses and is also sometimes called human herpes virus 4. As other herpes viruses do, EBV remains in the body for the rest of a person's life, though it seems to cause no illness most of the time it is in the body. It is also the most prominent cause of mononucleosis in teenagers and CHILDREN. More than 90 percent of all people in the world have been exposed to EBV. OHL occurs in somewhere between 25 to 60 percent of HIV-positive people.

Symptoms and Diagnostic Path

OHL appears in the mouth and has a distinctive look of white "hairy" patches on the tongue, roof of the mouth, gums, or inner cheeks. It is at times difficult to distinguish from CANDIDIASIS. It does not cause pain, and people may not realize they have the infection if they are not paying close attention to their oral care. There is no associated swelling with OHL. On occasion, some patients report a lessening of taste or sensitivity to heat or cold when the lesions are present. The lesions can be biopsied to determine the nature of the oral lesion and will be used to differentiate OHL from other oral diseases. It is not considered a serious infection and does not develop beyond the mouth, nor does it lead to any other conditions.

Treatment Options and Outlook

OHL tends to wax and wane, resolving on its own, then reappearing. It is not a life-threatening illness, though it can cause some difficulties in eating and can be considered embarrassing by some people. If the lesions are bothersome to a person, he or she may be given a course of antiviral medications such as valacyclovir, acyclovir, or famciclovir, sometimes in combination with oral steroids. There are also topical ointments that can remove the lesions after a few applications. All of these options can remove the OHL, but studies of the illness indicate that it is likely to return.

Risk Factors and Preventive Measures

Some activities such as smoking and use of chewing tobacco can increase a person's chance of contracting OHL. Also, accidental scraping or biting of the tongue can lead to the development of leukoplakia in some people who are already susceptible. As the cause of OHL is the EBV and more than 90 percent of all people have been infected with EBV, it is difficult for an HIV-positive person to avoid having OHL. There is no prophylaxis for OHL at this time.

AIDSmeds. "Oral Hairy Leukoplakia (OHL): What Is It?" Available online. URL: AIDSmeds.com. http://www.aidsmeds.com/articles/OHL_6819.shtml. Accessed April 4, 2011.

Kozyreva, Olga. "Hairy Leukoplakia." eMedicine.com. Available online. URL: http://www.emedicine.com/MED/topic938.htm. Accessed April 4, 2011.

National Library of Medicine. "Leukoplakia." NLM. NIH.gov. Available online. URL: http://www.nlm. nih.gov/medlineplus/ency/article/001046.htm. Accessed April 4, 2011.

UCSF Center for HIV Information. "Epstein-Barr Virus (EBV)/Oral Hairy Leukoplakia (OHL)." Women ChildrenHIV.org. Available online. URL: http://womenchildrenhiv.org/wchiv?page=im-2-03-07. Accessed April 4, 2011.

Walling, Dennis M. "Oral Hairy Leukoplakia: An Epstein-Barr Virus–Associated Disease of Patients with HIV." FindArticles.com. Available online. URL: http://findarticles.com/p/articles/mi_m0EXV/is_4_6/ai_68951365. Accessed April 4, 2011.

organ transplantation Each year, more than 50,000 people receive organ transplantations. When people first became ill with HIV, all options for an HIV-positive person to receive an organ transplantation were stopped. The medical establishment and insurance corporations did not consider it worth the cost of the surgery or the difficulty of securing organs for transplantation into HIV-positive people. In the late 1990s, with the advent of antiretroviral medications and the extended lives HIV-positive people were attaining, this attitude began to change within the medical community.

In the era of HIGHLY ACTIVE ANTIRETROVIRAL THERAPY (HAART), HIV-positive people began to face problems that were not seen in the era of OPPORTUNISTIC INFECTIONS (OIs). For many HIV-positive people, this has meant becoming ill with liver or kidney disease. Many antiretroviral drugs can cause liver and kidney problems. Because HIV can be transmitted in the same manner as HEPATITIS B or HEPATITIS C, both of these liver illnesses have a high incidence within the HIV-positive population. Diabetes associated with HIV medications may cause kidney function problems. HIV itself can also cause kidney dysfunction as the illness progresses. When end-stage kidney or liver disease occurs, an organ transplant may be the only means to prevent a person from dying.

In the early days of the epidemic, when a person was initially diagnosed with HIV, survival times were often not long. As antiretroviral therapy has become the standard of care, life expectancies for people who have HIV have been lengthening considerably. It is believed that the average HIV-positive person's life expectancy increased by 13 years between 1996 and 2006. In 2000, studies at two transplant centers—University of California, San Francisco, and the University of Pittsburgh—began studying transplants in HIV-positive people. The results of studies there and then later at several other transplant centers showed that survival rates of HIV-positive people who had received transplants were comparable to those of HIV-negative patients. Survival rates were similar in patients with kidney and liver transplants, as 90 percent of kidney transplant and 80 percent of liver transplant patients were still alive after three years. The success of liver transplants was lower in people who also had hepatitis C and HIV in comparison to HIV-negative people who had hepatitis C. HIV-positive people who had hepatitis B had the same survival rates as HIV-negative transplant patients.

The United Network of Organ Sharing (UNOS), which maintains all waiting lists for organ donations around the United States, has never forbidden the listing of HIV-positive people as candidates to receive organs. The National Organ Transplant Act (NOTA) specifically states that HIV-positive people should not be barred from being candidates to receive a transplant. A person who needs a transplant must complete paperwork with his or her doctor that discusses the patient's specific condition and the urgency, health status, and information needed to match a potential donor organ to the patient. Waiting lists are maintained by UNOS so that the right organ goes to the person with the most serious need that matches all the specifics of the donated organ. Each transplant center around the country accepts patients for its own transplant list, and not everybody qualifies for each list, as some centers specialize in particular treatments but may not have the necessary expertise in dealing with other conditions, such as HIV. An HIV-positive person will want to find a transplant center that understands both illnesses well. The noted HIV-positive author Larry Kramer received a liver transplant in 2001 at the University of Pittsburgh Medical Center. In 2001, just 11 of 4,954 liver transplants in the United States were done with HIV-positive people. The number today is much higher.

One of the reasons that HIV-positive people were for years seen as unable to undergo transplantation is the need to take immunosuppressive drugs to prevent the rejection of a donated organ. However, as HIV-positive people's immune systems were restored through HAART and the virus was kept under control, it was learned that these immunosuppressive drugs worked no differently in HIV-positive people than they did in HIV-negative people.

HIV-positive people have never been allowed to donate organs or other tissue that is used in surgery. The virus, even though it may be controlled through medications, is still alive and active in the body and particularly in organs that are transplanted. In a 2007 case in which four people received transplants from one donor who had not known he was HIV-positive when he died, the recipients all became HIV-positive after the transplants. Tests run on the individual did not detect the virus, and the organs were received and transplanted with no knowledge of the presence of the virus. All people who wish to be organ donors are screened thoroughly prior to donation, and though this case made headlines, it was the first case of such seroconversion from a transplant in more than 20 years.

In South Africa, where nearly 20 percent of adults are HIV positive, it has become difficult to locate organ donors with such a large percentage of the population ineligible to donate organs when they die. In 2008, doctors in Cape Town, South Africa, became the first to transplant organs from one HIV-positive person to two other HIV-positive people. Two kidneys were transplanted during the operation. Although some physicians believe that this might encourage the spread of HIV that is resistant to some drugs to a person who may not have those resistance mutations, these physicians considered the risks worth the ability to save the lives of two people. Since then, other kidney transplants have been done. In the United States, it is currently illegal to transplant organs from an HIV-positive person knowingly. Use of potential HIV-positive donors would increase the opportunities of other HIV-positive people to receive a necessary transplant. A Johns Hopkins University study in 2011 indicated that ending the organ donation ban would allow many HIV-positive people the opportunity to receive needed organs.

AIDSmeds. "Ending HIV Organ Donation Ban Could Eliminate Transplant Waiting List for People with HIV." AIDSmeds.com. Available online. URL: http://www.aidsmeds.com/articles/hiv_transplant_organ _1667_20165.shtml. Accessed April 4, 2011.

The Body. "Organ Transplants and HIV/AIDS." The Body.com. Available online. URL: http://www.thebody.com/index/treat/transplant.html. Accessed April 4, 2011.

Centers for Disease Control and Prevention. "New Life-Saver for HIV Patients: Transplants." TheBody.com. Available online. URL: http://www.thebody.com/content/treat/art54149.html. Accessed April 4, 2011.

———. "South Africa Pioneers HIV-Positive Transplants." TheBody.com. Available online. URL: http://www.thebody.com/content/treat/art49282.html. Accessed April 4, 2011.

Hindery, Robin. "HIV and Organ Transplants Can Coexist, UCSF Research Shows." UCSF.edu. Available online. URL: http://www.ucsf.edu/science-cafe/conversations/hiv-and-organ-transplants-can-coexist-ucsf-research-shows/. Accessed April 4, 2011.

Steenhuysen, Julie. "Four Chicago Transplant Recipients Contract HIV." Reuters.com. Available online. URL: http://www.reuters.com/article/2007/11/13/us-hiv-transplant-idUSN1363004720071113. Accessed April 4, 2011.

Stock, Peter G., and John Fung. "Viable Strategies to Facilitate Liver Transplantation for HIV/HCV Coinfection." NATAP.org. Available online. URL: http://www.natap.org/2009/HIV/090309_06.htm. Accessed April 4, 2011.

Vazquez, Enid. "Organ Transplants: Promising News for Positive People." TheBody.com. Available online. URL: http://www.thebody.com/content/treat/art1035.html. Accessed April 4, 2011.

penicilliosis marneffei This is a geographically limited OPPORTUNISTIC INFECTION (OI) that is seen in HIV-positive patients with greater frequency than in the general population because of their weakened immune system. Penicilliosis marneffei (penicilliosis) is caused by a fungus, *Penicillium marneffei,* that is endemic to regions of southeast ASIA. Thailand, southern China, Myanmar, Vietnam, Laos, Cambodia, Indonesia, and eastern India have all had outbreaks among HIV-positive people. HIV-positive travelers to this region need to be aware of the fungus and any potential infection risks.

P. marneffei is carried and spread by the several species of wood rat in the region. It is not clear whether the wood rats are infected by the fungus or whether they are simply carriers of the fungus, which is found on their fur and in their feces. The illness is most common during the rainy season and infects people when they inhale the spores of the fungus. It is the third-most diagnosed OI in Southeast Asia among HIV-positive people. In people who have healthy immune systems it is rare.

Symptoms and Diagnostic Path

Common symptoms include fever, weight loss, anemia, and skin infections that appear centralized initially and then seem to spread, often resembling MOLLUSCUM CONTAGIOSUM. Lesions can appear on the face, ears, genitals, and extremities. Infection of bone marrow, liver, lungs, lymph nodes, and intestines have been reported in studies. Liver infection is particularly dangerous and can cause liver swelling, pain in the abdomen, fever, and marked increases in blood liver markers. (see BLOOD WORK/BLOOD TESTS). Penicilliosis most often appears in HIV-positive people who have extremely low CD4 T lymphocyte counts, usually fewer than 100 T cells/μL. Prior to HIV, very few cases of penicilliosis were seen by doctors in the countries where it is endemic. Recent medical literature also has described penicilliosis in people who have lupus and other immune system illnesses. *P. marneffei* is the only known member of the penicillin family of fungi that causes illness in humans.

Diagnosis is done through isolation of the fungus from the blood or biopsy of the suspected lesions. Although culturing of the virus can take several days, the fungus can be identified from tissue samples. No blood assay test is currently available to aid diagnosis at this time.

Treatment Options and Outlook

The recommended treatment is intravenous amphotericin B for two weeks, followed by oral itraconazole for a period of 10 weeks. The fungus is highly treatable if diagnosed and treated early. If not diagnosed early enough, the illness can be fatal in a large number of immune-compromised people. It is considered to be a defining illness of AIDS, and often it is the presenting illness for people who are unaware they are HIV positive. Other medications used to treat penicilliosis include miconazole, 5-flucytosine, and ketoconazole.

After initial treatment of the illness, a study in Thailand showed prophylaxis treatment for patients with T cell counts below 200 can prevent recurrence of the fungal infection, which occurs in 50 percent of patients naturally. A low dose of itraconazole orally was used as prophylaxis in the study.

Risk Factors and Preventive Measures

Again, studies from Thailand have shown success in treating HIV-positive people with weakened immune systems through prophylaxis. U.S. doctors may consider prophylactic treatment with itraconazole for HIV-positive people visiting areas of endemic penicilliosis infection. Otherwise, risk in the United States, Canada, and Western Europe is minimal except for individuals who travel to the area of the world where the fungus is found.

Chariyalertsak, S., K. Supparatpinyo, T. Sirisanthana, and K. E. Nelson. "A Controlled Trial of Itraconazole as Primary Prophylaxis for Systemic Fungal Infections in Patients with Advanced Human Immunodeficiency Virus Infection in Thailand." *Clinical Infectious Diseases* 34, no. 2 (15 January 2002): 277–284.

Di-Qing, Luo, et al. "Disseminated *Penicillium marneffei* Infection in an SLE Patient: A Case Report and Literature Review." *Mycopathologia* 171, no. 3 (15 September 2010): 191–196.

Roy, Sampurna. "Penicilliosis (*Penicillium marneffei* Infection)." Histopathology-India.net. Available online. URL: http://www.histopathology-india.net/Penic.htm. Accessed April 4, 2011.

Sy Wong, Samson. "*Penicillium marneffei.*" Gov.hk. Available online. URL: http://www.info.gov.hk/aids/pdf/g190htm/28.htm. Accessed April 4, 2011.

Tantisiriwat, Woraphot, M.D., and Judith A. Aberg, M.D. "Penicilliosis and HIV." HIVInSite.ucsf.edu. Available online. URL: http://hivinsite.ucsf.edu/InSite?page=kb-05-02-07. Accessed April 4, 2011.

University of Adelaide. "Penicilliosis marneffei." *Mycology Online.* Adelaide.edu.au. Available online. URL: http://www.mycology.adelaide.edu.au/Mycoses/Opportunistic/Penicilliosis_marneffei/. Accessed April 4, 2011.

PEPFAR PEPFAR is the acronym for a U.S. government organization created by George W. Bush early in his administration. It stands for the President's Emergency Plan for AIDS Relief. PEPFAR was initially announced in a 2003 speech as a promise by President Bush that the U.S. government would do more in the worldwide fight against AIDS. The program is headed by the U.S. global AIDS coordinator, an individual appointed by the president of the United States and approved by the U.S. Senate. President Barack Obama nominated Dr. Eric Goosby, a physician from the University of California, San Francisco, to be the next coordinator.

Initial reaction to PEPFAR was varied. It was hailed by many people as a much-needed U.S. response to the world epidemic that many HIV activists thought had been missing for many years. It was also received with a great deal of skepticism by many, as people questioned why the United States did not simply use the already available United Nations (UN)–backed GLOBAL FUND TO FIGHT AIDS, TUBERCULOSIS, AND MALARIA. The United States was already the main contributor to the fund, but the Bush administration was politically opposed to contributing any further money that would be spent under UN regulations, and thus created its own government entity to deliver funding.

When announcing the creation of PEPFAR, Bush wanted to allocate $15 billion through the 2008 budget year. PEPFAR received initial funding of approximately $2 million in 2004, with increases over the next four years, eventually allocating $6 billion for the budget year 2008, exceeding the requested funding for the first five years by nearly $4 billion. PEPFAR was funded for another five-year cycle running through 2013 under a reauthorization act that increased funding to $48 billion for that period.

PEPFAR is run by the U.S. global AIDS coordinator, who reports directly to the secretary of the state, currently Hillary Rodham Clinton. PEPFAR does not run any of the individual programs, but oversees the coordination of the many programs administered through several government offices already in existence, and coordinates with other national governments to maximize the effectiveness of the monies put toward the AIDS epidemic. PEPFAR and the U.S. global coordinator oversee programs of several different federal agencies, including the Department of Health and Human Services, U.S. Agency for International Development, Peace Corps, and even some Department of Defense programs.

Although PEPFAR oversees funding that goes toward any AIDS program funded outside the United States, the initial funding for the program called for 15 target countries. These countries were specifically designated to receive a majority of direct funding for treatment of people with antiretroviral medications. The 15 target countries are Botswana, Côte d'Ivoire, Ethiopia, Guyana, Haiti, Kenya, Mozambique, Namibia, Nigeria, Rwanda, South Africa, Tanzania, Uganda, Vietnam, and Zambia. Other countries have also received PEPFAR aid, though not all of the following countries have received direct antiretroviral funding: Angola, Cambodia, China, Ghana, India, Indonesia, Lesotho, Malawi, Russia, Sudan, Swaziland, Thailand, Ukraine, and Zimbabwe. In the reauthorization bill passed in 2008, EASTERN EUROPE AND CENTRAL ASIA and LATIN AMERICA were listed as areas of alarming spread of the virus that threatens security, development, and global health, potentially causing a crisis. This enlarged the area of concern discussed in the previous bill, which mentioned sub-Saharan AFRICA, the CARIBBEAN, and developing countries in general.

PEPFAR had paid the cost of prescription coverage for more than 2 million people at the end of 2008. Goals for the reauthorized plan call for treatment of 3 million people by the end of 2013. PEPFAR has been very successful in getting antiretrovirals into countries that had not previously been able to provide such treatment to their citizens. It has not reached everyone in those countries, however, as medical facilities, doctors, and nurses are often unavailable in many rural or extremely poor regions of a country. In addition, individuals who need treatment have no way to travel to the care they may need on a regular basis, thereby making their treatment useless, as

consistent treatment is the key to maintaining health for an HIV-positive person.

One initial problem with providing antiretrovirals was the U.S. government's insistence that the U.S. FOOD AND DRUG ADMINISTRATION (FDA) approve any medication provided. Exceptions were allowed for medications approved by Western European, Canadian, and Japanese governmental organizations. Most countries do not recognize FDA guidelines, choosing to recognize World Health Organization–approved medications. By requiring FDA approval, the PEPFAR dollars were tied to foreign pharmaceutical companies seeking a lengthy approval process within the United States before their medications would be paid for under PEPFAR. This also excluded generic medications produced in several countries. These generic medications could have saved the PEPFAR program large amounts of money, as PEPFAR chose to support the program by funding the exorbitant cost of U.S. pharmaceutical company medications instead of the cost of the same generic medications produced in India or Brazil. It also initially prevented the use of fixed-dose combination (FDC) medications, pills that combine more than one drug to reduce the amount of pills a person takes. When generic antiretroviral drugs were first approved by the FDA, African governments did not approve them, as the drugs often had not received approval from the WHO, which was the preferred agency for drugs in those countries. Activist protests in the United States as well as abroad eventually led to agreements whereby the FDA approved several generic medications as well as several FDC drugs, which have produced savings and allowed the distribution of medications to more people in the targeted countries.

One of the chief criticisms of the funding for PEPFAR has been the limitations placed on the money. Half of all money spent on preventing AIDS TRANSMISSION in the reauthorized bill had to be spent on programs advocating ABSTINENCE, monogamy, and partner reduction. This was an increase from the initial bill, which specified that one-third of prevention dollars were to be spent on abstinence programs. This was later increased to two-thirds, but the term *being faithful* was added to the funding language in addition to *abstinence*. No funding was to be allotted for needle exchange programs of any variety. This prohibition prevented education and prevention activities from including this highly successful means of AIDS prevention. Condom programs were limited to those at high risk such as SEX WORKERS and INJECTION DRUG USE(R)S, as well as people in serodiscordant relationships. Condom education and distribution were not to be funded for youths at all. No discussion of education for gay males was mentioned either. Although President Obama ended funding of abstinence-only education programs shortly after he became president, this applies only to U.S. programs and not international programs as funded in the PEPFAR bill passed in 2008. Whether this decision will carry over to the international programs has yet to be seen.

Another restriction on funds was that no monies were to be given to countries, agencies, or entities that did not have explicit statements prohibiting prostitution or preventing sex trafficking. This led to Brazil's refusing PEPFAR dollars because they feared possibly reducing the effectiveness of reaching sex workers or their clients with prevention information or treatment. Tanzania was refused money by PEPFAR for education programs because that country wanted to contact sex workers through nonjudgmental television programming that was deemed unacceptable to PEPFAR guidelines. It was also unclear whether PEPFAR monies could be granted to countries or agencies that provided abortion counseling or services, as U.S. rules prevented any funding of countries or agencies that discussed such topics. This particular rule was called the global gag order and was designed to refuse funding to groups in several situations regarding anything to do with education, legal advocacy, or research into unsafe abortions. This rule was reversed shortly after President Obama took office in 2009, though recently elected Republican congressional leaders have attempted to reinstate the regulations in funding bills and have tried to refuse funding for the United Nations agency that pays for family planning education around the globe.

President Obama continued the funding of PEPFAR, despite the economic crisis. PEPFAR funding was initially flat during the Obama administration, though small increases were made in the 2011 budget, although HIV treatment activists stated that these increases did not match the rises in expenses due to inflation. The results from PEPFAR programs have been considered good by most observers in the HIV community. More than 2 million people are receiving treatment now in the targeted countries, though some countries such as Ethiopia have fallen short of their targets of the number of people treated. Other countries that have exceeded treatment targets, such as Uganda and Zambia, counter this. Prevention goals are also tracked. According to statistics derived from treatment of infected WOMEN, it is known that more than 240,000 CHILDREN born to these women have been prevented from contracting HIV. Because their mother received treatment during pregnancy, mother-to-child transmission of the virus was averted. It remains to be seen whether other preventive measures will be allowed so that prevention can be encouraged in populations that have not been reached because of current funding limitations.

PEPFAR is widely seen as President George Bush's chief success during his time in office. Despite the downsides to the funding, the program has been largely responsible for treatment and prevention of HIV across a large portion of the developing world.

AIDS Healthcare Foundation. "AHF Lauds Obama's Appointment of Dr. Eric Goosby at PEPFAR." AIDS Health.org. Available online. URL: http://www.aidshealth.org/news/press-releases/ahf-lauds-obamas-appointment.html. Accessed April 5, 2011.
AVERT: AVERTing HIV and AIDS. "The U.S. President's Emergency Plan for AIDS Relief (PEPFAR)." AVERT.org. Available online. URL: http://www.avert.org/pepfar.htm. Accessed April 5, 2011.

PEPFAR. "U.S. President's Emergency Plan for AIDS Relief." PEPFAR.gov. Available online. URL: http://www.pepfar.gov/index.htm. Accessed April 5, 2011.

PEPFARWatch: The Global AIDS Relief Monitor. "PEPFAR Watch." PEPFARWatch.org. Available online. URL: http://www.pepfarwatch.org/. Accessed April 1, 2011.

Richards, Cecile, and Amy Goodman. "Right Wing Republicans Are on the Verge of Voting to Defund Planned Parenthood." AlterNet.org. Available online. URL: http://www.alternet.org/reproductivejustice/149945/right-wing_republicans_are_on_the_verge_of_voting_to_defund_planned_parenthood/. Accessed April 5, 2011.

Savage, Dan. "The End of Abstinence-Only Sex 'Education.'" TheStranger.com. Available online. URL: http://slog.thestranger.com/slog/archives/2009/05/07/the-end-of-abstinence-only-sex-education. Accessed April 5, 2011.

United States Congress. "Public Law 108-25." GPO.gov. Available online. URL: http://frwebgate.access.gpo.gov/cgi-bin/getdoc.cgi?dbname=108_cong_public_laws&docid=f:publ025.108.pdf. Accessed April 5, 2011.

White House Press Office. "Statement by the President on Global Health Initiative." WhiteHouse.gov. Available online. URL: http://www.whitehouse.gov/the_press_office/Statement-by-the-President-on-Global-Health-Initiative/. Accessed April 5, 2011.

Pneumocystis pneumonia (PCP) *Pneumocystis carinii* pneumonia (PCP) is the most common OPPORTUNISTIC INFECTION (OI) in HIV-positive patients in the United States. It is a fungal pneumonia that was first noted during World War II in malnourished refugees in Europe. PCP was discovered in rats by Dr. Carlos Chagas and Dr. Antonio Carini, well-known Brazilian physicians. Carini believed the organism to be a trypanosome, from the same family of parasites that causes Chagas disease and African sleeping sickness. Then research led by Drs. Delanoë at the Pasteur Institute led to renaming what they believed to be a protozoan, *Pneumocystis carinii*, after Dr. Carini. For many years, it was assumed that the *Pneumocystis* in one mammal was the same as another, but further study showed that each species of *Pneumocystis* was host specific, meaning each mammal had a species that was adapted to its own environment. Therefore, a rat *Pneumocystis* could not infect a mouse or human, and the human variety could not infect a mouse or rat. In the late 1980s, deoxyribonucleic acid (DNA) analysis showed that *Pneumocystis* was a unicellular fungus, and a decision was eventually made to reclassify the human species of it as *Pneumocystis jirovecii* after the Czech researcher Otto Jirovec, who first studied *Pneumocystis* in humans.

Until the advent of HIV, *Pneumocystis* was seen in fewer than 100 patients annually in the United States. They were individuals who had suppressed immune systems a result of ORGAN TRANSPLANTATION or treatment of various cancers, or CHILDREN who did not have strong immune systems because of illness or malnourishment. Antibodies to *Pneumocystis* fungi are seen in two-thirds of American children by age four. Although the means of human TRANSMISSION is not absolutely clear, it is believed that humans become infected and clear the infection at different rates and times of their healthy life, depending on where they live in the world and their exposure to the fungi. It has been shown that the fungi can be spread through the air in rodents, and some studies indicate that airborne transmission by humans is possible. The common abbreviation PCP is still used for *Pneumocystis jirovecii* pneumonia.

Symptoms and Diagnostic Path

PCP infection is a generally slow progression of symptoms arising from the infection by the fungi. Progressive difficulty in breathing, persistent fever, nonproductive cough, and chest discomfort can be evident for a few days to a few weeks. Fatigue, weight loss, and diarrhea may also accompany the onset. CANDIDIASIS is a common coinfection with PCP. Disseminated PCP is possible in HIV patients, and any internal organ can become a possible infection site.

The infection attacks the interstitial, fibrous tissue of the lungs, causing inflammation and thickening of the alveoli, the small structures in the lungs involved in allowing the blood and body to receive oxygen during breathing. PCP patients will have marked drops in blood oxygen levels that can cause life-threatening situations if not treated immediately at that point.

Diagnosis of PCP is generally begun through a chest X-ray and blood gas measurements. The chest X-ray will show areas of increased whiteness in the image during PCP infection. Blood gas measurements will show a lack of oxygen and an increase in carbon dioxide levels. This can cause insufficient levels of oxygen in patients, leading to rapid, continuous breathing as patients try to draw acceptable levels of oxygen into the body. If not treated aggressively, this lack of oxygen can eventually lead to a collapsed lung and cause other medical complications for the patient.

Definitive means of testing for PCP include a bronchoscopy so the presence of the fungi can be measured in tissue or sputum retrieved during the test. Both sputum, the clear or white mucous fluid generated by the body to clear an infection, and tissue can be used in various lab tests to determine whether PCP is present in the lungs.

Treatment Options and Outlook

Treatment is generally begun immediately if the doctor presumes that PCP is the cause of the patient's discomfort. The lab tests and bronchoscopy will be completed as treatment is ongoing, as it takes several days to clear the lungs of infection. Because the disease can cause many complications if not treated quickly, it is not unusual for tests to be delayed until the patient has begun treatment.

Trimethoprim/sulfamethoxazole (TMP-SMX), known as co-trimoxozole in Europe, a combination of two sulfa antibiotics, is the standard of treatment for PCP. Oral medications are used unless the infection is severe, in which case intravenous TMP-SMX is used. Dosage depends on the weight of the patient. Treatment will switch to oral medication after a few days if the patient improves. Steroids will also be given in severe cases to prevent inflammation. These drugs have been shown to increase the success of treatment in severe cases.

Alternatives to this regimen for those allergic to TMP-SMX include a combination of intravenous clindamycin and oral primaquine. Intravenous pentamadine is also a standard treatment in severe cases. Aerosolized pentamadine is not used for treatment of active cases of PCP, as it is not effective in the long term in preventing relapse of the illness. A liquid form of atovaquone can also be used in mild cases of PCP but is less effective than TMP-SMX.

Risk Factors and Preventive Measures

At one time, this was the most common OI found among HIV infected individuals in the United States and WESTERN AND CENTRAL EUROPE. When HIV first attracted the attention of doctors, 70–80 percent of all people who had HIV developed *Pneumocystis* pneumonia. Approximately 90 percent of those people had CD4+ T lymphocyte cell counts of fewer than 200 cells per microliter (200/µL) of blood. The probability of acquiring the infection also increased if the CD4+ T lymphocyte cell percentage was less than 15 percent, viral load was high, or the patient had previous cases of bacterial pneumonia, a history of CANDIDIASIS, or unintentional excessive weight loss.

Since the development of HIGHLY ACTIVE ANTIRETROVIRAL THERAPY (HAART), *Pneumocystis* cases have fallen dramatically. The rate of infection among HIV-positive people is now somewhere in the 2–3 percent range. Cases of PCP occur primarily among people who had been unaware of their HIV status or had not been receiving HAART or PCP preventive treatment.

PCP can be prevented by treatment with TMP-SMX if a patient's CD4 T lymphocyte count falls below 200/µL. It is standard care to prescribe preventive medication for PCP. One or two single strength pills daily are standard, depending on the patient's ability to take the drug. Patients who are allergic to TMP-SMX will be prescribed dapsone or a combination of dapsone with other drugs such as pentamadine and pyrimethamine. Atovaquone is also as effective as dapsone or aerosolized pentamidine but is a more expensive alternative. Prophylaxis can be stopped if a person's immune system recovers and has more than 200/μL CD4 T lymphocytes for longer than three months.

Bennett, Nicholas John. *"Pneumocystis (carinii) jiroveci* Pneumonia.*"* Medscape.com. Available online. URL: http://emedicine.medscape.com/article/225976-over view. Accessed April 5, 2011.

Hughes, W. T. *"Pneumocystis carinii* Pneumonitis.*"* *Chest* 85, no. 6 (June 1984): 810–813.

Miller, R., and Laurence Huang. *"Pneumocystis jirove-cii* Infection.*"* *Thorax* 59, no. 9 (September 2004): 731–733.

Morris, Alison, et al. "Current Epidemiology of *Pneumo-cystis* Pneumonia.*"* *Emerging Infectious Diseases* (October 2004). Available online. URL: http://www.cdc.gov/ NCIDOD/EID/vol10no10/03-0985.htm#cit. Accessed April 5, 2011.

post-exposure prophylaxis (PEP) PEP is the acronym for post-exposure prophylaxis, a preventive treatment for something that a person may have been exposed to in a medical or social situation. A common PEP is the use of the drug Tamiflu to treat people who have had contact with someone who has the flu virus, to prevent them from becoming ill. In the case of HIV, PEP refers to the use of a combination of antiretroviral medications to prevent the TRANSMISSION of HIV, after an exposure may have taken place. The most common situation in which this occurs is at hospitals or health clinics where a health care worker is accidentally stuck by a needle after it has been used. Needlesticks occur occasionally in health care settings despite the many precautions that are taken to prevent them.

PEP for HIV has been approved since 1996. A study published in 1997 showed that health care workers who had been stuck by needles used in treating HIV-positive patients were 81 percent less likely to contract HIV if they used antiretroviral medications for one month after the exposure to the virus at their job. It is common practice in health care settings that a person who has been stuck with a needle be given the option of PEP treatment if there is good reason to think that the needle was used for a patient who has HIV or a person who has unknown HIV status. The PEP involves taking a multidrug course of HIGHLY ACTIVE ANTIRETROVIRAL THERAPY (HAART) much as a person who is HIV positive does for a month after the potential exposure. It is important that a person begin the PEP as soon as possible after the exposure but not later than 72 hours after exposure to the virus, as it is believed the PEP will not be helpful at that point.

PEP has also been studied in the context of preventing HIV after unsafe sexual activity, unsafe injection drug use, or other potential nonoccupational exposure to HIV. In a South African study of rape survivors who were provided PEP only one individual seroconverted after taking PEP, among nearly 500 people. That individual had started the PEP treatment 96 hours after the rape. Studies of 350 gay men in several locations around the world demonstrated no seroconversion after treatment with PEP. There was, however, some question in those studies whether actual exposure had taken place or whether the exposure was not high-risk enough for seroconversion. Other cases were also presented in the U.S. government report, including the case of a woman who took PEP after receiving a blood donation from an individual who was later found to be HIV positive. After nine months of PEP, she was determined not to be HIV positive despite the extremely high risk for seroconversion.

Despite these positive reports in the use of PEP, there are currently only five states (California, Massachusetts, New Mexico, New York, and Rhode Island) that allow the general public to request and receive PEP after potential exposure to HIV. Although the U.S. CENTERS FOR DISEASE CONTROL and Prevention (CDC) encourages doctors to prescribe PEP in such cases, they recommend that it be done on a case-by-case basis and not as a general rule of practice. Doctors in the United States have been generally unwilling to prescribe such medicines, and public health authorities have been unwilling as a rule to take on the costs of the prescriptions for such post-exposure treatment. Politically, it is seen as similar to the morning-after pill that can prevent pregnancy. Politicians seem unwilling to support legislation for such treatment when they believe abstinence or condom use is the answer to preventing TRANSMISSION of the virus. Popular press stories about PEP highlight the lack of public knowledge about the option to prescribe PEP or about the potential benefits in preventing transmission. Concern also exists that wide availability of PEP might simply stop people from using condoms or stopping drug use as a way of preventing exposure.

Many drawbacks to PEP as a means of transmission prevention exist. The first is the cost of the medications. For the uninsured, a month of treatment on antiretrovirals can run $1,000 or more. There are also side effects of the drugs, which are the same as for anyone taking the medications: headache, nausea, diarrhea, and others. These side effects are cited in several PEP articles as reasons for study participants, even health care workers stuck by needles, to discontinue treatment with antiretrovirals as a preventive measure.

There are also popular press reports about a trend in party-going circles for people to take antiretroviral medications—in particular, TENO-FOVIR DISOPROXIL FUMARATE—as a way to prevent someone exposed to HIV from becoming infected. Some people report taking tenofovir as a preexposure treatment, meaning they intend to engage in unsafe sexual activity and are using the drug in what they believe is a way to prevent getting the virus. It is highly unlikely that taking one pill prior to exposure to the virus will prevent HIV transmission.

A study called the Pre-exposure Prophylaxis (PrEP) is already under way around the world to test whether the administration of antiretrovirals on a regular basis can prevent someone from becoming infected with HIV. One of the driving reasons behind this study and another study testing a gel microbicide with tenofovir

as the main ingredient is that people continue to become HIV positive despite years of prevention education. Each year in the United States alone, 50,000 people become HIV positive. These studies attempt to show that the virus can be prevented even among people who cannot or will not change their behavior to prevent contracting HIV. These studies are ongoing in the United States as well as India, Thailand, and Botswana.

Many social, political, and medical arguments both for and against the idea of PrEP have been analyzed. In the current U.S. political and economic climate, cost is a primary deterrent to this use of antiretroviral medications. The average cost of more than $1,000 a month for antiretrovirals makes the prevention of HIV very expensive. It is unclear whether insurance companies or the government would be willing to cover the expense of prevention if the trials were to prove successful in preventing HIV. There is also the cost to the person taking the medication from a health standpoint. Antiretroviral medications have numerous side effects. In addition to minor side effects such as nausea, diarrhea, and gas, long-term side effects of some drugs can include loss of bone density, increase in cardiovascular problems, and potential liver or kidney damage. It has been proven that people do not always take their medications because of the side effects, even when they are HIV positive. To expect people who are not HIV positive to take medications regularly, given the potential side effects, may be expecting too much from people who do not understand the potential consequences fully. It is unclear whether the side effects of using a preventive microbicide will be the same as those of taking oral medications. It is unknown whether a microbicide will work for both men and women and whether they will have the opportunity to use the microbicide with regularity, or prior to sexual activity, to prevent the transmission of the virus.

Studies and experience have shown that brief doses of the drug can prevent the transmission of the virus from pregnant women to their infants during childbirth. Studies in animals have shown that periodic or regular use of antiretrovirals can prevent the transmission of HIV when the animals are purposefully exposed to the virus. These studies encouraged investigation into whether PrEP can succeed in humans. Preliminary results of at least one of the studies being conducted by the U.S. Department of Health and Human Services show that PrEP, when taken for at least 50 percent of the prescribed period, provides a 50 percent reduction in risk, while participants who took the medication at least 90 percent of the time showed a 73 percent lowered risk of transmission. This initial PrEP study was conducted among MEN WHO HAVE SEX WITH MEN (MSM) and transgender WOMEN who have sex with men, and the U.S. government has cautioned against drawing conclusions across all populations. Whether politics in the United States will allow the preventive use of expensive medications is not known. Studies under way also will be evaluating the cost-effectiveness of the preventive drugs versus the potential costs of treating someone who is HIV positive long term.

In July 2011, early results from two PrEP studies conducted in Africa demonstrated that PrEP was highly effective in preventing HIV conversion among couples where one person was HIV-positive and the other person was HIV-negative. In one of the studies conducted, Kenyan and Ugandan couples were given condoms and counseling on how to use them; one-third of those couples were given a placebo pill to take once a day, one-third were given the antiretroviral tenofovir disoproxil fumarate, and the final third of the couples studied were given the combination pill Truvada. The people in the Truvada arm of the study had a rate of infection 73 percent lower than those in the study using only condoms. A second study conducted in Botswana showed similar results. Participants who adhered to taking the drug regularly also fared better than those individuals who did not take the drug regularly.

Bowers, Dan, M.D. "A 'Morning After' Rescue Pill? No!" hivplusmag.com. Available online. URL: http://www.hivplusmag.com/Story.asp?id=1190&categoryid=4&issue_emi=current&jt=0. Accessed April 7, 2011.

Brown, David. "Two Studies Show That Drugs Used to Treat AIDS Can Prevent HIV Infection." *Washington Post.* Available online. URL: http://www.washingtonpost.com/national/two-studies-show-that-drugs-used-to-treat-aids-can-be-used-to-prevent-hiv-infection-too/2011/07/12/gIQAN51zBI_story.html. Accessed July 24, 2011.

Cardo, Denise, M.D., et al. "A Case-Control Study of HIV Seroconversion in Health Care Workers after Percutaneous Exposure." *New England Journal of Medicine* 337, no. 21 (20 November 1997): 1485–1490.

Centers for Disease Control and Prevention. "Antiretroviral Postexposure Prophylaxis after Sexual, Injection Drug Use, or Other Non-Occupational Exposure to HIV in the United States." CDC.gov. Available online. URL: http://www.cdc.gov/mmwr/preview/mmwrhtml/mm6003a1.htm?s_cid=mm6003a1_w. Accessed April 7, 2011.

———. "HIV/AIDS—Pre-Exposure Prophylaxis (PrEP)." CDC.gov. Available online. URL: http://www.cdc.gov/hiv/prep/. Accessed April 5, 2011.

Garcia-Lerma, J. Gerardo, et al. "Prevention of Rectal SHIV Transmission in Macaques by Daily or Intermittent Prophylaxis with Emtricitabine and Tenofovir." *PLoS Medicine* 5, no. 2 (February 2008): 30. Available online. URL: http://www.plosmedicine.org/article/info:doi/10.1371/journal.pmed.0050028. Accessed July 24, 2011.

Grant, Robert M., et al. "Preexposure Chemoprophylaxis for HIV Prevention in Men Who Have Sex with Men." NEJM.org. Available online. URL: http://www.nejm.org/doi/pdf/10.1056/NEJMoa1011205. Accessed April 7, 2011.

Hilton, Hilary. "Self-Medicating with AIDS Drugs." Time.com. Available online. URL: http://www.time.com/time/health/article/0,8599,1707417,00.html. Accessed April 5, 2011.

Panlilio, Adelisa L., M.D., et al. "Updated U.S. Public Health Service Guidelines for the Management of Occupational Exposures to HIV and Recommendations for Postexposure Prophylaxis." CDC.gov. Available online. URL: http://www.cdc.gov/mmwr/preview/mmwrhtml/rr5409a1.htm. Accessed April 5, 2011.

Project Inform. "PrEP (Pre-Exposure Prophylaxis)."
   TheBody.com. Available online. URL: http://
   www.thebody.com/content/treat/art52098.html.
   Accessed April 5, 2011.

Sharrock, Justine. "The HIV Morning-after Pill." *Mother
   Jones* (June 2008). Available online. URL: http://
   motherjones.com/politics/2008/05/hiv-morning
   -after-pill. Accessed April 5, 2011.

Suvash, Shrestha. "Tenofovir for HIV Prevention: Gel or
   Tablet." JYI.org. Available online. URL: http://www.
   jyi.org/news/nb.php?id=1559. Accessed April 7,
   2011.

prisons   Health problems—including HIV and AIDS, TUBERCULOSIS, and sexually transmitted infections (STIs)—that affect correctional inmate populations pose difficult programmatic and fiscal challenges for the administrators and staff of prisons and jails across the United States as well as the rest of the world. Populations continue to increase in U.S. federal and state facilities, while governmental budgets remain stagnant or shrinking. In addition, problems of substance abuse, high-risk sexual activity, poverty, and poor access to preventive and primary health care cause many problems not seen in typical medical settings.

Prisons consider themselves control facilities and not medical facilities, so concern is focused primarily on controlling the people within the walls. In studies published by the *American Journal of Public Health* and *Infectious Diseases in Corrections Report,* prisons are reported to be inefficient in providing prescriptions to the incarcerated and at times unhelpful in protecting those who are sick, as prisons are lacking in standard medical facilities and up-to-date equipment and technology. However, prisoners are the only people in the United States who have a constitutional right to medical care. A U.S. Supreme Court case decision, *Estelle v. Gamble* in 1976, stated that the "deliberate indifference to serious medical needs of prisoners" violates the eighth amendment to the constitution, which prohibits cruel and unusual punishment. So, despite the ruling that medical care is a constitutional right of prisoners, standards of care for prisoners or mandated guidelines for medical care of prisoners do not exist in many state and local correctional facilities.

By the end of 2006, the United States had more than 2.2 million people in a federal, state, or local prison. That is more than one in every 100 adult Americans, the highest rate of incarceration in the world. Prison populations have grown by 400 percent during the years that the HIV epidemic has been occurring because, beginning in the mid-1980s, the federal government and many states mandated minimum sentencing for drug offenses. This led to prison sentences for offenses that had previously not been punished by prison time. Offenses such as possession of small amounts of drugs or sex work resulted in sentencing. This effectively placed a large number of people who are at high risk for acquiring HIV in a closed setting. INJECTION DRUG USE(R)s (IDU) and SEX WORKERS have substantially higher rates of HIV infection than the general population. It is not surprising to find that rates of HIV and AIDS in the U.S. prison system are significantly higher than in the general population. According to the *HIV in Prisons, 2007–08* report issued by the U.S. Bureau of Justice Statistics, rates of HIV infection ranged from 0.3 percent of the prison population in Alaska and Wyoming, which is itself three times higher than the national average, to 5.8 percent in New York State.

The total rate of infection for men in all types of prison is 1.5 percent of the total population. Among WOMEN, that number is higher at 1.9 percent of the female prison population. Several states reported much higher rates of infection. In addition to New York State's high rate, in Florida 3.8 percent of the male prison population is HIV positive. Rates higher than 2 percent can be found in Connecticut, Louisiana, Maryland, Massachusetts, New Jersey, and North Carolina. Among women prisoners, 11.8 percent of female prisoners are HIV positive in New York; in Florida it is 4.8 percent; and in New Jersey, 4.2 percent. As with rates in the general U.S. population, the numbers of AIDS patients in prison have dropped significantly since the mid-1990s. The rates of HIV and AIDS in prisons also tend to reflect the numbers outside prisons. AFRICAN AMERICANS and LATINO/A AMERICANS make up larger numbers of HIV positive people both inside and outside prisons. African-American women represent the largest number of female HIV-positive prisoners.

Testing of prisoners for HIV upon entering a prison is mandatory in 21 of the U.S. states. Although the WORLD HEALTH ORGANIZATION (WHO) has made statements opposing mandatory testing, legislation in several other states regarding mandatory testing is pending. Some arguments against mandatory testing are based on the way the laws are enforced and the lack of control over the results of the tests. In some cases, prisoners are tested immediately upon entering the prison system. However, because of the length of the interval before results are received, often 10 days to two weeks in the best medical facility outside a prison, many prisoners have been transferred from the location where they first entered the prison system to one where they are housed on a more permanent basis. Prisoners are transferred for reasons of overcrowding, administrative purposes, or systems that have one processing point but many places to house prisoners. There are also concerns that state or federal prison regulations may not be applied to prisoners held in private, for-profit prisons with which state governments subcontract for prison services. Officially, the health information of a prisoner is to remain confidential in prisons, and officially prison staff and employees do not know a prisoner's HIV status. In reality, these regulations are ignored or circumvented, and a person's HIV status is often common knowledge through the medications that are given, unofficial or official segregation systems of HIV-positive prisoners, or guards' knowledge of prisoner status. All those factors serve to undermine the confidentiality of HIV status. In many instances, prisoners have been banned from certain prison jobs such as at the medical center or in the food handling areas because of their HIV status. In addition, some prisons, including all of those in the state of Alabama, ban HIV-positive prisoners from taking part in work-release programs in the community.

Prison HIV education programs are often poorly funded or nonexistent. For prisoners who change facilities between when they are tested and when results are known, the results often are not forwarded with them because of lack of administrative follow-up. Also, many prisons have the policy that a person who tested negative does not need to be informed of the results, as there is nothing to be treated. These times are lost opportunities to educate people who may never have received HIV education in the community. In addition, condoms are generally not allowed in prisons, as prison regulations generally oppose sexual relations of any kind. Other reasons cited in studies by AmFar state that condoms are banned for their potential use as weapons or drug-smuggling equipment. Lack of condoms simply ignores the fact that sexual relations happen in prison whether illegal or not. It can also encourage the spread of HIV and other STIs, eventually costing more in treatment than what might be saved by not distributing condoms. Only two states—Vermont and Mississippi—and five communities—New York City, Philadelphia, San Francisco, Los Angeles, and Washington, D.C.—provide condoms to prisoners upon request. Other localities or states may allow them to be distributed but do not pay for them, while in many instances condoms are simply banned. Studies have shown that where allowed, condoms are not used in any illegal activities such as drug smuggling or as weapons. However, even where they are available, only 30 percent of those having access to condoms use them, again showing the need for education in HIV prevention and harm reduction. Peer-education programs run by current or former prisoners have been very successful in reaching prison populations. Peers have an understanding of the situations and pressures that exist in prisons, and can offer suggestions and education to current prisoners. Studies of peer-education HIV programs have shown that after participating in such programs, prisoners were likely to request HIV testing, even if the prison had known segregation or discriminatory practices against HIV-positive people.

Sexual relations in prisons occur whether they are banned officially or not. They occur between prisoners, and they also occur between prisoners and guards or other prison employees. Some of the relations are consensual, and some are coerced relations. Because many people are imprisoned for various sexual actions such as prostitution, rape, pandering (pimping), or other similar crimes, the opportunities for these individuals to be HIV positive are considerably greater than among people in other settings. Sexual activity may be a means of survival, particularly for individuals who do not meet gender or sexual norms. It may be a means of trading for goods, such as illegal drugs, or for protection. Gay men and transgender individuals often face threats in jail because of their behavior or activities that set them apart from other prisoners. Recent studies of forced sexual activities in prisons show 20 percent of male prisoners and as many as 25 percent of female prisoners have faced sexual coercion in prison. A study by Grinstead and associates showed that people faced with future prison sentences as well as those recently released from prison engage in more frequent sex with multiple partners, thereby increasing the probability of HIV spread and infection. Prison-based HIV education and counseling may help stop the spread of HIV if offered effectively.

Drug use has been related in numerous studies to criminal acts and is often the cause of incarceration. Prisons officially ban such activity, but again, illegal drug use often continues once a person is in prison. The opportunities for INJECTION DRUG USE(R)s (IDU) in a prison are often more concentrated than outside prison and certainly less safe. Access to needles of any kind is difficult, and if needles are acquired, they are most often reused and unclean, as obtaining access to bleach and sterilization equipment is often more difficult than getting or creating a needle for injection. The incidence of HIV and other blood-borne viruses such as HEPATITIS B or HEPATITIS C is high in IDU populations if cleaning and sterilization materials are unavailable.

Tattooing is also a high-risk activity in prison life. Tattoos are etched into the skin and generally cause some bleeding and scabbing in clean and healthy settings. In prisons, where tattoos show individuality or membership in particular groups, tattooing can be dangerous for the same reasons that IDU is dangerous. Tattooing instruments made from guitar strings, pens, and pins are often reused by prison tattoo artists without bleaching or sterilization, leading to the spread of several viruses.

Issues can also arise when a prisoner is ready to be released. A person who has received health care in prison may not receive it after leaving prison. Former prisoners have a much higher rate of unemployment and a much lower income level than people who have never been in prison. In addition, people who have been in prison are automatically excluded from some governmental benefits such as food stamps by the Workfare laws passed in the late 1990s. Also, prisoners who have been on medication may not have access to HIV antiretrovirals immediately upon release. Medicaid is generally terminated by the state if a person is imprisoned, and it can take from two to 10 weeks to reestablish Medicaid for a person once it has been terminated. In that period, HIV can be reactivated, causing the virus to reproduce rapidly in some instances, making the just-released prisoner highly infectious at a time when he or she is seeing family or lovers for the first time in a long time and during a period that studies have shown involves frequent sex with multiple partners. Prerelease education, planning, and programming are essential not just for prisoners in general but for HIV-positive prisoners specifically so that they can continue to access needed medication to prevent other people from needlessly becoming infected. Studies of people who return to prison after their initial release have reported access to medical care as a reason for committing an offense and receiving prison time as a sentence. This further highlights the need for better pre-release education and services as well as easier access to medical care once a person is back in the community.

Aizenman, N. C. "New High in U.S. Prison Numbers." *WashingtonPost*. Available online. URL: http://www.washingtonpost.com/wp-dyn/content/story/2008/02/28/ST2008022803016.html. Accessed April 7, 2011.

AmFar: Foundation for AIDS Research. "HIV in Correctional Settings: Implications for Prevention and Treatment Policy." AmFar.org. Available online. URL: http://www.amfar.org/uploadedFiles/In_the_Community/Publications/HIV%20In%20Correctional%20Settings.pdf. Accessed April 7, 2011.

AVERT: AVERTing HIV and AIDS. "Prisons, Prisoners and HIV and AIDS." AVERT.org. Available online. URL: http://www.avert.org/prisons-hiv-aids.htm. Accessed April 7, 2011.

Bernard, K., et al. "Provider Perspectives about the Standards of HIV Care in Correctional Settings and Comparison to the Community Standard of Care: How Do We Measure Up?" IDCRonline.org. Available online. URL: http://www.idcronline.org/archives/march06/article.html. Accessed April 7, 2011.

Centers for Disease Control and Prevention. "HIV Transmission of Male Inmates in a State Prison System—Georgia, 1992–2005." *Morbidity and Mortality Weekly Report* 55, no. 15 (April 21, 2006): 421–426. Available online. URL: http://www.cdc.gov/mmwr/preview/mmwrhtml/mm5515a1.htm. Accessed April 7, 2011.

Cusac, Anne-Marie. "The Judge Gave Me Ten Years. He Didn't Sentence Me to Death." *Progressive* 64, no. 7 (July 2000): 22–27.

Grinstead, O. A., et al. "HIV, STD, and Hepatitis Risk to Primary Female Partners of Men Being Released from Prison." *Women & Health* 41, no. 2 (2005): 63–80.

Henry J. Kaiser Family Foundation. "Majority of Ex-Inmates in Texas Delay HIV Treatment, Study Finds." TheBody.com. Available online. URL: http://www.thebody.com/content/whatis/art50655.html. Accessed April 7, 2011.

Kantor, Elizabeth, M.D. "HIV Transmission and Prevention in Prisons." HIVInSite.org. April 2006. Available online. URL: http://hivinsite.ucsf.edu/InSite?page=kb-07-04-13. Accessed April 7, 2011.

Restrum, Z. G. "Public Health Implications of Substandard Correctional Health Care." *American Journal of Public Health* 95, no. 10 (October 2005): 1689–1691.

Strawn, Catherine. "Condoms Are a Rarity in U.S. Prisons." TheFrisky.com. Available online. URL: http://www.thefrisky.com/post/246-condoms-are-a-rarity-in-us-prisons/. Accessed April 7, 2011.

Sylla, Mary. "HIV Treatment in U.S. Jails and Prisons." TheBody.com. Available online. URL: http://www.thebody.com/content/art46432.html. Accessed April 7, 2011.

UNAIDS: Joint United Nations Programme on HIV/AIDS. "ICASA 2008: HIV in Prison Settings." UNAIDS.org. Available online. URL: http://www.unaids.org/en/KnowledgeCentre/Resources/FeatureStories/archive/2008/20081205_prisonsettings.asp. Accessed April 7, 2011.

United States Bureau of Justice Statistics. *HIV in Prisons, 2007–08*. Available online. URL: http://bjs.ojp.usdoj.gov/content/pub/pdf/hivp08.pdf. Accessed April 7, 2011.

United States Federal Bureau of Prisons. "Management of HIV: Federal Bureau of Prisons Clinical Practice Guidelines." BOP.gov. Available online. URL: http://www.bop.gov/news/PDFs/hiv.pdf. Accessed April 7, 2011.

progressive multifocal leukoencephalopathy (PML) Progressive multifocal leukoencephalopathy, or PML, is one of the fast-progressing OPPORTUNISTIC INFECTIONS (OIs) of the central nervous system (CNS). PML is caused by the JC virus, a polyomavirus named for the initials of the first patient diagnosed with the virus. The JC virus is distributed worldwide and is seen in approximately 85 percent of the world's population. People are generally infected as CHILDREN, and the virus seems to cause no illness unless it is reactivated at a point later in life. JC virus antibodies can be detected in healthy individuals' urine as well as tonsils. PML is the only disease associated with the JC virus at this time and is seen only in people who have severely compromised immune systems as a result of either ORGAN TRANSPLANTATION, HIV illness, or other immune system illnesses. It is known to be more common in HIV patients than in other immune-compromised individuals, though it is not understood why.

Symptoms and Diagnostic Path

PML is a demyelinating disease, meaning it causes the myelin, the protective layer of cells surrounding the neurons, to deteriorate. This in turn causes the signals that travel between neurons to stop functioning properly, causing impairment in movement, sensation, vision, thinking, or other activities, depending on which neurons may be involved. PML describes the action of the illness. It is progressive, usually quick, and people often die within one to six months after symptoms begin. It is multifocal, meaning it is seen in several areas of the brain. Leukoencephalopathy means that it affects the white matter (leuko) of the brain (encephalo), causing damage (pathy).

Initial symptoms can be vision changes, loss of hand coordination, clumsiness in walking, loss of memory, trouble in speaking, or problems in understanding what others say. The symptoms often appear quickly and progress steadily and rapidly. What starts as numbness in one leg can often progress to paralysis in a period of a couple of weeks. The JC virus becomes reactivated at some point in HIV illness, which is not well understood. At that point, lesions can appear in the brain in one or more locations; the resulting physical symptoms vary according to the location of the lesion(s).

Diagnosis is generally based on an examination by a doctor along with imaging of the brain. Other encephalopathies such as VZV infection or TOXOPLASMOSIS may initially be suspected; the imaging results for PML lesions are different in appearance, and the symptoms, though progressive, are slower than in an infection with either of those viruses. Another test that may be used for diagnosis is a spinal tap, which tests for JC viral load presence in the spinal fluid. Urinalysis can also show the presence of active JC virus;

however, this may not be helpful, as JC virus can be active in people who do not have PML.

If results of these tests are negative and PML involvement is still suspected, then a brain biopsy may be done to show JC virus activity in the visible lesions. A brain biopsy is the one sure way to diagnose PML, though many physicians or patients do not opt for this test as it can cause unneeded pain and is seen as too invasive. The biopsy will be able to rule out other possible infections and illnesses that may be causing the symptoms.

Most PML cases occur in those who have CD4 T lymphocyte counts below 100. Although PML is known to occur in patients with higher CD4 counts, it is unusual.

Treatment Options and Outlook

There is no approved treatment for PML. Prior to the advent of HIGHLY ACTIVE ANTIRETROVIRAL THERAPY (HAART), numerous drugs were tried unsuccessfully to stem the infection, but the progressive nature of the illness was nearly impossible to halt. Although one medication, cytarabine, a cancer chemotherapy, had been used in the belief that it inhibited the JC virus in vitro, subsequent studies have shown that cytarabine had no effect on JC viral load or long-term survival. It is no longer used to treat PML, as the drug has several serious side effects. Cidofovir was another drug that initially was believed to work against PML by preventing JC virus replication, but studies have again shown no difference in the outcome of patients treated with the drug. Other medications are being tested in studies for use with PML, but no current medications are known to be effective.

With the advent of HAART, changes in the nature of PML became apparent. Prior to HAART, 90 percent of PML patients died within the first six months. After HAART, patients began living longer, and more than 50 percent of patients showed an arrest of symptoms, meaning the infection was effectively stopped. Damage to the CNS functions did not reverse itself in all cases, but the progressive nature of the disease was stopped through the improvement in the immune system, allowing the immune system to fight the JC virus itself and preventing further deterioration. PML patients continue to have neurological problems after the illness has been actively stopped with HAART, although some have had some restoration of functions that had been previously lost to the illness.

IMMUNE RECONSTITUTION INFLAMMATORY SYNDROME (IRIS) is recognized as a side effect in some people who begin HAART. PML is one of the diseases that can go undiagnosed prior to a person's receiving HAART for the first time and become visibly activated when the person's immune system begins to function again. In cases of IRIS-induced PML, imaging can show inflammation and edema (abnormal fluid accumulation) around the sites of lesions. Some recommendations from studies suggest treatment with anti-inflammatory medications may help this condition, although there have been no definitive studies done at this time. Awareness of active JC virus prior to treatment with HAART can alert the patient and doctor to possible concerns as a patient begins HAART treatment for the first time.

Risk Factors and Preventive Measures

JC virus is seen worldwide and infects 85 percent of the population by the late teens; it is nearly impossible to avoid contact with this virus. What little is known about the virus is that it remains latent in the body, probably in the kidneys, until a person's immune system has weakened and the virus begins reproduction, generally in the CNS. Despite the widespread distribution of the virus and the immune system weakening, approximately 4 percent of HIV-positive people had PML prior to the HAART era. There has been no research into what causes some people and not others to be affected by the virus. As there is no certain remedy other than immune system health, the best way to prevent PML is to maintain a functioning immune system through the use of HAART.

Although there have been no studies to confirm observations, it is generally believed that once a patient's immune system has been restored to a functional level, PML does not recur. Remission seems to be maintained with HAART.

The Body. "Progressive Multifocal Leukoencephalopathy (PML) Fact Sheet." TheBody.com. Available online. URL: http://www.thebody.com/content/art 5041.html. Accessed April 7, 2011.

Jacewicz, Michael. "Progressive Multifocal Leukoencephalopathy (PML)." Merck.com. Available online. URL: http://www.merck.com/mmpe/sec16/ch217/ ch217f.html. Accessed April 7, 2011.

National Institute of Neurological Disorders and Stroke. "Progressive Multifocal Leukoencephalopathy Information Page." NIH.gov. Available online. URL: http://www.ninds.nih.gov/disorders/pml/pml.htm. Accessed April 7, 2011.

Simpson, David M. "PML, Despite Long-Term Virologic Suppression and High CD4 Count." Medscape.com. Available online. URL: http://www.medscape.com/ viewarticle/510060. Accessed April 7, 2011.

Singh, Niranjan N., M.D. "HIV-1 Associated Opportunistic Infections: PML." Medscape.com. Available online. URL: http://emedicine.medscape.com/ article/1167145-overview. Accessed April 7, 2011.

protease inhibitors (PIs)   Protease is an enzyme used in the reproduction of HIV. The protease functions as a cutting enzyme. Once the deoxyribonucleic acid (DNA) from the virus has infected the cell genetic structure, the cell begins making new copies of the virus ribonucleic acid (RNA). Protease is used to cut up the new virus RNA and make the particles that will leave the cell and infect other cells. The protease inhibitor works to block this chopping from happening or causes the chopping to make useless HIV particles that cannot infect other cells. PIs stop the virus from reproducing after it has infected the cell.

PIs are always used in conjunction with other medications. When PIs first came on the market, they were used in a three-drug combination, usually with one of two NUCLEOSIDE REVERSE TRANSCRIPTASE INHIBITORS (NRTIs). It was the first time that medications had been able to alter the survival of HIV-positive patients dramatically. Today, HIGHLY ACTIVE ANTIRETROVIRAL THERAPY (HAART) combinations can include one or two PIs in addition to other antiretroviral medications. Blocking the HIV reproduction in several different areas has proven very beneficial to patients' survival and the elimination of active virus from the body.

PIs currently available for use in the treatment of HIV include AMPRENAVIR, INDINAVIR, TIPRANAVIR, SAQUINAVIR, lopinavir, FOSAMPRENAVIR, ritonavir, NELFINAVIR, DARUNAVIR, and ATAZANAVIR SULFATE. A number of PIs are currently being tested but are not yet available for general use. There are several potential side effects from the use of PIs, including diarrhea, nausea, and redistribution of fat in the body. These side effects are detailed in the information for each individual drug.

AIDSmeds. "Protease Inhibitors (PIs)," AIDSmeds. com. Available online. URL: http://www.aidsmeds. com/archive/PIs_1068.shtml. Accessed April 7, 2011.

AIDS Treatment Data Network. "What Are Protease Inhibitors?" AEGIS.com. Available online. URL: http://www.aegis.com/factshts/network/simple/ protease.html. Accessed April 7, 2011.

Sullivan, Jim. "HIV Infection: Protease and Protease Inhibitors." CellsAlive.com. Available online. URL: http://www.cellsalive.com/hiv4.htm. Accessed April 7, 2011.

raltegravir Raltegravir is an INTEGRASE INHIBI-TOR drug used in combination with other medications in the treatment of HIV. It is manufactured by Merck and Company and was approved by the U.S. FOOD AND DRUG ADMINISTRATION (FDA) in late 2007. It was approved solely for use in highly treatment-experienced individuals. Raltegravir received accelerated approval from the FDA because of the high success rate the drug showed in decreasing viral load in highly-experienced patients during a phase II drug study. It is sold under the trade name Isentress and is abbreviated as RAL. The drug is the first integrase inhibitor approved by the FDA, and in early 2009 was given general approval for use in all treatment-experienced HIV-positive patients.

Raltegravir is still a very new drug. It works in a different way than other anti-HIV medications, and so far has shown few serious drug interactions and few side effects. It is not yet approved for treatment-naïve patients, those HIV-positive people who have not yet used antiretroviral medication. Long-term effects of the drug are not yet known, but short-term side effects have been much less significant than those of some other forms of anti-HIV medication. Raltegravir has not yet been studied in pregnant women or CHILDREN.

Dosage

Raltegravir is sold as a 400 mg tablet. One tablet is taken twice a day, with or without food.

Drug Interactions

Raltegravir does show some interactions with other HIV medications. When it is combined with tiranavir and ritonavir in a multidrug combination, levels of raltegravir in the blood were decreased, but no loss of effectiveness was seen, so no dosing changes have been recommended. When it was combined with ATAZANAVIR SULFATE and ritonavir, an increase in the level of raltegravir was seen. This did not seem to increase any side effects; again, dosing changes have not been recommended at this time.

Raltegravir interacts with the TUBERCULOSIS (TB) medication rifampin, as the body processes both in the same manner. A significant decrease in the amount of raltegravir was seen in studies in which both drugs were administered. Recent information suggests doubling the dosage of raltegravir to two 400 mg tablets twice a day if rifampin is also being taken.

Side Effects

Side effects in the studies have so far been minimal. Some side effects experienced include nausea, fever, diarrhea, headache, and dizziness. Some reports of depression have been seen in patients since accelerated approval was given.

Elevated levels of a muscle enzyme, creatine kinase, were seen in some patients using raltegravir. Someone taking raltegravir should report any unexplained muscle aches, pains, or weakness to the doctor.

Elevated liver enzyme levels on blood tests were seen in some patients, particularly those who were infected with HEPATITIS B and HEPATITIS C.

AIDS InfoNet. "Atazanavir (Reyataz)." AIDSInfoNet. org. Available online. URL: http://www.aidsinfo net.org/fact_sheets/view/471. Accessed March 11, 2011.

AIDSmeds. "Isentress (Raltegravir)." AIDSmeds.com. Available online. URL: http://www.aidsmeds.com/archive/Isentress_1639.shtml. Accessed March 11, 2011.

———. "Special Issues for Children with HIV." AIDS meds.com. Available online. URL: http://www.aids meds.com/articles/Children_7566.shtml. Accessed March 11, 2011.

The Body. "Isentress (Raltegravir)." TheBody.com. Available online. URL: http://www.thebody.com/index/treat/mk0518.html. Accessed March 11, 2011.

United States Department of Health and Human Services. "Atazanavir." aidsinfo.nih.gov. Available online. URL: http://www.aidsinfo.nih.gov/DrugsNew/Drug DetailNT.aspx?int_id=420. Accessed March 11, 2011.

resistance   Resistance in HIV discussions refers to the ability of the virus to resist treatment with antiretroviral medications. Over time, the virus can develop resistance to one or more of the drugs that are available to treat and control HIV. This can, at times, require a person to switch antiretrovirals in order to maintain suppression of the virus.

Drug resistance occurs because HIV reproduces itself continuously, millions of times a day. HIV does not contain the proper proteins in its structure necessary to make exactly the same copies of itself as it reproduces. Most of these random mutations are not harmful, and the new type of virus dies because it does not have the same abilities to infect as the original virus. However, there are mutations that can allow the virus to continue to infect cells and counteract the drugs that generally stop this. When a person develops drug resistance, it means that one of these mutations has been created that can overcome the drug's ability to stop the virus. Most of the virus that a person's body creates will continue to be the standard variety of HIV, and the drugs will continue to stop that virus, but as the mutated virus reproduces, more of it will become available to infect more cells and eventually will represent the majority of the virus a person is carrying. The original, or wild-type, virus, as it is called, does not disappear; it is just not reproducing at the same level as the mutated virus.

It is important that a person who begins taking antiretroviral drugs follow the directions provided by the doctor or pharmacist who prescribes them. Adherence to a schedule allows the drugs to work together properly to fight the virus. Because the virus reproduces millions of copies a day, experts stress adherence to a regular schedule of taking the drugs to keep the virus under control as much as possible. The antiretrovirals work against the wild-type virus, and if taken properly, keep the viral load extremely low. If adherence to taking the drugs is not consistent or if a person stops taking one or more of the drugs for another reason such as side effects, the virus has the opportunity to reproduce itself, and the opportunity for mutations to the wild-type virus increases. The standard antiretroviral treatment a person is using contains at least three different drugs from at least two different classes of antiretrovirals. This is because treatment early in the epidemic showed doctors that HIV could overcome antiretroviral treatment if only one drug or one class of drug were used. The virus could overcome such treatment by mutation. With three drugs and at least two different drug types, it is much more difficult for the virus to mutate and become resistant to treatment.

In addition to adherence, other factors can play a role in resistance. Absorption of the drug into the body is important in maintaining the right amount of the drug to fight the virus. Some drugs have special requirements regarding times when they can be taken. Some drugs require that food be eaten with the drug to help the body absorb the drug. Other antiretrovirals require that no food be taken at the same time or for some time after ingesting the drug. Diarrhea or vomiting can possibly cause the drug to be poorly absorbed. Some drugs require that they be combined with a second or third drug as part of the combination therapy. All of these factors can cause poor absorption of the antiretrovirals if a patient does not understand them. Many drugs interact with each other, causing changes in the amount of drug absorbed by the body. Some foods can cause changes in the absorption of a drug. Grapefruit juice, for instance, can interfere with the action of some antiretrovirals (INDINAVIR and SAQUINAVIR) in the body and thereby increase the chance that the virus will mutate and bring about resistance to the drug.

When resistance does occur, the first step in treatment is to see what type of resistance has developed. The virus is capable of becoming resistant to any of the antiretrovirals, though it is extremely unusual for the virus suddenly to become resistant to all of the drugs a person is taking. A doctor will order resistance testing, which is a series of tests on a person's blood to determine what mutation has occurred, what medication may need to be stopped or changed, and what combination of medications will work best to treat an individual's virus. Often a person will undergo resistance testing before any treatment is started a first time to see whether the virus he or she has is already resistant to some medications. The tests used to check for resistant virus are phenotype and genotype assays. Results for a genotype assay will take approximately two weeks and is the first test a doctor may use to determine the type of virus a person has and what drugs may not be effective. The second test, the phenotype assay, will take longer to produce results; approximately one month is normal. This test allows for more specific analysis of the virus and can be very helpful in allowing a doctor to understand which drugs are working and which ones are not, as well as what resistance patterns exist in the virus. Genotypic testing examines the genetic makeup of the virus, while phenotypic tests measure the behavior of the virus in relation to particular antiretrovirals.

A person can become infected with a virus that is already resistant to a particular drug or drugs. This can occur if he or she contracts the virus from a person who has developed such resistance. An example would be developing a virus resistant to ZIDOVUDINE (AZT), the first antiretroviral used in the treatment of HIV. Many people have taken AZT, and it was often prescribed as a single drug because it was the only drug known to work against HIV. If a person who has AZT-resistant virus has unprotected sex or shares a needle and infects someone else with HIV, it is possible that that individual will develop a virus that is AZT resistant. Researchers believe that 5–20 percent of new HIV infections spread are resistant to a drug or class of drugs.

It is possible that a person who has developed a virus resistant to one drug may be resistant to several drugs or a particular drug class. NON-NUCLEOSIDE REVERSE TRANSCRIPTASE INHIBITORS (NNRTIs) work against a specific process in the reproduction of the virus. Studies have shown that a virus can develop resistance against one NNRTI, and that resistance marker on the virus genome can cause resistance to more than one NNRTI. People who develop a virus resistant to EFAVIRENZ will, in most cases, also have a virus that is resistant to treatment with NEVIRAPINE and DELAVIRDINE. The genotype and phenotype assays will show which resistance patterns the virus has and what drugs will continue to work against it.

In 2005, several news stories highlighted a so-called HIV supervirus that was resistant to many of the drugs then available and had developed quickly into AIDS in a patient in New York City. However, afterward it became clear that this individual had simply acquired a virus resistant to some drugs and had not developed AIDS quickly, but had simply been examined while the virus was active during the initial infection. Multidrug-resistant strains of HIV can be spread between two people, but as of 2011, a superstrain had not been proven to exist. Researchers do refer to what they call superinfection, which is infection from more than one strain or subtype of HIV, but research into this effect is limited, as few cases are known positively to exist. It is also unclear whether reinfection with HIV can take place only within a limited time frame at the beginning of infection or whether it is possible to be reinfected beyond that. Analysis of known multi-infected people has shown that their reinfection occurred within three years of their first infection, and not after that point. Animal studies seem also to reflect that reinfection is possible early but not later beyond that time frame.

Some research has been done with HIV-positive male couples who do not use condoms. This study concluded that none of the couples had infected each other with new or resistant strains of the virus. They also found that these men who had been repeatedly exposed to the virus over time had a stronger T-cell response to the virus than men who had not been repeatedly exposed to HIV. This study is important in that there is a subculture of men engaged in sero-sorting, choosing to have unprotected sex but only with other men of the same HIV serosta-tus, meaning HIV-positive men will only have intercourse with other HIV-positive men, or HIV-negative men will only engage in intercourse with other HIV-negative men. The study did not rule out superinfection possibilities among men who engage in serosorting but did note the immune system response may be studied further for possible findings about continued exposure and superinfection.

AIDSmeds. "Understanding Drug Resistance." AIDS meds.com. Available online. URL: http://www.aids meds.com/articles/Resistance_7509.shtml. Accessed April 7, 2011.

AIDS Treatment Data Network. "Understanding Drug Resistance." AEGIS.com. Available online. URL: http://ww2.aegis.org/factshts/network/simple/resistance.html. Accessed April 7, 2011.

The Body. "A Guide to HIV Drug Resistance." The Body.com. Available online. URL: http://www.the body.com/content/art46018.html. Accessed April 7, 2011.

———. "HIV/AIDS Drug Resistance." TheBody.com. Available online. URL: http://www.thebody.com/index/treat/resistance.html. Accessed April 7, 2011.

Center for AIDS Information and Advocacy. "HIV Super Strain Revisited." *HIV Treatment Alerts,* (June 2007), 10–11. Available online. URL: http://www.centerfo raids.org/pdfs/alerts0607.pdf. Accessed April 7, 2011.

Cheonis, Nicholas. "Dual HIV Infection." TheBody. com. Available online. URL: http://www.thebody. com/content/treat/art2513.html. Accessed April 7, 2011.

Clavel, Francois, M.D., and Allan J. Hance, M.D. "HIV Drug Resistance." *New England Journal of Medicine* 350, no. 10 (4 March 2004): 1023–1035.

Shafer, Robert M., M.D., et al. "HIV Drug Resistance Database." Stanford.edu. Available online. URL: http://hivdb.stanford.edu/. Accessed April 7, 2011.

UCSF Center for HIV Information. "Database of Antiretroviral Drug Interactions." HIVInSite.ucsf. edu. Available online. URL: http://hivinsite.ucsf. edu/insite?page=ar-00-02&post=10&param=13. Accessed April 7, 2011.

Willberg, Christian B., et al. "Immunity to HIV-1 Is Influenced by Continued Natural Exposure to Exogenous Virus." *PLoS Pathogens* (October 2008). Available online. URL: http://www.plospathogens. org/article/info%3Adoi%2F10.1371%2Fjournal. ppat.1000185;jsessionid=4F9DE2ACF1800805CEC 872C5F67D9A18. Accessed April 8, 2011.

World Health Organization. "HIV Drug Resistance." WHO.int. Available online. URL: http://www.who. int/hiv/topics/drugresistance/en/index.html. Accessed April 7, 2011.

retrovirus A retrovirus is a virus that contains ribonucleic acid (RNA) as its genetic material, as opposed to most other viruses, which use deoxy-ribonucleic acid (DNA) to transmit genetic information. As all viruses do, a retrovirus makes copies of itself by inserting itself into a host's cells and then using the host's cells' genetic material to reproduce itself. A retrovirus is different in that it uses a particular enzyme known as reverse transcriptase to change its RNA into DNA once inside the host cell. Then the retrovirus inserts its DNA into the host cell's DNA, where it becomes part of the cell's reproductive mechanism. When the cell reproduces, so does the virus. The virus DNA is reproduced, and the various bits of virus DNA are reassembled to form new viral particles that go on to infect other cells.

The HUMAN IMMUNODEFICIENCY VIRUS (HIV) is a retrovirus. It predominantly infects human T cells and uses the reverse transcriptase enzyme to become part of the human host's body. RNA does not go through the type of self-check or proofreading system that DNA does. RNA is also more reactive chemically. Because of the lack of proofreading in RNA, and its higher reactivity, retroviruses are much more prone to mutation than other viruses. A mutation is a change, however minor, in the genome of any living organism. Retroviruses change all the time because of this manner of replication. This is why it is difficult to develop a vaccine for HIV or to treat a person with the same medication indefinitely, as the virus is able to mutate and become immune to the particular medication being used against it.

Including HIV, the confirmed retroviruses that affect humans currently number four distinct viruses. Human T-cell lymphotrophic virus 1 causes lymphomas and leukemia; human T-cell lymphotrophic virus 2 causes nerve problems leading to a spasming weakness in the feet and legs. HIV 1 and HIV 2 both cause loss of function in the HUMAN IMMUNE SYSTEM. Some recent work has claimed to show a fifth human retrovirus named XMRV, which scientists may have implicated in some prostate cancers.

In recent studies, it has been shown that the human genome contains numerous places where over many millennia retroviruses have inserted themselves into the DNA and remained, handed down from one person to his or her offspring. Retroviruses all have the reverse transcriptase enzyme in order to reproduce. Stopping this enzyme from working is the basis of several of the most successful antiretroviral medications. These medications are known as reverse transcriptase inhibitors.

Bio-Medicine.org. "Retrovirus." Bio-medicine.org. Available online. URL: http://www.bio-medicine.org/biology-definition/Retrovirus/. Accessed April 7, 2011.

Dartmouth Medical School. "Retroviruses." Epidemic.org. Available online. URL: http://www.epidemic.org/theFacts/viruses/retroviruses/. Accessed April 7, 2011.

Lerner, Brenda Wilmouth, and K. Lee Lerner, eds. *Infectious Diseases in Context.* Detroit: Thomson-Gale, 2008.

Science Daily. "Defensive Protein Killed Ancient Primate Retroviruses, Research Suggests." Science Daily.com. Available online. URL: http://www.sciencedaily.com/releases/2008/12/081227223102.htm. Accessed April 7, 2011.

———. "Links between XMRV and Human Disease Studied." ScienceDaily.com Available online. URL: http://www.sciencedaily.com/releases/2010/10/101012151246.htm. Accessed April 7, 2011.

rilpivirine Rilpivirine is a NON-NUCLEOSIDE REVERSE TRANSCRIPTASE INHIBITOR (NNRTI) that was approved for use in the United States in May 2011. It is the newest antiretroviral drug available for the treatment of HIV and the first approved in more than three years. It is manufactured by Tibotec Therapeutics, a division of Johnson & Johnson, and is sold under the trade name Edurant. It was known as TMC278 during experimental trials and testing.

Dosage

Rilpivirine is a 25 mg pill. It is taken once a day and must be taken with food. Rilpivirine is part of a multidrug regimen to combat HIV that includes at least two other drugs. The drug is approved only for people who are starting HIV therapy for the first time. Rilpivirine does not work as well against HIV if a person's viral load is above 100,000 copies per milliliter of blood.

Drug interactions

Rilpivirine is processed by the liver, like many medications used to treat HIV; therefore, it can interact with a number of other medications, causing the amount of rilpivirine in the body to be raised or lowered, depending on the interaction. For these reasons, rilpivirine should not be part of the same HIGHLY ACTIVE ANTIRETROVIRAL THERAPY (HAART) that already contains other NNRTIs.

PROTEASE INHIBITORS (PIs) can increase the level of rilpivirine in the blood. At this time, no recommendations have been made to adjust the dosage of rilpivirine because of this interaction. Rilpivirine is not known to increase or decrease the amount of PIs in the blood.

Some antibiotics can increase levels of rilpivirine. Clarithromycin and erythromycin are two common antibiotics that can cause this reaction. Use of other antibiotics is recommended when taking rilpivirine.

Methadone levels may decrease when using rilpivirine. People who are taking this medication may need to increase the dosage of methadone to maintain its effectiveness.

Antacids and acid reflux medications such as Tums, Pepto-Bismol, ranitidine, cimetidine, and nizatidine can all interfere with the absorption of rilpivirine into the blood. People taking these medications should be aware of possible complications. It is recommended that people take antacids and acid blockers 12 hours before or four hours after they take rilpivirine.

Anti-seizure medications may also cause dangerous interactions when used with rilpivirine.

Side Effects

In pre-approval drug studies, rilpivirine caused an increase in depression and mood changes among people taking the drug. Patients who have had issues with depression and sadness may not be the best candidates to take rilpivirine. Notify a doctor if mood changes occur after beginning rilpivirine.

People taking NNRTIs have reported issues with LIPODYSTROPHY, so it is possible that long-term use of rilpivirine may cause body fat changes in patients.

It is unknown at this time what effects rilpivirine may have on pregnant or nursing women or their babies. A doctor should discuss whether a woman is pregnant or nursing prior to prescribing rilpivirine.

Typical side effects found during clinical trials of rilpivirine include headache, rash, and insomnia.

AIDS InfoNet. "Rilpivirine (Edurant)." AIDSInfoNet. org. Available online. URL: http://www.aidsinfonet. org/fact_sheets/view/435. Accessed July 24, 2011.

AIDSmeds. "Edurant (rilpivirine, RPV, TMC-278)." AIDS meds.com. Available online. URL: http://www.aids meds.com/archive/Edurant_1619.shtml. Accessed July 24, 2011.

Helfand, Myles. "Edurant (Rilpivirine): The HIV Treatment Dating Game Just Got More Interesting." TheBody.com. Available online. URL: http://www. thebody.com/content/art62223.html. Accessed July 28, 2011.

Smith, Michael. "FDA Okays New HIV Drug." Med pagetoday.com. Available online. URL: http://www. medpagetoday.com/HIVAIDS/HIVAIDS/26604. Accessed July 28, 2011.

United States Department of Health and Human Services. "Rilpivirine." aidsinfo.nih.gov. Available online. URL: http://www.aidsinfo.nih.gov/DrugsNew/Drug DetailT.aspx?int_id=426. Accessed July 24, 2011.

S

safer sex   *Safer sex* is the term used to describe sexual activities that can, if done properly, protect a person from infection with HIV and a number or other sexually transmitted infections (STIs). Safer sex is sex in which there are no mucous membrane contact and no bodily fluid exchanged between partners during the sexual activity. The term *safer sex* is used because sexual activities can never be 100 percent absolutely safe. The only truly safe sexual practices are celibacy (no sexual activity) and masturbation.

The best way to engage in sex and to prevent HIV infection, as well as other STIs, is to have only one sexual partner, who is know to be HIV negative. Testing negative together twice, over a six-month period, is generally thought to indicate safety if neither person has been involved with others during that time frame. A person can take anywhere from three weeks to six months to develop antibodies to HIV. The current HIV tests measure antibodies to the virus, and this is the reason for the guidelines that were developed to encourage partners to test twice during a six-month period. At that point, if both partners have tested negative twice and they know that they are only engaging in sexual activity with each other, then there is no risk of infection with HIV.

The use of protection during sexual activity is the best way to prevent contact with body fluids that may contain HIV or other STIs. Protection can vary, depending on what the activity is, but it always involves placing a barrier between people. In most cases, that barrier is a condom. Studies of serodiscordant couples, in which one person is HIV positive and the other HIV negative, have shown that condom use, when done correctly and consistently, is highly effective in preventing the spread of HIV. Proper condom use involves several simple rules to remember and employ during every sexual encounter. Always use a new condom for each act of intercourse. Place the condom on as soon as erection occurs, before any intercourse, anal or vaginal, takes place. When placing the condom on the erect penis, hold the tip of the condom and unroll the condom onto the length of the penis. This prevents air from being trapped inside the condom. Use only water-based lubricants with a latex condom. Such gels and glycerin-type lubricants can be found with condoms in most pharmacies in the United States. Oil-based lubricants such as petroleum jelly, baby oil, hand lotions, or cold creams cause a breakdown of the latex in the condom and cause it to break. After ejaculation, hold the condom at the base and withdraw the penis from the sexual partner, ensuring the condom does not slip off. Never use two condoms at once. Double-bagging, as this act is known in slang terms, actually encourages breakage of the condoms as a result of friction of the latex during sexual intercourse.

There are different types of condoms, and the most researched type of condom is the latex condom. Lambskin, or natural, condoms are made from the intestinal lining of sheep. These condoms are effective in preventing pregnancy but have not been shown to be effective in preventing the spread of HIV or other STIs. Polyurethane condoms have been shown to be effective at preventing the spread of HIV and are an alternative to latex condoms if a person is allergic to latex. Latex allergies can be dangerous, and polyurethane is a safe replacement for latex in a number of medical products including condoms. Polyurethane also does not break down when used with oil-based lubricants and may be a better choice for some people for this reason.

In addition to male condoms, there are products called female condoms as well. The female condom is made of polyurethane and resembles a large sheath with two polyurethane rings, one at each end. The end of the device is inserted into the vaginal canal and the ring ensures that the ejaculate is collected in the end of the condom. The other ring remains outside the vagina and the penis is inserted into this end of the condom. It is not safe to use the female condom at the same time that a couple is using a male condom. The two sheaths rubbing against each other can cause friction and possibly tear one or both of the condoms, thereby making them ineffective. Water- or oil-based lubricants can be used with the polyurethane female condom. The original female condom was significantly more expensive than male condoms and this may be a deterrent for its use for some people. In March 2009, the U.S. Food and Drug Administration (FDA) approved a new version of the female condom, which is made with a different material and has been shown to be as effective as the first version of the condom as well as being 30 percent less expensive. The new condom can safely be used with water-based as well as oil-based lubricants.

Another barrier that can be used during sexual activity is called a dental dam. Originally used by dentists, this is a small square sheet of latex or polyurethane. A dental dam is used during oral-vaginal sex or oral-anal sex by people who wish to block direct contact with potential body fluids that may contain HIV. The dental dam creates a barrier between the mouth and the vagina or anus. Plastic wrap used to protect food in the refrigerator can also be used for the same purpose and has been found to be equally protective in maintaining a barrier between two people during these sexual activities.

Some HIV educators and medical specialists believe that people can make better decisions about sexual practices based on knowing the levels of risk of TRANSMISSION of HIV involved with various sexual activities.

Any sexual activity has the potential to transmit HIV or other STDs if the people involved do not know that they are infected. Regular testing for HIV and other STDs is effective in reducing the spread of illness in sexually active people. Knowledge of HIV status is important to share with sexual partners, as it allows those people to make decisions about risk reduction during sexual activity. The best decision is to be consistent in following safer sex guidelines that combine precautions based on what is known to be true and what seems reasonable in terms of the knowledge of the virus at this time.

AIDS.org. "Safer Sex Guidelines." AIDS.org. Available online. URL: http://www.aids.org/factSheets/151 -Safer-Sex-Guidelines.html. Accessed April 7, 2011.

The Body. "Fact Sheet: The Truth about Condoms." TheBody.com. Available online. URL: http://www. thebody.com/content/prev/art2436.html. Accessed April 7, 2011.

———. "Frequently Asked Questions (II)." TheBody. com. Available online. URL: http://www.thebody. com/content/art2309.html#wait. Accessed July 24, 2011.

Centers for Disease Control and Prevention. "Antiretroviral Postexposure Prophylaxis after Sexual, Injection-Drug Use, or Other Nonoccupational Exposure to HIV in the United States: Recommendations from the U.S. Department of Health and Human Services." CDC.gov. Available online. URL: http://www.cdc.gov/mmwr/preview/mmwrhtml/ rr5402a1.htm#tab1. Accessed April 7, 2011.

Citizen News Service. "Lower Cost Female Condom Gets FDA Approval." ThaIndian.com. Available online. URL: http://www.thaindian.com/newsportal/health 1/lower-cost-female-condom-gets-fda-approval _10 0166845.html. Accessed April 11, 2011.

Coalition for Positive Sexuality. "Just Say Yes: Safe Sex." Positive.org. Available online. URL: http://www. positive.org/JustSayYes/safesex.html. Accessed April 7, 2011.

Lane, Tim, and Herminia Palacio. "Safer-Sex Methods." HIVInSite.UCSF.edu. Available online. URL: http://hivinsite.ucsf.edu/InSite?page=kb-07-02-02#S3X. Accessed April 7, 2011.

MedlinePlus. "Safe Sex." NIH.gov. Available online. URL: http://www.nlm.nih.gov/medlineplus/ency/article/001949.htm. Accessed April 7, 2011.

saquinavir   Saquinavir is a PROTEASE INHIBITOR (PI) that was initially approved by the U.S. FOOD AND DRUG ADMINISTRATION (FDA) in 1995. Manufactured by Hoffman-Laroche, it was the first PI approved for the treatment of HIV. It is always prescribed as part of a multidrug treatment. It is currently sold under the trade name Invirase and is abbreviated as SQV.

The current formulation of the drug is chemically known as saquinavir mesylate, though most people simply call it saquinavir. This is a slightly different form of the medication than was originally formulated and used for many years as the preferred form of the drug. That drug was marketed under the name Fortovase. Although no longer available in the United States, Fortovase is still available in other countries. Fortovase requires more pills and larger dosages than Invirase, the current formulation of the drug sold in the United States, and therefore it was used less by patients and doctors and was eventually discontinued, in 2006.

Dosage

Saquinavir mesylate should always be taken with or immediately after a full meal. It is particularly effective when combined with a high-fat meal. Invirase is always prescribed along with ritonavir.

Invirase is available in 500 mg tablets or 200 mg gel capsules. The recommended dose is 1,000 mg taken with 100 mg of ritonavir twice a day. This translates to either two 500 mg tablets and one ritonavir capsule twice a day or five 200 mg capsules of Invirase and one ritonavir capsule twice a day. Dosing for Fortovase is 1,200 mg three times a day, which involves six 200 mg capsules three times a day. It was also prescribed at times with ritonavir at 1,000 mg two times a day. That equals five 200 mg capsules of Fortovase plus one 100 mg capsule of ritonavir twice a day.

Drug Interactions

Invirase is broken down by the body in the liver. This means that it can potentially interact with the metabolism of other drugs by the body. Some drugs will raise or lower the amount of Invirase in the body. Concentrations of other medications may be raised or lowered by their interactions with Invirase. Two NON-NUCLEOSIDE REVERSE TRANSCRIPTASE INHIBITORS (NNRTIs) that are known to decrease the amount of saquinavir are NEVIRAPINE and EFAVIRENZ. It is recommended that the PI TIPRANAVIR not be prescribed with saquinavir because of this same decrease in availability.

DIDANOSINE, an NNRTI, and INDINAVIR and NELFINAVIR, two PIs, all increase the amount of saquinavir in the body. No change in the dosage has been recommended.

Rifabutin and rifambin are two commonly used antibiotics that interact poorly with saquinavir. It is recommended that they not be used as they lower the amount of saquinavir significantly. A significant increase in transanimase levels during liver function testing has also been noted. Liver function returned to normal after discontinuation of the drugs. This combination may affect the ability to treat HIV and build resistance to saquinavir as well as other drugs in the protease inhibitor class of antiretrovirals, as well as harm the liver over the course of treatment.

Saquinavir interacts with a number of other medications including the cholesterol-lowering drugs simvastatin and lovastatin, antibiotics used to treat infections such as TUBERCULOSIS, antidepressant or antipsychotic medications, and medications for some fungal infections. It should not be taken with any drugs containing ergot, which is used in many migraine medications. It is important that a doctor know and understand all the medications and supplements a patient uses when prescribing saquinavir.

Methadone levels in the body decrease substantially while a person is taking saquinavir. People who use methadone for the treatment of opiate addiction should have dosages adjusted and monitored by a doctor.

St. John's wort, an herbal supplement, should never be taken with a PI, as it has been shown to reduce significantly the amount of PI in the body. Other supplements that may affect the level of saquinavir in the body include garlic pills and milk thistle. Saquinavir also increases the amount of the drugs sildenafil (Viagra), vardenafil (Levitra), and tadalafil (Cialis)—all erectile dysfunction medications—in the blood and thus can cause serious side effects. Lowering the dosage of these medications is recommended to prevent potential complications.

Grapefruit juice significantly increases levels of saquinavir in the body, thereby increasing the side effects of the drug. One should avoid consumption of grapefruit juice while using saquinavir formulations.

Side Effects

Saquinavir may cause some mild feelings of nausea, tiredness, headache, vomiting, and diarrhea. These are considered short-term effects and may disappear after the drug is used for a while. Other side effects reported include tingling feelings in the extremities (fingers, toes, lips), loss of taste, and loss of appetite.

The drug may cause an increase in bleeding in hemophiliac patients.

Protease inhibitors, as a class of drug, often increase the cholesterol and triglyceride levels of patients. High lipid levels have been recorded in some saquinavir patients. This side effect can be managed with appropriate cholesterol-lowering medications. Saquinavir has also been associated with treatment regimens that can cause LIPODYS-TROPHY, or the redistribution of fat within the body. Symptoms are increased fat around the neck and stomach area, facial wasting, breast enlargement, and peripheral wasting in the arms

and legs. Some of these changes appear when the drug is stopped.

Saquinavir may also increase the risk of worsening a person's diabetes or causing diabetes in people who were not diabetic prior to treatment.

AIDS InfoNet. "Saquinavir (Invirase)." AIDSInfoNet. org. Available online. URL: http://www.aidsinfo net.org/fact_sheets/view/443. Accessed March 11, 2011.

AIDSmeds. "Invirase (Saquinavir)." AIDSmeds.com. Available online. URL: http://www.aidsmeds.com/ archive/Invirase_1558.shtml. Accessed March 11, 2011.

———. "Special Issues for Children with HIV." AIDS meds.com. Available online. URL: http://www.aids meds.com/articles/Children_7566.shtml. Accessed March 11, 2011.

The Body. "Invirase (Saquinavir)." TheBody.com. Available online. URL: http://www.thebody.com/index/ treat/saquinavir.html. Accessed March 11, 2011.

United States Department of Health and Human Services. "Saquinavir Mesylate." aidsinfo.nih.gov. Available online. URL: http://www.aidsinfo.nih. gov/DrugsNew/DrugDetailNT.aspx?int_id=164. Accessed March 11, 2011.

sex workers A sex worker is someone who exchanges goods or money for sexual services. They are also known as prostitutes, porn actors, call girls/boys, gigolos, escorts, streetwalkers, and hookers. It is a profession that is generally discouraged by society, and it is illegal in most societies around the world. Many people view sex workers as being exploited by people or society in general, though often the sex workers themselves view their work as simply necessary or something they have chosen to perform. There is generally a distinction made between voluntary sex work and forced sex work, which is a form of sexual assault or, at times, imprisonment.

Sex workers represent a variety of people, from the extremely poor to the well off. Headlines in newspapers and online give an indication from time to time of the extent of sex work in the United States as politicians and famous individuals are occasionally reported to have visited or engaged in activities with sex workers. Sex workers represent all races and classes of people and serve all varieties of clients. Sex workers can be male, female, or transgender, and they can represent gay, straight, or bisexual orientations.

High HIV rates have been found among sex workers in many different countries. In nearly all countries, HIV rates are higher among sex workers than in the general population. Sex workers have, by nature of the business they are in, many different sexual partners in most cases. Large numbers of sex partners increase the opportunity both to become infected by the virus and to pass on the virus to other people. In many countries, those who practice injection drug use (IDU) (see INJECTION DRUG USE(R)) also are involved in sex work, often to support their drug use. Among many policy planners, the issue of whether it is IDU or sex work that drives the epidemic is a topic of frequent discussion.

In Russia, there is a high rate of HIV among sex workers. Some cities such as St. Petersburg and Irkutsk show rates of 20 percent or above according to the U.S. Agency for International Development. United Nations (UN) studies of these sex workers show that the majority became infected through IDU rather than sex work. Joint United Nations Programme on HIV/AIDS (UNAIDS) reports cite statistics showing that upward of 40 percent of sex workers are also IDUs in Russian cities. In Moscow, where sex work is more controlled and drug use is actively discouraged by sex workers, the HIV rate is only about 5 percent. UNAIDS reports from other parts of Europe show similarly low rates of HIV infection among sex workers. Sex work is more organized in WESTERN AND CENTRAL EUROPE and is legal in some of those countries. Rates of infection among sex workers who also use drugs are much higher than among sex workers who do not use drugs.

In AFRICA, many people turn to sex work to support themselves or their families. WOMEN in UN studies indicate they do not do sex work regularly, but many will do it as needed when food or money is in short supply. IDU is limited in Africa more than in other areas of the world, and sex work has driven the epidemic to a great degree there. When studies have been done, high rates of HIV have been shown among African sex workers. In sub-Saharan Africa, the average cited in the *AIDS Epidemic Update 2009* is 19 percent. UN studies show a rate of 0 percent in the Comoros and 49 percent in Guinea-Bissau. Local studies cited in the UN report show rates above 25 percent in Benin and Lesotho. A study of male sex workers conducted by the Population Council in Mombasa, Kenya, found that fewer than half used condoms. This is not uncommon among sex workers, as customers often do not have them nor want to use them, often paying more to the sex worker to forgo their use. Cost is an issue in condom use in many regions of the world.

In ASIA, sex work and drug use have led to large epidemics among populations in China, Kazakhstan, Indonesia, and Vietnam. Rates of HIV among sex workers who use drugs are significantly higher than among sex workers who do not use drugs. In Thailand, where sex work is more regulated, the government reacted quickly to HIV and began a campaign in 1992 to make sure that there was 100 percent use of condoms. Condom use increased from 14 percent of female sex workers in 1989 to more than 90 percent in 1994 according to UNAIDS studies. The government provided sex workers in brothels with free condoms, as well as education about how HIV spreads and proper use of condoms. Such successful programs have been seen in other Asian countries such as India and Cambodia, where prostitutes have been recruited to help run the programs. This sort of forward thinking has allowed the programs to reach into communities typically difficult to contact through government workers or others who might not understand or sympathize with the plight of women or men engaged in sex work.

Studies with male sex workers have been more difficult to conduct and less extensive than with female sex workers. In many places in the world, there is a denial of the existence of male sex workers; homosexual behavior is illegal in many places or highly taboo and not discussed. Although male sex work is known to occur, people do not want to volunteer that they participate in such activity and are often not reachable by people doing studies of their behavior or by people providing condoms or education. A study by Timpson and associates of male sex workers in Houston revealed that many of the men were bisexual, providing sexual services to both men and women for money or drugs. A study of similar male sex workers in Los Angeles by Gorbach and colleague revealed that many were homeless individuals who exchanged sex for drugs; again, many in the study reported providing sexual services for both men and women. Male sex workers are not limited to the United States. Some studies or news stories have been conducted with male sex workers in many countries, including very conservative nations such as Pakistan. One point that is fairly clear from the research is that male sex workers receive far less attention from governments and HIV education groups than female sex workers. The topic is avoided in many countries where the activity occurs, and people do not wish to risk acknowledging their work where it is illegal. Male sex workers are often left to their own initiative to educate themselves about HIV and other sexually transmitted illnesses.

One issue that concerns HIV educators and governments is the amount of sex trafficking being tracked among countries. In recent years, many WOMEN and CHILDREN have been sold or traded into sexual slavery. A study by Raymond and Hughes interviewed women who had been in the trafficking industry, and they reported becoming dependent on men for companionship or drugs, involvement that became overwhelming as the women could not escape the debt owed to a man or group. Among international women in the study, many were desperately poor in their home country and were forced into a situation in which they believed they

must make money, or tried to escape to a new life in another country; in some cases, families sell a child to pay a family debt. Especially when a group of people have been forced into migrations or have undergone trying economic times, these situations increase, and more women report being forced into sexual servitude to pay for living expenses. These populations in particular are at risk for HIV because they have no say in their living conditions, cannot negotiate condom use, cannot refuse to have sex, and are subject to forced sexual activities.

Another concern is sex tourism, which has become increasingly popular among wealthy travelers. This type of tourism has driven a demand for sex workers in some countries of the CARIBBEAN and Asia in particular. Thailand, Vietnam, the Dominican Republic, and Jamaica are but a few of the countries known to encourage or certainly not prohibit sex workers from earning a living among tourists. The tourists, mainly but not exclusively male, travel to these areas to engage in sex with local men and women, some of whom are underage. The opportunity for wealthy tourists to take advantage of the situation and forgo the use of condoms for the right price or to ignore or purposely avoid age of consent laws is all too common. HIV is very easily transmitted in such situations where ignorance and money prevail over education or common sense.

Another limiting factor in HIV education for sex workers around the world is that funding provided by the United States during the Bush administration could *not* be used on any program that included sex workers. Countries have had to fund their own programs or receive funding from other sources to reach these populations. The funding the United States provided both for internal programs and for programs abroad had zero tolerance for anything related to programs that officials felt encouraged or supported prostitution. This even included programs that educated or supported education for sex workers, which officials viewed as "supporting or promoting" prostitution. Although the rule was overturned for U.S. purposes in a federal district court decision in 2006, the Bush administration refused to change the policy, writing new rules that covered both public and private funds, even filing legal papers to protect this rule a week before President George W. Bush left office in 2009. The current U.S. administration has refused to continue Bush policies, fighting implementation of this rule in courts after the law was ruled as prohibiting free speech in 2006. The U.S. government has yet to repeal this rule or discuss ending it, though the Obama administration has not continued the court case since President Barack Obama took office. Although currently unenforced, the requirement that funding derived from U.S. sources refuse to assist sex workers in any way remains law.

Sex workers face very difficult lives in many parts of the world, including the United States, because of moral and legal prohibitions. Illegal trafficking in women and children makes reaching many people in this population extremely difficult. Providing education and outreach regarding HIV and prevention is difficult particularly when the issue is combined so frequently with IDU. Yet, as has been shown, effective HIV programs can be implemented when sex workers are recruited to participate in running the programs, and large decreases in HIV incidence have been seen in areas such as Thailand. Until this problem is addressed, there remains the potential for large outbreaks of HIV among sex workers, their clients, children, and families.

AVERT: AVERTing HIV and AIDS. "AIDS and Prostitution." AVERT.org Available online. URL: http://www.avert.org/prostitution-aids.htm. Accessed April 9, 2011.

———. "Sex Workers and HIV Prevention." AVERT.org. Available online. URL: http://www.avert.org/sex-workers.htm. Accessed April 9, 2011.

The Body. "Sex Workers and HIV/AIDS." TheBody.com. Available online. URL: http://www.thebody.com/index/whatis/sexwork.html. Accessed April 8, 2011.

Gorbach, Pamina M., et al. "Bridging Sexual Boundaries: Men Who Have Sex with Men and Women in a Street-Based Sample in Los Angeles." *Journal of Urban Health* 86, Suppl. 1 (July 2009): 63–76.

HIV AIDS Asia Pacific Research Statistical Data Information Resources. "Sex Workers and Clients." AIDSDataHub.org. Available online. URL: http://www.aidsdatahub.org/en/reference-materials/key-populations/cat_view/319-all-website-documents/40-reference-materials/63-key-populations--settings/167-sex-workers-and-clients?limit=10&limitstart=0&order=name&dir=DESC. Accessed April 9, 2011.

IRIN (Integrated Regional Information Networks), UN Office for the Coordination of Humanitarian Affairs. "Marginalised Male Sex Workers Vulnerable to HIV." IRINNews.org. Available online. URL: http://www.irinnews.org/report.aspx?reportid=61708. Accessed April 9, 2011.

Jacobson, Jodi. "DOJ Drops Appeal of 'Prostitution Pledge.'" RHRealityCheck.org. Available online. URL: http://www.rhrealitycheck.org/blog/2009/07/21/department-justice-withdraws-appeal-injunction-against-prostitution-pledge. Accessed April 8, 2011.

PEPFARWatch. "Anti-Prostitution Pledge." PEPFAR Watch.org. Available online. URL: http://www.pepfarwatch.org/the_issues/anti_prostitution_pledge/. Accessed April 9, 2011.

Population Council. "Vulnerable Populations: Sex Workers." PopCouncil.org. Available online. URL: http://www.popcouncil.org/topics/vulnerable_sexwork.asp. Accessed April 9, 2011.

Raymond, Janice G., and Donna M. Hughes. "Sex Trafficking of Women in the United States: International and Domestic Trends." URI.edu. Available online. URL: http://www.uri.edu/artsci/wms/hughes/sex_traff_us.pdf. Accessed April 9, 2011.

Scaccabarrozzi, Luis. "Sex Workers and HIV—ACRIA." TheBody.com. Available online. URL: http://www.thebody.com/content/whatis/art14140.html. Accessed April 8, 2011.

Talbott, John R. "Size Matters: The Number of Prostitutes and the Global HIV/AIDS Pandemic." PLoSone.org. Available online. URL: http://www.plosone.org/article/fetchArticle.action?articleURI=info:doi/10.1371/journal.pone.0000543. Accessed April 8, 2011.

Timpson, Sandra C., Michael W. Ross, Mark L. Williams, and John Atkinson. "Characteristics, Drug Use, and Sex Partners of a Sample of Male Sex

Workers." *American Journal of Drug and Alcohol Abuse* 33, no. 1 (2007): 63–69.

UNAIDS: Joint United Nations Programme on HIV/AIDS. *AIDS Epidemic Update 2009.* UNAIDS.org. Available online. URL: http://www.unaids.org/en/data-analysis/epidemiology/2009aidsepidemicupdate/. Accessed April 9, 2011.

———. "HIV and Sexually Transmitted Infection Prevention Among Sex Workers in Eastern Europe and Central Asia." UNAIDS.org. Available online. URL: http://data.unaids.org/publications/IRC-pub07/jc1212-hivpreveasterneurcentrasia_en.pdf. Accessed April 9, 2011.

———. "Sex Work and HIV/AIDS." UNAIDS.org. Available online. URL: http://www.unaids.org/en/media/unaids/contentassets/dataimport/publications/irc-pub02/jc705-sexwork-tu_en.pdf. Accessed April 8, 2011.

———. "Sex Workers and Clients." UNAIDS.org. Available online. URL: http://www.unaids.org/en/PolicyAndPractice/KeyPopulations/SexWorkers/default.asp. Accessed April 8, 2011.

United Nations Population Fund. "Working with Sex Workers to Stop the Spread of HIV in Russia." UNFPA.org. Available online. URL: http://eeca.unfpa.org/public/cache/offonce/pid/6208;jsessionid=7FEBF9A2B911419C81BC4361B736D511. Accessed April 9, 2011.

United States Agency for International Development. "Russia: HIV/AIDS Health Profile." USAID.gov. Available online. URL: http://www.usaid.gov/our_work/global_health/aids/Countries/eande/russia_profile.pdf. Accessed April 8, 2011.

stavudine   Stavudine is an antiretroviral used in the treatment of HIV. It is one of the NUCLEOSIDE REVERSE TRANSCRIPTASE INHIBITORS (NRTIs) and works to stop the reproduction of HIV that is already in the body. It is sold under the trade name Zerit and is also commonly called d4T. Three companies in India also manufacture it in generic form for use in developing countries. The generic forms were also approved for use in the United States in 2008. In 1994, it became the fourth antiretroviral approved for use in the treatment of HIV. It was at one time, because of its relatively low cost and the availability of generic forms, used by an estimated 80 percent of people on antiretroviral treatment around the world. That number has dropped in the past few years to about 50 percent according to the WORLD HEALTH ORGANIZATION (WHO).

Dosage

Stavudine is available in a variety of dosages: 15, 20, 30, and 40 mg capsules that are used according to body weight. Adults more than 130 pounds will take 40 mg twice a day. There is also a liquid formulation of the medication that is available to CHILDREN and infants. Dosage for the liquid variety of stavudine is also based on weight, and a doctor or medical specialist determines the proper dosage of liquid needed for infants and children. Dosages around the world are different from those in the United States, as the WHO recommends just 30 mg twice a day for adults taking stavudine.

Drug Interactions

Stavudine interacts with several different medications, so patients should check with their doctor prior to starting treatment with stavudine. Stavudine should not be taken at the same time as ZIDOVUDINE. These drugs are antagonistic, meaning they work against each other, decreasing the overall effectiveness of both medications. The side effects of both drugs can also increase if prescribed together.

Ribavirin is a drug used in the treatment of HEPATITIS C. If stavudine and ribavirin are prescribed together, the effectiveness of stavudine is greatly reduced.

Stavudine should also not be prescribed with the NRTI DIDANOSINE. Didanosine and stavudine both cause certain side effects. Use of the drugs together increases greatly the chance the patient will become affected by peripheral NEUROPATHY, one of the main side effects of stavudine. Other medications that can also increase the chance of peripheral neuropathy are dapsone, amphotericin B, and foscarnet, all of which can be used in treating various HIV-related OPPORTUNISTIC INFECTIONS (OIs).

Stavudine should not be prescribed with intravenous pentamadine, used in the treatment of MYCOBACTERIUM AVIUM COMPLEX (MAC). This combination of drugs increases the risk of pancreatitis in patients.

Side Effects

Stavudine was once considered an easy-to-take medication that caused few problems and was less toxic than other antiretroviral drugs. However, many years of use and many drug trials later, it has been shown to pose particularly difficult problems over the long term, with several potentially dangerous and long-lasting side effects.

Several of the initially recognized side effects of antiretroviral medications are linked with stavudine. LIPODYSTROPHY, the loss of fat or shifting of fat in the body, has been linked to stavudine through extended drug studies. Loss of fat in the face, arms, and buttocks can also be called lipoatrophy. In addition, buffalo hump, or the accumulation of fat in the shoulders and neck, as well as an increase in lipomas (benign fatty-tissue tumors) have been linked to the long-term use of stavudine.

Peripheral neuropathy, nerve damage that causes numbness in the feet, hands, and legs, has also been linked to the use of stavudine. The drug can also cause much more painful burning or tingling sensations in those areas, too, as the nerve damage worsens. The nerve damage can be temporary if the drug is stopped soon after the symptoms begin, but can be permanent or very long term depending on the length of time the drug is taken after the onset of symptoms.

Because of these significant side effects, the WHO recently issued a recommendation that stavudine be phased out as a first-line drug for the treatment of HIV and that other antiretrovirals replace the drug. Because of the dependence of many nations on the low cost of the drug, it may be several years before this occurs. Other side effects that have been seen in people using stavudine include pancreatitis and LACTIC ACIDOSIS. Symptoms of pancreatitis include stomach pain, nausea, and vomiting. Symptoms of lactic acidosis (the buildup of lactic acid in the blood) include nausea, vomiting, weakness in muscles, tiredness, pain in the stomach area, shortness of breath, and yellowing of the eyes or skin. Both of these side effects have been rare but are very serious. These conditions have been seen more often when stavudine has been combined with didanosine.

More common side effects that generally pass with time on the medication include headache, stomach upset, problems with sleeping, diarrhea, and muscle pain.

AIDS InfoNet. "Stavudine (Zerit, d4T)." AIDSInfoNet. org. Available online. URL: http://www.aidsinfo net.org/fact_sheets/view/414. Accessed March 11, 2011.

———. "Zerit (Stavudine, d4T)." AIDSInfoNet.org. Available online. URL: http://www.aidsmeds.com/ archive/Zerit_1588.shtml. Accessed March 11, 2011.

AIDSmeds. "Special Issues for Children with HIV." AIDSmeds.com. Available online. URL: http:// www.aidsmeds.com/articles/Children_7566.shtml. Accessed March 11, 2011.

The Body. "Zerit (Stavudine, d4T)." TheBody.com. Available online. URL: http://www.thebody.com/ index/treat/d4t.html. Accessed March 11, 2011.

Galli, Massimo, et al. "Brief Report: Gender Differences in Antiretroviral Drug–Related Adipose Tissue Alterations: Women Are at Higher Risk than Men and Develop Particular Lipodystrophy Patterns." NATAP.org. Available online. URL: http:// www.natap.org/2003/oct/101503_4.htm.

Nebehay, Stephanie. "UPDATE 2—New WHO Guidelines Urge Phaseout of Major HIV Drug: Reuters." Reuters.com. Available online. URL: http://www. reuters.com/article/idUSGEE5AT2F420091130. Accessed July 24, 2011.

United States Department of Health and Human Services. "Stavudine." aidsinfo.nih.gov. Available online. URL: http://www.aidsinfo.nih.gov/DrugsNew/Drug DetailNT.aspx?int_id=43. Accessed March 11, 2011.

syphilis Syphilis is a sexually transmitted disease caused by *Treponema pallidum,* a spirochete bacterium. The term *spirochete* refers to the shape of the bacterium, which resembles a spiral worm that trembles, when viewed by a microscope. Another type of spirochete is the bacterium that causes Lyme disease.

Syphilis is almost always spread through intimate sexual contact, particularly when a person has a sore, also called a chancre, which appears in the initial stage of the disease. Contact with the sore can pass the bacteria, which can then enter the bloodstream through minor cuts or through abrasions to the mucous membranes. It can also be passed through blood-to-blood contact and can be passed from a mother to a child during birth.

In HIV-positive people, syphilis has been reported to increase in severity of symptoms in both the primary and secondary phases of the illness. Because of the open sores that are part of primary and occasionally secondary syphilis, it also becomes much easier to spread HIV during sexual activity. Studies of HIV infection rates and syphilis infection rates during the 1990s showed that heterosexual spread of the two diseases was generally linked. That is, where large numbers of syphilis cases appeared, there were also relatively large numbers of HIV cases reported. Urban health clinics, particularly in the southern United States, reported similar rates of infection for both illnesses in the late 1990s.

Syphilis cases have been dramatically rising since 2000, particularly among MEN WHO HAVE SEX WITH MEN (MSM). In 2009, there were 13,066 cases of primary and secondary syphilis reported in the United States, up nearly 5.5 percent from the previous year. Total cases, which include tertiary and latent syphilis, were down more than 3 percent, to 44,828 in 2009. Cases among MSM now make up more than 60 percent of primary and secondary syphilis cases reported in the United States, from approximately 15 percent of the total number of cases in 1999. Men overall are 5.6 times more likely to be diagnosed with syphilis than WOMEN.

Symptoms and Diagnostic Path

Syphilis has three distinct phases of illness. The first phase is called primary syphilis, which presents with the appearance of usually one painless ulcer, also called a chancre (pronounced shanker), at the site of the initial infection. The chancre will appear approximately three weeks after initial infection but can occur anytime from a week to 10 weeks after initial infection. Depending on the sexual activity at the time of contact, that location can be the lips or mouth, penis, vagina, or anus. In HIV-infected individuals, there can be numerous chancres involved in the initial phase of infection, and the chancres may appear more rapidly than in an HIV-negative person. The chancre can appear inside the body in the anus or vagina and can often be unnoticed, as it is generally painless. The chancre will disappear after three to six weeks if left untreated.

Secondary syphilis will occur in a person if the initial phase of the illness is untreated. It involves numerous chancres or a general rash over much of the skin and mucous membranes of the body, as well as the palms of the hands and soles of the feet. The rash can be very widespread in HIV-positive people or limited to a few areas in HIV-negative people. Lymph glands are generally swollen and tender to the touch. It may also involve tiredness, headache, and sore throat. It can occur anywhere from two to 10 weeks after the initial chancre. As in primary syphilis, it will disappear over time if left untreated. People who have secondary syphilis are extremely infectious because the virus is being shed from the body through the rash or numerous chancres.

The stage of illness following secondary syphilis is known as latent syphilis. This occurs when the illness generally does not produce any symptoms, and it may be difficult to know that an infection exists. Some people will remain in a latent phase of the illness for many years, while others may only stay in this phase for a short time. The virus can still be passed to sexual partners during this time.

The third stage of syphilis, or tertiary syphilis, is the stage that causes most physical problems. Internal organs as well as the central nervous system (CNS) can be involved, leading to swelling of the aorta, lesions on the liver, large lesions of the skin called gummas, and several other complications. CNS involvement can lead to blindness, deafness, and loss of mental capacity. Researchers believe that HIV-positive people are at a higher risk for CNS complications when also ill with syphilis.

Untreated syphilis can also cause severe problems in WOMEN who are pregnant, as the bacteria pass to the child in the womb. Congenital syphilis can cause many birth defects, including mental retardation, blindness, and deafness.

Syphilis can be diagnosed through observation if the illness is seen during the primary or secondary phase of infection. BLOOD WORK/BLOOD TESTS are the general method of confirming the diagnosis. Biopsies of lesions or chancres may be necessary if the blood test results are inconclusive but syphilis is suspected. More extensive testing of patients with tertiary syphilis will be necessary to determine whether CNS involvement is present, as well as checking the health and function of the liver, heart, and other internal organs that syphilis can destroy.

Treatment Options and Outlook

Treatment for HIV-positive and -negative people is the same. First-line treatment is the intramuscular injection of benzathine penicillin. This single injection is generally enough to cure the illness, though some HIV specialists may opt to give two succeeding injections once a week. Including oral medications at this point has not been shown to increase the success of treatment, according to University of California, San Francisco, reports. Tertiary syphilis treatment is longer with, three-dose, once-a-week injections of penicillin.

People who have evidence of CNS involvement are most successfully treated with intravenous penicillin for a period of 10 days to two weeks to remove the bacteria from the eyes, ears, and CNS.

People who have an allergy to penicillin should be tested for skin reactions, undergo desensitization treatment, and then have treatment with penicillin. Other medications have been shown to be less effective in treatment of syphilis. Close monitoring of HIV-positive patients' medications and drug allergies is required to ensure elimination of the bacteria and to determine that the syphilis does not become resistant to the medication being used as an alternative.

Risk Factors and Preventive Measures

The best preventive measure for syphilis is the use of a condom and/or dental dam during sexual activities. Highly sexually active individuals may be helped with counseling regarding their behavior and the consequences of the illness. Sexually active individuals who are HIV positive should be tested annually to ensure that they have not contracted any new sexually transmitted infections.

Centers for Disease Control and Prevention. "Sexually Transmitted Diseases Surveillance: Syphilis." CDC.gov. Available online. URL: http://www.cdc.gov/std/stats09/Syphilis.htm. Accessed April 9, 2011.

———. "Sexually Transmitted Diseases Surveillance 2006 Supplement: Syphilis Surveillance Report." CDC.gov. Available online. URL: http://www.cdc.gov/std/Syphilis2006/Syphilis2006Short.pdf. Accessed April 9, 2011.

———. "Syphilis CDC Fact Sheet." CDC.gov. Available online. URL: http://www.cdc.gov/std/syphilis/STDFact-Syphilis.htm. Accessed April 9, 2011.

Hall, Christopher S., and Gail Bolan. "Syphilis and HIV." Available online. URL: http://hivinsite.ucsf.edu/InSite?page=kb-00&doc=kb-05-01-04. Accessed April 9, 2011

Mayo Clinic Staff. "Syphilis." MayoClinic.com. Available online. URL: http://www.mayoclinic.com/health/syphilis/DS00374. Accessed April 9, 2011.

National Institute of Allergy and Infectious Diseases. "Syphilis." NIH.gov. Available online. URL: http://www3.niaid.nih.gov/topics/syphilis/default.htm. Accessed April 9, 2011.

T

tenofovir disoproxil fumarate Tenofovir diso-proxil fumarate is a drug commonly called teno-fovir or tenofovir DF and sold under the trade name Viread. It is also one of the drugs in the anti-HIV combination pills TRUVADA and ATRI-PLA. The drug is manufactured by Gilead Sci-ences and was approved by the U.S. FOOD AND DRUG ADMINISTRATION (FDA) in 2001. It is one of the NUCLEOTIDE REVERSE TRANSCRIPTASE INHIBI-TORS (NtRTIs), the only one in this class of drugs approved for use against HIV. NtRTI drugs do not require the added step of being changed in the body, which NUCLEOSIDE REVERSE TRANSCRIPTASE INHIBITORS (NRTIs) require. It is still considered part of the "nuke" class of drugs and can have some of the same side effects and drawbacks that this class of drugs exhibits.

Dosage

The standard dose is one 300 mg tablet once a day. This may be decreased if a person has pre-existing kidney problems. It can be taken with or without food. When it is part of a three-drug combination pill, 300 mg of tenofovir is included in the combination. There is no liquid formula-tion available at this time.

Tenofovir has not been approved for use in CHILDREN or in WOMEN who are nursing. Stud-ies involving pregnant women have not been conducted. Tenofovir has also been shown to be highly active against HEPATITIS B (HBV) and is sometimes prescribed by doctors for this use for people who are coinfected with HIV and HBV. Tenofovir was not originally approved for use in the treatment of HBV, but received approval in late 2008 for treating chronic HBV. Tenofovir is always prescribed as part of a multidrug combi-nation in the treatment of HIV.

The drug is currently being tested in different sites around the world as a MICROBICIDE gel for the prevention of HIV TRANSMISSION. There are studies under way to test its use as both a vagi-nal and anal microbicide. Tenofovir pills are also being studied as an oral drug to be taken daily to prevent transmission of the virus. These uses had *not* been approved by the FDA as of early 2011, but studies have shown some effectiveness in the use of tenofovir as both a microbicide and an oral pre-exposure prophylaxis (PrEP) medication.

Drug Interactions

Tenofovir should not be taken at the same time as Atripla, Truvada, or the HBV drug adefovir. These medications contain the same or similar medicine and can cause problems when too much of the drug is in the body.

Tenofovir can cause an increase in the amount of DIDANOSINE, another HIV antiretroviral, in the body. The drugs should be prescribed together only with caution, as this increase can bring about an increased risk of didanosine side effects such as pancreatitis and drug-induced NEUROPATHY.

When tenofovir is given at the same time as KALETRA or ATAZANAVIR SULFATE with ritonavir, the amount of tenofovir is increased in the body. Increased signs of tenofovir side effects are pos-sible and require monitoring. At the same time, the amount of atazanavir sulfate in the body is decreased when combined with tenofovir, and atazanavir sulfate should always be given in combination with ritonavir, if this is the pre-ferred combination of anti-HIV medications.

Tenofovir is metabolized (processed in the body) differently than most antiretroviral drugs. As opposed to being metabolized by the liver, tenofovir is processed through the kidneys.

Side Effects

Cases of LACTIC ACIDOSIS, a serious blood buildup of lactic acid, and liver illness have been recorded while taking NRTIs. This occurs more often in pregnant women than other people taking NRTIs. Symptoms include nausea, vomiting, muscle soreness and weakness, shortness of breath, yellowing of the eyes and skin, and pain in the lower back. Any of these severe symptoms needs to be reported to a doctor immediately.

Tenofovir has been associated in at least one study with a loss of bone mineral density, known as osteopenia, in the hip and spine. Doctors may evaluate patients for this potential concern if patients have a preexisting history of bone fractures or ostopenia. It is not clear that mineral or vitamin supplementation with calcium or vitamin D is helpful to prevent this condition in patients taking Tenofovir.

There have been cases of kidney malfunction while taking tenofovir; doctors may periodically test a patient's kidney functioning. The most common short-term side effects are headache, nausea, tiredness, dizziness, vomiting, and flatulence (gas). These generally diminish as the body adjusts to the drug.

Doctors monitor liver function for any flare-ups of HBV viral activity in people who have HBV and are required to stop taking tenofovir. Stopping anti-HBV medicines can sometimes cause the disease activity to start up, causing potential liver problems and further damage.

AIDS InfoNet. "Tenofovir (Viread)." AIDSInfoNet.org. Available online. URL: http://www.aidsinfonet.org/fact_sheets/view/419. Accessed March 11, 2011.

AIDSmeds. "Special Issues for Children with HIV: Introduction." AIDSmeds.com. Available online. URL: http://www.aidsmeds.com/articles/Children_7566.shtml. Accessed April 9, 2011.

———. "Viread (Tenofovir)." AIDSmeds.com. Available online. URL: http://www.aidsmeds.com/archive/Viread_1587.shtml. Accessed April 9, 2011.

The Body. "Viread (Tenofovir)." TheBody.com. Available online. URL: http://www.thebody.com/content/art40488.html. Accessed April 9, 2011.

Rivera, Enrico. "Tenofovir Gel Protects Rectal Tissue against HIV, UCLA-Led Study Finds." UCLA.edu. Available online. URL: http://newsroom.ucla.edu/portal/ucla/tenofovir-gel-protects-rectal-193009.aspx. Accessed April 9, 2011.

Suvash, Shrestha. "Tenofovir for HIV Prevention: Gel or Tablet." JYI.org. Available online. URL: http://www.jyi.org/news/nb.php?id=1559. Accessed April 9, 2011.

United States Department of Health and Human Services. "Tenofovir Disoproxil Fumarate." aidsinfo.nih.gov.com. Available online. URL: http://www.aidsinfo.nih.gov/drugsNew/DrugDetailNT.aspx?int_id=290. Accessed March 11, 2011.

tipranavir Tipranavir is a PROTEASE INHIBITOR (PI) manufactured by the drug company Boehringer Ingelheim. The U.S. FOOD AND DRUG ADMINISTRATION (FDA) approved it for use in the treatment of HIV in 2005. It is used only in the treatment of patients for whom other HIGHLY ACTIVE ANTIRETROVIRAL TREATMENT (HAART) regimens that included other PIs have failed. The common term for drugs used only after others have failed is *salvage therapy*. Tipranavir has a different profile of action in the body and so can be used when other PI-based drug regimens have failed. It is approved for use in treatment-experienced adults, and the liquid formula is used for treatment-experienced CHILDREN. It is sold under the trade name Aptivus and is abbreviated as TPV.

Dosage

Tipranavir is available is 250 mg capsules that require refrigeration prior to being opened or in a liquid that also requires refrigeration prior to use. Once either is opened, room temperature is adequate for storage until the medicine is used up.

Tipranavir is always prescribed for use in conjunction with the PI ritonavir. The standard dose is two 250 mg capsules at the same time as two

100 mg capsules of ritonavir. This is taken twice a day. If the liquid form is used in adults, then 5 mL of tipranavir is given in place of the two tipranavir capsules. Dosage for children is based on the weight of the child and can be determined by a doctor.

Drug Interactions

As many PIs do, tipranavir interacts with the medications it is combined with and can cause increases or decreases in the amount of the drugs available in the body. It is recommended that tipranavir not be administered with other PIs, as the amount of other PIs in the body is decreased significantly while using tipranavir.

Tipranavir should not be taken at the same time as any antacids or acid-blocking drugs. Both magnesium- and aluminum-containing antacids reduce the absorption of tipranavir and should be taken at least two hours before or after administration of tipranavir.

The drug also interacts with NUCLEOSIDE REVERSE TRANSCRIPTASE INHIBITORS (NRTIs). Tipranavir should not be taken with ABACAVIR or ZIDOVUDINE, as both of these NRTIs are significantly reduced in effectiveness when combined with tipranavir. No studies have been completed to study proper dosage for these two drugs when combined with tipranavir. It also reduces the amount of DIDANOSINE in the body. It is recommended that when combining didanosine with tipranavir, the drugs be taken at least two hours before or after each other.

Tipranavir blood levels are decreased when it is combined with EFAVIRENZ, which is one of the NON-NUCLEOSIDE REVERSE TRANSCRIPTASE INHIBITORS (NNRTIs), or with the efavirenz-containing drug ATRIPLA. No recommendations have been made regarding this combination. Tipranavir interacts with a number of other medications including the cholesterol-lowering drugs simvastatin and lovastatin, antibiotics used to treat infections such as TUBERCULOSIS, antidepressant or antipsychotic medications, and medications to treat dysrhythmias of the heart. It should not be taken with any drugs containing ergot, which is used in many migraine medications. It is important that a doctor know and understand all the medications and supplements a patient is taking when prescribing tipranavir.

Tipranavir also increases the amount of the drugs sildenafil (Viagra), vardenafil (Levitra), and tadalafil (Cialis)—all erectile dysfunction medications—in the blood and therefore can cause serious side effects. Lowering the dosage of these medications is recommended to prevent potential complications.

Estrogen-based birth control methods are less effective when taking tipranavir. WOMEN who are using these forms of birth control may seek to use a barrier protection method such as condoms while taking tipranavir.

Methadone levels in the body decrease substantially while taking tipranavir. People who use methadone for the treatment of opiate addiction should have dosages adjusted and monitored by a doctor.

Antifungal medications such as ketoconazole, itraconazole, and voriconazole are affected by tipranavir and ritonavir. Amounts of ketoconazole and itraconazole are decreased in the blood, while voriconazole levels are increased. Care needs to be used in prescribing these antifungals so that the proper dosage to treat the fungal infection while not causing harm to the person taking tipranavir is found. St. John's wort, an herbal supplement, should never be taken with a PI, as it has been shown to reduce greatly the amount of PI in the body.

Increased levels of fluticasone, an inhaled steroidal allergy and asthma treatment, will occur while taking tipranavir. It is usually recommended not to combine these two drugs. Patients doing so must be monitored for serious increases in side effects of fluticasone.

Tipranavir contains small amounts of alcohol in the capsule formulation. It should not be prescribed to people who are taking either disulfuram, for the treatment of alcohol dependence, or metronidazole, used to treat parasite infections. These medications can make people who drink alcohol or take medications with any alcohol in them very sick. Tipranavir liquid contains vitamin E. People who are taking tipranavir should not use supplements for additional vitamin E.

Tipranavir is a sulfa drug. People who are allergic to sulfa medications should tell their doctor so that other medications are prescribed, or they are closely monitored while taking the drug.

Side Effects

Tipranavir may cause some mild nausea, tiredness, headache, vomiting, and diarrhea. These are considered short-term effects and may disappear after the person uses the drug for a while.

Tipranavir may cause an increase in bleeding in hemophiliac patients. Several cases of such bleeding have occurred

In studies before its approval, tipranavir was associated with some cases of stroke. Therefore, it may cause bleeding in the brain that could be fatal. Patients who use anticoagulants or other medicines that thin the blood, such as are used by some heart patients, should be careful when using this medication. BLOOD WORK/BLOOD TESTS should be considered to measure the decrease of the ability of the blood to clot when taking tipranavir.

Tipranavir has also been associated with some cases of liver failure. People who are chronic hepatitis carriers or those who have other liver disease problems need to be extremely careful if taking this medication to prevent liver failure or an increase in hepatitislike symptoms. It is not recommended for patients who already have some liver impairment.

PROTEASE INHIBITORS, as a class of drug, often increase the cholesterol and triglyceride levels of patients. High lipid levels have been recorded in some tipranavir patients. This side effect can be managed with appropriate cholesterol-lowering medications. Tipranavir has also been associated with treatment regimens that can cause LIPODYSTROPHY, or the redistribution of fat within the body. Symptoms are increased fat around the neck and stomach area, facial wasting, breast enlargement, and peripheral wasting in the arms

and legs. Some of these changes disappear when the drug is stopped.

Some people who take tipranavir develop a skin rash initially. It has been seen more in CHILDREN than adults and more in WOMEN who are taking birth control pills than in other women. In most people it is mild or moderate. There have been some serious skin reactions, or allergies, to the drug, so a doctor should monitor severe rashes. If the rash is accompanied by bone and muscle fatigue, tiredness, itchiness, throat tightening, or fever, the individual should stop taking tipranavir and notify a doctor. People who have used tipranavir also have noticed more sensitivity to the sun when taking the drug.

Tipranavir may also increase the risk of worsening diabetes or the onset of diabetes in people who were not previously diabetic.

AIDS InfoNet. "Tipranavir (Aptivus)." AIDSInfoNet.org. Available online. URL: http://www.aidsinfonet.org/fact_sheets/view/449. Accessed March 11, 2011.
AIDSmeds. "Aptivus (Tipranavir)." AIDSmeds.com. Available online. URL: http://www.aidsmeds.com/archive/Reyataz_1563.shtml. Accessed March 11, 2011.
———. "Special Issues for Children with HIV." AIDS meds.com. Available online. URL: http://www.aidsmeds.com/articles/Children_7566.shtml. Accessed March 11, 2011.
The Body. "Aptivus (Tipranavir)." TheBody.com. Available online. URL: http://www.thebody.com/index/treat/tipranavir.html. Accessed March 11, 2011.
United States Department of Health and Human Services. "Atazanavir." aidsinfo.nih.gov. Available online. URL: http://www.aidsinfo.nih.gov/DrugsNew/DrugDetailNT.aspx?int_id=351. Accessed March 11, 2011.

toxoplasmosis Toxoplasmosis is an illness caused by the parasitic protozoan *Toxoplasma gondii*. The parasite infects many warm-blooded animals, including humans. According to the U.S. CENTERS FOR DISEASE CONTROL and Prevention (CDC), nearly 20 percent of the adult U.S. population has been exposed to the parasite.

Most of these people will never know that they have been infected, as the illness is controlled by their healthy immune system. Worldwide, some areas show a 95 percent infection rate for humans. In humans, the parasite infects the brain and therefore can cause changes in the behavior of the person who has the parasite.

Toxoplasma gondii can grow in any of the host animals it invades but only reproduces through eggs laid in the intestinal linings of the cat family. These eggs then pass through the intestines of the cat through its excrement. Humans acquire the parasite through the ingestion of oocysts, eggs of the parasite, as well as the tissue cysts found in other animals. One common manner of ingestion occurs when people clean their cat's litter box. Oocysts from the cat's excrement become attached to the person's hands, and then either when they inadvertently wipe their hands on their mouth or handle something else that touches mouth, the parasite's eggs are ingested. The eating of undercooked or raw meat of an animal can also transfer tissue cysts of the *Toxoplasma* into a person. Other animals become infected through grazing of grass or material that has been contaminated with cat excrement. Once in the human body, the parasite transforms itself into further tissue cysts, often remaining in the human for the rest of the person's life.

Symptoms and Diagnostic Path

In a person who has a healthy immune system, toxoplasmosis appears as a mild flulike illness, if there are any symptoms at all. CHILDREN born with congenital toxoplasmosis can be severely ill and die shortly after birth, or they may have few symptoms until later in life. Typical symptoms in newborns can include inflammation of the eyes, called chorioretinitis, which can result in blindness. Other symptoms include swelling of the liver and spleen, seizures, a misshapen head, and developmental disabilities.

Among immune-compromised individuals, the most common symptoms are headache, confusion, motor weakness, and fever. Unless treated, the disease progresses to seizures, stu-

por, and coma. Although disseminated disease is possible, affecting the lungs, liver, and other organs, it generally does not happen in HIV-positive populations.

BLOOD WORK/BLOOD TESTS can determine whether a patient has positive findings for antitoxoplasma immunoglobulin G antibodies. Other tests that will be run to determine a toxoplasmosis diagnosis include a computed tomography (CT) scan, magnetic resonance imaging (MRI), or some similar computer imaging technique to look for lesions in the brain. After initiation of treatment, a person may undergo a brain biopsy during a CT scan to obtain tissue samples to ensure the correct diagnosis if the treatment appears to be ineffective. Images generally show several lesions, though just one lesion is sufficient to cause illness.

Toxoplasma gondii can also be passed from a woman to her unborn child. It does not happen if the woman has been infected prior to pregnancy, but if the woman becomes infected during pregnancy, the parasite can cause a miscarriage, stillbirth, or birth defects in children. If the child survives the infection in the womb, it will have congenital toxoplasmosis, which can lead to other health problems later in life. In rare instances, the parasite can be transmitted through blood transfusions or ORGAN TRANSPLANTATION. It is not spread person to person through sexual contact, sneezing, or coughing.

Treatment Options and Outlook

Treatment for toxoplasmosis is accomplished through a multidrug regimen over a course of at least six weeks. Once a patient has recovered from the acute illness, prophylaxis treatment continues until the patient has been in remission for at least three months with an immune system of at least 200 CD4 T lymphocytes per microliter (µL) of blood, at which time the prophylaxis may be stopped.

First-line treatment is with a combination of pyrimethamine, sulfadiazine, and leucovorin. The drug leucovorin is used to decrease toxicities in the blood often seen with pyrimethamine. Clindamycin may be substituted for sulfadiazine in those patients who are allergic to sulfadiazine. Trimethoprim/sulfamethoxazole (TMP-SMX) has also been used for treatment of acute toxoplasmosis infection. Other medications have shown effectiveness in trials but remain second-line treatments.

Corticosteroids are often administered to patients if inflammation is an issue in the infection. For patients who have had seizures from the infection, an anticonvulsant may be prescribed. All these medications will require monitoring of various blood measurements to determine whether the amount of medication is optimal and confirm that there are no adverse reactions to the medications.

Some studies of toxoplasmosis indicate that the parasite actually causes a change of behavior in the host. Novotna and colleagues in 2005 demonstrated that humans who had toxoplasmosis showed decreased novelty-seeking behavior compared to people never exposed to the parasite. Men infected with toxoplasmosis tended to be more reflective, required more input in decision making, and did not waste their energy or feelings. Research continues into the parasite and its effects on the brain.

Risk Factors and Preventive Measures

The chief risk factors for toxoplasmosis infection are eating undercooked meat and unintentionally ingesting infected cat feces. Pregnant women and HIV-positive individuals can avoid the parasite if they take care to cook meat properly. In particular, beef, pork, lamb, and venison (deer meat) should be cooked until no longer pink, or the meat reaches an internal temperature of 165–170°F. Meat thermometers can be purchased at many grocery stores to allow easy checking of internal cooking temperature. People preparing food should always wash their hands after handling raw meat to prevent any possible contamination.

Another way to avoid the parasite is to wash the hands after gardening, contact with soil, or cleaning a cat's litter box. People who have housecats can decrease the chance that their pet cat has *Toxoplasma gondii* by keeping the cat indoors and feeding it canned or dry food, not raw or undercooked meat. Cats that live or play outside can become infected with *Toxoplasma* by eating mice or other small animals or meat that is already infected. Individuals who have weakened immune systems or pregnant women should avoid emptying the litter box to be completely safe or wash their hands thoroughly after doing so. Keeping the litter box clean on a daily basis can also help to keep the contact with any potential parasite to a minimum.

HIV-positive patients who have fewer than 100 CD4 T lymphocytes per (μL) of blood should have prophylaxis for toxoplasmosis if they test seropositive for past exposure to *Toxoplasma gondii*. Standard preventive medication is TMP-SMX, one dual-strength pill daily or one dual-strength pill three times a week if the medication causes stomach distress. Other prophylaxis treatments, if the patient has an allergy to TMP-SMX, include dapsone-pyrimethamine plus leucovorin, which can also provide effective prophylaxis against PNEUMOCYSTIS PNEUMONIA.

Centers for Disease Control and Prevention. "Toxoplasmosis." CDC.gov. Available online. URL: http://www.cdc.gov/toxoplasmosis/. Accessed April 9, 2011.

Merck. "Toxoplasmosis." Merck.com. Available online. URL: http://www.merck.com/mmhe/sec17/ch196/ch196r.html. Accessed April 9, 2011.

Novotna, Martina, et al. "Probable Neuroimmunological Link between Toxoplasma and Cytomegalovirus Infections and Personality Changes in the Human Host." BioMedCentral.org. Available online. URL: http://www.biomedcentral.com/1471-2334/5/54. Accessed April 9, 2011.

Subauste, Carlos S. "Toxoplasmosis and HIV." HIVInSite.org. Available online. URL: http://hivinsite.org/InSite?page=kb-00&doc=kb-05-04-03. Accessed April 9, 2011.

transmission   Throughout the world, people can contract HUMAN IMMUNODEFICIENCY VIRUS (HIV) infection in three possible ways: through sexual contact, either homosexual or heterosexual;

through contact with blood or blood products or bloody body tissue of an HIV-positive person, including sharing contaminated needles; or through the transfer of the virus from an infected mother to her infant, shortly before or during birth, or through breast-feeding after birth. The transfer of a virus from one person to another in a population is known as horizontal transmission. This is distinguished from vertical transmission, which is the transfer of the virus from one generation to another. Sexual transmission and blood-to-blood transmission are examples of horizontal transmission. Perinatal transmission is an example of vertical transmission.

Transmission through Sexual Activity

Sexual transmission can occur through intercourse, both heterosexual and homosexual. Heterosexual transmission is the leading means of HIV transmission worldwide and the fastest-growing mode of transmission in the United States. HIV is transmitted bidirectionally; that is, it can be transmitted in two, usually opposite, directions. When referring to HIV transmission it means it can be passed from one person to the other in either direction. It can be spread from WOMEN to men, men to women, men to men, and potentially women to women. HIV is a virus that does not have sexual preferences. This is clear from the course of the epidemic in AFRICA, where the rate of infection is roughly equal for men and women and predominantly in the heterosexual community. It is also evident in the United States, where the profile of the disease has changed dramatically since the first decade of the epidemic. Additionally, it is clear from the continued evolution of the disease in the rest of the world in both developed and developing countries that cases of HIV transmission associated with heterosexual activity have been the predominant means of transmission since the 1990s. In the early years of the epidemic, it was assumed that the risk of transmission from an infected female to an uninfected male was lower than the risk of transmission from an infected male to an uninfected female. It was

also assumed that it was easier for a man to pass HIV to another man than it was for a woman to transmit HIV to another woman. It was assumed that it was easier for a woman to transmit HIV to her baby in her womb than it was to pass HIV to her baby after birth. Today, many of those initial assumptions about the transmission of HIV have been changed. Researchers know now that many factors may alter the susceptibility of an individual. The presence of either initial acute infection or advanced HIV disease in an infected partner increases the risk of sexual transmission.

The presence of genital tract infections in either partner increases the risk of HIV transmission. In particular, the risk is markedly increased if a partner has an active yeast infection or genital sores or ulcers. Such sores can be caused by ulcer-producing sexually transmitted infections (STIs) such as SYPHILIS, HERPES SIMPLEX VIRUS, and chancroid. Sores and ulcers in an uninfected partner facilitate contact between a positive person's bodily fluids and his or her own blood. Sores have many macrophages, lymphocytes, and other cells of the immune system trying to heal the area and increase the opportunity for infection to occur. Sores on an infected person increase the opportunity for HIV to be released and to have contact with the mucous membranes of an uninfected partner, exposing the uninfected partner to a greater quantity of virus.

STDs that do not produce ulcers, such as gonorrhea, chlamydia, and trichomoniasis, also increase the risk of acquiring HIV. This is thought to occur because these diseases cause inflammation of the mucous membranes of the genital tract. Inflammation is a normal immune response to infection or injury, but it activates and attracts a large number of white blood cells, including monocytes, macrophages, and lymphocytes, to the inflamed area. In the HIV-infected person, this increases the amount of free virus and the number of virus-infected cells in genital secretions. In the HIV-negative partner, the risk of acquiring HIV infection is increased because the inflammation of the genital tract concentrates cells susceptible to HIV infection in the genital tissues, giving the HIV-negative person contact with the potentially transmissible cells.

Anal intercourse and probably intercourse during menstruation also increase the risk of sexual transmission. The rectal lining is thin and contains many lymphocytes, macrophages, and other cells that HIV can infect. Anal intercourse can also cause small tears in the rectal lining that result in direct contact between infected semen and the blood of the receptive partner. It can also allow for the blood in an infected receptive partner to enter the mucous membranes of the insertive partner through the urethra or the foreskin. Intercourse during menstruation involves blood, which allows for easy access of the virus to either infect a partner or allow an infected partner to spread the virus more easily to the menstruating partner.

The number of instances of intercourse is related to risk. The greater the number of exposures to infected semen or vaginal secretions, the higher the risk of HIV transmission. Genetic characteristics of the particular HIV strain to which a person is exposed, as well as genetic characteristics of the exposed person, also affect the risk of HIV transmission.

Some studies have shown that the use of oral contraceptives, diaphragms, cervical caps, or intrauterine devices increases the risk of HIV transmission. Condoms, lubricants, or contraceptive devices that contain the spermicide nonoxynol-9 have been linked to increased chance of HIV transmission because of the irritating nature of nonoxynol-9 to the lining of the vagina and rectum. A risk of HIV transmission exists even during safe sex; minimizing this risk requires that condoms be used consistently and correctly.

Sexual Transmission from Men to Women This process is fairly well understood. Semen from an infected man contains HIV that is mostly associated with infected lymphocytes present in the semen. HIV introduced into the vagina must make its way into the bloodstream to initiate viral reproduction. Small breaks in the lining of the vagina are the presumed main route of entry into the bloodstream. HIV can also be directly absorbed through the mucous membranes that line the vagina and cervix.

Sexual transmission from men to women may be substantially more effective than transmission from women to men, particularly in the strains of HIV that are widespread in the developed nations. It has been estimated that there is anywhere from a three- to 19-fold excess risk for male-to-female over female-to-male sexual transmission among HIV-discordant couples. This difference has been documented in Africa, as well as Western countries, where more than 50 percent of those who have both HIV and AIDS are women, where heterosexual intercourse is the most common means of transmission of HIV for both sexes, and where homosexual sex is taboo. Other studies cited in United Nations (UN) reports indicate that women may be more susceptible to infection than men after a single exposure, a difference that may be attributable to the greater number of potential entry sites in the vagina than on the surface of the penis and to the fact that the vagina is exposed to a greater volume of infectious material during intercourse than the penis is.

Sexual Transmission from Women to Men Women can and do transmit STIs to men as well as to other women, and there are numerous documented cases of woman-to-man transmission of HIV. HIV, as with chlamydia, gonorrhea, herpes, syphilis, and other STIs, can thrive in the vaginal fluids, mucous tissues in the vagina, blood (including menstrual blood), and breast milk. STDs are readily passed between partners of either sex through open sores. Studies have also demonstrated a clear relationship between HIV infection in men and the presence of genital ulcers. Researchers hypothesize that genital ulcers in men serve the same function as breaks in the lining of the vagina by providing the virus a portal into the bloodstream. Men who have foreskins also have a higher risk, although slight, of acquiring HIV. A study from Rakai, Uganda, specifically related the increased risk to the size of the man's foreskin, rather than his being uncircumcised.

Other factors undoubtedly influence transmission during heterosexual genital intercourse. The presence of menstrual fluids, simultaneous infection with other organisms, skin conditions, prior exposure to chemicals that irritate the skin, and other conditions may all play a part.

Homosexual/Bisexual Transmission

For the first decade of the epidemic, male homosexuals and bisexuals, as well as INJECTION DRUG USE(R)s, were considered at high risk for HIV infection. Indeed, the growth of the epidemic in developed countries was often linked to gay and bisexual behavior. In the United States, the incidence rates among gay and bisexual men have declined, indicating changes in the epidemiology of AIDS. In the second decade of the epidemic, the focus shifted from designated high-risk groups to high-risk behavior. The sexual behavior between men most often related to HIV transmission is anal intercourse. The rectum is delicate and receives small tears through intercourse, placing the receptive partner at risk for infection from a positive insertive partner. There is also some risk involved in oral sex between men, as well as between men and women. Some cases of HIV transmission have been due to bleeding gums or sores in the mouth or throat that allowed HIV from semen to enter the blood system. This risk is acknowledged to be much lower than either receptive or insertive anal intercourse, in which mucous membranes from either partner are in potential contact with blood or semen.

Sexual Transmission from Women to Women As noted, women can and do transmit STDs to other women during sexual activity. Cases of woman-to-woman transmission of HIV have been reported, and it is now believed that the virus can indeed be transmitted in this way, although very little is known about the process. Researchers agree that while cervical secretions can carry HIV, menstrual blood does not carry it in the same potency as circulatory blood, which has a higher living cell density than other body fluids. The U.S. CENTERS FOR DISEASE CONTROL and Prevention (CDC) has so far not identified any particular high-risk sexual behavior between women and finds no reason to believe that lesbians are at a particularly high risk for transmitting HIV between partners.

Transmission via Contaminated Blood and Blood Products

HIV is present in the blood of both asymptomatic and symptomatic people as free virus particles and in infected cells. The number of free virus particles in the blood can rise to extremely high levels during the period of acute infection, shortly after a person has been exposed to the virus. Then, within weeks, viral levels decrease, and the virus nearly disappears from the blood. As the disease progresses, however, the number of T cells in the blood drops, and the number of free virus particles progressively rises again. In advanced HIV disease, there may be as many as a million free virus particles per milliliter of blood, as a large proportion of CD4 cells, each of which can produce thousands of virus particles daily, are infected.

Transmission by blood and body fluids can occur very efficiently through transfusion of HIV-contaminated blood or blood products or through the sharing of needles and other equipment used to inject drugs. Although safety has been a concern since the beginning of the era of transfusion medicine and although it is not unique to the AIDS epidemic, the advent of AIDS and HIV infection raised new concerns about the safety of the blood supply in the United States. Early in the epidemic, suspicions arose that AIDS could be transmitted by transfusion. In spring 1983, cases of AIDS diagnosed among hemophiliacs were believed to have been caused by clotting factor concentrates made from contaminated blood. Although the etiologic or causative agent of AIDS had not been identified in the early 1980s and no specific diagnostic tests were available, reports of cases among transfusion recipients and hemophiliacs eventually prompted blood banks to institute a variety of procedures to reduce the risk of AIDS associated with blood transfusions. Such procedures included efforts to exclude donors who were members of groups at high risk for the disease, studies of the use of tests that measured factors considered to be surrogate markers of AIDS (e.g., antibody to HEPATITIS B core antigen, T cell ratios), increased use of autologous donation (providing one's own blood for personal use), and reduction of unnecessary transfusions of blood and blood components.

After the virus, HIV, was identified and blood tests for the antibody to the virus became available in March 1985, blood collection organizations added this serologic test to their screening procedures. Despite the high sensitivity of HIV antibody tests, they do not detect all infected donors. A variable length of time elapses between acquisition of the virus and development of a detectable antibody response. Generally, this period is no more than a few months. During this so-called window period, the blood collected from an infected donor may test negative and infection thus will be undetected by the serologic screening mechanisms employed in most blood banks. Since the beginning of the testing of donated blood in the United States, cases of transfusion-related HIV have dropped to almost none. Despite this, gay and bisexual men are still banned from donating blood in the United States. Transfusion-related HIV transmission still occurs in some developing countries where extensive testing does not happen and where local needs for blood often outweigh the possibility of infection in an emergency.

Although HIV antibody tests cannot eliminate the possibility of transfusion-associated HIV infection, they have vastly improved the safety of the blood supply. Additional methods to detect infected units of blood are being explored to increase the sensitivity of serologic testing. These future methods include those based on recombinant deoxyribonucleic acid (DNA) technology, synthetic peptides, and gene-amplification techniques.

Injection drug users (IDUs) compose a population severely affected by AIDS. The spread of AIDS in the substance-abusing population occurs via two primary vectors. IDUs transmit HIV to other users through the use of unclean injection needles or other blood-contaminated drug apparatus. In addition, as with other populations at risk for AIDS, IDUs spread HIV to other drug users and nonusers alike through unsafe sexual activity. The use of injection drugs without disinfecting needles between uses and users is the prominent risk in the former category. Two drug injection practices in particular set the stage for HIV transmission during needle sharing: the initial drawing of blood into the barrel of the syringe to verify that the needle is inserted into a vein, and the practice of refilling the syringe repeatedly with blood after drug injection to rinse out any remaining drug. Hygienic needle use is hard to achieve for a variety of reasons, the two most obvious of which are the cost and availability of sterile needles and the lack of proper disinfecting after use. Hygienic needle use does not occur frequently enough to alter significantly the spread of HIV through blood and needles among IDUs. The AIDS risk-reduction message has, to date, not reached IDUs with the same impact as with gay and bisexual men. Many counselors and epidemiologists consider IDUs to be the second wave of the AIDS epidemic.

In China, HIV was transmitted to people who donated blood through unsafe donation practices used by the blood collection agencies. The poor were encouraged to sell their blood and plasma and often used the process to make money, pay taxes or school fees, and support their family financially. In the late 1980s, China banned imported blood and blood products, believing that HIV could be in the blood that had been imported into the country. Because the need for blood and blood plasma was still high, thousands of collection stations were set up around the country, particularly in the rural areas of China. When these collection stations collected plasma, they mixed the blood of all the local donors together, extracted the plasma, and then reinjected the remaining blood from the pooled donations into the donors to speed their recovery after the donation process. It is believed that a few HIV-positive injection drug users initially infected these pooled blood resources. By the early 2000s, China had blood donation HIV and AIDS cases in all provinces of the country, particularly centered in rural areas. The Chinese government has stated the number of HIV cases related to these procedures to be approximately 10 percent of the total number of HIV cases in the country, far surpassing transfusion or blood products cases in the rest of the world. United Nations (UN) estimates suggest a far higher number, closer to 30 percent. The UN still believes that there is reason for concern with the blood and blood products in China, as the pressure for supply often outweighs the availability of safely tested blood.

Transmission from Mother to Child during Pregnancy, Birth, and the Postpartum Period

In the mid-1980s, the idea that AIDS would become an epidemic of women and CHILDREN would have been met with considerable skepticism. But increasingly, women and children are becoming infected. Women are more vulnerable to HIV infection than men, in part because the direction of sexual spread favors male-to-female transmission. Worldwide HIV transmission to a child is the second most common mode of transmission after sexual transmission. About 25–35 percent of babies born to HIV-infected women have HIV infection, if HIV treatment is not available. The time from birth to the development of AIDS varies from weeks to years in a child, depending on the availability of medications, premature birth, and a variety of other factors.

The vast majority of AIDS cases in children are a result of transmission from mother to child during pregnancy or birth. Note that a woman can also transmit the virus to her infant during the postpartum period, the interval after birth, through BREAST-FEEDING. Clinical studies have found HIV in fetuses well before delivery, in umbilical cord blood obtained from the placenta, and in maternal blood lost during delivery.

Exposure to any of these sources of virus is a potential means of infection.

Transmission from Mother to Child during Pregnancy

It is possible to transmit the virus to the fetus in the uterus before birth. The virus has been isolated from the placenta, the amniotic fluid, and the fetal tissue. Infection may occur prenatally, at delivery, or through breast-feeding. The risk in each pregnancy may depend on such factors as whether the mother is undergoing acute HIV infection, how advanced the disease is, the woman's immunological state, or the gestational age of the infant at birth. The rate of transmission ranges widely. Studies have shown that women who have HIV base their reproductive choices on the same criteria used by noninfected women of similar socioeconomic and psychosocial status.

The question of whether infected mothers will give birth to infected infants has attracted enormous emotional attention in the HIV/AIDS pandemic. As early as 1982, only a few months after AIDS had been described as a new disease in adults by the CDC, children who had AIDS were reported in NORTH AMERICA and Europe. Even though the virus responsible for the disease had not yet been identified, the pediatricians involved were certain that the children had been infected either by their mother during pregnancy or through blood transfusions. Even though the description differed from that of genetic immune deficiencies, the medical community initially received these reports with skepticism, in part because these cases had been identified almost simultaneously in different geographical areas under widely differing circumstances. Today we know that factors associated with perinatal transmission include the characteristics of the mother's infection (her clinical status during pregnancy and her immune response to the virus), the integrity of the placental barrier, the virus itself, and the child's clinical status during exposure to HIV.

Studies show that fetuses can be infected with HIV as early as eight weeks after conception. By then, they already have the receptors that enable HIV to penetrate their T cells. However, HIV transmission also seems to occur at a later stage in pregnancy, as indicated by both the absence of clinical signs of infection in the newborn and the low number of virus particles in the blood, which therefore creates difficulties in detection by polymerase chain reaction or viral culture. By far, most children are infected during birth; studies demonstrate that 50–80 percent of vertical transmissions occurs at this point.

One of the central difficulties confronting researchers seeking to uncover how HIV passes from mother to child is the determination of whether or not HIV has passed. Babies do not enter this world complete with their own ready-made immune systems. They inherit some antibodies from their mothers; others, they develop themselves. A child's immune system takes more than a year to mature, and this process is by no means uniform. Some maternal antibodies disappear more quickly than others. Some of the child's own antibodies take longer to develop than others. Although a reliable indicator of HIV infection in an adult, the presence of HIV antibodies provides no reliable indication of an infant's HIV status. And because newborns lack fully developed immune systems, they naturally remain at high risk of contracting some of the OPPORTUNISTIC INFECTIONS (OIs) normally associated with HIV during the first 15 months of life.

The relationship between a pregnant woman's viral HIV levels and transmission of the virus to her child is important. A woman who is in the acute phase of HIV infection or later stages of infection has a higher rate of vertical transmission. A viral load less than 1,000 copies per mL has been shown to correlate to almost no risk of transmission regardless of whether a mother uses antiretroviral drugs prior to delivery or not. There is not, however, a viral load marker at which transmission never occurs or always occurs.

Transmission from Mother to Child during Birth While it is possible for HIV to pass from a pregnant woman to her fetus, a woman is most likely to transmit the virus to the fetus either immediately after she is infected or during childbirth. A low T cell count (below 300 per µL), anemia, inflammation of the placenta, the presence of other infections, and advanced AIDS in a woman may each increase the risk of transmission to the fetus and affect a woman's health and the progress of her pregnancy.

Every infant born to an HIV-positive woman will have its mother's antibodies in its blood and may test positive for HIV for a period of time even if it is not infected. Because the current standard antibody test cannot distinguish between the mother's and the infant's antibodies, it has been necessary to wait a few months to determine whether the infant is infected. New tests have been developed that can determine HIV infection in infants as young as three to six months, and researchers are seeking tests that can reliably detect infection in a fetus. Testing, however, is a complex issue. Some policy makers advocate routine testing of all newborns for HIV as a means of assessing the percentage of reproductive-age women who are infected with HIV. Those concerned with women's rights strenuously oppose any testing that is done without the informed consent of the mother. They argue persuasively that the time and money involved in widespread testing could be better spent on prevention, education, and treatment of HIV disease.

It is believed that the level of HIV in vaginal secretions and the birth canal increases the opportunity for vertical transmission. Studies have shown that different conditions can lead to higher HIV levels in the birth canal, such as smoking, vitamin A deficiencies, vaginal discharge, and open sores or ulcerations. Other conditions that can expose the child to more blood during birth include membrane ruptures, episiotomy, placental tearing, and amniocentesis. Cesarean sections have been recommended in some cases for HIV-positive women to reduce the amount of blood and vaginal secretions the child is exposed to, though use of antiretrovirals prior to birth have proven most effective when available. A research report published in the

July 26, 1997, issue of the *British Medical Journal* noted that cleansing the birth canal with an inexpensive antiseptic solution dramatically reduced postbirth infections, hospitalizations, and deaths. The investigators report that washing the birth canal with a very safe solution—0.25 percent chlorhexidine in sterile water—at each vaginal examination before delivery and then wiping the babies with the solution after delivery significantly reduced postpartum infection problems in both mothers and babies. Perhaps most significant was their finding that infant deaths related to sepsis, or bacteria in the bloodstream, were reduced threefold among babies in the intervention phase of the trial. Chlorhexidine has a long track record of safety, and the investigators noted no adverse reactions to the solution among mothers or babies. Chlorhexidine may also impede trasmission of HIV. The low cost, simplicity, and safety of this approach suggest that it may have a role in reducing illness and death associated with perinatal bacterial infections, which exact a considerable toll among women and neonates, especially in the developing world. Specifically, the cost of the antiseptic solution used in the study and the cotton to apply it was less than 10 cents per patient, making this a feasible approach for the most resource-poor settings.

Transmission from Mother to Child during Breast-Feeding BREAST-FEEDING has been a poorly understood and often ignored way that HIV can be passed to children. It was discovered in the mid-1980s that several mothers who became infected with HIV while breast-feeding had passed the virus onto their children. The WORLD HEALTH ORGANIZATION (WHO) passed guidelines stating that it was possible to transmit HIV in this manner but that it did not view breast milk as a major issue in the transmission of the virus. However, by the early 1990s, studies conducted predominantly in sub-Saharan Africa were showing the rates of infection for children who were breast-fed were significantly higher than for babies who were formula fed. Further studies in the late 1990s suggested that babies breast-fed for longer periods were more suscep-

tible to transmission of HIV than those breast-fed for shorter duration. Studies early in the 2000s showed that babies raised with mixed feeding were at higher risk for HIV transmission through breast-feeding than either babies exclusively breast-fed or those who were only formula fed. A study completed in 2006 in Botswana determined that during an outbreak of diarrhea in the country, babies of HIV-positive mothers who were breast-fed survived at a higher rate than did formula-fed babies of HIV-positive mothers. A study completed in 2008 highlighted the potential for a lactobacillus found in yogurt to prevent the spread of HIV by binding to the virus and preventing transmission. A study is under way in Tanzania to test this possibility.

Current WHO guidelines leave the choice to the mother but strongly encourage counseling prior to initiation of breast-feeding. The only sure, and completely safe, method to ensure HIV is not spread to a baby through breast-feeding is to use formula for the entirety of the process. WHO guidelines are expressed in the acronym AFASS, which stands for acceptability, feasibility, affordability, sustainability, and safety. *Acceptability* is important because in most cultures breast-feeding is the norm and expected. If a woman decides to formula feed, people in her family or community may assume she is HIV positive, and she, her child, or other family members may face discrimination and isolation. If formula feeding is not acceptable in her community, then it may not be practiced properly, and this will harm the baby more than not doing it at all. *Feasibility* refers to the time, skills, and knowledge required to formula feed. It takes a good amount of time to build a charcoal fire, heat the formula, allow it to cool, and follow the guidelines of the formula manufacturer to store the mixed formula properly. Mixed formula only stores for two hours in any condition without a refrigerator. A mother must be able to handle these various tasks, which involve large quantities of her time, to ensure proper feeding using formula. *Affordability* refers to the cost of the fuel, either wood or bottled gas, to have a fire; the cost of the formula itself;

and the cost of water to the mother to make the formula properly. In most countries, the cost of formula exceeds the minimum wage of the family and must be supplemented through programs that pay for the formula. *Sustainability* refers to the ability to maintain access to the water and formula for six months, as the baby needs this amount of time on formula to develop properly. Any disruption to the water supply or availability of formula can have serious consequences for the baby. *Safety* speaks to the need for a safe, secure water supply. It also refers to the need to boil the water and the utensils used in the preparation of the formula to prevent any germs from causing illness in the baby. This is one of the most important issues in formula preparation in resource-poor areas of the world.

Transmission from HIV-Positive Patients to Health Care Workers

The transmission of HIV from an infected patient to an uninfected health care worker is possible if the health care worker accidentally cuts himself or herself during surgery or is stuck by a needle that contains infected blood from the patient. This kind of on-the-job exposure to HIV is known as occupational exposure. It can also occur if a health care worker has open wounds or skin abrasions that have contact with an infected patient's blood or other virus-laden body fluids. Exposure to any infectious agent that involves a cut, abrasion, or break in the skin—including a break caused by a needlestick—is referred to as percutaneous exposure.

Transmission of HIV in this manner is rare but does occur. Treatment with antiretrovirals has proven to be useful for health care workers. This is called POST-EXPOSURE PROPHYLAXIS (PEP). It is readily available to any health care worker who feels his or her safety has been compromised through a needlestick accident, surgical accident, or even incidents involving difficult-to-restrain patients when, for instance, biting or scratching of the health care worker has occurred. Although PEP can last from one month to a year, depending on the need, it must be remembered that it is the same antiretroviral treatment an HIV-positive person would use, with all the side effects as possibilities.

Transmission from HIV-Positive Health Care Workers to Patients

In the United States, the only verified case of transmission from a health care worker to patients involved a dentist who infected six of his patients. The mode of transmission in this case remains unknown. Testing of the dentist's 1,100 patients by the CDC revealed nine who were HIV infected. Infections in three of them proved to be unrelated to the dentist: Not only did all three have a history of recognized risk factors, but molecular analyses showed that the viral strains present in these three patients were only distantly genetically related to the viral strain present in the dentist. Viruses isolated from the remaining six patients, however, were closely related to the virus from the dentist. Studies of other HIV-positive health care workers have shown no cases of transmission from doctors, nurses, or aides to patients.

Secondary Routes of Transmission

Aside from the three primary routes of transmission, HIV may be transmitted through nonsexual contact with body fluids and secretions other than blood, including cerebrospinal fluid, donated sperm, transplanted organs, and vaginal and cervical secretions. Other body fluids such as tears and urine are as yet unproven routes of transmission. Transmission via saliva may be possible through deep kissing—French or tongue kissing—which could possibly lead to infection, especially if open sores are present on the lips, tongue, or mouth. Note that, to date, this route of transmission has not been confirmed; only one case of such a transmission has been investigated by the CDC, and no proof found.

HIV has been transmitted in rare instances in the home among family members, outside sexual activity. All cases involved family members responsible for the care of an HIV-positive individual. However, simple precautions can reduce these occurrences. Latex or polyure-thane gloves should be worn during any injection or other event in which blood is present, such as changing bandages, stopping bleeding after a wound has been sustained, or disposing of bloody materials. Hands should be washed after any incident involving blood. Personal care items should never be shared, particularly those that may unintentionally involve blood contact, such as a toothbrush or razor.

It is theoretically possible to transmit HIV through activities such as body piercing, tattooing, or acupuncture. No cases of HIV transmission from body piercing or tattooing have ever been recorded, though cases of HEPATITIS B have been reported, and it is possible that this could happen. People who choose to have tattooing or body piercing need to select the tattoo or piercing location based on cleanliness, use of sterile needles and equipment, and use of latex gloves during the process by the tattoo or piercing employee. Any questions about the sterilization of equipment must be asked prior to choosing the business for the piercing or tattoo. One confirmed case of HIV transmission has occurred during an acupuncture treatment. Although acupuncture involves the insertion of needles into a patient, it is generally not to a depth that would draw blood. However, it is possible for any number of needle pricks to occur to a patient or an acupuncturist.

How HIV Is Not Transmitted

The major myth is that HIV infection is easy to contract. This is not the case, as the virus is vulnerable to the air and is killed by household cleaning products if, for instance, blood from a cut spills onto a kitchen counter. HIV is not found in human sweat. Having casual contact with an HIV-positive person does not allow the virus to spread. Hugging, touching, and holding hands cannot spread the virus.

HIV is found in very low quantities in the saliva and tears of HIV-positive people during the acute and final phases of the illness. The amount found in these substances has never been proven to be enough to transmit the infection. Kissing on the cheek, crying on a person's shoulder, or doing anything similar will not transmit the virus. Spitting has occasionally been in the news, particularly in the setting of police activities. No cases of HIV have been spread in this manner, as the saliva does not contain enough of the virus to cause infection. Despite the high-profile reports of prisoners spitting at guards or police officers, this is considered a no-risk event.

Insects do not spread HIV, unlike plague or MALARIA. HIV particles have not been found in biting insects, and the virus dies quickly once an insect has bitten a human. Studies of biting insects show that an insect rests between meals of human blood, and the virus dies during this digestion time.

Unlike the common cold, sneezing does not spread HIV. It is not spread by water, as is cholera. If it were spread in any of these ways, the pattern of the epidemic would be far different from what it is: Either entire households would be affected, or individuals would be affected randomly, or the epidemic's spread would be determined by climate, altitude, quality of the water supply, and other such environmental factors. That is not the case for the epidemic of HIV.

HIV is spread in specific ways: sexual contact, blood-to-blood contact, and mother-to-infant transmission. These modes were established early in the epidemic, and continuing surveillance over a period of more than 30 years (ca. 1980 to date) has revealed no additional routes of transmission. There is no evidence that HIV is transmitted by casual contact, including talking, shaking hands, hugging, or ordinary kissing; sharing kitchens, lunchrooms, dishes, or eating utensils; touching floors, walls, doorknobs, or toilet seats; sharing offices, restrooms, computers, telephones, or writing utensils; being bitten by mosquitoes, fleas, bedbugs, and other insects. Note that if precautions are taken to prevent blood-to-blood contact, there is no evidence that HIV transmission occurs in a nonsexual, nonneedle-sharing relationship with a person who is HIV positive.

AVAC: Global Advocacy for HIV Prevention. "HIV Prevention News." AVAC.org. Available online. URL: http://www.avac.org/. Accessed April 9, 2011.

AVERT: AVERTing HIV and AIDS. "Becoming Infected, Transmission and Testing." AVERT.org. Available online. URL: http://www.avert.org/transmission. htm. Accessed April 9, 2011.

———. "HIV and AIDS in China." AVERT.org. Available online. URL: http://www.avert.org/aidschina. htm. Accessed April 9, 2011.

———. "HIV and Breastfeeding." AVERT.org. Available online. URL: http://www.avert.org/hiv-breast feeding.htm. Accessed April 9, 2011.

Centers for Disease Control and Prevention. "Basic Information about HIV and AIDS." CDC.gov. Available online. URL: http://www.cdc.gov/hiv/topics/ basic/index.htm. Accessed April 9, 2011.

———. "HIV Transmission." CDC.gov. Available online. URL: http://www.cdc.gov/hiv/resources/ qa/transmission.htm. Accessed April 9, 2011.

Hafez, S., H. El Tonsi, and M. Lofty. "Contraceptives, HIV Infections and Heterosexual Transmission." *International Conference on AIDS 1989.* Abstract. Available online. URL: http://gateway.nlm.nih.gov/Meet ingAbstracts/ma?f=102178391.html. Accessed April 9, 2011.

HIVInSite. "Sexual Transmission of HIV: Related Resources." HIVInSite.ucsf.edu. Available online. URL: http://hivinsite.ucsf.edu/InSite?page=kbr-07 -02-01. Accessed April 9, 2011.

Hofmeyr, G. Justus, and James McIntyre. "Preventing Perinatal Infections." *BMJ* 315 (26 July 1997): 199–200.

Kantor, Elizabeth, M.D. "HIV Transmission and Prevention in Prisons." HIVInSite.ucsf.edu. Available online. URL: http://hivinsite.ucsf.edu/InSite ?page=kb-07-04-13. Accessed April 9, 2011.

McGowan, Joseph P., and Sanjiv S. Shah. "Prevention of Perinatal HIV Transmission during Pregnancy." *Journal of Antimicrobial Chemotherapy* 46, no. 5 (2000): 657–668.

Minnesota AIDS Project. "HIV Transmission." MN AIDSProject.org. Available online. URL: http:// www.mnaidsproject.org/learn/transmission.htm. Accessed April 9, 2011.

San Francisco AIDS Foundation. "How HIV Is Spread." SFAF.org. Available online. URL: http://www.sfaf. org/aids101/transmission.html#assessment. Accessed April 9, 2011.

Tanya. "Foreskin Surface Area and HIV Acquisition: It's the Size That Matters." MedIndia.net. Available online. URL: http://www.medindia.net/news/ Foreskin-Surface-Area-and-HIV-Acquisition-Its-the-Size-That-Matters-60237-1.htm. Accessed April 9, 2011.

UNAIDS: Joint United Nations Programme on HIV/AIDS. "HIV Transmission in Intimate Partner Relationships in Asia." UNAIDS.org. Available online. URL: http:// www.unaids.org/en/Resources/PressCentre/Feature stories/2009/August/20090811Intimatepartners/. Accessed April 9, 2011.

United States Department of Health and Human Services. "Perinatal Guidelines." www.aidsinfo.nih. gov. Available online. URL: http://www.aidsinfo. nih.gov/Guidelines/GuidelineDetail.aspx?Guide lineID=9. Accessed April 9, 2011.

U.S. News and World Report. "Circumcision Doesn't Lessen HIV Transmission." USNews.com. Available online. URL: http://www.usnews.com/health/family -health/womens-health/articles/2009/07/16/cir cumcision-doesnt-lessen-hiv-transmission.html. Accessed April 9, 2011.

Triomune Triomune is the trade name for the generic pill that contains NEVIRAPINE, LAMIVUDINE, and STAVUDINE. Triomune is probably the most common generic antiretroviral combination pill used in the treatment of HIV. Cipra Limited, a large Indian generic drug manufacturer, initially manufactured the medication. It is also sold under other trade names and manufactured by other companies. It was the first generic combination therapy pill approved by the President's Emergency Plan for AIDS Relief (PEPFAR), the U.S. program established to pay for antiretroviral medications for people in other countries. This combination is *not* approved for use in the United States.

Dosage

Triomune and other generic brands of this combination are manufactured to be taken as one pill, twice a day. Triomune for adults contains 40 mg of stavudine, 150 mg of lamivudine, and 200 mg of nevirapine. There are also formulations for adolescents and CHILDREN as well as a liquid formulation for babies.

There has been concern whether the three drugs combined into one pill would be as effective as the three drugs taken individually. There has also been concern that the combination pill created by a generic manufacturer from three generic pills would be as effective as the three patented medications individually or combined. Studies conducted in Uganda and Malawi have shown that Triomune has good efficacy over a long period in HIV patients who take the medication as required. Although there is some difference in the levels of stavudine in the body between the combination pill and those when taken individually, this has proven not to be a complication to the pill's working well in preventing HIV replication. It has also been shown that generic drug manufacturers can and do maintain proper levels of the required drug in their medications to ensure effectiveness in treating HIV. The U.S. FOOD AND DRUG ADMINISTRATION (FDA) has approved more than 100 generic formulations of individual drugs or combination pills by various manufacturers in India, China, and South Africa for use in the PEPFAR program. One of the major advantages of generic pills is the cost savings to patients. A standard treatment of the three drugs in Triomune would cost an uninsured person approximately US $1,500 a month. The generic combination pill costs a patient about US $35 each month.

Drug Interactions

Drug interactions for Triomune are the same potential interactions that would occur if a person took the three drugs individually.

Nevirapine, one of the drugs in Triomune, can interact with some PROTEASE INHIBITORS (PIs) and significantly reduce their effectiveness in treating HIV infection. It does not affect the PIs NELFINAVIR and ritonavir. People who use methadone may need to have their dosage of that drug adjusted, as nevirapine can reduce the amount of methadone in the blood, causing withdrawal

symptoms in patients. The herbal supplement St. John's wort should not be taken while on Triomune, as it reduces the amount of nevirapine in the body. Antifungal drugs such as ketoconazole and antibiotics such as clarithromycin also interact with nevirapine, and a doctor will need to evaluate these types of drugs before prescribing them at the same time as Triomune.

Stavudine, one of the drugs in Triomune, interacts with several different medications, so patients should check with a doctor prior to starting treatment with stavudine. Stavudine should not be taken at the same time as ZIDOVUDINE. These drugs are antagonistic, meaning they work against each other, decreasing the overall effectiveness of both medications. The side effects of both drugs can also increase if prescribed together. Ribavirin is a drug used in the treatment of HEPATITIS C. If Triomune and ribavirin are prescribed together, the effectiveness of Triomune is greatly reduced.

Triomune should also not be prescribed with DIDANOSINE; didanosine and stavudine both cause certain side effects. Use of the drugs together increases greatly the chance that the patient will become affected by peripheral NEUROPATHY, one of the main side effects of stavudine. Other medications that can also increase the chance of peripheral neuropathy are dapsone, amphotericin B, and foscarnet, all of which can be used in treating various HIV-related OPPORTUNISTIC INFECTIONS (OIs).

Triomune should not be prescribed with intravenous pentamadine, used in the treatment of *MYCOBACTERIUM AVIUM* COMPLEX (MAC). The stavudine in Triomune increases the risk of pancreatitis.

Side Effects

Side effects of Triomune are the same potential side effects that would occur if a person took the three drugs contained in the pill individually.

The most common potential side effects when taking Triomune include headache, nausea, fever, rash, and vomiting. Nevirapine is often the cause of these initial side effects, and people are often given a start-up dose of nevirapine, which increases over a period of two weeks, to reduce the potential initial side effects. After the start-up dose, a switch to the combination pill can occur. If a rash develops and becomes more severe over time, a person will need to stop taking Triomune. A potentially fatal reaction known as Stevens-Johnson syndrome has been recorded in people taking nevirapine. Stevens-Johnson syndrome is a severe allergic reaction to a medication. Symptoms of the syndrome include inflammation and redness of the eyes, blistering rashes, aching muscles and joints, prolonged fever, and general exhaustion. Cases of liver toxicity have also occurred. WOMEN who have CD4 counts greater than 250 per μL of blood and men who have CD4 counts greater than 400 are at greatest risk of liver problems, but this reaction can potentially happen to anyone. People starting Triomune will need to be monitored for any liver problems during the course of treatment.

Triomune can cause the same side effects as stavudine, one of three drugs found in the combination pill, whose use can lead to peripheral neuropathy as well as LIPODYSTROPHY. Peripheral neuropathy is nerve damage that can cause mild pain and tingling in the hands, feet, and legs and can become quite severe over time. Lipodystrophy is the loss or shifting of fat in the body. People who have lipodystrophy can suffer from facial wasting; loss of fat in the arms, buttocks, and legs; accumulation of fat in the breasts and shoulder areas; as well as lipomas, fatty deposits, generally in the trunk of the body.

Alcorn, Keith. "Triomune Approved for PEPFAR Use." AIDSmap.com. Available online. URL: http://www.aidsmap.com/en/news/2A58F359-908B-433E-945C-A45ECC176AD4.asp. Accessed April 9, 2011.

Barlow-Mosha, L., et al. "Early Effectiveness of Triomune in HIV Infected Ugandan Children." AEGIS.com. Available online. URL: http://www.aegis.com/conferences/iashivpt/2005/WeOa0103.html. Accessed April 9, 2011.

Hosseinpour, Mina C., et al. "Pharmacokinetic Comparison of Generic and Trade Formulations of Lamivudine, Stavudine and Nevirapine in HIV-Infected Malawian Adults." *AIDS* 21, no. 1 (3 January 2007): 59–64.

Oyugi, J. H., et al. "Treatment Outcomes and Adherence to Generic Triomune and Maxivir Therapy in Kampala, Uganda." NIH.gov. Available online. URL: http://gateway.nlm.nih.gov/MeetingAbstracts/ma?f=102283470.html. Accessed April 9, 2011.

United States Food and Drug Administration. "President's Emergency Plan for AIDS Relief." FDA.gov. Available online. URL: http://www.fda.gov/internationalprograms/fdabeyondourbordersforeignoffices/asiaandafrica/ucm119231.htm. Accessed April 9, 2011.

Trizivir   Trizivir is the trade name for a multidrug combination antiretroviral pill. It is composed of three other antiretrovirals, LAMIVUDINE, ZIDOVUDINE, and ABACAVIR. All of these drugs are NUCLEOSIDE REVERSE TRANSCRIPTASE INHIBITORS (NRTIs), and therefore Trizivir is also an NRTI. It is manufactured by GlaxoSmithKline and was approved by the U.S. FOOD AND DRUG ADMINISTRATION (FDA) in 2000. It is not approved for use in CHILDREN less than 12 years of age.

Dosage

One Trizivir tablet two times a day is the recommended dose. Each Trizivir tablet contains 300 mg of abacavir, 150 mg of lamivudine, and 300 mg of zidovudine. Trizivir is generally prescribed in combination with at least one other antiretroviral because all of the drugs in Trizivir are in the same class of drugs, NRTIs. Research has shown that generally it is best to combine at least two classes of antiretrovirals to suppress HIV in the body.

Drug Interactions

Trizivir has the same drug interactions that lamivudine, zidovudine, and abacavir have individually. Trizivir is never prescribed with lamivudine, zidovudine, abacavir, COMBIVIR, or EPZICOM. Because Trizivir is a combination of lamivudine, zidovudine, and abacavir, it would be dangerous to increase the doses of any of these drugs. Epzicom and Combivir are combination drugs that also contain abacavir, zidovudine, and/

or lamivudine and would not be prescribed at the same time for the same reasons. The drugs EMTRICITABINE and TRUVADA, which contains emtricitabine, are not generally prescribed at the same time as Trizivir, as emtricitabine is very similar to lamivudine, and it is not believed that prescribing them at the same time offers any benefit to the patient.

Abacavir decreases the amount of the drug methadone in the body. People who are taking methadone to manage the symptoms of heroin withdrawal may need to have the dosage of that medication increased by a physician. Using any type of alcohol while taking Epzicom increases the amount of abacavir in the body. This can increase the side effects of abacavir and raise the probability of suffering one of those side effects.

Lamivudine increases in concentration in the body of a person who is taking trimethoprim/sulfamethoxazole (TMP-SMX), an antibiotic used for prevention and treatment of PNEUMOCYSTIS PNEUMONIA (PCP). People who are using Epzicom may need to adjust the dosage of TMP-SMX if their doctor believes this could cause problems.

Zidovudine interacts with several other drugs. It is not generally prescribed with either ZALCITABINE or STAVUDINE, two other NRTIs, as they have been shown in lab testing to interact negatively with each other. Because they are processed in the liver in the same manner, aspirin, acetaminophen, and benzodiazepines (Valium and others) present risk of increased zidovudine concentrations in the body, which may increase side effects of the drug, particularly anemia. Check with a physician regarding all of the potential drug interactions of zidovudine.

Side Effects

Trizivir contains abacavir. Between 3 percent and 8 percent of people who take abacavir have an allergic reaction to the drug. Research into the reaction has shown that this is caused by an inherited genetic marker named *HLA-B*5701*. There is an inexpensive test that is recommended for all people who are planning to take abacavir or one of the multidrug combination pills that contain abacavir. This test will determine whether a person carries this genetic marker. If it is determined that someone carries the *HLA-B*5701* marker, he or she will not be prescribed abacavir in any form. *HLA-B*5701* is one of the numerous genes that play a role in the HUMAN IMMUNE SYSTEM, allowing the body to fight off viruses and other pathogens. HLA stands for human leukocyte antigen. The allergic reaction occurs less often among men and people of African descent.

Signs of an allergic reaction to Trizivir can include fever, rash, headache, stomach pain, vomiting, diarrhea, coughing, or respiratory illness. People who suspect that they are having a reaction should immediately talk to a physician about their symptoms, as in some cases the reaction can lead to severe illness or death. The reaction most often occurs within the first two weeks of beginning Trizivir. A person who is having such a reaction should never use abacavir in any form again, as the reaction will worsen the next time the medication is taken. Some people who have stopped taking Trizivir for reasons other than the allergic reaction have suffered the reaction when they restarted Trizivir. It is generally recommended that a person who stops taking Trizivir for any reason consult a physician before restarting the drug.

Common side effects, not related to the potential allergic reaction, include stomach upset, headache, tiredness, and loss of appetite. These lessen over time while taking the drug. NRTIs have been implicated in increased fat levels in the blood as well as LIPODYSTROPHY, changes in fat in the body, .

NRTIs have also been shown to cause LACTIC ACIDOSIS and liver disease in a small number of people. Severe pain in the upper abdomen and lower back, as well as severe nausea, can be signs of lactic acidosis. Enlarged spleen, pancreas, or liver can also be a sign of the condition. It is important that all medications be stopped if a physician diagnoses this condition. Liver markers in the blood are always monitored during regular BLOOD WORK/BLOOD TESTS to watch for these conditions, but any symptoms should be reported to a doctor. This reaction to NRTIs is more prevalent among WOMEN, obese people, and people who have advanced HIV disease but can occur at any time.

An increase in heart attacks among people taking abacavir has also been noted in studies, particularly among those already at risk for heart attacks. Those risk factors include being male, having high cholesterol, having high blood pressure, being obese, and smoking.

Abacavir is listed as a pregnancy category C drug. It has been shown to cause death or birth defects in laboratory animals. No studies of abacavir have been done among pregnant women, and it is unknown whether abacavir causes changes in breast milk for women who are BREAST-FEEDING babies. It is only recommended for pregnant or breast-feeding women if the benefits clearly outweigh the potential risks of the drug.

A rare side effect of zidovudine is muscle deterioration, myopathy, including of the heart muscle. People who have taken zidovudine for long periods are at greatest risk of developing myopathy. Severe anemia and bone marrow suppression can also occur in some people taking zidovudine. Signs of this condition are unusual weakness or exhaustion, paler skin tone than normal, fevers, or chills. A physician should be notified if these symptoms occur.

AIDS InfoNet. "Trizivir (Zidovudine + Abacavir + Lamivudine)." AIDSInfoNet.org. Available online. URL: http://www.aidsinfonet.org/fact_sheets/view/418. Accessed March 11, 2011.

AIDSmeds. "Special Issues for Children with HIV." AIDSmeds.com. Available online. URL: http://www.aidsmeds.com/articles/Children_7566.shtml. Accessed March 11, 2011.

———. "Trizivir (Abacavir + Zidovudine + Lamivudine)." AIDSmeds.com. Available online. URL: http://www.aidsmeds.com/archive/Trizivir_1583.shtml. Accessed March 11, 2011.

The Body. "Trizivir (AZT/3TC/Abacavir)." TheBody.com. Available online. URL: http://www.thebody.com/index/treat/trizivir.html. Accessed March 11, 2011.

Highleyman, Liz. "HLA-B*5701 Screening for Abacavir (Ziagen) Hypersensitivity." HIVandHepatitis.com. Available online. URL: http://www.hivandhepatitis.com/recent/2008/022608_c.html. Accessed April 9, 2011.

United States Department of Health and Human Services. "Abacavir/Lamivudine/Zidovudine." aidsinfo.nih.gov. Available online. URL: http://www.aidsinfo.nih.gov/DrugsNew/DrugDetailNT.aspx?int_id=325. Accessed March 11, 2011.

Truvada Truvada is the brand name of the combination pill that contains EMTRICITABINE and TENOFOVIR DISOPROXIL FUMARATE. It is manufactured by Gilead Sciences. The U.S. FOOD AND DRUG ADMINISTRATION (FDA) approved it in 2004, as a combination, once-a-day pill to be used in the treatment of HIV. It must be taken in combination with at least one other antiretroviral, as it contains just two medications. Truvada, like both the drugs it contains, is effective against the HEPATITIS B virus (HBV). Although not approved by the FDA for the treatment of HBV, this drug can effectively control the viral load of a person who has HBV and may be used by some doctors for this purpose. Truvada has not been studied extensively for use in people who are both HBV and HIV positive.

Dosage

It is prescribed in a pill form and contains 200 mg of emtricitabine and 300 mg of tenofovir disoproxil fumarate. One pill is taken each day. People who have limited kidney function may be prescribed a lower dosage and monitored closely while taking Truvada. Truvada can be taken with or without food, as absorption is not affected by food.

Drug Interactions

Both emtricitabine and tenofovir disoproxil fumarate have some drug interactions, and both sets of those interactions apply to Truvada. Emtricitabine and tenofovir will not be prescribed at the same time as Truvada. ATRIPLA, a multidrug combination pill, contains both emtricitabine and tenofovir disoproxil fumarate and will not be prescribed concurrently with Truvada. Another medication used in the treatment of HBV is adefovir. It is similar in structure to tenofovir and is not prescribed at the same time as Truvada. LAMIVUDINE is similar in structure to emtricitabine and any combination pill of lamivudine, such as EPZICOM, COMBIVIR, or TRIZIVIR, will not be prescribed at the same time as Truvada.

Tenofovir can increase the amount of DIDANOSINE in the body. People who are taking didanosine and Truvada may need to adjust the dosage of didanosine and have their blood levels of the drug monitored to prevent any potential side effects of too much didanosine.

ATAZANAVIR SULFATE, DARUNAVIR, and KALETRA (ritonavir and lopinavir) can all increase the amount of tenofovir in the body. This may increase liver function problems in some patients. Close monitoring of blood work may need to accompany prescribing these drugs and Truvada at the same time. Patients who do take atazanavir and Truvada concurrently will need to take ritonavir to boost the amount of atazanavir in the blood to correct treatment levels, as atazanavir levels are lowered when combined with Truvada.

Side Effects

Because Truvada is effective against HBV, stopping the drug will have the potential effect of allowing the HBV to reactivate and begin reproducing again. This can cause a rebound of hepatitis symptoms and potentially life-threatening liver problems. A person who is taking this medication who also has HBV needs to be monitored by a doctor before stopping this drug or switching to another treatment for HIV. HBV viral rebound can be a serious condition if not monitored closely. A different HBV medication may be prescribed to fight the HBV if Truvada is no longer an optimal treatment for HIV.

LACTIC ACIDOSIS is a serious condition of the blood in which lactic acid builds up, at times fairly quickly. Cases of lactic acidosis have been recorded in conjunction with use of an antiretroviral combination that contains any NUCLEOSIDE REVERSE TRANSCRIPTASE INHIBITORS (NRTIs). Lactic acidosis can overwhelm the liver and spleen, causing life-threatening failure of those organs. WOMEN are more likely to develop lactic acidosis. Obesity and length of time a person is on a HIGHLY ACTIVE ANTIRETROVIRAL THERAPY (HAART) regimen containing an NRTI are also believed to be factors.

Some drug studies have indicated that the tenofovir in Truvada may lead to a lessening of bone density in people taking the drug. It has not been linked with assurance to the drug, but many reports conclude that this is a side effect of tenofovir. Older patients taking Truvada may need to be monitored for bone density problems. Patients who have low-impact fracturing of bones may need to be taken off Truvada if this is the case. Research is continuing to examine the potential effect of tenofovir on bone density.

Side effects that are commonly reported with Truvada include diarrhea, gas, bloating, and nausea. Many of these symptoms lessen with time on the drug. Truvada is generally well tolerated, and the side effects discussed are generally rare. It is one of the medications listed as preferred for use by the U.S. government treatment guidelines.

AIDS InfoNet. "Truvada (Tenofovir + Emtricitabine)." AIDSInfoNet.org. Available online. URL: http://www.aidsinfonet.org/fact_sheets/view/421. Accessed March 11, 2011.

AIDSmeds. "Special Issues for Children with HIV." AIDSmeds.com. Available online. URL: http://www.aidsmeds.com/articles/Children_7566.shtml. Accessed March 11, 2011.

———. "Truvada (Tenofovir + Emtricitabine)." AIDS meds.com. Available online. URL: http://www.aids meds.com/archive/Truvada_1584.shtml. Accessed March 11, 2011.

The Body. "Truvada (Tenofovir/FTC)." TheBody.com. Available online. URL: http://www.thebody.com/index/treat/truvada.html. Accessed March 11, 2011.

United States Department of Health and Human Services. "Emtricitabine/Tenofovir Disoproxil Fumarate." aidsinfo.nih.gov. Available online. URL: http://www.aidsinfo.nih.gov/drugsNew/DrugDetailNT.aspx?int_id=406. Accessed March 11, 2011.

tuberculosis Tuberculosis (TB) is a bacterial infection, predominantly caused by the *Mycobacterium tuberculosis* bacteria in the United States. Sometimes it may be referred to as the *M. tuberculosis* complex, as other *Mycobacterium* species can cause tuberculosis, though these are most often found outside the United States. Other varieties include *M. africanum,* a common cause of TB in parts of AFRICA; *M. canetti*, rarely seen but mainly found in the Horn of Africa; and *M. bovis*, a common form of TB that in the past spread to humans from cows through their milk but has become less common in the Western world since the advent of pasteurization of milk. All can cause TB in humans.

Statistics show that approximately one-third of all humans have been infected with TB. Nearly one-third of HIV-positive people in the world have been infected with TB. TB is the leading killer of HIV-infected people in the world today. In the United States, 9 percent of HIV-positive people and 16 percent of HIV-positive people between the ages of 25 and 44 years old are infected with TB. U.S. CENTERS FOR DISEASE CONTROL and Prevention (CDC) statistics show that 63 percent of these HIV/TB-infected people in the United States are non-Hispanic black individuals, making this a serious dual infection among AFRICAN AMERICANS in the United States.

Symptoms and Diagnostic Path

TB is a relatively slow-growing bacterium that divides only once every 16–20 hours. Most bacteria divide about once every hour. TB is spread predominantly through the air. Once a bacterium is inhaled, it settles into the lung. TB first infects the alveoli, the small cavities in the lungs that allow gases such as oxygen and carbon dioxide to be exchanged in the blood. The macrophages in the alveoli ingest the bacteria, and often granulomas form around the bacteria as the body's immune system attempts to fight the infection. From the lungs, the bacteria are transported via the lymph system to other parts of the body, where they also reproduce. Common areas of secondary infection can be the bones, brain, kidneys, and lymph nodes. Once infected, approximately 10 percent of people with TB will develop an active infection; the other 90 percent will not. An active infection means that someone who has TB can spread the illness to others. Someone who has an inactive TB infection is said to have latent TB infection (LTBI).

Symptoms of an active TB infection include a prolonged cough that is racking in nature and produces sputum and occasionally blood; other symptoms include fever, chills, night sweats, fatigue, weight loss, and pain with the coughing. TB that has spread to other areas of the body can produce a variety of symptoms that may not be initially recognized, including localized pain, stiffness if it involves the bones, and swelling of the lymph nodes if it involves them.

The standard test in the United States to determine whether a person has been infected with TB is called the Mantoux test. A doctor inserts a needle that contains an extract of the TB bacteria under the skin. After two days, the doctor examines the spot where the injection was done. If a small, hard bump appears, then it may mean that a person has been infected with TB. There are some people for whom the test does not work or who may register a false-positive result, meaning the test result looks positive but there is no TB infection. This can occur in anyone who has received the bacille Calmette-Guérin (BCG) vaccine against TB or who has an active *Mycobacterium avium* infection that is not TB related. A new test called the QuantiFERON®-TB Gold test (QFT) has been approved by the United States and other countries as a simple blood test that can produce accurate results within 24 hours.

After a positive result from a skin or blood test, the patient will probably be given a chest X-ray to look for lung infection or nodes in the lungs that may suggest a disseminated infection. Sputum will also be gathered to try to culture the *M. tuberculosis* in a lab to show the type of infection involved. Other tissue samples, such as biopsies of a lymph node, skin lesion, or lung fluid, may be taken to try to culture the bacteria if the doctor thinks the infection may be disseminated.

All HIV-positive people should receive a TB skin test and a chest X-ray upon their initial diagnosis to determine whether they already have had TB or might have an LTBI. Because of the grave nature of a dual diagnosis of TB and HIV, precaution warrants these tests. Ongoing yearly skin tests are recommended for any HIV-positive persons, particularly those who travel extensively, work in close settings with large numbers of people, or work in prisons, hospitals, or social service professions.

HIV-positive people who are diagnosed with severe immunodeficiency will need to be tested for TB prior to starting HIGHLY ACTIVE ANTIRETROVIRAL THERAPY (HAART). Many cases of people who had unknown TB results or LTBIs, started HAART, and had a severe reaction to the restoration of the immune system have been recorded. This reaction is called IMMUNE RECONSTITUTION INFLAMMATORY SYNDROME (IRIS). The body suddenly has a functioning immune system again and, in a sense, overreacts to a previous infection and causes a worsening of the symptoms of the detected infection. This generally occurs with TB within the first two months of a patient's starting HAART. The treatment most often involves the addition of corticosteroids in severe cases or nonsteroidal anti-inflammatory drugs, such as acetaminophen, in nonsevere cases.

Treatment Options and Outlook

Since treatments for TB first were found in the early 1940s, TB has proven remarkably fast at developing resistance to the medications used in treatment. Initial treatment was done with only one drug. Currently, three or four drugs are given to a person who has active TB. Because treatment lasts a long time, generally at least a

year in length, people often forget to take their medications or simply stop because of the cost or other factors. This tendency has led to the development of multiple-drug-resistant tuberculosis (MDR TB), which cannot be treated with the most common first-line drugs (rifampin and isoniazid), and extensively drug-resistant tuberculosis (XDR TB), which cannot be treated with first- or second-line anti-TB drugs (rifampin, isoniazid, and other drugs used to treat MDR TB). First-line drugs are those that are generally used first in the treatment of a particular illness. *Second-line* refers to those drugs used when the first-line drugs cannot be. Testing for drug resistance in lab samples will reveal the drugs that are best suited to fight the infection in a person. MDR TB and XDR TB have been found in the United States and every other region of the world. XDR TB has been especially virulent among HIV-positive people in southern Africa and large urban areas of the world such as Delhi and New York City.

Because of the severity of TB in conjunction with HIV, all HIV-positive individuals who are suspected of having LTBI need to have a chest X-ray and clinical tests to rule out possible active infection and to confirm a latent diagnosis. If the tests show LTBI and rule out active TB, then all HIV-positive people should begin treatment for the TB. The first line of treatment for people with LTBI is isoniazid given daily if the patient is able to handle the dosage, or twice weekly if there is some concern about the ability to manage the dosage. Patients also receive pyridoxine to prevent possible NEUROPATHY as a side effect of the isoniazid. This medication will be given for nine months, at which time the treatment is considered complete. People who have LTBI that is resistant to isoniazid should receive rifampin. HIV-positive people who have XDR LTBI should receive a course of drug therapy that includes one or two drugs that will be chosen according to the resistance tests conducted on the TB bacteria.

For active TB in an HIV-positive individual, treatment should be started immediately with a multidrug regimen. This can begin killing the TB bacteria and prevent drug resistance. What is known as directly observed therapy (DOT) is also practiced during the treatment of an HIV-positive TB-infected person. This means that the infected person is observed taking the medication on a regular basis by the doctor or other medical personnel so that the medication can work and the patient does not forget to take or stop taking the medication, which would increase the chance that TB would transform into MDR TB or XDR TB.

The first line of drug therapy for someone who is HIV positive involves the use of isoniazid, rifampin (or rifabutin), ethambutol, and pyrazinamide for a period of two months, followed by four months of isoniazid and rifampin (or rifabutin), for a total of six months of drug therapy. The ethambutol may be discontinued if resistance testing of the TB bacteria shows a response to treatment by the other drugs. If after the initial two months of treatment the HIV-positive person still has positive culture results and lung disease, an additional three months on the isoniazid and rifampin will be prescribed, totaling nine months of TB therapy. Intermittent dosage, meaning taking drugs only three or four times a week, is possible after the first two months of daily treatment.

If the *M. tuberculosis* strain is shown in resistance testing to be immune to isoniazid, then that drug may be dropped from treatment and the other previously mentioned drugs continued. A fluoroquinolone drug (moxifloxacin, gatifloxacin, levofloxacin, ofloxacin, or ciprofloxacin) may be added to the drug regimen. Fluoroquinolones of some nature will used in conjunction with antimycobacterial drugs to treat MDR TB, depending on the resistance testing pattern of the strain of the bacteria. At least four medications will be used in MDR TB to treat this serious illness so it does not develop further resistance to medications. Other medications used in the treatment of MDR or XDR TB include streptomycin, capreomycin, amikacin, kanamycin, ethionimide, cycloserine, protionamide, and *p*-aminosalicylic acid. A specific treatment regimen would be designed for the patient on the basis of previous treatment for TB resistance testing that determines which drugs the bacteria is immune to and any previous reactions to medications the patient may have had. Treatment of MDR and XDR TB is much more complicated than treatment for standard TB. There are more possible side effects of medications, difficulty in controlling the infection, and lower recovery rates for these versions of TB than for standard TB. Approximately 30 percent of XDR TB patients recover from the infection according to CDC reports.

Risk Factors and Preventive Measures

TB is predominantly spread through the air in Western countries. When a person actively infected with TB sneezes, laughs, or coughs, aerial droplets of the bacteria are released into the air. A sneeze can release up to 40,000 of such droplets. A person in close contact with the person who has active TB could breathe in the droplets and become infected with TB. TB infects people who are in regular close contact with an infected person, and it spreads most readily in enclosed spaces. So family members, health care workers, friends, and coworkers can all be susceptible to TB infection if they are in contact with an infected person. Cases of TB have also, on rare occasions, been associated with airline travel, though exposure most often takes a longer contact period than the length of an airplane trip.

Other risk factors are more associated with geography. If an HIV-positive person lives in a country or area where TB is endemic, then the patient needs to know that he or she is at a higher risk of contracting TB from friends and family who may have the disease. In health care or other environments of close required contact such as a prison, HIV-positive patients should be physically separated from patients or prisoners who have or are thought to have active TB infections. Testing of all HIV-positive people in such settings as hospitals, prisons, and endemic areas of TB should be considered to reduce the risk of the spread of TB.

There is a vaccine against TB called the bacille Calmette-Guérin (BCG). The BCG is available in many countries around the world and is mandatory for children below the age of three in South Africa. However, in the United States, the BCG vaccine is not recommended for a child unless he or she is repeatedly in an environment where there is exposure to TB-infected people, nor is it recommended for health care workers who work in an area where they are continually exposed to TB-infected individuals. The BCG vaccine is *not* recommended for anyone who is already HIV positive because it contains TB virus that may cause an active disseminated disease in the immune-compromised person. It is effective in more than 80 percent of children but is less effective in preventing TB in adolescents or adults, with an efficacy range of 0–80 percent. New vaccines for the prevention of TB are currently being tested in clinical trials in the United States and in other parts of the world.

Centers for Disease Control and Prevention. "Extensively Drug-Resistant TB (XDR-TB)." Available online. URL: http://www.cdc.gov/tb/publications/factsheets/drtb/xdrtb.htm. Accessed April 11, 2011.
———. "Reported HIV Status of Tuberculosis Patients—United States, 1993–2005." CDC.gov. Available online. URL: http://www.cdc.gov/MMWR/preview/mmwrhtml/mm5642a2.htm. Accessed April 11, 2011.
———. "TB and HIV/AIDS." CDC.gov. Available online. URL: http://www.cdc.gov/hiv/resources/factsheets/hivtb.htm. Accessed April 11, 2011.
———. "Tuberculosis." CDC.gov. Available online. URL: http://www.cdc.gov/tb/topic/basics/default.htm. Accessed April 11, 2011.
Goozé, Lisa, M.D., and Charles L. Daley, M.D. "Tuberculosis and HIV." HIVInSite.ucsf.edu. Available online. URL: http://hivinsite.ucsf.edu/InSite?page=kb-05-01-06. Accessed April 11, 2011.
Mohapatra, Prasanta Raghab. "Fluoroquinolones in Multidrug-Resistant Tuberculosis." *American Journal of Respiratory and Critical Care Medicine* 170, no. 8 (2004): 920. Available online. URL: http://ajrccm.atsjournals.org/cgi/content/full/170/8/920-a. Accessed April 11, 2011.
New Jersey Medical School Global Tuberculosis Institute. "History of TB." UMDNJ.edu. http://www.umdnj.edu/globaltb/tbhistory.htm. Accessed April 11, 2011.
Smart, Theo. "Failure to Suppress Viral Load More Likely with Nevirapine than Efavirenz If ART Started during TB Treatment." AIDSmap.com. Available online. URL: http://www.aidsmap.com/en/news/692482A3-2FAD-48EE-B928-0073D67B4CDE.asp. Accessed April 11, 2011.
UNAIDS: United Nations Joint Programme on HIV/AIDS. "Tuberculosis and HIV." UNAIDS.gov. Available online. URL: http://www.unaids.org/en/PolicyAndPractice/HIVTreatment/Coinfection/TB/default.asp. Accessed April 11, 2011.
World Health Organization. "TB/HIV." WHO.int. Available online. URL: http://www.who.int/tb/challenges/hiv/en/index.html. Accessed April 11, 2011.
———. "Treatment of Tuberculosis: Guidelines for National Programmes." WHO.int. Available online. URL: http://whqlibdoc.who.int/hq/2003/WHO_CDS_TB_2003.313_eng.pdf. Accessed April 11, 2011.

U

UNAIDS (Joint United Nations Programme on HIV/AIDS) UNAIDS is an agency of the United Nations (UN) that merges the resources of 10 separate UN organizations to fight the HIV epidemic. Those 10 organizations are the United Nations High Commissioner for Refugees (UNHCR), United Nations Children's Fund (UNICEF), World Food Programme (WFP), United Nations Development Programme (UNDP), United Nations Population Fund (UNFPA), United Nations Office on Drugs and Crime (UNODC), International Labour Organization (ILO), United Nations Educational, Scientific and Cultural Organization (UNESCO), World Health Organization (WHO), and World Bank. It was founded in 1996 when several agencies agreed not to work against each other's efforts trying to fight AIDS, and to prevent duplication of effort and the waste that the UN had often been accused of in their AIDS programs.

UNAIDS controls a huge budget of more than $400 million with which to implement AIDS education, medical assistance, treatment, and prevention. It is the main coordinating program for most of the world in fighting HIV and AIDS. It funds and executes programs, drawing money from the world's governments and using its own staff to coordinate and execute the programs. It is second to the U.S. President's Emergency Plan for AIDS Relief (PEPFAR) in the amount of money available to fight the epidemic. Michel Sidibé is currently secretary of UNAIDS. He began his term in January 2009. He has worked for the UN for more than 20 years and with UNAIDS since 2001. He is originally from Mali.

The agency's plan called for full access to antiretroviral treatment for all people by the year 2010. This fell within a broader goal of UNAIDS to halt the spread and reverse the effects of HIV by 2015, as part of the UN's Millennium Goals program. The goal was ridiculed by activists and viewed as unrealistic by many since it was implemented several years ago. Many activists question whether there is a need for UNAIDS, in the long run, as there are two large funding organizations—PEPFAR and the Global Fund to Fight AIDS, Tuberculosis, and Malaria (Global Fund)—currently working to provide funding to nongovernmental organizations (NGOs) and resource-poor countries. UNAIDS has not received the funding it had hoped for from the U.S. government, though that country remains one of the largest funders of the group, because the U.S. government has viewed some UN policies as unsupportable, owing to the opposition of conservative politicians. These include needle exchange programs, programs that encouraged condom distribution as opposed to abstinence education, and others to which conservative politicians objected. In early 2011, the secretary general issued a report stating that although funding was flat and not expected to meet the original goals, treatment for all was possible despite the global economic downturn. However, activists quickly protested the secretary general's message, noting that the numbers outlined in his plan for treatment over the next five years fall short of the numbers of people who will need HIV antiretrovirals. Activists' estimates fall in the range of proposed funds' meeting only one-third of antiretroviral needs by 2015.

UNAIDS runs programs across the globe in all areas of concern in HIV and AIDS. Research in labs around the world, sponsorship of numerous international conferences on HIV and related issues, education on injection drug use (see INJECTION DRUG USE(R)), surveys of SEX WORKERS and the status of WOMEN in the HIV epidemic, and basic health education programs make up the majority of its work. Without the role that the UN has played in the epidemic, it is doubtful whether some of the other programs such as PEPFAR or the Global Fund would exist as they are today.

African Press International. "UNAIDS Executive Director Peter Piot Defies Critics and Prints US$1 Million UNAIDS 'History' Book." Wordpress.com. Available online. URL: http://africanpress.wordpress.com/2008/06/04/unaids-executive-director-peter-piot-defies-critics-and-prints-us1-million-unaids-history-book/. Accessed April 11, 2011.

Akukwe, Chinua. "The Future of UNAIDS." Worldpress.org. Available online. URL: http://www.worldpress.org/Americas/3278.cfm. Accessed April 11, 2011.

England, Roger. "It's Time to Dismantle UNAIDS." PolicyNetwork.net. Available online. URL: http://www.policynetwork.net/health/media/it%E2%80%99s-time-dismantle-unaids. Accessed April 11, 2011.

HealthGap. "HealthGap at the 2011 UN High Meeting on AIDS." HealthGap.org. Available online. URL: http://www.healthgap.org/unhlm2011/index.html. Accessed April 11, 2011.

Merson, Michael. "HIV/AIDS: A Truly Global Response Needed for a Global Scourge." Yale.edu. Available online. URL: http://yaleglobal.yale.edu/content/hivaids-truly-global-response-needed-global-scourge. Accessed April 11, 2011.

UNAIDS: Joint United Nations Programme on HIV/AIDS. "General Assembly—Implementation of the Declaration of Commitment on HIV/AIDS and the Political Declaration on HIV/AIDS—Secretary General's Report." UNAIDS.org. Available online. URL: http://www.unaids.org/en/media/unaids/contentassets/documents/document/2011/20110331_SG_report_en.pdf. Accessed April 11, 2011.

———. "UNAIDS: The Joint United Nations Programme on HIV/AIDS." UNAIDS.org Available online. URL: http://www.unaids.org/en/default.asp. Accessed April 11, 2011.

vaccinations Vaccinations, also sometimes called immunizations, are preventive treatments to prevent a particular illness or infection. Many people have yearly flu shots, which are vaccinations against particular types of influenza virus. Most vaccinations are injectable, though there are some that are nasal sprays and some that are taken orally.

There are broadly two different types of vaccines, one using an attenuated, or live, virus or bacterium, and the other using inactivated vaccine, which is made of parts or pieces of the germ but does not contain a living virus or bacterium. Inactivated vaccines are safe for most HIV-positive people. Live vaccines are not always safe for people who have a compromised immune system, and an HIV-positive person should always notify the doctor of his or her HIV status prior to receiving a vaccine. Vaccines are generally safe for people who are not immunocompromised. HIV can weaken the immune system; a physician will evaluate the overall health of the individual before recommending a live vaccination, or will discuss the concerns of not having a particular vaccine.

Vaccinations are known to increase the HIV viral load for a short time in most HIV-positive people; however, this is a temporary effect, and the viral load will drop again. It is not clear what exactly causes the brief rise in viral load in HIV-positive patients, but it has not been shown to cause a failure in HIGHLY ACTIVE ANTIRETROVIRAL THERAPY (HAART) treatment nor to cause general problems in receiving any of the vaccines. A person should wait a month after any vaccination to have the viral load measured so it can return to normal levels after the vaccination.

Vaccines have been studied in HIV-positive people, and it is known that not all vaccines will work as well in HIV-positive people as they do in HIV-negative people. For instance, the HEPATITIS B vaccine is known not to confer immunity in HIV-positive people at the same level of effectiveness that it does in HIV-negative people. This is because the person's immune system cannot force a response to the inactivated particles that compose the vaccine, therefore no immunity can be built. Some vaccines for HIV-positive people may need to be given with a stronger dosage or may need to be repeated to attempt to spur the body to produce antibodies for the pathogen, indicating that the vaccine has worked properly. Not all vaccines become effective in HIV-positive people. Standard vaccines also may not confer immunity for as long a duration as vaccines in an HIV-negative person.

In HIV-positive people who have CD4 T cell count of less than 200 per μL of blood, vaccinations with live vaccines are generally not recommended. This is because the immune system is weakened already, and the live vaccine may cause the person to become ill from the vaccine. In particular, vaccines for anthrax, smallpox, and herpes zoster (shingles) are not recommended for *any* HIV-positive people. In countries where the bacille Calmette-Guérin (BCG) vaccine for TUBERCULOSIS is given, it is also not recommended for any HIV-positive person. People who have CD4 T cell count of less than 200 per μL are advised *not* to have the following vaccines: chickenpox; measles, mumps, and rubella (MMR); and yellow fever.

HIV-positive CHILDREN should follow the usual childhood vaccination process if their immune systems are functional. All inactivated vaccines can be used safely. Children should receive the MMR and chickenpox vaccine, because these illnesses can be particularly dangerous in HIV-positive children. They are regarded as safe and generally effective in children unless the immune system is severely compromised. HIV-positive children and adults should receive only the inactivated polio vaccine that is available as an injection, not the oral live vaccine. In addition, any annual influenza vaccine should also be given in injection form and not the nasal spray formula, as the nasal spray is a live vaccine.

Pregnant women also should not have specific live vaccinations, as the vaccinations can affect the unborn child in unintended ways. Specifically, vaccinations against HPV, chickenpox, and measles, mumps, and rubella are not recommended for pregnant women.

People traveling to different parts of the world often are required to have vaccines that are not always given in the United States. The vaccine for yellow fever is one of those required for entry in several nations in the tropics. It is a live attenuated vaccine. Studies of inoculation with the yellow fever vaccine in HIV-positive people show it to be safe to administer to people who have CD4 T cell counts greater than 200 per μL, though it is more likely to offer fewer years of protection or less be effective than in people who are HIV-negative. Currently, research and testing are being conducted on an inactivated yellow fever vaccine. Phase I trials of the vaccine proved effective and safe in the general population. Further studies are being planned to test the length of time immunity is given by the new vaccine.

Other vaccines an HIV-positive person may need and that are safe for HIV-positive people include meningitis; bacterial meningitis; pneumonia; hepatitis A; hepatitis B; tetanus, diptheria, and pertussis (Tdap); influenza (all varieties); and human papillomavirus (HPV), which has now been approved for use in boys. It is important for HIV-positive adults to maintain good health, and vaccination is a particularly good way to avoid illnesses through prevention. All of these illnesses can be serious in HIV-positive people if their immune system is weakened in any way.

AETC: AIDS Education & Training Centers. "Immunizations for HIV-Infected Adults and Adolescents." AETC.org. Available online. URL: http://www.aidsetc.org/aidsetc?page=cm-201_immune. Accessed April 11, 2011.

Bhadelia, Nahid, Mary Klotman, and Daniel Caplivski. "The HIV-Positive Traveler." *American Journal of Medicine* 120, no. 7 (July 2007): 574–580.

Monath, Thomas P., et al. "An Inactivated Cell-Culture Vaccine against Yellow-Fever." NEJM.org. Available online. URL: http://www.nejm.org/doi/full/10.1056/NEJMoa1009303. Accessed April 11, 2011.

New Mexico AIDS Education and Training Center. "Vaccinations and HIV." AIDSInfoNet.org. Available online. URL: http://www.aidsinfonet.org/fact_sheets/view/207. Accessed April 11, 2011.

Rodriguez, Carina A. "Update on Immunizations in HIV-Infected and Exposed Children and Adolescents." Available online. URL: http://www.faetc.org/PDF/Newsletter/Newsletter-Volume10-2009/HIVCareLink-08-21-09-v10_i11-Immunizations_HIV-Infected_Children-Adolescents.pdf. Accessed April 11, 2011.

ScienceDaily. "HPV Vaccine Works for Boys: Study Shows First Clear Benefits." ScienceDaily.com. Available online. URL: http://www.sciencedaily.com/releases/2011/02/110204142257.htm. Accessed April 11, 2011.

Thaczuk, Derek. "Yellow Fever Vaccine in HIV-Positive People: Safe, but Not Always Effective." AIDSmap.com. Available online. URL: http://www.aidsmap.com/en/news/8DE2A1DD-E8F2-491B-B103-D361FD6CA493.asp. Accessed April 11, 2011.

United States Department of Health and Human Services. "Recommended Immunizations for HIV Positive Adults." aidsinfo.nih.gov. Available online. URL: http://www.aidsinfo.nih.gov/contentfiles/Recommended_Immunizations_FS_en.pdf. Accessed April 11, 2011.

vaccines against HIV/AIDS   A vaccine is a suspension of potentially infectious agents, or some noninfectious part of those agents, given for the purpose of establishing resistance to an infectious disease. Vaccines stimulate an immune response in the body by creating antibodies or activated T cells capable of controlling the organism. The result is more or less permanent protection against a disease. There are four general classes of vaccines: those containing living attenuated infectious organisms, those containing infectious agents killed by physical or chemical means, those containing living fully virulent organisms, and those containing soluble parts of microorganisms. Vaccines are given by mouth, injection, or nasal spray. Cholera, DPT (diphtheria, pertussis, tetanus), *Haemophilus influenzae* B, HEPATITIS B, influenza, measles, mumps, plague, pneumococcal, polio, rabies, rubella (German measles), smallpox, typhoid, and yellow fever are examples of vaccines. The age when they are administered and booster schedule vary for each vaccine.

In 1984 Margaret Heckler, then secretary of the Department of Health and Human Services under the U.S. president Ronald Reagan, made the overly optimistic announcement that there would be an "AIDS" vaccine ready for the public within two years. She made this announcement the day after the alleged discovery by Robert Gallo of the virus that caused AIDS. In 1997, then-president Bill Clinton started a significant funding and research effort to create a vaccine to prevent HUMAN IMMUNODEFICIENCY VIRUS (HIV) spread within 10 years. Dr. Jonas Salk, the famous polio researcher, was one of the first investigators to suggest vaccination of HIV-infected people with HIV vaccine products, in order to spur immune system response to the virus. Today, most doctors, researchers, and scientists would agree that a preventive HIV vaccine is the world's best hope of ending the AIDS epidemic. Many scientists currently believe that finding a safe and effective vaccine is possible, though they are unsure when some substantive development might occur. The need for an HIV vaccine is most acute in developing countries, where 90 percent of all new HIV infections are occurring, and the epidemic is expanding rapidly in many of those countries. For worldwide use, researchers and activists agree an anti-HIV vaccine should be inexpensive and easy to administer; should be easy to transport and store; should include long-lasting immunity with a single immunization and require few, if any, booster doses; should be compatible with other vaccines; and should provide protection against the many strains of HIV.

Diverse approaches to vaccine design have been actively pursued and are continuing, including vaccines based on HIV surface proteins, deoxyribonucleic acid (DNA) vaccines, vaccines using HIV functional proteins, combination vaccines, and novel vaccines that stimulate both components of the HUMAN IMMUNE SYSTEM (antibody and cell-mediated responses). The pipeline of innovative concepts continues to generate new possibilities for a preventive vaccine. Several approaches have shown some promise in animal model tests; several of these candidates have moved into phase I safety trials in humans or have gone through phase I trials with disappointing results. Approaches continue on many different fronts in an attempt to work beyond initial trials to large phase III trials to determine whether the potential vaccines can work.

The Challenge

HIV is very different from other viruses against which vaccines have been developed, and HIV infection is different in important ways from other viral infections. Since the immune system of an HIV-infected individual does not spontaneously clear the virus from his or her body, the question of what constitutes an effective immune response to HIV is unanswered. Cell-mediated immunity is thought to be more important than antibody-mediated immunity in controlling HIV infection. In contrast, existing vaccines primarily stimulate antibody-mediated immunity and only to a lesser degree cell-mediated immunity. Furthermore, there is no ideal animal model that exactly mimics the human immune response.

Compared to most other viral infections, HIV infection establishes itself quickly in the body, producing high viral loads during an initial infection. A successful HIV vaccine will have to prepare the immune system to respond exceptionally quickly to the virus. HIV mutates frequently. This means that although all HIV particles have the same basic structure, their various proteins can differ slightly from one virus particle to the next. Whereas the immune responses generated by a vaccine would recognize the proteins of the HIV strain(s) used to make the vaccine, they might not recognize all the genetic variants of HIV.

There are two varieties of HIV, plus four strains and multiple subtypes of HIV-1 worldwide. It is unlikely that a single vaccine will protect against all of them. Thus, several vaccines may be needed, each protective against a few subtypes or perhaps even only one of them.

Other than the rare, protected, impractical, and costly chimpanzee, no animal has yet been found to experience an AIDS-like immune deficiency when given HIV. The best animal model currently available is the macaque infected with the simian immunodeficiency virus (SIV), which produces an AIDS-like disease. SIV is closely related to HIV, but it is nevertheless a different virus. So although vaccine experiments with SIV are useful, they cannot indicate the safety or effectiveness of a vaccine designed for use in humans.

In addition to these difficulties, ethical, legal, and economic hurdles have dampened the pharmaceutical industry's interest in development of an HIV vaccine. To date, some of the most central issues remain unsolved. Researchers have yet to agree on the so-called correlates of protection, what sort of measurable immune response—blood-borne versus mucosal, antibody versus cellular—a vaccine should trigger to confer protective immunity to HIV. Vaccines against other diseases have been developed without settling the correlates question, but human testing of HIV vaccines is bogged down by this controversy. Additionally, scientists have not created a generally accepted animal model for more direct testing of vaccine-generated protection.

There are several obstacles in developing a vaccine to prevent AIDS. One obstacle is that HIV is genetically diverse in populations and mutates within infected individuals. This means that a vaccine will need to protect a person against many different strains of the virus. In addition, HIV infects helper T cells, the immune cells that orchestrate the immune response. It is very difficult to design a vaccine that to be effective must activate the very cells that are infected by the virus.

A second obstacle is that HIV is transmitted both as free virus as well as by infected cells. This suggests that both arms of the immune system—antibodies that clear free virus and cell-mediated responses that kill HIV-infected cells—may have to be stimulated to provide protection. More information on the immunological characteristics of HIV infection and ways to induce broadly reactive immune responses is needed.

A third problem is that the most common means of human infection is sex. During sex, the virus directly infects cells in the mucous membranes of the sexual organs. It is likely that cytotoxic lymphocytes (CTLs) in the bloodstream are not sufficient to produce full protection from sexual exposure of HIV. The activation of specific mucosal responses will also be required. Stopping this route of infection—ensuring mucosal protection whether through vaccines or topical anti-HIV MICROBICIDES—calls for cellular immunity, a quite distinct arm of the immune system that employs antibodies in the fluid surrounding mucous membranes as well as white blood cells called killer T cells. (Virus that is transmitted directly into the bloodstream as a free-floating particle is easier to stop: An effective vaccine must produce the kind of antibodies that circulate in the blood, ready to neutralize the invader before it infects cells.)

Fourth, scientists do not know at this point whether a vaccine that works in the United States will also work in other countries. To develop a vaccine to prevent HIV transmission, studies need to include populations around the world with the same candidate vaccines or strategies. Clinical studies need to include participants of different races and ethnicities reflective of not only the U.S. population but global populations. Recruitment efforts for an efficacy trial must therefore include various racial and ethnic populations, various groups who represent the way HIV is transmitted, and people in a range of geographic locations around the globe.

A final obstacle is a risk inherent to all killed-virus vaccines. Suppose by accident some virus escapes being killed? The 1950s witnessed such a catastrophe when a manufacturing error loosed into the population a number of doses of Salk vaccine that contained live virus; they caused a rash of vaccine-induced polio that almost derailed the fight against the disease. With AIDS, the consequences of such a mistake could even be more devastating. All viruses subvert cells by ordering them to make new viral offspring instead of new cells. But the AIDS virus takes subdivision one step further: It not only invades the cell, it splices the genes into those in the cell and then hides there indefinitely, invisible to the immune system. All it might take to cause disease, then, is a single escapee, just one live virus.

To learn more about HIV current vaccine clinical trials, go to http://www3.niaid.nih.gov/topics/HIVAIDS/Research/vaccines/clinical/, the National Institutes of Health Web site.

Vaccine Development

Participants in AIDS vaccine development have included researchers who focus on primates as well as those who focus on people already infected with the virus. In 1986, Daniel Zagury of Pierre and Marie Curie University in Paris and Robert Gallo of the National Cancer Institute began a series of experiments to try to immunize humans against HIV. Their experiments involved injecting people who already had symptoms with a genetically engineered vaccine containing an HIV envelope protein. The vaccine incorporated the HIV protein in the harmless vaccinia virus, originally used in smallpox inoculations, which has become an all-purpose carrier for engineered

vaccines. Soon afterward, Zagury expanded the study to include uninfected volunteers. One year later, albeit with the help of an impractical regimen of booster shots, it was clear that the vaccine could indeed beef up immune defenses against HIV. Zagury himself served as one of the volunteers in the experiment. Although Zagury ran into trouble with U.S. officials during his initial vaccine trials because of alleged ethical violations in the treatment of his patient volunteers, he continues his development work on HIV vaccines.

Jonas Salk, who died in 1995, took a similar tack, arguing that since AIDS symptoms typically do not develop until years after the initial infection, there may be a way to augment the body's immune defenses before it is too late. He called this approach immunotherapy, to distinguish it from what people conventionally think of as vaccination. Salk began with the premise that once in the body, HIV has as its main mode of spread not the bloodstream but movement from cell to cell. Infected cells often fuse with healthy ones to form unwieldy clumps filled with virus. By destroying diseased cells, much of the resident virus may also be destroyed. Salk's team, who continue his research, thus hope to prevent disease in people already infected by shoring up their immune system's ability to destroy infected cells—so-called cellular immunity. The researchers are relying on the proven techniques that served Salk so well with his polio vaccine. In contrast to Zagury and others, who are using genetically engineered vaccines containing pieces of HIV, Salk's preparation contains the actual killed virus. In a further departure from the approach favored by others, Salk's killed virus contains no envelope proteins. Salk's team is seeking the destruction of infected cells rather than free-floating virus, so the loss of the outer proteins may not be crucial. The company Salk created to work on HIV vaccines filed for bankruptcy in 2008, after failing to advance their vaccine beyond phase I trials.

Two African doctors have worked on vaccine development that uses the blood of an individual patient to create an immune-boosting vaccine. Jeremiah Abalaka of Nigeria and Victor Ngu of Cameroon have independently developed therapeutic vaccines that use the blood of the patient. Abalaka's vaccine, named THIVAC, and Ngu's vaccine, called VANHIVAX, have attracted attention on the African continent but have not received funding from Western companies. Both vaccines use the core of the virus derived from the patient, which is then transfused back into the individual. Although these vaccines have been tested locally, large-scale tests have not occurred, and some researchers doubt the efficacy of such an approach. Similar vaccine development is also occurring in Australia and India.

Over the course of the HIV epidemic, more than 30 different vaccines have entered some type of phase I clinical trial, but only three have entered a phase III trial, which is a long-term study with a large number of human participants. Two of the studies were stopped because of the lack of benefit demonstrated during the trial. In particular, one study of a potential vaccine candidate, HVTN 502, was stopped in South Africa after the results showed that participants in the study who received the vaccine had higher rates of HIV seroconversion than participants in the study who had not received the vaccine.

During preclinical testing, researchers give the candidate vaccine to animals and study the strength and durability of the resulting immune response. They wait weeks, months, or even years and then expose vaccinated and unvaccinated animals to a live form of the microbe to measure the candidate vaccine's success in protecting the animal against the specific disease. Scientists refer to this step as challenging the animals.

If animal testing shows that a candidate vaccine is safe and effective, a vaccine developer (in the United States it is usually a pharmaceutical company) applies to the U.S. FOOD AND DRUG ADMINISTRATION (FDA) for approval to begin testing in humans. The pharmaceutical company must also develop a safe, efficient, and cost-effective method for manufacturing the candidate vaccine in large quantity. No effective vaccine against HIV/AIDS has yet been developed. Developing one is a particularly difficult challenge because the virus is constantly mutating. To be effective, a vaccine would have to protect against a variety of types. One obstacle to developing a vaccine is the lack of a laboratory animal that develops AIDS after infection with HIV. Such an animal would make it much easier to test potential vaccines. Since that animal has not been found yet, scientists have to rely on human volunteers. Moreover, the major scientific obstacle faced in developing an HIV vaccine is that the correlates of immunity—the specific immune responses that might protect an individual from HIV—have thus far proven elusive. Tough questions such as "What if a flawed vaccine caused a volunteer to develop AIDS?" and "How do you determine whether a vaccine works?" raise serious barriers to research, and many fear that there may never be an effective vaccine against HIV. Each separate vaccine can require years to be developed to the point it would be safe to use in humans.

Developing a vaccine against the HIV has been the chief goal of AIDS vaccine science. The traditional view of an HIV/AIDS vaccine was that it would provide sterilizing immunity, which means that it would prevent an individual from becoming infected with the virus. Over time, scientists developed other ideas of what a vaccine against HIV could potentially do. Some vaccines may be able to produce what is known as a transient infection. This means that although infection with HIV would occur, the immune system would fight off the virus, resulting in a clearance of the illness after a period of a month or two, while preventing the spread of the virus or limiting the time the virus could be spread to the initial infection period. Such a scenario would not allow the virus to advance to a serious disease. Another type of vaccine would keep HIV under control, maintaining a low level of virus but no decrease in CD4 cell counts or in the passing of the virus to others. Another goal of vaccine research is the development of vaccinelike agents designed to boost the defenses of people who are already infected. An altruistic vaccine is also another possibility. This scenario would prevent the virus from being passed on to others but might have no known benefit to the person receiving the vaccine, perhaps by lowering the viral load in mucosal secretions.

Current Strategies

Investigators have observed that a high HIV set point (the HIV level attained after primary infection) is associated with rapid disease progression, while a low set point is associated with slow progression. If a drug or vaccine is developed that can push down this initial steady state, disease progression might be slowed to a very low rate, even though an individual would remain chronically infected. Since viral load also is associated with infectiousness, a vaccine that merely limited the HIV set point would have substantial epidemiological impact by reducing the rate of HIV transmission. The most immediate implication for HIV vaccine research is the possibility of using plasma viral load as an end point measurement for vaccine evaluation studies in primates. Several approaches have been used in the preparation of the various candidate vaccines that have undergone testing in humans—subunit vaccines based on HIV envelope proteins, synthetic peptide vaccines, recombinant subunit vaccines, and live recombinant vector vaccines.

Two candidate vaccines based on the gpl20 envelope protein were among the most widely tested initially. Two of them went through phase I and phase II testing, but, in June 1994, the National Institutes of Health decided not to proceed with phase III testing. The vaccines were faulted for their inability to produce neutralizing antibodies and to elicit cell-mediated immune responses.

Synthetic peptide candidate vaccines consist of short chains of amino acids, peptides, which are assembled by machines. The structure of the synthetic peptides mimics that of small fragments of certain HIV proteins. These fragments are believed to be those to which neutralizing antibodies bind. The so-called V3 loop, for example, is a fragment of the HIV gpl20 envelope protein that is important to that protein's function. At least two candidate synthetic peptide vaccines mimicking portions of the V3 loop that are common to several strains of HIV have undergone early testing in humans. However, this type of vaccine has elicited only weak antibody responses and has not stimulated cell-mediated immunity.

Recombinant subunit vaccines use viral proteins produced by using recombinant deoxyribonucleic acid (DNA) technology. Recombinant gpl60 proteins and p24 proteins have been tested in early clinical trials. Their apparent drawback resides in a component of the recombinant product that is subtly different from that of the natural HIV proteins. As a result, the antibodies elicited by the recombinant proteins did not effectively neutralize strains of HIV that are commonly transmitted.

Live recombinant vector vaccines use a non-disease-causing virus—an avirulent virus other than HIV—in which certain genes from HIV have been inserted through recombinant DNA technology. The avirulent virus serves merely as a vehicle, or vector, that carries the HIV genes, along with its own, into body cells. There, the avirulent virus replicates harmlessly but produces both its own proteins and those encoded by the HIV genes. In theory, all the viral proteins should elicit an immune response, including a response against HIV proteins. Vaccinia and canarypox viruses are two live recombinant vector vaccines currently undergoing development and early testing. The STEP trial (HVTN 502), which ended in 2007, was a vaccine of this nature. It was stopped when more people in the vaccination arm of the study seroconverted to HIV positive than people in the control arm who did not receive the real vaccine.

Vaccine strategies undergoing laboratory study include attenuated live-HIV vaccines, DNA vaccines, and pseudovirions. Attenuated live-virus vaccines use a weakened form of the virus. The virus actually replicates within cells of the host, but without causing disease. In this way, attenuated live-virus vaccines imitate a natural infection and activate both cell-mediated and antibody-mediated arms of the immune system. As a result, these vaccines are very effective—attenuated live-virus vaccines are used to protect children against measles, mumps, rubella, and polio and were successful in eradicating smallpox. The feasibility of an attenuated live-HIV vaccine has been tested by using SIV in macaques. Attenuated live-virus vaccines carry an important risk: They can sometimes mutate back to a virulent form.

DNA vaccines are made up of rings of harmless bacterial DNA that also include one or two viral genes. The viral genes are spliced into the rings of bacterial DNA by recombinant techniques. When the vaccine is injected into muscle tissue, the DNA rings are taken up by body cells. If all goes well, the cells begin producing the viral proteins, which then elicit immune responses that will protect against the virus. Furthermore, because the cells that have taken up the DNA produce viral proteins, the proteins are displayed on the cell surface, which activates the cell-mediated immune response. Thus, they can elicit both cell-mediated and antibody-mediated immune responses. DNA vaccines have a number of advantages over other types of vaccines: They may be safer for individuals with a compromised immune system, they are easier to prepare, and they do not require refrigeration. For these reasons, DNA vaccines could potentially be produced in large quantities and distributed worldwide at a reasonable cost.

Research on attenuated live-virus HIV candidate vaccines has led to the finding that the *gag* gene of HIV may itself direct the assembly of viruslike particles. These particles—known as pseudovirions, or false viruses—have much of the outer structure of a normal HIV particle but do not contain genetic material. Pseudovirions, therefore, cannot replicate, but they do display many important HIV antigens.

The phase III trial that has generated most press coverage was the vaccine trial started in 2003 in Thailand, sponsored by the Thai health ministry and managed by the U.S. Army. This trial involved a combination of four injections of an attenuated canarypox vaccine and two injections of a recombinant vaccine. This combination of two different types of potential vaccines proved to be 30 percent more effective in preventing HIV transmission than not receiving a vaccine. Although that number is in itself not a large improvement, it is an improvement over not having any means of prevention at all. Researchers were hopeful that the experience would provide many insights into development of vaccines.

Today, there are numerous groups involved in vaccine advocacy. These include community groups, such as the AIDS Vaccine Advocacy Coalition (AVAC); government agencies, such as the CENTERS FOR DISEASE CONTROL and Prevention (CDC), the Food and Drug Administration (FDA), the National Institutes of Health (NIH), and the U.S. Agency for International Development (USAID); and international agencies, such as the Global Alliance for Vaccines and Immunizations; the GLOBAL FUND TO FIGHT AIDS, TUBERCULOSIS, AND MALARIA; the International AIDS Vaccine Initiative; and the United Nations Programme on HIV/AIDS (UNAIDS). Other key players include various bodies of the National Institutes of Health (NIH), such as the AIDS Vaccine Research Committee (an advisory group); the Comprehensive International Program of Research on AIDS (a program); the HIV Vaccine Trials Network (an NIH-funded trial network); the National Cancer Institute (an NIH institute) the Global HIV Vaccine Enterprise; and the Office of AIDS Research (an NIH office); as well as the Vaccine Research Center, an NIH center. Note, too, the involvement of the U.S. military at the Walter Reed Army Institute of Research.

AVERT: AVERTing HIV and AIDS. "History of AIDS up to 1986." AVERT.org. Available online. URL: http://www.avert.org/aids-history-86.htm. Accessed April 11, 2011.

Barouch, Dan H. "Challenges in the Development of an HIV-1 Vaccine." *Nature* 455 (2 October 2008): 613–619.

The Body. "Vaccines for HIV/AIDS Prevention." The Body.com. Available online. URL: http://www.the body.com/index/treat/vaccines.html. Accessed April 11, 2011.

Boseley, Sarah, and Haroon Siddique. "HIV Breakthrough as Scientists Discover New Vaccine to Prevent Infection." Guardian.co.uk. Available online. URL: http://www.guardian.co.uk/world/2009/sep/24/hiv-infection-vaccine-aids-breakthrough. Accessed April 11, 2011.

Butler, Declan. "Jury Still Out on HIV Vaccine Results." Nature.com. Available online. URL: http://www.nature.com/news/2009/091028/full/4611187a.html. Accessed April 11, 2011.

Global HIV Vaccine Enterprise. "Global HIV Vaccine Enterprise." Available online. URL: http://www.hivvaccineenterprise.org/. Accessed April 11, 2011.

Metadilogkul, Orapun, Vichai Jirathitikal, and Aldar S. Bourinbaiar. "Serodeconversion of HIV Antibody-Positive AIDS Patients Following Treatment with V-1 Immunitor." Hindawi.com. Available online. URL: http://www.hindawi.com/journals/jbb/2009/934579.html. Accessed April 11, 2011.

National Institute of Allergy and Infectious Diseases. "HIV/AIDS Vaccines." NIH.gov. Available online. URL: http://www.niaid.nih.gov/topics/hivaids/research/vaccines/Pages/default.aspx. Accessed April 11, 2011.

NMAC: National Minority AIDS Council. "Introduction to AIDS Vaccines." NMAC.org. Available online. URL: http://nmac.org/vt/en/AVAC_pt1.html. Accessed April 11, 2011.

vacuolar myelopathy Myelopathy is disease or deterioration of the spinal cord. In HIV, there can be different types of myelopathy arising from different causes. The most common is vacuolar myelopathy. Vacuolar myelopathy is the deterioration of the myelin sheath, a fatty covering around the nerve cells that connect to the spinal cord, thereby connecting to the brain. The myelin deteriorates, causing holes, called vacuoles, to appear. This can lead to miscommunication from the brain to the nerves, causing a loss of control of the body by the person suffering from vacuolar myelopathy. Vacuolar myelopathy often occurs with peripheral NEUROPATHY and HIV ENCEPHALOPATHY.

The causes of HIV vacuolar myelopathy are not fully understood but relate to some of the same causes as HIV encephalopathy and neuropathy. HIV itself infects the macrophages in the brain, including microglial cells. As these cells die off, it is believed that they release toxins that interfere with the neurons of the brain and the signals being sent between the neurons and the nerves. It is also thought possible that HIV directly infects the neurons; however, this possibility has not been substantiated yet. It is also possible that HIV activity in the body interferes with the way some people process vitamin B_{12} and in turn interrupts the ability to produce the necessary protection for the myelin, thereby leading to its deterioration.

Symptoms and Diagnostic Path
Symptoms of vacuolar myelopathy include leg weakness, leg stiffness, numbness in the arms and legs, jerky reflexes, difficulty in coordinating movements, spasticity in movement, impotence, frequent urination, and incontinence. If the problems progress undiagnosed, patients can lose the use of their legs as they become more numb and unable to control movement. Symptoms do not generally involve back pain.

Diagnosis is based upon observation of reflexes as well as blood and cerebrospinal fluid testing and imaging. These all are used to eliminate other potential causes as well as look for markers of vacuolar myelopathy. BLOOD WORK/BLOOD TESTS look for other possible causes of myelopathies, such as late-stage syphilis or potential spinal cancers. Testing of the cerebrospinal fluid will look for CYTOMEGALOVIRUS infection, shingles, or a HERPES SIMPLEX VIRUS infection. These can all cause nerve inflammation and deterioration in some instances. A person who has vacuolar myelopathy will typically have normal cerebrospinal fluid test results. Blood tests can also determine levels of vitamin B_{12}. Deficiencies in vitamin B_{12} can cause symptoms similar to those seen in myelopathy. Computed axial tomography (CAT or CT scan) or magnetic resonance imaging (MRI) can also be used to rule out such abnormalities as herniated disk problems, degenerative spinal problems, or tumors of the spine. A type of MRI referred to as a T2-weighted MRI can reveal some evidence of vacuolation of the myelin surrounding the nerves.

Treatment Options and Outlook

The best treatment to date has been the administration of HIGHLY ACTIVE ANTIRETROVIRAL THERAPY (HAART) for patients who have vacuolar myelopathy. By starting a patient on HAART and controlling the viral load of HIV-positive patients, it is possible that the deterioration of the myelin can be stopped, and possibly the patient will have remission of the disease process. Stories about this process occurring have been recorded in patient blogs, but extensive research studies have not been conducted.

Supplementation with injection shots of vitamin B_{12} has been suggested, but no studies have been done to determine its effectiveness. In addition, studies have been proposed that would attempt to find other means for the body to absorb vitamin B_{12} properly, such as through nutrient-based amino acids necessary for improvement and proper protection of the myelin. One such nutrient, methionine, did not prove useful when it was studied. Pain medication can be used to reduce pain if that is involved. Antispasticity drugs can provide some reduction of the jerky movements seen in myelopathy patients. Physical therapy and exercise can build muscle strength and flexibility and increase control of muscles.

Risk Factors and Preventive Measures

Patients who have low CD4 counts and high viral loads are more likely to have neurologic complications of HIV than those who have strong CD4 counts and low or controlled viral load counts. Vacuolar myelopathy was seen in 5–25 percent of all HIV patients prior to the development of antiretroviral treatments. It was also seen in 25–55 percent of tissue samples at autopsies of AIDS patients prior to the introduction of HAART. Since use of

HAART began, vacuolar myelopathy incidence has dropped to less than 10 percent of all HIV-positive people.

Bizaare, Maresce, Halima Dawood, and Anand Moodley. "Vacuolar Myelopathy: A Case Report of Functional, Clinical, and Radiological Improvement after Highly Active Antiretroviral Therapy." *International Journal of Infectious Diseases* 12, no. 4 (July 2008): 442–444.

Di Rocco, Alessandro, M.D. "Alessandro Di Rocco, MD Comments on the Future of HIV/AIDS Research." TheBody.com. Available online. URL: http://www.thebody.com/content/art14317.html. Accessed April 11, 2011.

James, John S. "Frequent Urination, Leg Cramps, Leg Weakness, Erection Difficulties: HIV Myelopathy Amino Acid Study." TheBody.com. Available online. URL: http://www.thebody.com/content/art32125.html. Accessed July 24, 2011.

McGuire, Dawn, M.D. "Neurologic Manifestations of HIV." HIVInSite.org. Available online. URL: http://www.hivinsight.com/InSite?page=kb-04-01-02#S3.2X. Accessed July 24, 2011.

Singh, Niranjan N., M.D., and Florian P. Thomas, M.D. "HIV-1 Associated Vacuolar Myelopathy: eMedicine Neurology." eMedicine. Available online. URL: http://emedicine.medscape.com/article/1167064-overview. Accessed July 11, 2011.

Singh, Niranjan N., M.D., Florian P. Thomas, M.D., and R. Charles Callison, M.D. "HIV-1 Associated CNS Complications (Overview): eMedicine Neurology." eMedicine. Available online. URL: http://emedicine.medscape.com/article/1167008-overview. Accessed April 11, 2011.

Uthman, Olalekan A., and Rashidah T. Uthman. "What Do We Currently Know about Treatment of AIDS-Related Myelopathy?" *Neurology Asia* 12 (2007): 77–80. Available online. URL: http://www.neurology-asia.org/articles/20072_077.pdf. Accessed April 11, 2011.

varicella-zoster virus (VZV) Also known as VZV, varicella, chickenpox, herpes zoster, and shingles, VZV has the same properties as all herpes viruses in that it causes some initial disease followed by long periods of latency in the body with reactivation at some future point. Around

95 percent of all adults in the United States have had primary VZV infection leading to chickenpox; usually this has occurred by the time a person is a teenager. A further 15–20 percent of all Americans then become ill with herpes zoster or shingles as adults, the greatest number of whom are immune compromised and elderly individuals. It is not limited to but occurs most often in HIV-positive people with fewer than 200 CD4 T cells per μL of blood. HIGHLY ACTIVE ANTIRETROVIRAL THERAPY (HAART) seems to have no effect on the appearance of shingles.

After a person has recovered from chickenpox, the virus stays in the body and becomes latent. It primarily lives in nerve cells along the spine. When shingles occurs, the virus travels down the length of the nerve to cause painful ulcers at the ends of the nerves wherever the nerve focuses on the skin. This area is called a dermatome. The dermatomes most often affected usually are on the trunk of the body. This is where shingles occurs in about half of all cases: the back, chest, or shoulder area. It can also occur on one side of the face or the other, often involving the eye, ear, or mouth. Most cases of shingles involve only one area, or dermatome, in the body.

Symptoms and Diagnostic Path

Chickenpox, or varicella, appears first on the head, then later on the trunk, arms, and legs of the person infected. Initially, raised red bumps appear; then these become itchy and filled with pus, and then they heal over to scabs. Bumps spread quickly over the course of the first couple of days of infection. Other symptoms include fever, lack of appetite, tiredness, and headache, as well as the well-known itching. The rash can last from five days to two weeks in CHILDREN, who are the typical victims of the illness. Primary infection with VZV for an HIV-positive adult can be dangerous, causing VZV pneumonitis and other disseminated illness. There is a relatively high death rate among these individuals.

The first sign of shingles is a sharp, stabbing pain in a particular area of the body; then, within a few days a rash erupts on the skin in that same area. The rash changes to blisters, which rupture, itch, and continue to cause pain. The rash can spread from the eruptions to other areas of the skin near the initial rash. Shingles generally occurs in older individuals or people who have a weakened immune system. Most cases occur in individuals with fewer than 200 CD4 T cells per μL of blood. Shingles can recur in people who have weak immune systems, though in most cases, once a person has had a shingles outbreak it will not recur. The pain often lingers after the rash and ulcers have cleared and scabbed over, sometimes for several months after the rash first appears. Other symptoms besides the rash and the strong pain are fever, tiredness, and partial loss of hearing, taste, or sight if those areas of the face are involved.

Both chickenpox and shingles have a distinctive appearance and can be diagnosed visually by a medical professional. If there are unusual appearances to the rash, a test can be run to look for the virus from swabs of the skin lesions. BLOOD WORK/BLOOD TESTS can also determine whether a person is displaying antibodies to the virus.

There are a variety of complications of shingles infections in HIV-positive people who have low CD4 T cell counts. They include vasculitis (inflammation of the blood vessel walls, particularly in the central nervous system [CNS]), myelitis (inflammation of the spinal cord), and meningitis (inflammation of the meninges, the lining around the brain). Two particularly dangerous infections of the eye, acute retinal necrosis (ARN) and progressive outer retinal necrosis (PORN), can lead to blindness, and are associated with herpes infections of the eye. PORN is closely associated with VZV and HIV in particular and needs to be closely watched for in people who have low T cell counts.

Treatment Options and Outlook

Treatment for active VZV infection, whether chickenpox or shingles, should begin as soon as possible in HIV-infected adults. Oral medication is generally used for cases in which the person's immune system is functioning well. Treatment of disseminated or severe VZV in HIV-positive people requires intravenous (IV) medication.

Acyclovir is the IV medication most often used in VZV when the skin involvement is extensive or VZV is believed to be disseminated. Inpatient treatment often occurs when the disease is disseminated. Treatment begins with IV acyclovir but can be switched to oral acyclovir if the lesions stop forming during treatment. IV treatment can be used in both chickenpox and shingles forms of VZV if the patient requires it. The course of treatment can range from one to two weeks, depending on the individual symptoms.

Oral medications used for chickenpox or shingles treatment on an outpatient basis are valacyclovir or famciclovir in addition to oral acyclovir. The amount of medication used is greater with VZV than in the treatment of HERPES SIMPLEX VIRUS.

The best treatment for PORN has yet to be identified through studies. The ability to preserve vision once the illness has spread to the eyes is not good even with treatment of the illness. A combination of drugs including IV ganciclovir, foscarnet, and injections into the eye of ganciclovir and foscarnet are the current recommendations of the CENTERS FOR DISEASE CONTROL and Prevention (CDC). IV cidofovir is another treatment option.

ARN can be better controlled with antiretroviral drugs, and vision loss can be minimalized with treatment. IV acyclovir and long-term valacyclovir are the recommended medications.

Risk Factors and Preventive Measures

VZV VACCINATIONS can prevent chickenpox. They are safe and effective; two shots are given three months apart. HIV-positive children who are more than eight years old and have CD4 T cell counts greater than 200 per μL should receive the vaccine. It is possible that in a small number of patients, the vaccine will cause the disease. Treatment with acyclovir can be given in those

cases. Adults who have not had VZV as children may also consider the vaccine, if they have a CD4 T cell count greater than 200 per μL. People who have more highly compromised immune systems should not receive the vaccine.

There is also a VZV immune globulin that has been shown to protect adults and children exposed to VZV if given within 96 hours of exposure. Exposure to chickenpox entails a much higher risk of spread than exposure to shingles, and the immune globulin has been shown to be more effective than pretreatment with antiviral medications.

Once shingles has occurred in an HIV-positive patient, there is no drug that has been shown to reduce recurrence. A vaccine to prevent shingles in older adults, those older than 60 years of age, does exist, but trials of the vaccine in HIV-positive people have not been done, and the vaccine is not recommended currently, as it is a live-virus vaccine. Trials of the vaccine are still being planned for HIV-positive people.

AIDSmap. "Varicella Zoster Virus." AIDSmap.com. Available online. URL: http://www.aidsmap.com/iVaricella-zosteri-virus/page/1731748/. Accessed April 11, 2011.

Centers for Disease Control and Prevention. "Shingles (Herpes Zoster)." CDC.gov. Available online. URL: http://www.cdc.gov/vaccines/vpd-vac/shingles/dis-faqs.htm. Accessed April 11, 2011.

Copeland, Robert. "Ocular Manifestations of HIV." Medscape.com. Available online. URL: http://emedicine.medscape.com/article/1216172-overview. Accessed April 11, 2011.

Erlich, Kim S., M.D., and Sharon Safrin, M.D. "Varicella-Zoster Virus and HIV." HIVInSite.org. Available online. URL: http://www.hivinsite.org/InSite?page=kb-05-03-01. Accessed April 11, 2011.

Project Inform. "Shingles." ProjectInform.org. Available online. URL: http://www.projectinform.org/info/shingles/index.shtml. Accessed April 11, 2011.

University of Maryland Medical Center. "Varicella-Zoster Virus." UMM.edu. Available online. URL: http://www.umm.edu/altmed/articles/varicella-zoster-000080.htm. Accessed April 11, 2011.

Western and Central Europe In sheer numbers, the HIV epidemic in Western and Central Europe is minor in comparison to that in southern AFRICA and the CARIBBEAN. According to the latest United Nations (UN) statistical reports on HIV, France, Italy, and Spain have the largest numbers of adult HIV-positive people: 130,000 in Spain, 140,000 in Italy, and 150,000 in France. Portugal has an estimated infection rate of 0.6 percent of the total population. France, Spain, and Switzerland have estimated infection rates of 0.4 percent, while Iceland and Italy have rates of 0.3 percent. Those rates of infection are the highest in the region but are lower than the rates seen in parts of Eastern Europe. Overall, the rate of infection in Western and Central Europe is 0.2 percent. There are approximately 820,000 people living with HIV in Western Europe.

In Western Europe, the HIV epidemic has followed the same pattern as in NORTH AMERICA. The epidemic began in the early 1980s as OPPORTUNISTIC INFECTIONS (OIs) that were seen at first almost exclusively in MEN WHO HAVE SEX WITH MEN (MSM). It spread out of control to the INJECTION DRUG USE(R) (IDU) community, as well as showing up in hemophiliacs, blood donation recipients, and SEX WORKERS. After testing for the virus became common and testing of blood and blood products was established, rates of infection among transfusion recipients and hemophiliacs dropped to nearly zero. SAFER SEX education produced a drop in MSM infection rates, and with the advent of HIGHLY ACTIVE ANTIRETROVIRAL THERAPY (HAART), death rates of opportunistic infections dropped. According to UN reports, in 1985, approximately 63 percent of cases in

Western Europe were among MSM, but by 1992, that number was 42 percent, as safer sex education had brought about a decrease in the spread of the virus. Among IDUs, the percentage of total cases increased from 5 percent in the mid-1980s to 36 percent in the early 1990s.

The UN reports show that in the early part of the 21st century, the epidemic in Western Europe has shown an increase in cases among MSM in countries such as Switzerland, the United Kingdom, and the Netherlands. Countries such as Spain, Portugal, and Italy show more recent cases in IDU populations and in heterosexual spread in the immigrant populations from Africa. The largest increases in HIV cases have resulted from heterosexual sex, which now represents the main cause of the spread of the virus, at 42 percent of new cases in 2006 for Western Europe. The United Kingdom showed a doubling of new HIV cases, in all populations, between the years 2001 and 2007. The largest numbers of those cases were in London. Germany also had a large increase in cases among the MSM population in these years, with new diagnoses rising 87 percent. The number of new HIV cases among the IDU population has fallen in much of northern Europe. It is believed that the increase in unsafe sex practices among MSM, as well as good education programs among IDUs and the government's making available clean injection equipment, have brought about the changes in the epidemic in recent years.

In Central Europe, the epidemic did not begin until the late 1980s and early 1990s. The IDU population initially drove the epidemic in the majority of the countries. Poland, Romania, and

Estonia in particular had large concentrations of HIV-positive IDUs early in the epidemic. In the late 1980s, Romania also had a large number of CHILDREN who had HIV. This was in large part due to the reuse of needles for transfusions and injections in Romanian hospitals and orphanages. The UN reports show that new cases in recent years continue to be predominantly IDU-driven in Albania, Bosnia, Bulgaria, Romania, and Turkey. Croatia, the Czech Republic, Hungary, and Slovenia show unsafe sex between men as the main cause of spread of the virus currently. The number of annually reported HIV cases has doubled in Central Europe in the early 21st century according to the United Nations.

Conditions of the epidemic in Central and southeastern Europe are not as clear as in Western Europe, as cases were not monitored until recently in many countries, and HAART is less available there than in Western Europe. The majority of diagnoses in Central Europe are not made until a person has AIDS, and education about the virus and means of transmission is more limited than in Western Europe. Generally, most of the countries in Western and Central Europe provide centralized health care through the government. This has allowed easy access to treatment for most, if not all, people who have sought it. It also means that a greater portion of a country's budget is spent on health care and on HIV specifically.

Across Europe, rates of infection are relatively low, and many countries register 0.10 percent or less of the population as HIV positive. Albania, Bulgaria, the Czech Republic, Finland, Germany, Greece, Hungary, Lithuania, Macedonia, Malta, Norway, Poland, Serbia, Slovakia, Slovenia, and Sweden all report prevalence rates in this range. Belgium, Denmark, Ireland, the Netherlands, and the United Kingdom report prevalence rates of 0.20 percent.

Western and Central Europe do not have the double epidemics of MALARIA and TUBERCULOSIS that are seen in many areas of the world. In recent years, however, cases of LEISHMANIASIS have increased in France, Italy, Portugal, and

Spain. Leishmaniasis has been endemic in southern Europe for many years, and the opportunity for this vector-borne disease to spread remains a concern for epidemiologists. The dual health problems of HIV and leishmaniasis may increase the virulence of both illnesses, especially among people who do not receive treatment for either illness.

AVERT: AVERTing HIV and AIDS. "Injecting Drugs, Drug Users, HIV & AIDS." AVERT.org. Available online. URL: http://www.avert.org/injecting.htm. Accessed April 13, 2011.

Centers for Disease Control and Prevention. "Spread of Vector-Borne Diseases and Neglect of Leishmaniasis, Europe." CDC.gov. Available online. URL: http://www.cdc.gov/eid/content/14/7/1013.htm. Accessed April 12, 2011.

Dente, Karen, M.D., and Jamie Hess III. "Pediatric AIDS in Romania." Medscape.com. Available online. URL: http://www.medscape.com/viewarticle/528693. Accessed April 13, 2011.

UNAIDS: Joint United Nations Programme on HIV/AIDS. "AIDS Epidemic Update, 2009." UNAIDS.org. Available online. URL: http://www.unaids.org/en/media/unaids/contentassets/dataimport/pub/report/2009/jc1700_epi_update_2009_en.pdf. Accessed April 12, 2011.

———. "North America, Western and Central Europe: AIDS Epidemic Update Regional Summary, 07." UNAIDS.org. Available online. URL: http://data.unaids.org/pub/Report/2008/jc1532_epibriefs_namerica_europe_en.pdf. Accessed April 12, 2011.

———. "UNAIDS Report on the Global AIDS Epidemic, 2010." UNAIDS.org. Available online. URL: http://www.unaids.org/globalreport/. Accessed April 12, 2011.

women   HIV/AIDS in women has long been a neglected aspect of the HIV epidemic. Until recently, little scientific attention was paid to many fundamental questions about HIV disease in women. Reading articles in newspapers or magazines about HIV-positive women or seeing them on television is still an uncommon event. Yet despite the availability of antiretroviral medications, HIV remains the third-largest killer of African American women ages 35–44, and the fourth leading killer of Hispanic women of the same age group, according to 2006 death data from the CENTERS FOR DISEASE CONTROL and Prevention (CDC). In the early 1980s, women represented just 7 percent of all HIV and AIDS cases. Now, nearly 30 years into the epidemic, women represent the fastest-growing number of HIV-positive people and nearly 27 percent of all people who are HIV-positive in the United States, according to CDC statistics for 2008.

HIV infection among women often represents a threat to two or more people—a mother and her CHILDREN. Indeed, the growing HIV case rate in women has implications for children, since the overwhelming majority of HIV-positive children have acquired the virus from the mother. The incidence of HIV infection continues to grow among women, and the rate at which it is growing is now higher than that among men. In the United States in 1995, heterosexual transmission overtook injection drug use (IDU) (see INJECTION DRUG USE(R)) as the leading cause of HIV infection in women. Today, HIV infection has increased among women in the United States, and in many developing countries it is even more prevalent in women than in men. In the United States, HIV infection is more likely to occur among women of color, particularly African-American and Hispanic women, who make up more than 80 percent of all women who are HIV positive in this country.

Many factors affect women's vulnerability to HIV infection: the prevention of HIV TRANSMISSION in women, the course of HIV infection in women, differences in the "natural history" of HIV infection in women and people of color, biologically unique aspects of HIV disease in women, and the medical management of women who have HIV disease.

Both biological and psychosocial factors place women at higher risk of acquiring HIV infection than men. In biological terms, when an HIV-infected male ejaculates during intercourse, the several milliliters of semen he releases are rich in both free virus (virus circulating in the semen before it integrates with various immune cells) and virus-infected lymphocytes and macrophages. This semen is in contact with a broad surface of mucosal tissue in the vagina and the cervix. These tissues contain high numbers of T cell lymphocytes, which can become infected by HIV from the semen. When an HIV-infected woman has intercourse with an uninfected man, the primary sources of transmission from her to him are free virus and virus-infected cells present in the vaginal and cervical secretions. These secretions mainly have contact with the skin of the penis. If the skin is intact, the virus cannot penetrate it. HIV-infected vaginal secretions have little access to the mucosal tissue lining the male's urethral canal, making transmission of the virus a less likely event. Contact with the uncircumcised penis increases the amount of mucosal tissue exposed to the vaginal secretions. Studies have shown that men who have larger areas of foreskin are more likely than circumcised men or those who have smaller foreskin area to become HIV positive. Note, too, that sexual intercourse is rarely a single event for two members of a sexually active couple. Each instance of unprotected sexual intercourse with an infected female statistically increases the risk that an uninfected male will acquire HIV. Thus, in the long run, the rate of female-to-male HIV transmission becomes similar to the rate of male-to-female transmission. This explains why the prevalence of HIV infection is similar in men and women in the developing world today.

A number of psychosocial factors also increase a woman's vulnerability to HIV infection. Some women have little or no control over the means to practice low-risk sexual behavior. There is nothing they can do to protect themselves without the knowledge and consent of their male sexual partner. In addition, because of their lesser social standing in relation to men virtually worldwide, women are generally unable to negotiate the frequency and nature of sexual interactions. Sometimes they are not even able to choose who their partner will be. Women around the world need methods to prevent heterosexual HIV transmission that are under their own control. Condoms are considered a male-controlled method, and men often refuse to use condoms in situations where women do not have the power to make decisions about sex. Female SEX WORKERS in particular often have no say in whether condoms are used. Although a number of MICROBICIDES are under development and testing, none has so far been shown to be 100 percent effective, and at best it will be several years before any are licensed and widely available to women around the world.

Other important sources of HIV infection for women living in developing countries include transfusions with untested or poorly tested blood, unsterile medical equipment used during childbirth, and reused, unsterilized needles and syringes used to inject medications.

Lesbian and bisexual women are also at risk for HIV/AIDS. Transmission of HIV during homosexual sex between women is uncommon (although it has been documented) and remains poorly researched. However, lesbians may engage in the same high-risk behavior as heterosexual women, and because they often socialize with bisexual and gay men, they may be at higher risk than heterosexual women when having unprotected sex with an infected man.

All sexually active women, including pregnant women, should consider themselves at risk for HIV infection. The level of risk for a woman who is not an injection drug user varies greatly, depending on her sexual practices and the risk factors of the men with whom she engages in sexual relations. For a woman who has no sexual relations, the risk is virtually nil. For a woman in a stable monogamous relationship, the risk is small, although it depends on her partner's faithfulness. For a woman who engages in casual sex with multiple partners, the risk can be very high. Here, the level of risk rises with the prevalence of HIV infection in her social circles and geographic area. The safest course for a woman who wants to be sexually active is to enter into a monogamous, committed, and mutually faithful

relationship. Before entering such a relationship, both the woman and her partner should have HIV testing twice, over the course of six weeks to three months (completely abstaining from risky sexual behavior and drug use in the interval), and receive negative results on both blood tests. Only after both partners have tested negative for HIV, and after sufficient trust in fidelity has been established between them, can they forgo safe-sex practices and engage in unprotected sex with each other and only with each other. Under all other circumstances, sexually active women should always practice SAFER SEX—by using a male latex or polyurethane condom or a female condom during every act of vaginal or rectal intercourse. To avoid potential sexually transmitted infections (STIs) completely during oral-penile sex, a male condom should be worn; during oral-vaginal sex, a latex or polyurethane barrier such as a condom split lengthwise to form a sheet should be used.

In general, with regard to the course of HIV disease in women, several studies cited by the CDC have shown that women have poorer survival rates than men. Some investigators have speculated that this might be due to social factors such as limited access to health care and lower socioeconomic status, including homelessness, depression, domestic violence, and lack of social support. The rates of disease progression do not appear to differ significantly in men and women. Psychological factors play a significant role in the course of HIV disease in women. For example, women who are not pregnant are usually diagnosed later in the disease than men, largely because HIV infection is still regarded by many, particularly in American minority communities, as a disease of drug users and gay men. This delays the start of antiretroviral therapies and the use of prophylaxis for OPPORTUNISTIC INFECTIONS (OIs) in women. Older women are usually diagnosed and treated even later because they and their doctors have still lower expectations of HIV infection; their way of life is assumed to present none of the risk factors associated with HIV infection. Women also have less access than men to routine and state-of-the-art HIV/AIDS care. They are often less mobile than men and more likely to face language and cultural barriers, all of which reduce access to health care and interfere with their ability to comply with demanding treatment regimens. Women often neglect their own health care to take care of others. More than 70 percent of women in the United States who have HIV had children below the age of 18 in their homes according to data collected in one study. Additionally, to this day, the number of women enrolled in HIV clinical drug and treatment trials is often low, sometimes too low to allow statistical calculations that might reveal whether the response of women to a treatment is different from the response of men.

Reports from the National Institute of Allergy and Infectious Diseases show that the normal T cell levels in women and men are different. In people who do not have HIV infection, the T cell levels are about 100 cells higher in women than in men. The differences in T cell counts may matter if they mean that women can acquire AIDS- or HIV-related diseases at higher T cell counts than men. A study released in 2009 indicated that women's immune systems reacted more chronically to HIV infection, particularly women who were premenstrual. This was caused, researchers believed, by higher levels of progesterone in women, which in turn created more levels of a protein that turned on their immune systems full force in the presence of the virus. The study authors also noted that while this may be good initially when first infected by the virus, over the long term, the chronic nature of the illness wears the person down more rapidly and may be the reason that women progress faster to AIDS illnesses than men. Other studies, including one conducted in 14 countries in AFRICA, found that there was no correlation between women's progesterone levels, particularly when using birth control, and time to disease.

T cell counts do not appear to differ by race, at least among white Americans, AFRICAN AMERICANS, and LATINO/A AMERICANS in the United

States. One recent study of female sex workers in Kenya revealed that approximately 7 percent of the women in the study seemed to be resistant to HIV infection. An analysis of their vaginal secretions showed a highly variant grouping of proteins in the secretions in comparison to those of other women. Ongoing studies of these secretions and larger studies looking at differences in vaginal mucosa have been started. This information will be useful in developing both MICROBICIDES and, potentially, VACCINES AGAINST HIV/AIDS.

These findings have led some physicians and scientists to question whether it is appropriate to assume that the information gained from studies of white men should be used to develop the treatment recommendations for women. There are three major measures that physicians and other health care providers use to recommend treatment to HIV-infected individuals: clinical disease, T cell count, and viral load. It is clear that HIGHLY ACTIVE ANTIRETROVIRAL THERAPY (HAART) should be recommended and provided to any person who has clinical disease. It is less clear at what T cell or viral load level treatment should first be recommended. Because of recent information suggesting gender differences in T cells and viral load, there has been concern that the current treatment recommendations may not be correct for women and people of color; the scientific community is currently trying to determine their applicability.

Some treatment differences are known to exist between men and women. Women on HAART are more likely to have allergic reactions and skin reactions to medications than men. In addition, women suffer from severe liver reactions to HAART more often than men. The reactions are different enough that women who have T-cell counts greater than 250 per microliter (µL) of blood are advised *not* to use NEVIRAPINE because of dangerous liver reactions that occur. Women also are known to start treatment later during the course of HIV infection than men, thereby causing the medicines to be less effective than in men. Studies expressly starting women at the same level of illness or viral load as men have shown no differences in the effectiveness of antiretrovirals between them.

There are several biologically unique aspects of HIV disease in women, many of which stem from the fact that the HIV-related conditions that occur uniquely in women involve infections or malignancy of the female reproductive tract. Most of these gynecological problems also occur in HIV-negative women. They include certain vaginal infections (genital ulcers of unknown origin; vaginal CANDIDIASIS, or yeast infection, of the vagina; and bacterial vaginosis and trichomoniasis), severe pelvic inflammatory disease, precancerous cellular changes of the cervix, and menstrual disorders. Cervical cancers progress more rapidly to invasive cervical cancer in women infected with HIV. Note that cervical cancer occurs less frequently in women in developed countries, as a result of more widespread medical management, among other factors. Since few studies have compared the incidence of these conditions in women with and without HIV disease, a debate continues over whether they actually occur more frequently in women who are HIV infected. It is agreed, however, that these diseases are more aggressive in women infected with HIV.

Considerations of gynecological and family planning needs are often a component of the medical management of women who have HIV disease. Women who are HIV positive should receive a complete gynecological exam, including a Pap smear test, during their initial medical visit. A second Pap test should be done six months later. If both tests reveal no sign of cervical changes, women who have symptomatic HIV disease can later be given annual Pap tests. However, HIV-positive women should receive subsequent Pap tests every six months if they have symptomatic HIV disease or if they show evidence of HIV infection, as suggested by the presence of cervical changes through a positive Pap smear test result or the finding of genital warts. The initial medical evaluation of HIV-positive women should also include the following: a complete menstrual, sexual, obstetrical, and gynecological history; breast and pelvic exams; and screening for vaginitis, urinary tract infection, syphilis, gonorrhea, and chlamydia.

Nonpregnant HIV-positive women should receive counseling regarding pregnancy and potential concerns involved with transmission of the virus to a child. In addition, certain opportunistic infection prophylactic drugs must be prescribed with caution during pregnancy because of risks to the fetus. Women should be offered antiretroviral therapy with the same standards of care that are used for men; they must also have the same opportunities as men to participate in clinical trials.

Weight loss and wasting are common complications of HIV disease. Wasting is a life-threatening condition that results in the loss not only of fat tissue but also of muscle. Differences between women and men with wasting syndrome do exist. HIV-positive women lose more of their body fat and HIV-positive men tend to lose more of their muscle. Use of the male sex hormone testosterone has been studied in both men and women and has proven helpful in both groups to control wasting and restore body mass. The drug Marinol is also used to increase a person's appetite and decrease nausea. Marinol is a derivative of the active ingredient in marijuana. If marijuana is legal in a particular state or locality, a doctor may also prescribe it for wasting treatment.

In recent years, consideration of menopausal issues has become more important as HIV-positive women live longer and as more women who are nearing menopause or are postmenopausal become infected. To date, there has been no documented association between HIV disease and premature ovarian failure. Menopause is defined as the permanent cessation of menstruation caused by the loss of ovarian function. Women who are HIV positive can receive hormone replacement therapy for managing the symptoms of natural or premature menopause. There are several alternatives to hormone replacement therapy that are also available to HIV-positive women, including progestin-only regimens, nonhormonal lubricants and/

or moisturizers or Estring for the management of urogenital atrophy, bisphosphonates for the prevention or treatment of osteoporosis, and selective estrogen receptor modulators that offer bone and cardiovascular benefit. Symptoms of menopause can be overlooked in HIV-positive women or can be attributed to the symptoms of HIV infection. Menopausal symptoms include hot flashes, sweating, cystitis, atrophic vaginitis, urethritis, vaginal dryness and itching, and discomfort during urination or intercourse.

Another issue concerning HIV/AIDS in women is the importance of enrollment in both pharmaceutical and government-sponsored HIV clinical trials. To date, women remain underrepresented in clinical trials. It has been established that both structural and attitudinal barriers prevent women from enrolling in clinical trials. Recent studies have identified reasons for not participating, including lack of information about clinical trials, lack of interest in participating, and fear of side effects. Studies have also shown that lack of child care, lack of transportation, and amount of time required for participation were less frequently cited as reasons for not participating. Additionally, studies have shown that among the women enrolled in clinical trials, the greatest facilitator to participation in a trial was the support and/or recommendation of the primary care provider. Women enrolled in clinical trials have also identified the support of the research staff as a major facilitator to participation. Finally, studies have shown perceived barriers to participation from the provider's side—gender prejudice in the medical profession, lack of knowledge of available studies, and lack of coordinated care. Representation in clinical research ensures equal access to investigational medications; it also ensures the availability of accurate information regarding side effects and pharmacokinetics in women as the face of the epidemic changes.

AVERT: AVERTing HIV and AIDS. "Women, HIV and AIDS." AVERT.org. Available online. URL: http://www.avert.org/women-hiv-aids.htm. Accessed April 13, 2011.

The Body. "Women and HIV/AIDS—Overview." The Body.com. Available online. URL: http://www.the body.com/content/art45915.html. Accessed April 13, 2011.

Burgener, Adam, et al. "Identification of Differentially Expressed Proteins in the Cervical Mucosa of HIV-1-Resistant Sex Workers." *Journal of Proteome Research* 7, no. 10 (2008): 4446–4454. Available online. URL: http://pubs.acs.org/doi/full/10.1021/pr800406r. Accessed April 13, 2011.

Centers for Disease Control and Prevention. "Deaths: Leading Causes for 2006." *National Vital Statistics Report* 58, no. 14 (21 March 2010): 1–100. Available online. URL: http://www.cdc.gov/nchs/data/nvsr/nvsr58/nvsr58_14.pdf. Accessed April 13, 2011.

Global Coalition on Women and AIDS. "Resource Centre." WomenandAIDS.net. Available online. URL: http://www.womenandaids.net/resource-centre.aspx. Accessed April 13, 2011.

Henry J. Kaiser Family Foundation. "HIV/AIDS Policy Fact Sheet: Women and HIV/AIDS in the United States." KFF.org. Available online. URL: http://www.kff.org/hivaids/upload/6092-07.pdf. Accessed April 13, 2011.

Hosein, Sean R. "Troubling Trends in American Women with HIV." catie.ca. Available online. URL: http://www.catie.ca/catienews.nsf/00a48c8905294f0b8525717f00661eb8/84ef295c04e191bd852575f90052e515!OpenDocument. Accessed April 13, 2011.

Keller, Daniel M. "Tenofovir Vaginal Gel First Microbicide to Prevent HIV, HSV Infections." Medscape.com. Available online. URL: http://www.medscape.com/viewarticle/725583. Accessed April 13, 2011.

National Institute of Allergy and Infectious Diseases. "HIV Infection in Women." NIH.gov. Available online. URL: http://www.niaid.nih.gov/topics/hivaids/understanding/population%20specific%20information/pages/womenhiv.aspx. Accessed April 13, 2011.

Pauktuutit. "Fact Sheet HIV Wasting Syndrome." pauktuutit.ca. Available online. URL: http://www.pauktuutit.ca/hiv/downloads/FactSheets/HIV%20Wasting%20Syndrome.pdf. Accessed April 13, 2011.

ScienceDaily. "Study Documents Initial Differences in Sexual Transmission of HIV between Males and Females." ScienceDaily.com. Available online. URL: http://www.sciencedaily.com/releases/2005/02/050228122946.htm. Accessed April 13, 2011.

————. "Vaginal Proteins in HIV-Resistant Prostitutes Suggest New Prevention Measures." ScienceDaily. com. Available online. URL: http://www.science daily.com/releases/2008/09/080901205622.htm. Accessed April 13, 2011.

————. "Why HIV Progresses Faster in Women Than in Men with Same Viral Load." ScienceDaily. com. Available online. URL: http://www.science daily.com/releases/2009/07/090713131549.htm. Accessed April 13, 2011.

Society for Women's Health Research. "Barriers to Women's Participation in Clinical Trials and SWHR Proposed Solutions." WomensHealthResearch.org. Available online. URL: http://www.womenshealth research.org/site/PageServer?pagename=policy _issues_clintrials_barriersandreccommendations. Accessed April 13, 2011.

Stringer, Elizabeth et al. "Effect of Hormonal Contraception on HIV Disease Progression: A Multi-Country Cohort Analysis." NATAP.org. Available online. URL: http://www.natap.org/2009/CROI/croi_33.htm. Accessed April 13, 2011.

UNAIDS: Joint United Nations Programme on HIV/ AIDS. "UNAIDS Report on the Global AIDS Epidemic 2010." UNAIDS.org. Available online. URL: http://www.unaids.org/globalreport/. Accessed April 13, 2011.

United States Department of Health and Human Services. "Women and HIV/AIDS—Treatment." WomensHealth.gov. Available online. URL: http://www.womenshealth.gov/hiv/treatment/. Accessed April 13, 2011.

World Health Organization. "Gender Inequalities and HIV." WHO.int. Available online. URL: http://www.who.int/gender/hiv_aids/en/. Accessed April 13, 2011.

World Health Organization (WHO)   The World Health Organization (WHO) is the public health agency of the United Nations (UN). It is responsible for coordinating UN action in the area of public health as well as setting norms and standards for countries, setting a research agenda, providing public policy leadership and guidance for countries and nongovernmental organizations, and providing technical assistance in developing countries.

The WHO came into being on April 7, 1948, and that date is celebrated as World Health Day each year. It is considered one of the charter organizations of the UN, named and described in the UN constitution adopted in 1946. There are currently 193 members of the WHO, all UN members except Liechtenstein plus the self-governing nations of Niue and Cook Islands. Associate members can be territories that are not responsible for their foreign relations if approved by the UN general assembly. Currently, these are Puerto Rico and Tokelau. Other groups can be accorded observer status; these include Chinese Taipei, Palestine, and the Vatican.

The WHO constitution, adopted by all countries and territories that are members, states that "enjoyment of the highest attainable standard of health is one of the fundamental rights of every human being without distinction of race, religion, political belief, economic or social condition." The constitution also states that health is "fundamental to the attainment of peace and security and is dependent upon the fullest cooperation of individuals and States." Using these statements as their mandate, the WHO monitors and tracks all diseases and illnesses to try to implement programs and policies to affect and promote the health of all peoples around the world. In 1969, the WHO implemented specific International Health Regulations; among these are guidelines for international aircraft, VACCINATIONS, and statistical compilation. This background in organization and leadership allowed the WHO to be at the forefront of working in HIV and AIDS when the epidemic became known in the 1980s. The WHO, both before and after the formation of the Joint United Nations Programme on HIV/ AIDS (UNAIDS), has been instrumental in providing HIV and AIDS education and prevention in many countries that otherwise could not afford those types of programs.

In 1985, the WHO, in conjunction with several other organizations such as the U.S. CENTERS FOR DISEASE CONTROL and Prevention (CDC), met in Bangui, Central African Republic, to discuss how AIDS could be defined where testing for the virus could not be done. A test for the virus had been developed, and wealthier countries were using the test to define HIV infection. Poorer countries did not always have the ability to test individuals early in the epidemic, and definitions were needed to allow for a solid measurement of the spread of HIV across AFRICA in particular. The Bangui definition for AIDS, as the document that emerged from the meeting, gave a definition to AIDS outside being tested for the virus. The definition drew criticism from many people for the generalized nature of the illnesses included that helped define the syndrome. Studies that tested the definition in clinical settings found it useful and able to predict well, but predominantly in adults, not in CHILDREN. In 1994, the WHO met in Geneva and expanded their AIDS definition to include testing for the virus, but continued to support the Bangui definition where testing was not an option. Today testing is available in the majority of the world's countries, but not always in specific localities.

The WHO still maintains an active role in HIV education, clinical assistance to countries, statistical compilations, as well as technical knowledge. However, much of the UN activity on AIDS is managed through the UNAIDS organization.

WHO AIDS Case Definition for Surveillance Purposes (Bangui Definition)

A person is considered to have AIDS if at least two of the following major signs are present in combination with at least one of the minor signs listed, and if these signs are not known to be due to a condition unrelated to HIV infection.

Major signs:
Weight loss greater than 10 percent of body weight
Chronic diarrhea for longer than one month
Prolonged fever for longer than one month

Minor signs:
Persistent cough for longer than one month
Generalized pruritic dermatitis (itchy skin rashes)
History of herpes zoster
Oropharyngeal CANDIDIASIS (thrush in the mouth and throat)
Chronic progressive or disseminated HERPES SIMPLEX VIRUS infection
Generalized lymphadenopathy (lymph node swelling)

The presence of either generalized Kaposi's sarcoma or cryptococcal meningitis is sufficient for the diagnosis of AIDS for surveillance.

Expanded WHO Case Definition for AIDS Surveillance (Geneva Definition)

A person is considered to have AIDS if a test for HIV antibody gives a positive result, and one or more of the following conditions are present:

- Ten percent body weight loss or cachexia (loss of body mass that cannot be regained through proper nutrition), with diarrhea or fever, or both, intermittent or constant, for at least one month, not known to be due to a condition unrelated to HIV infection
- Cryptococcal meningitis
- Pulmonary or extrapulmonary TUBERCULOSIS
- Kaposi's sarcoma
- Neurological impairment that is sufficient to prevent independent daily activities, not known to be due to a condition unrelated to HIV infection (for example, trauma or cerebrovascular accident)
- Candidiasis of the esophagus (which may be assumed on the basis of the presence of oral candidiasis accompanied by difficulty in swallowing)
- Clinically diagnosed life-threatening or recurrent episodes of pneumonia, with or without laboratory confirmation
- Invasive cervical cancer

Grant, Alison D., and Kevin M. De Cock. "ABC of AIDS: HIV Infection and AIDS in the Developing World." *BMJ* 322, no. 7300 (16 June 2001): 1475–1478.

Keou, F. X., et al. "World Health Organization Clinical Case Definition for AIDS in Africa: An Analysis of Evaluations." Abstract. NIH.gov. Available online. URL: http://www.ncbi.nlm.nih.gov/pubmed/1335410. Accessed April 13, 2011.

World Health Organization. "Bangui Report 1985." WHO.int. Available online. URL: http://www.who.int/hiv/strategic/en/bangui1985report.pdf. Accessed April 13, 2011.

———. "WHO: World Health Organization." WHO.int. http://www.who.int/en/. Accessed April 13, 2011.

zalcitabine Zalcitabine, also known as dideoxycytidine, or ddC, was the third antiretroviral approved for use in the treatment of HIV by the U.S. FOOD AND DRUG ADMINISTRATION (FDA). It was initially approved after clinical trials showed that when it was used in combination with ZIDOVUDINE, patients gained more T cells than when they were treated with zidovudine alone. It was not used as a monotherapy, as zidovudine had been, as those studies showed less improvement than zidovudine. The trade name for the drug was Hivid. Zalcitabine is one of the NUCLEOSIDE REVERSE TRANSCRIPTASE INHIBITORS (NRTIs). In 2006, the manufacturer, Roche Pharmaceuticals, discontinued production and distribution of the drug. It is no longer available for use in the treatment of HIV.

Dosage

Zalcitabine was available in pill form for adults. Although the drug was not officially approved for use in CHILDREN, it was used at times, with amounts used based on a child's weight.

Drug Interactions

Zalcitabine could not be combined with several other antiretrovirals that were available at the early stage of treatments. DIDANOSINE, STAVUDINE, and LAMIVUDINE did not combine well with the drug. Zalcitabine could not be used by people being treated with radiation therapy for cancer, as it broke down too quickly in that environment. Many HIV patients had different cancers at that time in the epidemic. Food decreased the absorption of the drug, and antacids also interfered with proper absorption.

Side Effects

Side effects with zalcitabine were numerous and probably led to its removal from the market. Zalcitabine was directly linked to the development of NEUROPATHY in patients. It could not be used with stavudine, as that drug also causes neuropathy, and together they were a particularly bad combination.

Cases of LACTIC ACIDOSIS were linked to the use of zalcitabine. People who had kidney impairment were at greater risk of kidney function problems when taking zalcitabine.

Common side effects were nausea, fever, rashes, chancre sores, and skin eruptions around the mouth. Pancreatitis was a condition that people on zalcitabine would be monitored for by a doctor.

Although this drug was one of the first on the market for HIV, it was proven over time to be less beneficial than initially hoped. The treatment guidelines issued by the CENTERS FOR DISEASE CONTROL and Prevention (CDC) had stopped recommending zalcitabine for use in several treatment options, and some options discouraged its use. The manufacturer decided to pull the drug from the market at the end of 2006, though it had become infrequently used long before that time.

AIDSInfoNet. "Zalcitabine (Hivid, ddC)." AIDSInfo Net.org. Available online. URL: http://www.aidsinfo net.org/fact_sheets/view/412. Accessed April 13, 2011.

Birgerson, Lars E., M.D. "M.D./alert." FDA.gov. Available online. URL: http://www.fda.gov/downloads/ Drugs/DrugSafety/DrugShortages/ucm086099.pdf. Accessed April 13, 2011.

Coffey, Susa, M.D. "Zalcitabine (Hivid)." HIVInSite. org. Available online. URL: http://www.hivinsite. org/InSite?page=ar-01-03. Accessed April 13, 2011.

Mayo Clinic Staff. "Zalcitabine (Oral Route)." Mayo Clinic.com. Available online. URL: http://www. mayoclinic.com/health/drug-information/DR 601447. Accessed April 13, 2011.

MedicineNet.com. "Zalcitabine (DDC)—Oral (HIVID)." medicinenet.com. Available online. URL: http:// www.medicinenet.com/zalcitabine_ddc-oral/article. htm. Accessed April 13, 2011.

zidovudine (AZT) AZT was the first drug approved by the U.S. FOOD AND DRUG ADMINISTRATION (FDA) for the treatment of HIV and AIDS, in 1987. It is known by several different names. Azidothymidine, source of the abbreviation AZT, was the original common name for the drug. Later, that common name was changed to zidovudine, abbreviated ZDV, as the previous name was close to another named substance that had come into use. Generally, people refer to it as AZT to this day. The trade name for the drug is Retrovir.

It had originally been created in the 1960s as an anticancer drug but had proven ineffective in treating various cancers, and had more side effects than other available drugs. It was created under a U.S. National Institutes of Health (NIH) grant by a scientist at Wayne State University in Detroit. After HIV was found to be a retrovirus in the mid-1980s, the drug company Burroughs Wellcome and the NIH were looking at a variety of substances in the laboratory that might be effective against HIV and came across AZT, which some research had suggested was effective against retroviruses found in mice. When it proved successful in the laboratory, Burroughs-Wellcome claimed and was granted a patent on the chemical, though many lawsuits were filed against the company and its successor, GlaxoSmithKline, because the drug was developed under a governmental grant, meaning the product was believed to be public property and therefore not patentable by a private institution. The patent on AZT expired in 2004, and since then several generic versions have been approved by the FDA for sale in the United States and abroad.

When AZT was found to have activity against the virus, it was moved through the regulatory pipeline quickly, as HIV advocates were calling for the government to do something to stop the death of people from this poorly understood illness. Once initial studies showed it worked on people, delaying the progression of HIV to AIDS, AZT was put on the market. The clamor was so great that Burroughs Wellcome stock jumped 32 percent the day it was approved by the FDA. Burroughs Wellcome initially priced the drug at $10,000 a year. Protests, led by the activist group ACT UP, over such high pricing for a drug that had been invented more than 20 years earlier forced the company to lower costs soon afterward by 20 percent, leaving the cost at $8,000 for a year's supply. GlaxoSmithKline, the successor company of Burroughs Wellcome, currently charges around $2,200 a year. The cost of generic versions of AZT is approximately $100 a year in many countries.

Initially, AZT was given every four hours. People who took the drug when it first came out would often set alarms to wake themselves up to take the scheduled dose, an unavoidable inconvenience, as this was the only available medication to prevent AIDS from advancing. Side effects were common. People quickly developed anemia or neutropenia; digestive problems such as nausea, gas, and diarrhea; and headaches, all frequently talked about at HIV support groups. It was also soon learned that AZT did not work well over an extended period and that the drug could make people quite sick in the amounts at which it was being administered. But this was a new disease and a new drug that had been moved quickly through the approval process. There was much left to learn in the field, as people took the drug, that had not been learned in clinical trials.

Dosage

The current dosage is generally one 300 mg tablet, two times a day. There are also 100 mg capsules, the well-known blue-and-white capsules that were the available pills when it first appeared. Two 100 mg capsules can be taken three times a day. The 100 mg capsules also allow for easier prescribing in younger CHILDREN. AZT can be taken with or without food.

There is also a liquid formulation that infants and children, unable to swallow pills, can use. There is in addition an intravenous formula that is often used for newborn infants, for WOMEN who are delivering babies, and for people too sick to swallow medications. Zidovudine is also part of the combination pills COMBIVIR and TRIZIVIR.

Drug Interactions

Zidovudine should not be taken at the same time as any other medication containing zidovudine. This includes the combination pills Combivir and Trizivir.

This medication should not be taken at the same time as ribavirin, a drug used in the treatment of HEPATITIS C. Zidovudine and ribavirin interact and cause a decrease in the availability of zidovudine in the body while increasing its potentially dangerous side effects. Methadone can cause an increase in the amount of zidovudine in the body, thereby increasing the side effects of the drug. People taking some medications for the treatment of TUBERCULOSIS (TB) and *Mycobacterium avium* COMPLEX (MAC) as well as other antibacterial medications may need to switch HIV antiretrovirals, as the amount of zidovudine in the body can drop below levels optimal for controlling HIV.

Zidovudine should not be taken at the same time as STAVUDINE. Zidovudine and stavudine are antagonistic, meaning they do not work together in the body and can cause more side effects when combined. There are also some PROTEASE INHIBITORS (PIs) that can cause levels of zidovudine to drop in the body. The FDA has not made recommendations on dosage adjustments in some of these instances, but a doctor can weigh the benefits of potential HIGHLY ACTIVE ANTIRETROVIRAL THERAPY (HAART) combinations to use with zidovudine.

Side Effects

Zidovudine has a host of side effects including cramps, diarrhea, headache, tiredness, gas, trouble in sleeping, and rash. Long-term use of zidovudine has on rare occasions been known to cause the development of myopathy, a weakness of the muscles including the heart. Symptoms include a general weakness of muscles, particularly those closest to the trunk of the body. Bone marrow problems can also occur with long-term use of zidovudine. This results in anemia (decreased production of red blood cells) or neutropenia (decreased production of white blood cells) and occurs more frequently with people who are taking certain antibiotics such as ganciclovir and trimethoprim/sulfamethoxazole (TMP-SMX), among the most common. It also occurs more often when people are just starting zidovudine and have never used HAART before.

Zidovudine is one of the NUCLEOSIDE REVERSE TRANSCRIPTASE INHIBITORS (NRTIs). There are several potential serious side effects that can occur with NRTI use. These drugs have been linked to LIPODYSTROPHY, the loss of fat from some areas of the body and the accumulation of fat in others. NRTI usage can also cause a rise in cholesterol and triglyceride levels.

LACTIC ACIDOSIS has also been linked to NRTIs. It is a rare condition but can occur with greater frequency in women and obese individuals. Lactic acidosis is a very dangerous condition and should be monitored closely. Hyperlactemia, higher than normal levels of lactate in the blood, can be a way to determine that someone might be at risk for the more serious lactic acidosis. If symptoms of nausea, stomach pain, shortness of breath, irregular heartbeat, vomiting, weakness, and tiredness occur while taking zidovudine, the patient should consult a doctor immediately. Although other NRTIs are more often associated with lactic acidosis, zidovudine has been believed to be the cause of some cases of this condition.

AZT initially caused many side effects at the large dosages at which it was originally prescribed. Many people often became more sick when they took AZT than when they took nothing. Many gay men, in particular, saw what happened when their friends took the medication and decided against taking it because of their friends' complaints. Some activists began referring to the drug as a way to poison gay men and minorities. To this day, the stories of people who became more ill on antiretroviral medication prevent some people from taking antiretrovirals. AZT as prescribed today is much safer and has fewer side effects than when it was first introduced.

AIDSInfoNet. "Zidovudine (Retrovir, AZT)." AIDSInfo Net.org. Available online. URL: http://www.aidsinfo net.org/fact_sheets/view/411. Accessed April 13, 2011.

The Body. "Retrovir (Zidovudine, AZT)." TheBody. com. Available online. URL: http://www.thebody. com/index/treat/azt.html. Accessed April 13, 2011.

AIDSmeds. "Retrovir." AIDSmeds.com. Available online. URL: http://www.aidsmeds.com/archive/ Retrovir_1582.shtml. Accessed April 13, 2011.

————. "Special Issues for Children with HIV: NRTIs." AIDSmeds.com. Available online. URL: http:// www.aidsmeds.com/articles/Children_4935.shtml. Accessed April 13, 2011.

O'Connor, Chris. "A Bitter-Sweet Pill." PositiveNation. co.uk. Available online. URL: http://www.positive nation.co.uk/issue120/treatments/treatment3/ treatment3.htm. Accessed April 13, 2011.

Test Positive Aware Network. "Retrovir." TheBody.com. Available online. URL: http://www.thebody.com/ content/art1326.html. Accessed April 13, 2011.

United States Department of Health and Human Services. "Zidovudine." aidsinfo.nih.gov. Available online. URL: http://www.aidsinfo.nih.gov/DrugsNew/Drug DetailNT.aspx?MenuItem=Drugs&Searc h=On&int _id=4. Accessed April 13, 2011.

APPENDIXES

APPENDIX I
FREQUENTLY USED ABBREVIATIONS

3TC	lamivudine (Epivir)
ADAP	AIDS Drug Assistance Program
AIDS	acquired immune deficiency syndrome
ARC	AIDS-related complex
ART	antiretroviral treatment
ASO	AIDS Service Organization
AZT	Azidothymidine (zidovudine)
CBO	community based organization
CCR5	chemokine receptor 5
CD4	CD4 lymphocyte, helper T cell
CDC	U.S. Centers for Disease Control and Prevention
CMV	cytomegalovirus
CXCR4	chemokine receptor 4, fusin
D4T	stavudine (Zerit)
DDC	dideoxycytodine (zalcitabine, Hivid)
DDI	dideoxyinosine (didanosine, Videx)
dL	deciliter
DNA	deoxyribonucleic acid
ELISA	enzyme-linked immunosorbent assay
FDA	U.S. Food and Drug Administration
GLBT	gay, lesbian, bisexual, and transgender
Global Fund	The Global Fund to Fight AIDS, Tuberculosis, and Malaria
GRID	gay-related immune deficiency
HAART	highly active antiretroviral treatment
HBV	hepatitis B virus
HCV	hepatitis C virus
HHV	human herpes virus
HIV	human immunodeficiency virus
HSV	herpes simplex virus
IDU	injection drug user, injection drug use
IRIS	immune reconstitution inflammatory syndrome
IV	intravenous
KS	Kaposi's sarcoma
MAC	*Mycobacterium avium* complex
μL	microliter
mL	milliliter
MRI	magnetic resonance imaging
MTCT	mother-to-child transmission
NGO	nongovernmental organization
NIAID	National Institute of Allergy and Infectious Diseases
NIH	National Institutes of Health
NNRTI	non-nucleoside reverse transcriptase inhibitor
NNtRTI	non-nucleotide reverse transcriptase inhibitor
NRTI	nucleoside reverse transcriptase inhibitor
NSAIDs	nonsteroidal anti-inflammatory drugs
OI	opportunistic infection
PCP	*Pneumocystis jirovecii* pneumonia
PEP	post-exposure prophylaxis
PEPFAR	President's Emergency Plan for AIDS Relief
PI	protease inhibitor
PWA	person with AIDS
PWHIV	person with human immunodeficiency virus
RNA	ribonucleic acid
STD	sexually transmitted disease

STI	sexually transmitted infection	U.S.	United States
T20	enfuvirtide (Fuzeon)	VZV	varicella-zoster virus, chicken pox, shingles
TB	tuberculosis		
TMP-SMX	trimethoprim/sulfamethoxazole	WHO	World Health Organization
UN	United Nations	XDR TB	extensively drug-resistant tuberculosis
UNAIDS	Joint United Nations Programme on HIV/AIDS		

APPENDIX II
HIV AND AIDS STATISTICS, UNITED STATES

TABLE 1. REPORTED AIDS CASES AND ANNUAL RATES (PER 100,000 POPULATION),
BY AREA OF RESIDENCE, 2006, 2007, AND CUMULATIVE—UNITED STATES AND DEPENDENT AREAS

Area of residence	2006		2007		Cumulative[a]		
	No.	Rate	No.	Rate	Adults or adolescents	Children (<13 yrs)	Total
Alabama	462	10.1	391	8.4	9,015	76	9,091
Alaska	39	5.8	32	4.7	682	7	689
Arizona	511	8.3	585	9.2	10,929	46	10,975
Arkansas	253	9.0	196	6.9	4,083	36	4,119
California	3,990	11.0	4,952	13.5	148,274	675	148,949
Colorado	320	6.7	355	7.3	9,098	31	9,129
Connecticut	410	11.7	528	15.1	15,216	183	15,399
Delaware	117	13.7	171	19.8	3,715	26	3,741
District of Columbia	820	140.1	871	148.1	18,008	188	18,196
Florida	4,922	27.3	3,961	21.7	107,980	1,544	109,524
Georgia	1,589	17.0	1,877	19.7	33,607	240	33,847
Hawaii	89	7.0	78	6.1	3,002	17	3,019
Idaho	25	1.7	23	1.5	626	2	628
Illinois	1,341	10.5	1,348	10.5	34,783	283	35,066
Indiana	344	5.5	329	5.2	8,572	56	8,628
Iowa	84	2.8	76	2.5	1,802	13	1,815
Kansas	121	4.4	132	4.8	2,919	14	2,933
Kentucky	203	4.8	292	6.9	4,869	35	4,904
Louisiana	819	19.3	879	20.5	18,480	132	18,612
Maine	68	5.2	46	3.5	1,156	7	1,163
Maryland	1,615	28.8	1,394	24.8	31,611	320	31,931
Massachusetts	530	8.2	612	9.5	19,819	218	20,037
Michigan	661	6.5	628	6.2	15,558	114	15,672
Minnesota	211	4.1	197	3.8	5,016	28	5,044
Mississippi	358	12.3	352	12.1	6,976	56	7,032
Missouri	464	7.9	542	9.2	11,585	61	11,646

Area of residence	2006		2007		Cumulative[a]		
	No.	Rate	No.	Rate	Adults or adolescents	Children (<13 yrs)	Total
Montana	7	0.7	25	2.6	401	3	404
Nebraska	119	6.7	80	4.5	1,561	11	1,572
Nevada	292	11.7	335	13.1	6,095	29	6,124
New Hampshire	54	4.1	51	3.9	1,124	10	1,134
New Jersey	1,063	12.3	1,164	13.4	49,907	787	50,694
New Mexico	93	4.8	113	5.7	2,712	9	2,721
New York	5,473	28.4	4,810	24.9	179,116	2,345	181,461
North Carolina	1,243	14.0	1,024	11.3	17,007	120	17,127
North Dakota	6	0.9	8	1.3	151	2	153
Ohio	760	6.6	703	6.1	15,698	140	15,838
Oklahoma	203	5.7	264	7.3	5,079	26	5,105
Oregon	278	7.5	239	6.4	6,229	19	6,248
Pennsylvania	1,887	15.2	1,750	14.1	35,120	369	35,489
Rhode Island	112	10.5	66	6.2	2,648	28	2,676
South Carolina	704	16.3	742	16.8	14,055	108	14,163
South Dakota	18	2.3	15	1.9	270	5	275
Tennessee	679	11.2	658	10.7	13,114	59	13,173
Texas	2,958	12.6	2,964	12.4	72,434	394	72,828
Utah	57	2.2	68	2.6	2,363	20	2,383
Vermont	19	3.1	6	1.0	468	6	474
Virginia	599	7.8	634	8.2	17,431	177	17,608
Washington	377	5.9	427	6.6	12,202	35	12,237
West Virginia	65	3.6	76	4.2	1,575	11	1,586
Wisconsin	216	3.9	199	3.6	4,716	33	4,749
Wyoming	8	1.6	13	2.5	242	2	244
Subtotal	37,656	12.6	37,281	12.4	989,099	9, 156	998,255
U.S. dependent areas							
American Samoa	0	0.0	0	0.0	1	0	1
Guam	0	0.0	0	0.0	68	1	69
Northern Mariana Islands	0	0.0	0	0.0	3	0	3
Puerto Rico	844	21.5	847	21.5	30,333	403	30,736
U.S. Virgin Islands	32	29.5	34	31.4	663	18	681
Other[b]	0	0.0	0	0.0	3	0	3
Total[c]	**38,751**	**12.8**	**38,384**	**12.5**	**1,021,242**	**9,590**	**1,030,832[d]**

[a] From the beginning of the epidemic through 2007.
[b] Persons reported from areas with confidential name-based AIDS reporting but who are residents of other areas.
[c] Includes persons whose state or area of residence is unknown.
[d] Includes 1,084 persons whose state or area of residence is unknown.

TABLE 2. REPORTED AIDS CASES AND ANNUAL RATES (PER 100,000 POPULATION),
BY METROPOLITAN STATISTICAL AREA OF RESIDENCE, 2006, 2007, AND CUMULATIVE—
UNITED STATES AND PUERTO RICO

| | 2006 | | 2007 | | Cumulative[a] | | |
Area of residence	No.	Rate	No.	Rate	Adults or adolescents	Children (<13 yrs)	Total
MSA (population > 500,000)							
Akron, OH	32	4.6	23	3.3	786	1	787
Albany—Schenectady—Troy, NY	106	12.5	67	7.9	2,325	24	2,349
Albuquerque, NM	51	6.2	65	7.8	1,470	3	1,473
Allentown—Bethlehem—Easton, PA—NJ	118	14.8	91	11.3	1,441	17	1,458
Atlanta—Sandy Springs—Marietta, GA	991	19.3	1,216	23.0	23,106	135	23,241
Augusta—Richmond County, GA—SC	35	6.7	77	14.6	1,937	24	1,961
Austin—Round Rock, TX	193	12.6	210	13.1	5,042	26	5,068
Bakersfield, CA	141	18.2	164	20.7	1,739	9	1,748
Baltimore—Towson, MD	998	37.5	791	29.6	21,153	218	21,371
Baton Rouge, LA	230	30.1	242	31.4	3,971	20	3,991
Birmingham—Hoover, AL	111	10.1	89	8.0	2,701	25	2,726
Boise City—Nampa, ID	14	2.5	12	2.0	293	0	293
Boston, Mass—NH[a]	353	7.9	371	8.3	13,864	149	14,013
Boston Division	183	9.9	229	12.3	8,697	91	8,788
Cambridge Division	103	7.0	93	6.3	3,220	36	3,256
Essex Division	51	7.0	39	5.3	1,617	21	1,638
Bridgeport—Stamford—Norwalk, CT	136	15.2	140	15.6	3,865	57	3,922
Buffalo—Niagara Falls, NY	98	8.6	102	9.0	2,578	20	2,598
Cape Coral—Fort Myers, FL	88	15.4	84	14.2	1,773	24	1,797
Charleston—North Charleston, SC	89	14.4	99	15.7	2,135	18	2,153
Charlotte—Gastonia—Concord, NC—SC	285	18.0	259	15.7	3,502	22	3,524
Chattanooga, TN—GA	49	9.6	47	9.1	1,034	3	1,037
Chicago, IL—IN—WI	1,127	11.9	1,254	13.2	31,226	262	31,488
Chicago Division	1,043	13.2	1,152	14.5	29,314	249	29,563
Gary Division	49	7.1	71	10.2	1,109	8	1,117
Lake Division	35	4.0	31	3.6	803	5	808
Cincinnati—Middletown, OH—KY—IN	196	9.2	132	6.2	2,868	18	2,886
Cleveland—Elyria—Mentor, OH	168	8.0	135	6.4	4,368	48	4,416
Colorado Springs, CO	21	3.5	23	3.8	599	5	604
Columbia, SC	200	28.4	181	25.3	3,457	24	3,481
Columbus, OH	163	9.4	146	8.3	3,268	16	3,284
Dallas, TX	920	15.4	806	13.1	20,960	63	21,023
Dallas Division	709	17.7	618	15.0	16,597	37	16,634
Fort Worth Division	211	10.7	188	9.2	4,363	26	4,389
Dayton, OH	55	6.6	65	7.8	1,286	15	1,301

Area of residence	2006		2007		Cumulative[a]		
	No.	Rate	No.	Rate	Adults or adolescents	Children (<13 yrs)	Total
Deltona—Daytona Beach—Ormond Beach, FL	88	17.7	63	12.6	1,519	16	1,535
Denver—Aurora, CO	237	9.8	271	11.0	7,174	22	7,196
Des Moines, IA	23	4.3	26	4.8	556	4	560
Detroit, MI	438	9.7	413	9.2	10,778	74	10,852
Detroit Division	323	16.1	294	14.8	8,554	58	8,612
Warren Division	115	4.6	119	4.8	2,224	16	2,240
El Paso, TX	40	5.5	135	18.4	1,609	10	1,619
Fresno, CA	66	7.5	98	10.9	1,544	11	1,555
Grand Rapids—Wyoming, MI	50	6.5	39	5.0	854	6	860
Greensboro—High Point, NC	66	9.6	64	9.2	1,328	14	1,342
Greenville, SC	67	11.2	50	8.1	1,343	4	1,347
Harrisburg—Carlisle, PA	69	13.2	78	14.7	1,330	8	1,338
Hartford—West Hartford—East Hartford, CT	127	10.7	202	17.0	5,317	46	5,363
Honolulu, HI	66	7.3	55	6.1	2,175	14	2,189
Houston—Baytown—Sugar Land, TX	1,097	19.9	1,001	17.8	26,782	172	26,954
Indianapolis, IN	147	8.8	121	7.1	3,944	25	3,969
Jackson, MS	115	21.6	139	26.0	2,555	30	2,585
Jacksonville, FL	310	24.2	301	23.1	6,316	76	6,392
Kansas City, MO—KS	161	8.2	297	15.0	4,984	15	4,999
Knoxville, TN	35	5.2	45	6.6	927	5	932
Lakeland, FL	113	20.3	77	13.4	1,890	21	1,911
Las Vegas—Paradise, NV	256	14.4	278	15.1	4,923	28	4,951
Little Rock—North Little Rock, AR	76	11.6	74	11.1	1,460	14	1,474
Los Angeles, CA	1,667	13.0	1,927	15.0	60,289	294	60,583
Los Angeles Division	1,472	14.9	1,638	16.6	53,183	250	53,433
Santa Anna Division	195	6.5	289	9.6	7,106	44	7,150
Louisville, KY—IN	96	7.9	177	14.3	2,451	25	2,476
Madison, WI	29	5.3	30	5.4	550	4	554
McAllen—Edinburg—Pharr, TX	44	6.4	55	7.7	688	12	700
Memphis, TN—MS—AR	345	27.1	255	19.9	5,382	19	5,401
Miami, FL	2,284	42.2	1,792	33.1	57,554	1,000	58,554
Fort Lauderdale Division	769	43.4	642	36.5	17,045	263	17,308
Miami Division	1,162	48.9	846	35.4	30,522	514	31,036
West Palm Beach Division	353	27.9	304	24.0	9,987	223	10,210
Milwaukee—Waukesha—West Allis, WI	109	7.1	110	7.1	2,621	18	2,639
Minneapolis—St Paul—Bloomington, MN—WI	184	5.8	168	5.2	4,431	22	4,453
Modesto, CA	22	4.3	36	7.0	711	6	717

(continues)

TABLE 2. *(continued)*

Area of residence	2006		2007		Cumulative[a]		
	No.	Rate	No.	Rate	Adults or adolescents	Children (<13 yrs)	Total
Nashville—Davidson—Murfreesboro, TN	172	11.6	223	14.7	4,071	20	4,091
New Haven—Milford, CT	106	12.6	142	16.8	4,707	73	4,780
New Orleans—Metairie—Kenner, LA	271	27.4	325	31.5	9,158	69	9,227
New York, NY—NJ—PA	5,469	29.1	5,095	27.1	199,402	2,903	202,305
Edison Division	131	5.7	166	7.2	6,871	140	7,011
Nassau Division	253	9.1	213	7.7	8,404	111	8,515
New York Division	4,672	40.3	4,249	36.6	163,738	2,313	166,051
Newark Division	413	19.4	467	21.9	20,389	339	20,728
Ogden—Clearfield, UT	7	1.4	8	1.5	273	4	277
Oklahoma City, OK	89	7.6	112	9.4	2,365	5	2,370
Omaha—Council Bluffs, NE—IA	82	10.0	60	7.2	1,097	3	1,100
Orlando, FL	517	25.9	461	22.7	9,108	94	9,202
Oxnard—Thousand Oaks—Ventura, CA	19	2.4	34	4.3	1,046	3	1,049
Palm Bay—Melbourne—Titusville, FL	61	11.5	45	8.4	1,556	11	1,567
Philadelphia, PA—NJ—DE—MD	1,364	23.5	1,275	21.9	29,476	315	29,791
Camden Division	112	9.0	96	7.7	3,217	42	3,259
Philadelphia Division	1,157	29.8	1,053	27.1	23,144	252	23,396
Wilmington Division	95	13.8	126	18.2	3,115	21	3,136
Phoenix—Mesa—Scottsdale, AZ	355	8.8	452	10.8	7,883	31	7,914
Pittsburgh, PA	134	5.7	145	6.2	3,322	20	3,342
Portland—South Portland, ME	34	6.6	24	4.7	586	0	586
Portland—Vancouver—Beaverton, OR—WA	212	9.9	186	8.6	5,006	10	5,016
Poughkeepsie—Newburgh—Middletown, NY	109	16.4	67	10.0	3,231	24	3,255
Providence—New Bedford—Fall River, RI—MA	155	9.7	104	6.5	4,007	44	4,051
Raleigh—Cary, NC	205	20.5	153	14.6	2,153	13	2,166
Richmond, VA	121	10.1	97	8.0	3,465	35	3,500
Riverside—San Bernardino—Ontario, CA	319	8.0	427	10.5	9,078	61	9,139
Rochester, NY	132	12.8	122	11.8	3,267	13	3,280
Sacramento—Arden-Arcade—Roseville, CA	166	8.0	131	6.3	4,155	26	4,181
St. Louis, MO—IL	364	12.9	233	8.2	6,220	40	6,260
Salt Lake City, UT	40	3.7	48	4.4	1,792	10	1,802
San Antonio, TX	246	12.7	239	12.0	5,223	30	5,253
San Diego—Carlsbad—San Marcos, CA	380	12.9	478	16.1	13,489	65	13,554

Area of residence	2006		2007		Cumulative[a]		
					Adults or	Children	
	No.	Rate	No.	Rate	adolescents	(<13 yrs)	Total
San Francisco, CA	705	16.9	1,091	26.0	41,498	98	41,596
Oakland Division	250	10.2	373	15.0	9,987	50	10,037
San Francisco Division	455	26.7	718	41.7	31,511	48	31,559
San Jose—Sunnyvale—Santa Clara, CA	145	8.2	152	8.4	3,924	15	3,939
San Juan—Caguas—Guaynabo, PR	571	22.0	590	22.7	21,993	279	22,272
Sarasota—Bradenton—Venice, FL	105	15.4	61	8.9	2,040	28	2,068
Scranton—Wilkes-Barre, PA	46	8.4	47	8.6	587	5	592
Seattle, WA	271	8.3	312	9.4	9,468	28	9,496
Seattle Division	248	9.9	277	10.9	8,423	19	8,442
Tacoma Division	23	3.0	35	4.5	1,045	9	1,054
Springfield, MA	46	6.7	106	15.5	2,189	27	2,216
Stockton, CA	54	8.1	60	8.9	1,142	16	1,158
Syracuse, NY	51	7.9	44	6.8	1,369	9	1,378
Tampa—St. Petersburg—Clearwater, FL	603	22.4	469	17.2	11,639	115	11,754
Toledo, OH	66	10.1	40	6.1	855	14	869
Tucson, AZ	95	10.0	84	8.7	2,075	10	2,085
Tulsa, OK	62	6.9	103	11.4	1,594	10	1,604
Virginia Beach—Norfolk—Newport News, VA—NC	131	7.9	211	12.7	4,923	63	4,986
Washington, DC—VA—MD—WV	1,643	31.2	1,618	30.5	32,494	315	32,809
Bethesda Division	172	15.0	185	16.0	2,956	24	2,980
Washington Division	1,471	35.8	1,433	34.5	29,538	291	29,829
Wichita, KS	38	6.4	30	5.0	880	2	882
Worcester, MA	77	9.9	62	7.9	1,840	21	1,861
Youngstown—Warren—Boardman, OH—PA	28	4.9	54	9.5	576	0	576
Subtotal for MSAs (population > 500,000)	31,261	15.8	31,088	15.6	862,954	8,238	871,192
Metropolitan areas (population of 50,000–499,999)	4,331	7.8	4,295	7.7	96,828	830	97,658
Nonmetropolitan areas	2,753	5.5	2,555	5.1	57,151	454	57,605
Total[b]	**38,500**	**12.7**	**38,128**	**12.5**	**1,019,432**	**9,559**	**1,028,991**

Note. Because of the lack of U.S. census information for all U.S. dependent areas, includes data for only the 50 states, the District of Columbia, and Puerto Rico.

MSA, metropolitan statistical area.

MSA definitions for this report can be found at http://www.census.gov/population/www/estimates/metrodef.html.

[a] Reported case counts for the metropolitan divisions do not sum to the MSA total. MSA total includes data from 1 metropolitan division with population of <500,000.

[b] Includes persons whose county of residence is unknown.

TABLE 3. REPORTED AND DIAGNOSED CASES OF HIV INFECTION (NOT AIDS),
BY AREA OF RESIDENCE, 2007 AND CUMULATIVE—47 STATES, THE DISTRICT OF COLUMBIA,
AND FIVE U.S. DEPENDENT AREAS WITH CONFIDENTIAL NAME-BASED HIV INFECTION REPORTING

Area of residence (date HIV reporting initiated)	Reported[b]	Diagnosed	Cumulative[a]		
			Adults or adolescents	Children (<13 yrs)	Total
Alabama (January 1988)	529	447	6,380	50	6,430
Alaska (February 1999)	27	21	308	2	310
Arizona (January 1987)	771	488	6,329	89	6,418
Arkansas (July 1989)	206	180	2,487	18	2,505
California (April 2006)	17,588	2,687	24,199	195	24,394
Colorado (November 1985)	382	274	6,334	31	6,365
Connecticut (January 2005)[c]	932	259	3,178	109	3,287
Delaware (February 2006)	480	88	1,270	18	1,288
District of Columbia (November 2006)	1,629	483	1,871	10	1,881
Florida (July 1997)[d]	5,165	3,982	39,393	541	39,934
Georgia (December 2003)	3,204	1,059	11,039	218	11,257
Idaho (June 1986)	39	17	377	5	382
Illinois (January 2006)	3,576	936	9,763	190	9,953
Indiana (July 1988)	406	313	4,260	42	4,302
Iowa (July 1998)	93	82	658	4	662
Kansas (July 1999)	110	79	1,330	16	1,346
Kentucky (October 2004)	414	218	1,631	22	1,653
Louisiana (February 1993)	797	642	8,450	167	8,617
Maine (January 2006)	46	36	420	3	423
Massachusetts (January 2007)	777	181	881	29	910
Michigan (April 1992)	623	498	6,996	133	7,129
Minnesota (October 1985)	289	224	3,550	40	3,590
Mississippi (August 1988)	471	411	4,892	61	4,953
Missouri (October 1987)	460	353	5,239	54	5,293
Montana (September 2006)	92	5	118	2	120
Nebraska (September 1995)	78	52	716	11	727
Nevada (February 1992)	369	299	3,827	28	3,855
New Hampshire (January 2005)	52	32	509	9	518
New Jersey (January 1992)	1,571	693	18,297	314	18,611
New Mexico (January 1998)	92	80	997	4	1,001
New York (June 2000)	5,197	2,836	45,786	1,765	47,551
North Carolina (February 1990)	1,746	1,465	15,325	154	15,479
North Dakota (January 1988)	9	3	88	2	90
Ohio (June 1990)	852	600	8,760	112	8,872

Area of residence (date HIV reporting initiated)	Reported[b]	Diagnosed	Cumulative[a]		
			Adults or adolescents	Children (<13 yrs)	Total
Oklahoma (June 1988)	199	172	2,449	29	2,478
Oregon (April 2006)	1,477	134	1,565	27	1,592
Pennsylvania (October 2002)[e]	3,694	1,007	12,162	243	12,405
Rhode Island (July 2006)	130	67	146	5	151
South Carolina (February 1986)	542	451	7,147	94	7,241
South Dakota (January 1988)	17	16	226	6	232
Tennessee (January 1992)	841	708	7,602	92	7,694
Texas (January 1999)[f]	3,495	2,507	26,030	430	26,460
Utah (April 1989)	92	73	953	14	967
Virginia (July 1989)	823	560	10,790	97	10,887
Washington (March 2006)	620	386	4,423	42	4,465
West Virginia (January 1989)	55	50	689	8	697
Wisconsin (November 1985)	220	181	2,593	30	2,623
Wyoming (June 1989)	15	12	103	2	105
Subtotal	61,292	26,347	322,536	5,567	328,103
U.S. dependent areas					
American Samoa (August 2001)	0	0	1	0	1
Guam (March 2000)	1	1	67	0	67
Northern Mariana Islands (October 2001)	0	0	7	0	7
Puerto Rico (January 2003)	1,450	580	6,693	108	6,801
U.S. Virgin Islands (December 1998)	20	17	253	7	260
Persons reported from areas with confidential name-based HIV infection reporting but who were residents of other areas	151	54	1,016	87	1,103
Total	**63,230**	**27,126**	**331,768**	**5,822**	**337,590**

Note. Includes data from 47 states, the District of Columbia, and 5 U.S. dependent areas with confidential name-based HIV infection reporting as of December 2007.

[a] From the beginning of the epidemic through 2007.

[b] Cases of HIV infection (not AIDS) reported in 2007 include cases diagnosed during earlier years.

[c] Beginning in 1992, Connecticut had name-based HIV reporting for cases in children only. From January 2002 through December 2004, Connecticut had name- or code-based HIV reporting for cases in adolescents and adults. As of January 2005, Connecticut had name-based reporting of all cases of HIV infection.

[d] Florida has confidential name-based HIV infection reporting for only the diagnoses made during July 1997 or later.

[e] On October 18, 2002, Pennsylvania initiated confidential name-based HIV infection reporting in all areas except Philadelphia. Code-based reporting was implemented in Philadelphia in March 2004, and the switch to name-based reporting was made in October 2005. From February 1994 through December 1998, Texas reported HIV infection in children only.

[f] Includes 1,248 persons reported from areas with confidential name-based HIV infection reporting but whose area of residence is unknown.

TABLE 4. REPORTED AIDS CASES, BY TRANSMISSION CATEGORY AND SEX,
2007 AND CUMULATIVE—UNITED STATES AND DEPENDENT AREAS

	Males				Females				Total			
	2007		Cumulative[a]		2007		Cumulative[a]		2007		Cumulative[a]	
Transmission category	No.	%	No.	%	No.	%	No.	%	No.	%	No.	%
Adult or adolescent												
Male-to-male sexual contact	14,383	51	445,645	54	—	—	—	—	14,383	38	445,645	44
Injection drug use	3,103	11	166,251	20	1,633	16	69,591	35	4,736	12	235,842	23
Male-to-male sexual contact and injection drug use	1,514	5	67,797	8	—	—	—	—	1,514	4	67,797	7
Hemophilia/coagulation disorder	37	0	5,212	1	9	0	355	0	46	0	5,567	1
High-risk heterosexual contact[b]	2,791	10	52,623	6	4,713	47	90,229	45	7,504	20	142,852	14
Sex with injection drug user	281	1	11,941	1	704	7	26,825	13	985	3	38,766	4
Sex with bisexual male	—	—	—	—	233	2	5,415	3	233	1	5,415	1
Sex with person with hemophilia	4	0	90	0	10	0	513	0	14	0	603	0
Sex with HIV-infected transfusion recipient	31	0	584	0	25	0	819	0	56	0	1,403	0
Sex with HIV-infected person, risk factor not specified	2,475	9	40,008	5	3,741	37	56,657	28	6,216	16	96,665	9
Receipt of blood transfusion, blood components, or tissue[c]	50	0	5,181	1	59	1	4,134	2	109	0	9,315	1
Other/risk factor not reported or identified[d]	6,442	23	77,328	9	3,563	36	36,896	18	10,005	26	114,224	11
Subtotal	28,320	100	820,037	100	9,977	100	201,205	100	38,297	100	1,021,242	100
Child (<13 yrs at diagnosis)												
Hemophilia/coagulation disorder	0	0	222	5	0	0	7	0	0	0	229	2
Mother with documented HIV infection or one of the following risk factors:	30	77	4,333	89	43	90	4,464	95	73	84	8,797	92
Injection drug use	8	21	1,675	34	10	21	1,673	36	18	21	3,348	35
Sex with injection drug user	2	5	783	16	3	6	752	16	5	6	1,535	16
Sex with bisexual male	1	3	103	2	1	2	111	2	2	2	214	2
Sex with person with hemophilia	0	0	20	0	0	0	16	0	0	0	36	0
Sex with HIV-infected transfusion recipient	0	0	11	0	0	0	15	0	0	0	26	0
Sex with HIV-infected person, risk factor not specified	8	21	746	15	8	17	804	17	16	18	1,550	16
Receipt of blood transfusion, blood components, or tissue	0	0	70	1	0	0	82	2	0	0	152	
Has HIV infection, risk factor not specified	11	28	925	19	21	44	1,011	21	32	37	1,936	20

Transmission category	Males				Females				Total			
	2007		Cumulative[a]		2007		Cumulative[a]		2007		Cumulative[a]	
	No.	%	No.	%	No.	%	No.	%	No.	%	No.	%
Receipt of blood transfusion, blood components, or tissue[e]	1	3	242	5	0	0	141	3	1	1	383	4
Other/risk factor not reported or identified[f]	8	21	87	2	5	10	94	2	13	15	181	2
Subtotal	39	100	4,884	100	48	100	4,706	100	87	100	9,590	100
Total	28,359	100	824,921	100	10,025	100	205,911	100	38,384	100	1,030,832[g]	100

[a] From the beginning of the epidemic through 2007.
[b] Heterosexual contact with a person known to have, or to be at high risk for, HIV infection.
[c] AIDS developed in 43 adults/adolescents after they received transfusion of HIV-infected blood that had tested negative for HIV antibodies. AIDS developed in 13 additional adults after they received tissue, organs, or artificial insemination from HIV-infected donors.
[d] Includes 37 adults/adolescents who were exposed to HIV-infected blood, body fluids, or concentrated virus in health care, laboratory, or household settings, as supported by seroconversion, epidemiologic, or laboratory evidence. One person was infected after intentional inoculation with HIV-infected blood. Includes an additional 908 persons who acquired HIV infection perinatally but who were more than 12 years of age when AIDS was diagnosed. These 908 persons are not counted in the values for the pediatric transmission category.
[e] AIDS developed in 3 children after they received transfusion of HIV-infected blood that had tested negative for HIV antibodies.
[f] Includes 25 children who had sexual contact with an HIV-infected man and an additional 4 children who were exposed to HIV-infected blood in household, health care, or other settings, as supported by seroconversion, epidemiologic, or laboratory evidence.
[g] Includes 2 persons of unknown sex.

TABLE 5. REPORTED CASES OF HIV INFECTION (NOT AIDS), BY TRANSMISSION CATEGORY AND SEX, 2007 AND CUMULATIVE—47 STATES, THE DISTRICT OF COLUMBIA, AND FIVE U.S. DEPENDENT AREAS WITH CONFIDENTIAL NAME-BASED HIV INFECTION REPORTING

Transmission category	Males 2007 No.	%	Cumulative[a] No.	%	Females 2007 No.	%	Cumulative[a] No.	%	Total 2007 No.	%	Cumulative[a] No.	%
Adult or adolescent												
Male-to-male sexual contact	29,713	61	129,915	54	—	—	—	—	29,713	47	129,915	39
Injection drug use	3,653	8	27,158	11	2,041	14	15,509	17	5,694	9	42,667	13
Male-to-male sexual contact and injection drug use	2,298	5	12,920	5	—	—	—	—	2,298	4	12,920	4
Hemophilia/coagulation disorder	65	0	560	0	8	0	79	0	73	0	639	0
High-risk heterosexual contact[b]	3,333	7	19,490	8	6,528	46	43,517	47	9,861	16	63,007	19
Sex with injection drug user	345	1	2,825	1	863	6	7,353	8	1,208	2	10,178	3
Sex with bisexual male	—	—	—	—	299	2	2,491	3	299	0	2,491	1
Sex with person with hemophilia	4	0	32	0	15	0	207	0	19	0	239	0
Sex with HIV-infected transfusion recipient	28	0	155	0	54	0	276	0	82	0	431	0
Sex with HIV-infected person, risk factor not specified	2,956	6	16,478	7	5,297	37	33,190	36	8,253	13	49,668	15
Receipt of blood transfusion, blood components, or tissue	64	0	510	0	71	0	545	1	135	0	1,055	0
Other/risk factor not reported or identified	9,221	19	49,207	21	5,578	39	32,354	35	14,799	24	81,565	25
Subtotal	48,347	100	239,760	100	14,226	100	92,004	100	62,573	100	331,768	100
Child (<13 yrs at diagnosis)												
Hemophilia/coagulation disorder	7	2	108	4	0	0	1	0	7	1	109	2
Mother with documented HIV infection or one of the following risk factors:	254	81	2,397	85	283	82	2,669	89	537	82	5,066	87
Injection drug use	44	14	556	20	61	18	615	20	105	16	1,171	20
Sex with injection drug user	22	7	226	8	14	4	223	7	36	5	449	8
Sex with bisexual male	2	1	39	1	7	2	33	1	9	1	77	1
Sex with person with hemophilia	0	0	3	0	1	0	9	0	1	0	12	0
Sex with HIV-infected transfusion recipient	0	0	4	0	1	0	5	0	1	0	9	0
Sex with HIV-infected person, risk factor not specified	76	24	600	21	89	26	698	23	165	25	1,298	22
Receipt of blood transfusion, blood components, or tissue	1	0	17	1	0	0	19	1	1	0	36	1
Has HIV infection, risk factor not specified	109	35	952	34	110	32	1,062	35	219	33	2,014	35

Transmission category	Males				Females				Total			
	2007		Cumulative[a]		2007		Cumulative[a]		2007		Cumulative[a]	
	No.	%	No.	%	No.	%	No.	%	No.	%	No.	%
Receipt of blood transfusion, blood components, or tissue	1	0	25	1	2	1	25	1	3	0	50	1
Other/risk factor not reported or identified	50	16	290	10	60	17	307	10	110	17	597	10
Subtotal	312	100	2,820	100	345	100	3,002	100	657	100	5,822	100
Total	**48,659**	**100**	**242,580**	**100**	**14,571**	**100**	**95,006**	**100**	**63,230**	**100**	**337,590**[c]	**100**

Note. See Table 3 for the list of 47 states and 5 U.S. dependent areas with confidential name-based HIV infection reporting as of December 2007.

[a] From the beginning of the epidemic through 2007.

[b] Heterosexual contact with a person known to have, or to be at high risk for, HIV infection.

[c] Includes 4 persons of unknown sex.

TABLE 6. REPORTED AIDS CASES FOR MALE ADULTS AND ADOLESCENTS, BY TRANSMISSION CATEGORY AND RACE/ETHNICITY, 2007 AND CUMULATIVE—UNITED STATES AND DEPENDENT AREAS

Transmission category	2007		Cumulative[a]	
	No.	%	No.	%
American Indian/Alaska Native				
Male-to-male sexual contact	71	54	1,473	55
Injection drug use	18	14	410	15
Male-to-male sexual contact and injection drug use	15	11	477	18
Hemophilia/coagulation disorder	0	0	25	1
High-risk heterosexual contact[b]	6	5	119	4
Sex with injection drug user	1	1	31	1
Sex with person with hemophilia	0	0	0	0
Sex with HIV-infected transfusion recipient	0	0	3	0
Sex with HIV-infected person, risk factor not specified	5	4	85	3
Receipt of blood transfusion, blood components, or tissue	1	1	8	0
Other/risk factor not reported or identified	20	15	171	6
Total	**131**	**100**	**2,683**	**100**
Asian[c]				
Male-to-male sexual contact	216	57	4,154	67
Injection drug use	16	4	299	5
Male-to-male sexual contact and injection drug use	10	3	260	4
Hemophilia/coagulation disorder	1	0	63	1
High-risk heterosexual contact[13]	34	9	378	6
Sex with injection drug user	4	1	49	1
Sex with person with hemophilia	0	0	1	0
Sex with HIV-infected transfusion recipient	2	1	12	0
Sex with HIV-infected person, risk factor not specified	28	7	316	5
Receipt of blood transfusion, blood components, or tissue	4	1	104	2
Other/risk factor not reported or identified	96	25	973	16
Total	**377**	**100**	**6,231**	**100**
Black/African American				
Male-to-male sexual contact	4,497	39	108,134	37
Injection drug use	1,391	12	84,645	29
Male-to-male sexual contact and injection drug use	460	4	22,917	8
Hemophilia/coagulation disorder	9	0	614	0
High-risk heterosexual contact[b]	1,677	15	31,669	11
Sex with injection drug user	149	1	6,949	2
Sex with person with hemophilia	2	0	41	0

Sex with HIV-infected transfusion recipient	11	0	249	0
Sex with HIV-infected person, risk factor not specified	1,515	13	24,430	8
Receipt of blood transfusion, blood components, or tissue	20	0	1,195	0
Other/risk factor not reported or identified	3,497	30	42,527	15
Total	**11,551**	**100**	**291,701**	**100**
Hispanic/Latino[d]				
Male-to-male sexual contact	2,926	48	68,278	44
Injection drug use	903	15	47,344	30
Male-to-male sexual contact and injection drug use	297	5	11,366	7
Hemophilia/coagulation disorder	4	0	468	0
High-risk heterosexual contact[b]	626	10	11,698	8
Sex with injection drug user	67	1	2,489	2
Sex with person with hemophilia	1	0	12	0
Sex with HIV-infected transfusion recipient	8	0	133	0
Sex with HIV-infected person, risk factor not specified	550	9	9,064	6
Receipt of blood transfusion, blood components, or tissue	8	0	663	0
Other/risk factor not reported or identified	1,350	22	15,743	10
Total	**6,114**	**100**	**155,560**	**100**
Native Hawaiian/Other Pacific Islander				
Male-to-male sexual contact	39	70	430	76
Injection drug use	2	4	26	5
Male-to-male sexual contact and injection drug use	3	5	29	5
Hemophilia/coagulation disorder	0	0	5	1
High-risk heterosexual contact[b]	1	2	28	5
Sex with injection drug user	0	0	5	1
Sex with person with hemophilia	0	0	0	0
Sex with HIV-infected transfusion recipient	0	0	0	0
Sex with HIV-infected person, risk factor not specified	1	2	23	4
Receipt of blood transfusion, blood components, or tissue	0	0	3	1
Other/risk factor not reported or identified	11	20	42	7
Total	**56**	**100**	**563**	**100**
White				
Male-to-male sexual contact	6,490	66	260,797	73
Injection drug use	737	8	32,425	9
Male-to-male sexual contact and injection drug use	711	7	32,325	9

(continues)

TABLE 6. *(continued)*

Transmission category	2007		Cumulative[a]	
	No.	%	No.	%
White				
Hemophilia/coagulation disorder	23	0	4,013	1
High-risk heterosexual contact[b]	417	4	8,260	2
Sex with injection drug user	56	1	2,348	1
Sex with person with hemophilia	1	0	36	0
Sex with HIV-infected transfusion recipient	10	0	183	0
Sex with HIV-infected person, risk factor not specified	350	4	5,693	2
Receipt of blood transfusion, blood components, or tissue	17	0	3,176	1
Other/risk factor not reported or identified	1,410	14	17,302	5
Total	**9,805**	**100**	**358,298**	**100**
Total				
Male-to-male sexual contact	14,383	51	445,645	54
Injection drug use	3,103	11	166,251	20
Male-to-male sexual contact and injection drug use	1,514	5	67,797	8
Hemophilia/coagulation disorder	37	0	5,212	1
High-risk heterosexual contact[b]	2,791	10	52,623	6
Sex with injection drug user	281	1	11,941	1
Sex with person with hemophilia	4	0	90	0
Sex with HIV-infected transfusion recipient	31	0	584	0
Sex with HIV-infected person, risk factor not specified	2,475	9	40,008	5
Receipt of blood transfusion, blood components, or tissue	50	0	5,181	1
Other/risk factor not reported or identified	6,442	23	77,328	9
Total	**28,320[e]**	**100**	**820,037[f]**	**100**

[a] From the beginning of the epidemic through 2007.

[b] Heterosexual contact with a person known to have, or to be at high risk for, HIV infection.

[c] Includes Asian/Pacific Islander legacy cases.

[d] Hispanics/LATINOS/AS can be of any race.

[e] Includes 286 males of unknown race or multiple races.

[f] Includes 5,001 males of unknown race or multiple races.

TABLE 7. REPORTED CASES OF HIV INFECTION (NOT AIDS) FOR MALE ADULTS AND ADOLESCENTS,
BY TRANSMISSION CATEGORY AND RACE/ETHNICITY, 2007 AND CUMULATIVE—47 STATES,
THE DISTRICT OF COLUMBIA, AND FIVE U.S. DEPENDENT AREAS
WITH CONFIDENTIAL NAME-BASED HIV INFECTION REPORTING

Transmission category	2007		Cumulative[a]	
	No.	%	No.	%
American Indian/Alaska Native				
Male-to-male sexual contact	123	61	614	58
Injection drug use	13	6	106	10
Male-to-male sexual contact and injection drug use	21	10	130	12
Hemophilia/coagulation disorder	1	0	1	0
High-risk heterosexual contact[b]	10	5	63	6
Sex with injection drug user	1	0	16	2
Sex with person with hemophilia	0	0	0	0
Sex with HIV-infected transfusion recipient	0	0	0	0
Sex with HIV-infected person, risk factor not specified	9	4	47	4
Receipt of blood transfusion, blood components, or tissue	0	0	1	0
Other/risk factor not reported or identified	33	16	143	14
Total	**201**	**100**	**1,058**	**100**
Asian[c]				
Male-to-male sexual contact	596	77	1,362	68
Injection drug use	11	1	56	3
Male-to-male sexual contact and injection drug use	22	3	46	2
Hemophilia/coagulation disorder	0	0	1	0
High-risk heterosexual contact[b]	41	5	120	6
Sex with injection drug user	0	0	6	0
Sex with person with hemophilia	0	0	0	0
Sex with HIV-infected transfusion recipient	3	0	5	0
Sex with HIV-infected person, risk factor not specified	38	5	108	5
Receipt of blood transfusion, blood components, or tissue	4	1	9	0
Other/risk factor not reported or identified	102	13	400	20
Total	**776**	**100**	**1,994**	**100**
Black/African American				
Male-to-male sexual contact	7,320	45	36,389	39
Injection drug use	1,510	9	13,189	14
Male-to-male sexual contact and injection drug use	526	3	3,958	4
Hemophilia/coagulation disorder	13	0	120	0
High-risk heterosexual contact[b]	2,009	12	12,470	13
Sex with injection drug user	180	1	1,662	2
Sex with person with hemophilia	1	0	16	0
Sex with HIV-infected transfusion recipient	10	0	83	0

(continues)

TABLE 7. *(continued)*

Transmission category	2007		Cumulative[a]	
	No.	%	No.	%
Black/African American				
Sex with HIV-infected person, risk factor not specified	1,818	11	10,709	11
Receipt of blood transfusion, blood components, or tissue	24	0	228	0
Other/risk factor not reported or identified	4,877	30	27,421	29
Total	**16,279**	**100**	**93,775**	**100**
Hispanic/Latino[d]				
Male-to-male sexual contact	6,077	60	21,173	51
Injection drug use	1,115	11	7,327	17
Male-to-male sexual contact and injection drug use	401	4	1,825	4
Hemophilia/coagulation disorder	3	0	32	0
High-risk heterosexual contact[b]	677	7	3,557	8
Sex with injection drug user	98	1	534	1
Sex with person with hemophilia	2	0	8	0
Sex with HIV-infected transfusion recipient	5	0	23	0
Sex with HIV-infected person, risk factor not specified	572	6	2,992	7
Receipt of blood transfusion, blood components, or tissue	16	0	67	0
Other/risk factor not reported or identified	1,768	18	7,931	19
Total	**10,057**	**100**	**41,912**	**100**
Native Hawaiian/Other Pacific Islander				
Male-to-male sexual contact	69	76	161	74
Injection drug use	4	4	7	3
Male-to-male sexual contact and injection drug use	4	4	10	5
Hemophilia/coagulation disorder	0	0	0	0
High-risk heterosexual contact[b]	5	5	13	6
Sex with injection drug user	1	1	3	1
Sex with person with hemophilia	0	0	0	0
Sex with HIV-infected transfusion recipient	0	0	0	0
Sex with HIV-infected person, risk factor not specified	4	4	10	5
Receipt of blood transfusion, blood components, or tissue	0	0	1	0
Other/risk factor not reported or identified	9	10	27	12
Total	**91**	**100**	**219**	**100**
White				
Male-to-male sexual contact	15,345	74	69,234	70
Injection drug use	978	5	6,247	6
Male-to-male sexual contact and injection drug use	1,307	6	6,827	7

TABLE 7. *(continued)*

Transmission category	2007		Cumulative[a]	
	No.	%	No.	%
White				
Hemophilia/coagulation disorder	48	0	403	0
High-risk heterosexual contact[b]	571	3	3,075	3
Sex with injection drug user	62	0	577	1
Sex with person with hemophilia	1	0	8	0
Sex with HIV-infected transfusion recipient	10	0	44	0
Sex with HIV-infected person, risk factor not specified	498	2	2,446	2
Receipt of blood transfusion, blood components, or tissue	19	0	197	0
Other/risk factor not reported or identified	2,393	12	12,541	13
Total	**20,661**	**100**	**98,524**	**100**
Total				
Male-to-male sexual contact	29,713	61	129,915	54
Injection drug use	3,653	8	27,158	11
Male-to-male sexual contact and injection drug use	2,298	5	12,920	5
Hemophilia/coagulation disorder	65	0	560	0
High-risk heterosexual contact[b]	3,333	7	19,490	8
Sex with injection drug user	345	1	2,825	1
Sex with person with hemophilia	4	0	32	0
Sex with HIV-infected transfusion recipient	28	0	155	0
Sex with HIV-infected person, risk factor not specified	2,956	6	16,478	7
Receipt of blood transfusion, blood components, or tissue	64	0	510	0
Other/risk factor not reported or identified	9,221	19	49,207	21
Total	**48,347[e]**	**100**	**239,760[f]**	**100**

Note. See Table 3 for the list of 47 states and 5 U.S. dependent areas with confidential name-based HIV infection reporting as of December 2007.
[a] From the beginning of the epidemic through 2007.
[b] Heterosexual contact with a person known to have, or to be at high risk for, HIV infection.
[c] Includes Asian/Pacific Islander legacy cases.
[d] Hispanics/Latinos can be of any race.
[e] Includes 282 males of unknown race or multiple races.
[f] Includes 2,278 males of unknown race or multiple races.

TABLE 8. REPORTED AIDS CASES FOR FEMALE ADULTS AND ADOLESCENTS, BY TRANSMISSION CATEGORY
AND RACE/ETHNICITY, 2007 AND CUMULATIVE—UNITED STATES AND DEPENDENT AREAS

Transmission category	2007		Cumulative[a]	
	No.	%	No.	%
American Indian/Alaska Native				
Injection drug use	8	18	286	40
Hemophilia/coagulation disorder	0	0	3	0
High-risk heterosexual contact[b]	22	50	299	42
Sex with injection drug user	7	16	115	16
Sex with bisexual male	1	2	28	4
Sex with person with hemophilia	0	0	2	0
Sex with HIV-infected transfusion recipient	0	0	6	1
Sex with HIV-infected person, risk factor not specified	14	32	148	21
Receipt of blood transfusion, blood components, or tissue	1	2	18	3
Other/risk factor not reported or identified	13	30	105	15
Total	**44**	**100**	**711**	**100**
Asian[c]				
Injection drug use	2	2	95	9
Hemophilia/coagulation disorder	0	0	7	1
High-risk heterosexual contact[b]	47	53	540	54
Sex with injection drug user	5	6	92	9
Sex with bisexual male	2	2	74	7
Sex with person with hemophilia	0	0	3	0
Sex with HIV-infected transfusion recipient	0	0	18	2
Sex with HIV-infected person, risk factor not specified	40	45	353	35
Receipt of blood transfusion, blood components, or tissue	3	3	87	9
Other/risk factor not reported or identified	36	41	274	27
Total	**88**	**100**	**1,003**	**100**
Black/African American				
Injection drug use	817	13	39,793	33
Hemophilia/coagulation disorder	7	0	149	0
High-risk heterosexual contact[b]	2,928	46	52,928	44
Sex with injection drug user	345	5	13,871	12
Sex with bisexual male	139	2	2,498	2
Sex with person with hemophilia	3	0	122	0
Sex with HIV-infected transfusion recipient	17	0	297	0
Sex with HIV-infected person, risk factor not specified	2,424	38	36,140	30
Receipt of blood transfusion, blood components, or tissue	33	1	1,517	1
Other/risk factor not reported or identified	2,516	40	25,761	21
Total	**6,301**	**100**	**120,148**	**100**

Transmission category	2007		Cumulative[a]	
	No.	%	No.	%
Hispanic/Latino[d]				
Injection drug use	313	18	13,298	35
Hemophilia/coagulation disorder	0	0	68	0
High-risk heterosexual contact[b]	894	52	18,991	50
Sex with injection drug user	152	9	6,705	17
Sex with bisexual male	33	2	857	2
Sex with person with hemophilia	1	0	46	0
Sex with HIV-infected transfusion recipient	3	0	142	0
Sex with HIV-infected person, risk factor not specified	705	41	11,241	29
Receipt of blood transfusion, blood components, or tissue	8	0	613	2
Other/risk factor not reported or identified	490	29	5,370	14
Total	1,705	100	38,340	100
Native Hawaiian/Other Pacific Islander				
Injection drug use	2	14	22	19
Hemophilia/coagulation disorder	0	0	0	0
High-risk heterosexual contact[b]	8	57	63	54
Sex with injection drug user	1	7	23	20
Sex with bisexual male	1	7	7	6
Sex with person with hemophilia	0	0	1	1
Sex with HIV-infected transfusion recipient	0	0	2	2
Sex with HIV-infected person, risk factor not specified	6	43	30	26
Receipt of blood transfusion, blood components, or tissue	1	7	6	5
Other/risk factor not reported or identified	3	21	25	22
Total	14	100	116	100
White				
Injection drug use	471	28	15,473	40
Hemophilia/coagulation disorder	2	0	125	0
High-risk heterosexual contact[b]	756	45	16,541	42
Sex with injection drug user	188	11	5,839	15
Sex with bisexual male	55	3	1,915	5
Sex with person with hemophilia	6	0	336	1
Sex with HIV-infected transfusion recipient	5	0	344	1
Sex with HIV-infected person, risk factor not specified	502	30	8,107	21
Receipt of blood transfusion, blood components, or tissue	12	1	1,858	5
Other/risk factor not reported or identified	452	27	5,046	13
Total	1,693	100	39,043	100

(continues)

TABLE 8. *(continued)*

Transmission category	2007		Cumulative[a]	
	No.	%	No.	%
Total				
Injection drug use	1,633	16	69,591	35
Hemophilia/coagulation disorder	9	0	355	0
High-risk heterosexual contact[b]	4,713	47	90,229	45
Sex with injection drug user	704	7	26,825	13
Sex with bisexual male	233	2	5,415	3
Sex with person with hemophilia	10	0	513	0
Sex with HIV-infected transfusion recipient	25	0	819	0
Sex with HIV-infected person, risk factor not specified	3,741	37	56,657	28
Receipt of blood transfusion, blood components, or tissue	59	1	4,134	2
Other/risk factor not reported or identified	3,563	36	36,896	18
Total	**9,977[e]**	**100**	**201,205[f]**	**100**

[a] From the beginning of the epidemic through 2007.
[b] Heterosexual contact with a person known to have, or to be at high risk for, HIV infection.
[c] Includes Asian/Pacific Islander legacy cases.
[d] Hispanics/Latinos can be of any race.
[e] Includes 132 females of unknown race or multiple races.
[f] Includes 1,844 females of unknown race or multiple races.

TABLE 9. REPORTED CASES OF HIV INFECTION (NOT AIDS) FOR FEMALE ADULTS AND ADOLESCENTS, BY TRANSMISSION CATEGORY AND RACE/ETHNICITY, 2007 AND CUMULATIVE—47 STATES, THE DISTRICT OF COLUMBIA, AND FIVE U.S. DEPENDENT AREAS WITH CONFIDENTIAL NAME-BASED HIV INFECTION REPORTING

Transmission category	2007		Cumulative[a]	
	No.	%	No.	%
American Indian/Alaska Native				
Injection drug use	18	26	121	28
Hemophilia/coagulation disorder	0	0	0	0
High-risk heterosexual contact[b]	27	39	204	47
Sex with injection drug user	5	7	56	13
Sex with bisexual male	1	1	16	4
Sex with person with hemophilia	0	0	2	0
Sex with HIV-infected transfusion recipient	0	0	0	0
Sex with HIV-infected person, risk factor not specified	21	30	130	30
Receipt of blood transfusion, blood components, or tissue	0	0	1	0
Other/risk factor not reported or identified	24	35	109	25
Total	**69**	**100**	**435**	**100**
Asian[c]				
Injection drug use	7	4	19	4
Hemophilia/coagulation disorder	1	1	2	0
High-risk heterosexual contact[b]	88	54	235	47
Sex with injection drug user	6	4	17	3
Sex with bisexual male	4	2	12	2
Sex with person with hemophilia	0	0	0	0
Sex with HIV-infected transfusion recipient	7	4	7	1
Sex with HIV-infected person, risk factor not specified	71	44	199	40
Receipt of blood transfusion, blood components, or tissue	3	2	7	1
Other/risk factor not reported or identified	63	39	233	47
Total	**162**	**100**	**496**	**100**
Black/African American				
Injection drug use	894	11	7,781	14
Hemophilia/coagulation disorder	2	0	36	0
High-risk heterosexual contact[b]	3,561	44	26,378	46
Sex with injection drug user	358	4	3,660	6
Sex with bisexual male	123	2	1,357	2
Sex with person with hemophilia	8	0	75	0
Sex with HIV-infected transfusion recipient	18	0	138	0
Sex with HIV-infected person, risk factor not specified	3,054	38	21,148	37
Receipt of blood transfusion, blood components, or tissue	40	0	325	1
Other/risk factor not reported or identified	3,622	45	22,212	39
Total	**8,119**	**100**	**56,732**	**100**

(continues)

TABLE 9. *(continued)*

Transmission category	2007		Cumulative[a]	
	No.	%	No.	%
Hispanic/Latino[d]				
Injection drug use	375	13	2,578	18
Hemophilia/coagulation disorder	2	0	13	0
High-risk heterosexual contact[b]	1,470	53	7,587	52
Sex with injection drug user	233	8	1,519	10
Sex with bisexual male	63	2	323	2
Sex with person with hemophilia	1	0	12	0
Sex with HIV-infected transfusion recipient	15	1	53	0
Sex with HIV-infected person, risk factor not specified	1,158	41	5,680	39
Receipt of blood transfusion, blood components, or tissue	7	0	56	0
Other/risk factor not reported or identified	941	34	4,374	30
Total	**2,795**	**100**	**14,608**	**100**
Native Hawaiian/Other Pacific Islander				
Injection drug use	3	16	9	18
Hemophilia/coagulation disorder	0	0	0	0
High-risk heterosexual contact[b]	13	68	28	56
Sex with injection drug user	3	16	5	10
Sex with bisexual male	0	0	4	8
Sex with person with hemophilia	0	0	0	0
Sex with HIV-infected transfusion recipient	0	0	0	0
Sex with HIV-infected person, risk factor not specified	10	53	19	38
Receipt of blood transfusion, blood components, or tissue	0	0	0	0
Other/risk factor not reported or identified	3	16	13	26
Total	**19**	**100**	**50**	**100**
White				
Injection drug use	733	25	4,819	26
Hemophilia/coagulation disorder	3	0	26	0
High-risk heterosexual contact	1,326	45	8,644	46
Sex with injection drug user	246	8	2,024	11
Sex with bisexual male	105	4	756	4
Sex with person with hemophilia	6	0	116	1
Sex with HIV-infected transfusion recipient	14	0	78	0
Sex with HIV-infected person, risk factor not specified	955	32	5,670	30
Receipt of blood transfusion, blood components, or tissue	17	1	150	1
Other/risk factor not reported or identified	892	30	5,041	27
Total	**2,971**	**100**	**18,680**	**100**

Transmission category	2007		Cumulative[a]	
	No.	%	No.	%
Total				
Injection drug use	2,041	14	15,509	17
Hemophilia/coagulation disorder	8	0	79	0
High-risk heterosexual contact[b]	6,528	46	43,517	47
Sex with injection drug user	863	6	7,353	8
Sex with bisexual male	299	2	2,491	3
Sex with person with hemophilia	15	0	207	0
Sex with HIV-infected transfusion recipient	54	0	276	0
Sex with HIV-infected person, risk factor not specified	5,297	37	33,190	36
Receipt of blood transfusion, blood components, or tissue	71	0	545	1
Other/risk factor not reported or identified	5,578	39	32,354	35
Total	**14,226[e]**	**100**	**92,004[f]**	**100**

Note. See Table 3 for the list of 47 states and 5 U.S. dependent areas with confidential name-based HIV infection reporting as of December 2007.
[a] From the beginning of the epidemic through 2007.
[b] Heterosexual contact with a person known to have, or to be at high risk for, HIV infection.
[c] Includes Asian/Pacific Islander legacy cases.
[d] Hispanics/Latinos can be of any race.
[e] Includes 91 females of unknown race or multiple races.
[f] Includes 1,003 females of unknown race or multiple races.

TABLE 10. REPORTED CASES OF HIV/AIDS IN INFANTS BORN TO HIV-INFECTED MOTHERS, BY YEAR OF REPORT AND SELECTED CHARACTERISTICS, 1994–2007—25 STATES WITH CONFIDENTIAL NAME-BASED HIV INFECTION REPORTING

	Year of report													
	1994	1995	1996	1997	1998	1999	2000	2001	2002	2003	2004	2005	2006	2007
Child's race/ethnicity														
American Indian/Alaska Native	5	1	0	1	0	1	0	0	1	1	0	1	2	0
Asian[a]	1	0	0	1	1	0	1	0	0	1	0	2	2	2
Black/African American	215	200	158	120	94	77	77	84	66	62	61	70	47	57
Hispanic/Latino[b]	31	20	19	14	10	11	15	13	18	10	15	18	8	9
Native Hawaiian/ Other Pacific Islander	0	0	0	0	0	0	0	0	0	0	0	0	0	0
White	76	73	45	25	27	18	10	17	20	15	10	15	11	9
Perinatal transmission category														
Mother with documented HIV infection or 1 of the following risk factors:														
Injection drug use	120	90	77	49	23	23	24	21	13	9	6	18	7	11
Sex with injection drug user	65	43	40	27	19	21	8	9	11	7	5	8	6	5
Sex with bisexual male	8	11	5	5	2	5	3	5	2	5	4	6	2	0
Sex with person with hemophilia	2	2	0	0	1	1	1	1	0	1	0	0	0	0
Sex with HIV-infected transfusion recipient	1	0	0	0	0	0	0	0	0	0	0	0	0	1
Sex with HIV-infected person, risk factor not specified	82	86	49	53	46	29	42	47	40	40	33	35	24	15
Receipt of blood transfusion, blood components, or tissue	6	4	3	2	2	1	0	2	1	0	0	0	0	0
Has HIV infection, risk factor not specified	46	59	50	30	39	29	25	30	40	32	38	40	35	47
Child's diagnosis[c]														
HIV infection	123	130	114	89	90	68	73	74	71	76	68	88	58	64
AIDS	207	165	110	77	42	41	30	41	36	18	18	19	16	15
Total[d]	**330**	**295**	**224**	**166**	**132**	**109**	**103**	**115**	**107**	**94**	**86**	**107**	**74**	**79**

Note. Since 1994, the following 25 states have had laws and regulations requiring confidential name-based HIV infection reporting: Alabama, Arizona, Arkansas, Colorado, Idaho, Indiana, Louisiana, Michigan, Minnesota, Mississippi, Missouri, Nevada, New Jersey, North Carolina, North Dakota, Ohio, Oklahoma, South Carolina, South Dakota, Tennessee, Utah, Virginia, West Virginia, Wisconsin, and Wyoming.

Data include children with a diagnosis of HIV infection (not AIDS), a diagnosis of HIV infection and a later diagnosis of AIDS, or concurrent diagnoses of HIV infection and AIDS.
[a] Includes Asian/Pacific Islander legacy cases.
[b] Hispanics/Latinos can be of any race.
[c] In the surveillance system as of June 2008.
[d] Includes children of unknown race or multiple races.

Source: Centers for Disease Control and Prevention. *HIV/AIDS Surveillance Report, 2007.* Vol. 19. Atlanta: U.S. Department of Health and Human Services, Centers for Disease Control and Prevention; 2009: 32–54. http://www.cdc.gov/hiv/topics/surveillance/resources/reports/.

APPENDIX III
HIV AND AIDS STATISTICS, GLOBAL
2009 AND 2001*

* These data were reported in the 2010 UNAIDS report. At the time of production of the current report, analyses incorporating new data from a population-based survey with data from other sources were ongoing. This is why only ranges based on preliminary analysis are published. As soon as updated final estimates are available, they will be published on the UNAIDS Web site.

ESTIMATED NUMBER OF PEOPLE LIVING WITH HIV

	2009 Adults + Children		2001 Adults + Children		2009 Adults (15+)	
	estimate	[low – high estimate]	estimate	[low – high estimate]	estimate	[low – high estimate]
GLOBAL	33 300 000	[31 400 000 – 35 300 000]	28 600 000	[27 100 000 – 30 300 000]	30 800 000	[29 200 000 – 32 600 000]
SUB-SAHARAN AFRICA	22 500 000	[20 900 000 – 24 200 000]	20 300 000	[18 900 000 – 21 700 000]	20 300 000	[19 000 000 – 21 600 000]
Angola	200 000	[160 000 – 250 000]	140 000	[110 000 – 190 000]	180 000	[140 000 – 220 000]
Benin	60 000	[52 000 – 69 000]	50 000	[42 000 – 62 000]	55 000	[48 000 – 63 000]
Botswana	320 000	[300 000 – 350 000]	270 000	[250 000 – 290 000]	300 000	[280 000 – 330 000]
Burkina Faso	110 000	[91 000 – 140 000]	140 000	[120 000 – 180 000]	93 000	[77 000 – 120 000]
Burundi	180 000	[160 000 – 190 000]	170 000	[160 000 – 190 000]	150 000	[130 000 – 160 000]
Cameroon	610 000	[540 000 – 670 000]	480 000	[430 000 – 530 000]	550 000	[500 000 – 610 000]
Central African Republic	130 000	[110 000 – 140 000]	180 000	[160 000 – 220 000]	110 000	[98 000 – 120 000]
Chad	210 000	[170 000 – 300 000]	140 000	[99 000 – 180 000]	180 000	[150 000 – 280 000]
Comoros	<500	[<200 – <500]	<100	[<100 – <200]	<500	[<200 – <500]
Congo	77 000	[68 000 – 87 000]	69 000	[61 000 – 80 000]	69 000	[61 000 – 78 000]
Côte d'Ivoire	450 000	[390 000 – 510 000]	630 000	[560 000 – 710 000]	380 000	[340 000 – 440 000]
Democratic Republic of the Congo	...	[430 000 – 560 000]	...	[310 000 – 420 000]	...	[380 000 – 490 000]
Equatorial Guinea	20 000	[14 000 – 26 000]	5700	[3900 – 9100]	18 000	[13 000 – 23 000]
Eritrea	25 000	[18 000 – 33 000]	26 000	[19 000 – 34 000]	22 000	[16 000 – 29 000]
Ethiopia	...	...	...	...	...	...
Gabon	46 000	[37 000 – 55 000]	36 000	[29 000 – 46 000]	43 000	[35 000 – 51 000]
Gambia	18 000	[12 000 – 26 000]	4300	[2400 – 8400]	17 000	[11 000 – 24 000]
Ghana	260 000	[230 000 – 300 000]	250 000	[220 000 – 280 000]	240 000	[210 000 – 260 000]
Guinea	79 000	[65 000 – 95 000]	78 000	[57 000 – 120 000]	70 000	[58 000 – 84 000]
Guinea Bissau	22 000	[18 000 – 26 000]	14 000	[12 000 – 17 000]	20 000	[16 000 – 24 000]
Kenya	1 500 000	[1 300 000 – 1 600 000]	1 500 000	[1 400 000 – 1 600 000]	1 300 000	[1 200 000 – 1 400 000]
Lesotho	290 000	[260 000 – 310 000]	240 000	[220 000 – 270 000]	260 000	[240 000 – 280 000]
Liberia	37 000	[32 000 – 43 000]	51 000	[36 000 – 70 000]	31 000	[27 000 – 37 000]
Madagascar	24 000	[19 000 – 30 000]	18 000	[15 000 – 22 000]	23 000	[18 000 – 28 000]
Malawi	920 000	[830 000 – 1 000 000]	860 000	[770 000 – 960 000]	800 000	[730 000 – 890 000]
Mali	76 000	[61 000 – 96 000]	89 000	[72 000 – 110 000]	66 000	[52 000 – 84 000]
Mauritania	14 000	[11 000 – 17 000]	8900	[7300 – 11 000]	13 000	[11 000 – 16 000]
Mauritius	8800	[6400 – 12 000]	3100	[2 100 – 4 200]	8700	[6300 – 12 000]
Mozambique	1 400 000	[1 200 000 – 1 500 000]	850 000	[760 000 – 940 000]	1 200 000	[1 100 000 – 1 400 000]
Namibia	180 000	[150 000 – 210 000]	160 000	[140 000 – 200 000]	160 000	[140 000 – 190 000]
Niger	61 000	[50 000 – 77 000]	53 000	[43 000 – 67 000]	53 000	[43 000 – 67 000]
Nigeria	3 300 000	[2 900 000 – 3 600 000]	2 700 000	[2 300 000 – 3 100 000]	2 900 000	[2 600 000 – 3 200 000]
Rwanda	170 000	[140 000 – 190 000]	170 000	[150 000 – 210 000]	140 000	[120 000 – 160 000]
Senegal	59 000	[50 000 – 69 000]	33 000	[29 000 – 38 000]	54 000	[46 000 – 63 000]
Sierra Leone	49 000	[40 000 – 63 000]	25 000	[13 000 – 39 000]	46 000	[38 000 – 59 000]
South Africa	5 600 000	[5 400 000 – 5 900 000]	4 600 000	[4 500 000 – 4 700 000]	5 300 000	[5 100 000 – 5 500 000]
Swaziland	180 000	[170 000 – 200 000]	130 000	[120 000 – 150 000]	170 000	[160 000 – 180 000]
Togo	120 000	[99 000 – 150 000]	100 000	[82 000 – 130 000]	110 000	[91 000 – 140 000]
Uganda	1 200 000	[1 100 000 – 1 300 000]	980 000	[870 000 – 1 100 000]	1 000 000	[940 000 – 1 100 000]
United Republic of Tanzania	1 400 000	[1 300 000 – 1 500 000]	1 400 000	[1 200 000 – 1 500 000]	1 200 000	[1 100 000 – 1 400 000]
Zambia	980 000	[890 000 – 1 100 000]	830 000	[750 000 – 900 000]	860 000	[800 000 – 940 000]
Zimbabwe	1 200 000	[1 100 000 – 1 300 000]	1 700 000	[1 600 000 – 1 800 000]	1 000 000	[950 000 – 1 200 000]

	2001 Adults (15+)		2009 Adult (15–49) prevalence percent		2001 Adult (15–49) prevalence percent	
	estimate	[low – high estimate]	estimate	[low – high estimate]	estimate	[low – high estimate]
GLOBAL	26 700 000	[25 400 000 – 28 000 000]	0.8	[0.7 – 0.8]	0.8	[0.7 – 0.8]
SUB-SAHARAN AFRICA	18 500 000	[17 500 000 – 19 700 000]	5.0	[4.7 – 5.2]	5.9	[5.6 – 6.1]
Angola	130 000	[100 000 – 170 000]	2.0	[1.6 – 2.4]	1.9	[1.4 – 2.4]
Benin	47 000	[40 000 – 56 000]	1.2	[1.0 – 1.3]	1.4	[1.2 – 1.7]
Botswana	260 000	[240 000 – 280 000]	24.8	[23.8 – 25.8]	26.3	[25.5 – 27.4]
Burkina Faso	120 000	[99 000 – 150 000]	1.2	[1.0 – 1.5]	2.1	[1.7 – 2.5]
Burundi	150 000	[140 000 – 160 000]	3.3	[2.9 – 3.5]	5.0	[4.8 – 5.1]
Cameroon	440 000	[400 000 – 490 000]	5.3	[4.9 – 5.8]	5.5	[5.1 – 6.0]
Central African Republic	170 000	[150 000 – 200 000]	4.7	[4.2 – 5.2]	8.9	[8.1 – 10.6]
Chad	130 000	[91 000 – 170 000]	3.4	[2.8 – 5.1]	3.2	[2.3 – 4.0]
Comoros	<100	[<100 – <100]	0.1	[<0.1 – 0.1]	<0.1	[<0.1 – <0.1]
Congo	61 000	[54 000 – 71 000]	3.4	[3.1 – 3.8]	3.8	[3.4 – 4.4]
Côte d'Ivoire	570 000	[510 000 – 640 000]	3.4	[3.1 – 3.9]	6.5	[5.9 – 7.1]
Democratic Republic of the Congo	...	[270 000 – 360 000]	...	[1.2 – 1.6]	...	[1.1 – 1.5]
Equatorial Guinea	5400	[3700 – 8700]	5.0	[3.5 – 6.6]	1.9	[1.3 – 3.1]
Eritrea	23 000	[18 000 – 31 000]	0.8	[0.6 – 1.0]	1.2	[0.9 – 1.5]
Ethiopia	...	...	...	...	...	...
Gabon	34 000	[27 000 – 43 000]	5.2	[4.2 – 6.2]	5.3	[4.3 – 6.8]
Gambia	3900	[2200 – 7500]	2.0	[1.3 – 2.9]	0.6	[0.3 – 1.1]
Ghana	230 000	[200 000 – 260 000]	1.8	[1.6 – 2.0]	2.3	[2.0 – 2.5]
Guinea	70 000	[52 000 – 100 000]	1.3	[1.1 – 1.6]	1.7	[1.2 – 2.4]
Guinea-Bissau	13 000	[11 000 – 16 000]	2.5	[2.0 – 3.0]	2.0	[1.7 – 2.4]
Kenya	1 300 000	[1 200 000 – 1 400 000]	6.3	[5.8 – 6.5]	8.4	[8.1 – 9.0]
Lesotho	230 000	[210 000 – 250 000]	23.6	[22.3 – 25.2]	24.5	[23.1 – 26.1]
Liberia	46 000	[33 000 – 63 000]	1.5	[1.3 – 1.8]	3.1	[2.2 – 4.1]
Madagascar	17 000	[14 000 – 20 000]	0.2	[0.2 – 0.3]	0.2	[0.2 – 0.3]
Malawi	760 000	[690 000 – 840 000]	11.0	[10.0 – 12.1]	13.8	[12.7 – 15.1]
Mali	80 000	[66 000 – 98 000]	1.0	[0.8 – 1.3]	1.6	[1.3 – 1.9]
Mauritania	8600	[7100 – 11 000]	0.7	[0.6 – 0.9]	0.6	[0.5 – 0.7]
Mauritius	3100	[2100 – 4200]	1.0	[0.7 – 1.3]	0.4	[0.3 – 0.5]
Mozambique	800 000	[720 000 – 870 000]	11.5	[10.6 – 12.2]	9.4	[8.7 – 10.3]
Namibia	150 000	[130 000 – 180 000]	13.1	[11.1 – 15.5]	16.1	[13.6 – 19.0]
Niger	49 000	[40 000 – 61 000]	0.8	[0.7 – 1.0]	1.0	[0.8 – 1.3]
Nigeria	2 400 000	[2 100 000 – 2 700 000]	3.6	[3.3 – 4.0]	3.8	[3.4 – 4.2]
Rwanda	150 000	[140 000 – 170 000]	2.9	[2.5 – 3.3]	3.7	[3.4 – 4.4]
Senegal	31 000	[26 000 – 35 000]	0.9	[0.7 – 1.0]	0.6	[0.6 – 0.7]
Sierra Leone	24 000	[13 000 – 38 000]	1.6	[1.4 – 2.1]	1.1	[0.6 – 1.7]
South Africa	4 400 000	[4 300 000 – 4 500 000]	17.8	[17.2 – 18.3]	17.1	[16.7 – 17.5]
Swaziland	130 000	[120 000 – 140 000]	25.9	[24.9 – 27.0]	23.6	[22.4 – 24.8]
Togo	98 000	[76 000 – 120 000]	3.2	[2.5 – 3.8]	3.6	[2.8 – 4.3]
Uganda	840 000	[760 000 – 920 000]	6.5	[5.9 – 6.9]	7.0	[6.4 – 7.4]
United Republic of Tanzania	1 200 000	[1 100 000 – 1 300 000]	5.6	[5.3 – 6.1]	7.1	[6.7 – 7.7]
Zambia	730 000	[670 000 – 790 000]	13.5	[12.8 – 14.1]	14.3	[13.7 – 15.0]
Zimbabwe	1 500 000	[1 400 000 – 1 700 000]	14.3	[13.4 – 15.4]	23.7	[22.8 – 24.9]

ESTIMATED NUMBER OF PEOPLE LIVING WITH HIV *(continued)*

	2009 Women (15+)		2001 Women (15+)		2009 Children (0–14)	
	estimate	[low – high estimate]	estimate	[low – high estimate]	estimate	[low – high estimate]
GLOBAL	15 900 000	[14 800 000 – 17 200 000]	13 600 000	[12 900 000 – 14 700 000]	2 500 000	[1 600 000 – 3 400 000]
SUB-SAHARAN AFRICA	12 100 000	[11 100 000 – 13 200 000]	10 900 000	[10 100 000 – 11 700 000]	2 300 000	[1 400 000 – 3 100 000]
Angola	110 000	[85 000 – 130 000]	77 000	[59 000 – 100 000]	22 000	[12 000 – 35 000]
Benin	32 000	[27 000 – 37 000]	27 000	[23 000 – 33 000]	5400	[2900 – 7800]
Botswana	170 000	[160 000 – 190 000]	150 000	[140 000 – 160 000]	16 000	[9900 – 20 000]
Burkina Faso	56 000	[44 000 – 70 000]	73 000	[60 000 – 92 000]	17 000	[8100 – 25 000]
Burundi	90 000	[78 000 – 100 000]	90 000	[81 000 – 99 000]	28 000	[17 000 – 40 000]
Cameroon	320 000	[290 000 – 370 000]	260 000	[230 000 – 290 000]	54 000	[29 000 – 78 000]
Central African Republic	67 000	[57 000 – 78 000]	99 000	[86 000 – 120 000]	17 000	[8200 – 25 000]
Chad	110 000	[88 000 – 160 000]	76 000	[54 000 – 98 000]	23 000	[12 000 – 35 000]
Comoros	<100	[<100 – <100]	<100	[<100 – <100]	...	...
Congo	40 000	[35 000 – 47 000]	36 000	[31 000 – 42 000]	7900	[4000 – 12 000]
Côte d'Ivoire	220 000	[190 000 – 260 000]	320 000	[280 000 – 370 000]	63 000	[32 000 – 91 000]
Democratic Republic of the Congo	...	[220 000 – 300 000]	...	[160 000 – 220 000]	...	[33 000 – 86 000]
Equatorial Guinea	11 000	[7600 – 14 000]	3100	[2100 – 5100]	1600	[<1000 – 2600]
Eritrea	13 000	[9800 – 18 000]	14 000	[11 000 – 19 000]	3100	[1500 – 5000]
Ethiopia	...	...	...	...	...	...
Gabon	25 000	[20 000 – 30 000]	20 000	[16 000 – 25 000]	3200	[1700 – 4800]
Gambia	9700	[6200 – 14 000]	2300	[1300 – 4400]	...	...
Ghana	140 000	[120 000 – 160 000]	130 000	[120 000 – 150 000]	27 000	[14 000 – 41 000]
Guinea	41 000	[34 000 – 50 000]	41 000	[30 000 – 61 000]	9000	[4300 – 14 000]
Guinea-Bissau	12 000	[9300 – 14 000]	7800	[6400 – 9300]	2100	[1100 – 3200]
Kenya	760 000	[650 000 – 860 000]	780 000	[700 000 – 870 000]	180 000	[98 000 – 260 000]
Lesotho	160 000	[140 000 – 180 000]	140 000	[130 000 – 160 000]	28 000	[17 000 – 37 000]
Liberia	19 000	[16 000 – 22 000]	27 000	[19 000 – 37 000]	6100	[3000 – 9900]
Madagascar	7300	[5800 – 9000]	5400	[4500 – 6400]	...	...
Malawi	470 000	[410 000 – 530 000]	440 000	[390 000 – 500 000]	120 000	[68 000 – 170 000]
Mali	40 000	[31 000 – 52 000]	48 000	[40 000 – 59 000]	...	...
Mauritania	4000	[3200 – 4900]	2600	[2100 – 3200]	...	...
Mauritius	2500	[1800 – 3400]	<1000	[<1000 – 1200]	...	...
Mozambique	760 000	[680 000 – 840 000]	470 000	[430 000 – 530 000]	130 000	[70 000 – 180 000]
Namibia	95 000	[79 000 – 110 000]	90 000	[76 000 – 110 000]	16 000	[9100 – 23 000]
Niger	28 000	[23 000 – 36 000]	25 000	[20 000 – 32 000]	...	...
Nigeria	1 700 000	[1 500 000 – 1 900 000]	1 400 000	[1 200 000 – 1 600 000]	360 000	[180 000 – 520 000]
Rwanda	88 000	[76 000 – 98 000]	91 000	[83 000 – 110 000]	22 000	[11 000 – 34 000]
Senegal	32 000	[27 000 – 38 000]	18 000	[16 000 – 21 000]	...	...
Sierra Leone	28 000	[22 000 – 35 000]	14 000	[7500 – 23 000]	2900	[1500 – 4500]
South Africa	3 300 000	[3 000 000 – 3 500 000]	2 600 000	[2 500 000 – 2 700 000]	330 000	[190 000 – 440 000]
Swaziland	100 000	[91 000 – 110 000]	74 000	[69 000 – 82 000]	14 000	[8300 – 18 000]
Togo	67 000	[54 000 – 83 000]	57 000	[45 000 – 72 000]	11 000	[3700 – 18 000]
Uganda	610 000	[540 000 – 680 000]	490 000	[430 000 – 560 000]	150 000	[80 000 – 210 000]
United Republic of Tanzania	730 000	[650 000 – 830 000]	720 000	[640 000 – 800 000]	160 000	[83 000 – 240 000]
Zambia	490 000	[440 000 – 550 000]	420 000	[380 000 – 470 000]	120 000	[64 000 – 160 000]
Zimbabwe	620 000	[530 000 – 710 000]	890 000	[800 000 – 990 000]	150 000	[92 000 – 200 000]

	2001 Children (0–14)		2009 Young women (15–24) prevalence (%)		2009 Young men (15–24) prevalence (%)	
	estimate	[low – high estimate]	estimate	[low – high estimate]	estimate	[low – high estimate]
GLOBAL	2 000 000	[1 200 000 – 2 700 000]	0.6	[0.5 – 0.7]	0.3	[0.2 – 0.3]
SUB-SAHARAN AFRICA	1 800 000	[1 100 000 – 2 500 000]	3.4	[3.0 – 4.2]	1.4	[1.2 – 1.7]
Angola	14 000	[6900 – 24 000]	1.6	[1.1 – 2.2]	0.6	[0.4 – 0.9]
Benin	3100	[1600 – 6600]	0.7	[0.5 – 1.1]	0.3	[0.2 – 0.4]
Botswana	14 000	[7800 – 19 000]	11.8	[9.0 – 15.9]	5.2	[3.7 – 7.3]
Burkina Faso	24 000	[12 000 – 37 000]	0.8	[0.6 – 1.2]	0.5	[0.3 – 0.6]
Burundi	26 000	[16 000 – 36 000]	2.1	[1.6 – 2.7]	1.0	[0.8 – 1.2]
Cameroon	33 000	[18 000 – 50 000]	3.9	[3.1 – 5.4]	1.6	[1.2 – 2.1]
Central African Republic	17 000	[8600 – 25 000]	2.2	[1.4 – 3.1]	1.0	[0.6 – 1.4]
Chad	13 000	[6400 – 22 000]	2.5	[1.7 – 5.2]	1.0	[0.7 – 2.0]
Comoros	…	…	<0.1	[<0.1 – <0.1]	<0.1	[<0.1 – 0.1]
Congo	8300	[4200 – 12 000]	2.6	[2.1 – 3.6]	1.2	[0.9 – 1.6]
Côte d'Ivoire	59 000	[31 000 – 95 000]	1.5	[1.1 – 2.3]	0.7	[0.5 – 1.1]
Democratic Republic of the Congo	…	[26 000 – 70 000]	…	[0.9 – 1.5]	…	[0.4 – 0.6]
Equatorial Guinea	<500	[<200 – <1000]	5.0	[2.7 – 7.9]	1.9	[1.0 – 3.2]
Eritrea	2300	[1200 – 4100]	0.4	[0.2 – 0.7]	0.2	[0.1 – 0.3]
Ethiopia	…	…	…	…	…	…
Gabon	2000	[1200 – 3100]	3.5	[2.1 – 5.2]	1.4	[0.8 – 2.0]
Gambia	…	…	2.4	[1.4 – 4.0]	0.9	[0.5 – 1.6]
Ghana	18 000	[9900 – 29 000]	1.3	[0.9 – 1.8]	0.5	[0.4 – 0.7]
Guinea	8400	[3500 – 18 000]	0.9	[0.6 – 1.3]	0.4	[0.3 – 0.6]
Guinea-Bissau	<1000	[<1000 – 1400]	2.0	[1.5 – 2.9]	0.8	[0.5 – 1.1]
Kenya	170 000	[98 000 – 230 000]	4.1	[3.0 – 5.4]	1.8	[1.3 – 2.4]
Lesotho	18 000	[11 000 – 23 000]	14.2	[11.2 – 19.2]	5.4	[4.1 – 7.4]
Liberia	4600	[2100 – 8400]	0.7	[0.2 – 1.2]	0.3	[0.1 – 0.5]
Madagascar	…	…	0.1	[<0.1 – 0.1]	0.1	[0.1 – 0.4]
Malawi	100 000	[57 000 – 140 000]	6.8	[5.3 – 9.2]	3.1	[2.3 – 4.2]
Mali	…	…	0.5	[0.2 – 0.9]	0.2	[0.1 – 0.4]
Mauritania	…	…	0.3	[0.1 – 0.5]	0.4	[0.2 – 1.4]-
Mauritius	…	…	0.2	[0.1 – 0.3]	0.3	[0.2 – 0.4]
Mozambique	53 000	[30 000 – 77 000]	8.6	[7.0 – 12.1]	3.1	[2.4 – 4.4]
Namibia	7900	[4400 – 11 000]	5.8	[3.7 – 8.6]	2.3	[1.3 – 3.6]
Niger	…	…	0.5	[0.4 – 0.6]	0.2	[0.2 – 0.3]
Nigeria	270 000	[130 000 – 410 000]	2.9	[2.3 – 3.9]	1.2	[0.9 – 1.6]
Rwanda	23 000	[11 000 – 38 000]	1.9	[1.3 – 2.3]	1.3	[0.9 – 1.6]
Senegal	…	…	0.7	[0.5 – 1.0]	0.3	[0.2 – 0.4]
Sierra Leone	<1000	[<500 – 2100]	1.5	[0.9 – 2.5]	0.6	[0.3 – 1.0]
South Africa	170 000	[97 000 – 220 000]	13.6	[12.3 – 15.0]	4.5	[4.1 – 5.0]
Swaziland	7600	[4700 – 10 000]	15.6	[12.6 – 21.3]	6.5	[4.8 – 8.8]
Togo	6700	[2700 – 11 000]	2.2	[1.5 – 3.1]	0.9	[0.6 – 1.2]
Uganda	150 000	[84 000 – 210 000]	4.8	[4.0 – 6.4]	2.3	[1.8 – 2.8]
United Republic of Tanzania	150 000	[83 000 – 210 000]	3.9	[3.1 – 5.3]	1.7	[1.3 – 2.3]
Zambia	100 000	[57 000 – 140 000]	8.9	[7.3 – 12.0]	4.2	[3.2 – 5.5]
Zimbabwe	160 000	[100 000 – 210 000]	6.9	[5.3 – 9.3]	3.3	[2.5 – 4.4]

ESTIMATED NUMBER OF PEOPLE LIVING WITH HIV *(continued)*

	2009 Adult (15–49) incidence rate		2001 Adult (15–49) incidence rate		2009 Adults + children newly infected	
	estimate	[low – high estimate]	estimate	[low – high estimate]	estimate	[low – high estimate]
GLOBAL	<0.10	[<0.10 – <0.10]	<0.10	[<0.10 – <0.10]	2 600 000	[2 300 000 – 2 800 000]
SUB-SAHARAN AFRICA	0.41	[0.36 – 0.46]	0.61	[0.54 – 0.65]	1 800 000	[1 600 000 – 2 000 000]
Angola	0.21	[0.14 – 0.28]	0.22	[0.17 – 0.28]	22 000	[16 000 – 29 000]
Benin	0.10	[<0.10 – 0.13]	0.11	[<0.10 – 0.15]	4900	[3400 – 6500]
Botswana	1.56	[1.11 – 2.27]	3.03	[2.64 – 3.48]	14 000	[10 000 – 20 000]
Burkina Faso	<0.10	[<0.10 – 0.11]	0.11	[<0.10 – 0.16]	6800	[4300 – 11 000]
Burundi	...	[0.17 – 0.28]	...	[0.34 – 0.47]	...	[11 000 – 17 000]
Cameroon	0.53	[0.43 – 0.61]	0.59	[0.50 – 0.69]	58 000	[48 000 – 67 000]
Central African Republic	0.17	[<0.10 – 0.25]	0.56	[0.43 – 0.69]	5200	[3100 – 7100]
Chad	...	[0.15 – 0.87]	...	[0.39 – 0.55]	...	[12 000 – 47 000]
Comoros	...	[<0.10 – <0.10]	...	[<0.10 – <0.10]	...	[<100 – <100]
Congo	0.28	[0.23 – 0.35]	0.43	[0.36 – 0.51]	6500	[5200 – 7900]
Côte d'Ivoire	0.11	[<0.10 – 0.20]	0.39	[0.30 – 0.51]	17 000	[11 000 – 27 000]
Democratic Republic of the Congo	...	[0.13 – 0.18]	...	[0.13 – 0.18]	...	[49 000 – 67 000]
Equatorial Guinea	...	[0.23 – 1.20]	...	[0.38 – 0.83]	...	[1200 – 4500]
Eritrea	<0.10	[<0.10 – <0.10]	<0.10	[<0.10 – 0.14]	1300	[<1000 – 2300]
Ethiopia	...	...	...	...	...	...
Gabon	0.43	[0.10 – 0.61]	0.63	[0.46 – 0.85]	3600	[1300 – 5000]
Gambia	...	[0.21 – 0.83]	...	[<0.10 – 0.22]	...	[1900 – 6400]
Ghana	0.15	[0.12 – 0.19]	0.18	[0.15 – 0.22]	22 000	[17 000 – 27 000]
Guinea	0.10	[<0.10 – 0.13]	0.15	[0.11 – 0.21]	6200	[3800 – 8400]
Guinea-Bissau	0.21	[0.14 – 0.32]	0.32	[0.24 – 0.40]	2100	[1400 – 2900]
Kenya	0.53	[0.34 – 0.70]	0.55	[0.38 – 0.76]	110 000	[81 000 – 150 000]
Lesotho	2.58	[2.18 – 3.04]	2.88	[2.53 – 3.40]	23 000	[20 000 – 27 000]
Liberia	...	[<0.10 – 0.17]	...	[<0.10 – 0.22]	...	[<1000 – 3800]
Madagascar	...	[<0.10 – <0.10]	...	[<0.10 – <0.10]	...	[1800 – 3700]
Malawi	0.95	[0.67 – 1.23]	1.35	[1.15 – 1.61]	73 000	[57 000 – 91 000]
Mali	<0.10	[<0.10 – 0.12]	<0.10	[<0.10 – 0.14]	4600	[1300 – 8300]
Mauritania	...	[<0.10 – 0.11]	...	[<0.10 – 0.11]	...	[<1000 – 1900]
Mauritius	...	[<0.10 – 0.22]	...	[<0.10 – 0.12]	...	[<1000 – 1800]
Mozambique	1.19	[0.99 – 1.35]	1.77	[1.56 – 1.96]	130 000	[110 000 – 150 000]
Namibia	0.43	[<0.10 – 0.93]	2.29	[1.77 – 2.90]	5800	[2100 – 11 000]
Niger	<0.10	[<0.10 – <0.10]	<0.10	[<0.10 – <0.12]	6100	[4300 – 8400]
Nigeria	0.38	[0.33 – 0.44]	0.39	[0.33 – 0.47]	340 000	[280 000 – 390 000]
Rwanda	0.18	[<0.10 – 0.32]	0.34	[0.26 – 0.41]	8800	[3800 – 15 000]
Senegal	<0.10	[<0.10 – 0.11]	0.10	[<0.10 – 0.12]	6000	[4100 – 7900]
Sierra Leone	0.14	[<0.10 – 0.35]	0.22	[0.16 – 0.29]	4700	[3000 – 9900]
South Africa	1.49	[1.27 – 1.76]	2.35	[2.14 – 2.60]	390 000	[340 000 – 440 000]
Swaziland	2.66	[2.19 – 3.14]	4.07	[3.72 – 4.46]	14 000	[12 000 – 16 000]
Togo	0.27	[0.15 – 0.39]	0.37	[0.28 – 0.48]	10 000	[6200 – 14 000]
Uganda	0.74	[0.62 – 0.85]	0.71	[0.61 – 0.82]	120 000	[100 000 – 140 000]
United Republic of Tanzania	0.45	[0.34 – 0.57]	0.64	[0.55 – 0.76]	100 000	[82 000 – 130 000]
Zambia	1.17	[0.96 – 1.40]	1.72	[1.52 – 1.95]	76 000	[62 000 – 89 000]
Zimbabwe	0.84	[0.54 – 1.19]	1.94	[1.62 – 2.36]	62 000	[45 000 – 80 000]

	2009		ESTIMATED AIDS-RELATED DEATHS			
	Adults newly infected		2009		2001	
			AIDS-related deaths in adults + children		AIDS-related deaths in adults + children	
	estimate	[low – high estimate]	estimate	[low – high estimate]	estimate	[low – high estimate]
GLOBAL	2 200 000	[2 000 000 – 2 400 000]	1 800 000	[1 600 000 – 2 100 000]	1 800 000	[1 600 000 – 2 100 000]
SUB-SAHARAN AFRICA	1 500 000	[1 300 000 – 1 600 000]	1 300 000	[1 100 000 – 1 500 000]	1 400 000	[1 200 000 – 1 600 000]
Angola	17 000	[12 000 – 23 000]	11 000	[7700 – 16 000]	10 000	[6500 – 14 000]
Benin	4000	[2700 – 5400]	2700	[1800 – 3700]	3100	[1900 – 5200]
Botswana	13 000	[9400 – 19 000]	5800	[2300 – 14 000]	15 000	[12 000 – 18 000]
Burkina Faso	5000	[2800 – 7900]	7100	[4800 – 9700]	15 000	[11 000 – 19 000]
Burundi	...	[7000 – 11 000]	15 000	[12 000 – 17 000]	14 000	[12 000 – 17 000]
Cameroon	48 000	[39 000 – 56 000]	37 000	[29 000 – 46 000]	31 000	[25 000 – 37 000]
Central African Republic	3600	[1800 – 5200]	11 000	[8800 – 13 000]	15 000	[12 000 – 20 000]
Chad	...	[8000 – 39 000]	11 000	[8100 – 15 000]	8900	[5400 – 13 000]
Comoros	...	[<100 – <100]	<100	[<100 – <100]	<100	[<100 – <100]
Congo	5100	[4100 – 6300]	5100	[4100 – 6400]	5800	[4800 – 7100]
Côte d'Ivoire	11 000	[5700 – 19 000]	36 000	[29 000 – 44 000]	51 000	[37 000 – 66 000]
Democratic Republic of the Congo	...	[38 000 – 52 000]	...	[26 000 – 40 000]	...	[24 000 – 34 000]
Equatorial Guinea	...	[<1000 – 3800]	<1000	[<1000 – 1400]	<500	[<200 – <500]
Eritrea	<1000	[<500 – 1700]	1700	[1000 – 2500]	1800	[1200 – 2600]
Ethiopia	...	...	...	...	...	...
Gabon	3100	[<1000 – 4300]	2400	[1600 – 3400]	2000	[1500 – 2800]
Gambia	...	[1600 – 5800]	<1000	[<500 – 1200]	<500	[<200 – <1000]
Ghana	18 000	[14 000 – 23 000]	18 000	[14 000 – 22 000]	16 000	[13 000 – 21 000]
Guinea	4800	[2600 – 6600]	4700	[3100 – 6900]	6300	[3000 – 14 000]
Guinea-Bissau	1600	[1100 – 2300]	1200	[<1000 – 1600]	<1000	[<1000 – <1000]
Kenya	92 000	[61 000 – 120 000]	80 000	[61 000 – 99 000]	120 000	[100 000 – 150 000]
Lesotho	20 000	[17 000 – 24 000]	14 000	[10 000 – 18 000]	14 000	[12 000 – 18 000]
Liberia	...	[<200 – 3100]	3600	[2800 – 4600]	3900	[2300 – 6200]
Madagascar	...	[1600 – 3400]	1700	[1400 – 2000]	1300	[1100 – 1600]
Malawi	56 000	[40 000 – 72 000]	51 000	[38 000 – 67 000]	68 000	[57 000 – 81 000]
Mali	3400	[<500 – 6800]	4400	[3000 – 6100]	7200	[4200 – 11 000]
Mauritania	...	[<1000 – 1700]	<1000	[<1000 – 1000]	<500	[<500 – <1000]
Mauritius	...	[<1000 – 1800]	<500	[<500 – <1000]	<200	[<100 – <200]
Mozambique	110 000	[91 000 – 120 000]	74 000	[57 000 – 92 000]	43 000	[34 000 – 53 000]
Namibia	4400	[<1000 – 9300]	6700	[2500 – 11 000]	8100	[6200 – 11 000]
Niger	4600	[3200 – 6100]	4300	[3300 – 5600]	3300	[2500 – 4500]
Nigeria	270 000	[230 000 – 310 000]	220 000	[170 000 – 260 000]	210 000	[130 000 – 260 000]
Rwanda	6000	[1100 – 12 000]	4100	[<1000 – 9700]	15 000	[12 000 – 21 000]
Senegal	4800	[3100 – 6300]	2600	[1900 – 3500]	1800	[1500 – 2300]
Sierra Leone	3900	[2300 – 8900]	2800	[2100 – 3700]	<1000	[<500 – 2200]
South Africa	340 000	[300 000 – 400 000]	310 000	[260 000 – 390 000]	220 000	[180 000 – 260 000]
Swaziland	12 000	[10 000 – 14 000]	7000	[4600 – 10 000]	6800	[5700 – 8400]
Togo	8700	[5100 – 12 000]	7700	[5300 – 10 000]	6400	[4600 – 8400]
Uganda	100 000	[84 000 – 120 000]	64 000	[49 000 – 80 000]	89 000	[75 000 – 100 000]
United Republic of Tanzania	88 000	[66 000 – 110 000]	86 000	[69 000 – 110 000]	110 000	[94 000 – 130 000]
Zambia	59 000	[48 000 – 71 000]	45 000	[30 000 – 60 000]	68 000	[57 000 – 78 000]
Zimbabwe	48 000	[31 000 – 66 000]	83 000	[70 000 – 97 000]	130 000	[110 000 – 160 000]

	ESTIMATED ORPHANS DUE TO AIDS				HIV PREVALENCE (%) IN MOST-AT-RISK GROUPS IN CAPITAL CITY					
	2009 Orphans (0–17) currently living		2001 Orphans (0–17)		Injecting drug users		Female sex workers		Men who have sex with men	
	estimate	[low – high estimate]	estimate	[low – high estimate]	Year	HIV (%)	Year	HIV (%)	Year	HIV (%)
GLOBAL	16 600 000	[14 400 000 – 18 800 000]	10 000 000	[7 900 000 – 12 500 000]	...	...	...	...	...	...
SUB-SAHARAN AFRICA	14 800 000	[12 800 000 – 17 000 000]	8 900 000	[6 900 000 – 11 200 000]	...	...	...	...	...	...
Angola	140 000	[95 000 – 200 000]	65 000	[30 000 – 110 000]	...	...	...	...	...	...
Benin	30 000	[18 000 – 53 000]	13 000	[5100 – 100 000]	2009	4.2	2009	24.7	...	...
Botswana	93 000	[71 000 – 120 000]	56 000	[45 000 – 72 000]	...	...	...	...	...	...
Burkina Faso	140 000	[100 000 – 170 000]	140 000	[100 000 – 190 000]	...	...	2005	16.3	...	...
Burundi	200 000	[170 000 – 230 000]	130 000	[110 000 – 160 000]	...	...	2007	39.8	...	...
Cameroon	330 000	[270 000 – 420 000]	140 000	[91 000 – 230 000]	...	...	2009	35.5	...	...
Central African Republic	140 000	[110 000 – 180 000]	82 000	[54 000 – 120 000]	...	...	...	...	...	...
Chad	120 000	[79 000 – 170 000]	50 000	[26 000 – 91 000]	...	...	2009	20.0	...	...
Comoros	<100	[<100 – <100]	<100	[<100 – <100]	...	...	...	...	...	...
Congo	51 000	[41 000 – 66 000]	51 000	[34 000 – 73 000]	...	...	...	...	...	...
Côte d'Ivoire	440 000	[330 000 – 550 000]	270 000	[170 000 – 440 000]	...	...	...	...	...	...
Democratic Republic of the Congo	...	[350 000 – 510 000]	...	[290 000 – 450 000]	...	...	...	...	...	...
Equatorial Guinea	4100	[2500 – 6400]	<1000	[<500 – <1000]	...	...	...	...	...	...
Eritrea	19 000	[12 000 – 28 000]	8 700	[4100 – 18 000]	...	...	2008	7.8	...	...
Ethiopia	...	...	...	...	...	...	...	...	...	...
Gabon	18 000	[12 000 – 25 000]	7 600	[5200 – 11 000]	...	...	2010	23.6	...	...
Gambia	2800	[1400 – 6500]	<1000	[<500 – 6400]	...	...	...	...	...	...
Ghana	160 000	[120 000 – 210 000]	60 000	[42 000 – 120 000]	...	...	2009	25.0	...	...
Guinea	59 000	[34 000 – 120 000]	40 000	[12 000 – 100 000]	...	...	2008	32.7	...	...
Guinea-Bissau	9700	[7700 – 12 000]	2800	[1800 – 3900]	...	...	2009	39.6	...	...
Kenya	1 200 000	[980 000 – 1 400 000]	820 000	[640 000 – 1 100 000]	...	...	...	...	...	...
Lesotho	130 000	[110 000 – 160 000]	52 000	[41 000 – 68 000]	...	...	...	...	...	...
Liberia	52 000	[34 000 – 76 000]	19 000	[9900 – 33 000]	...	...	...	...	...	...
Madagascar	11 000	[9 300 – 14 000]	9500	[7600 – 12 000]	...	...	2007	0.5	...	...
Malawi	650 000	[540 000 – 780 000]	430 000	[330 000 – 550 000]	...	...	2006	70.7	...	...
Mali	59 000	[36 000 – 93 000]	35 000	[15 000 – 89 000]	...	...	2006	35.3	...	...
Mauritania	3600	[2700 – 4800]	1500	[<1000 – 2200]	...	...	2007	7.6	...	...
Mauritius	<1000	[<500 – <1000]	<200	[<100 – <500]	2009	47.1	...	...	...	...
Mozambique	670 000	...	220 000	...	...	...	...	...	...	...
Namibia	70 000	[50 000 – 96 000]	30 000	[22 000 – 42 000]	...	...	...	...	...	...
Niger	57 000	[44 000 – 73 000]	17 000	[12 000 – 24 000]	...	...	2009	35.6	...	...
Nigeria	2 500 000	[1 800 000 – 3 100 000]	1 300 000	[420 000 – 1 900 000]	2007	5.6	2007	32.7	2007	13.5
Rwanda	130 000	[98 000 – 180 000]	170 000	[140 000 – 250 000]	...	...	...	...	...	...
Senegal	19 000	[15 000 – 25 000]	8700	[6600 – 11 000]	...	...	2006	19.8	2007	21.8
Sierra Leone	15 000	[9 200 – 26 000]	2100	[1000 – 7000]	...	...	2005	8.5	...	...
South Africa	1 900 000	[1 600 000 – 2 400 000]	580 000	[460 000 – 750 000]	...	...	...	...	2008	13.2
Swaziland	69 000	[55 000 – 86 000]	29 000	[23 000 – 37 000]	...	...	...	...	...	...
Togo	66 000	[47 000 – 89 000]	25 000	[12 000 – 45 000]	...	...	2005	44.5	...	...
Uganda	1 200 000	[1 000 000 – 1 400 000]	1 100 000	[860 000 – 1 400 000]	...	...	...	...	...	...
United Republic of Tanzania	1 300 000	[1 100 000 – 1 500 000]	840 000	[690 000 – 1 000 000]	...	...	...	...	...	...
Zambia	690 000	[570 000 – 810 000]	580 000	[410 000 – 770 000]	...	...	...	...	...	...
Zimbabwe	1 000 000	[910 000 – 1 200 000]	760 000	[630 000 – 940 000]	...	...	...	...	...	...

	2009 Adults + Children		2001 Adults + Children		2009 Adults (15+)	
	estimate	[low – high estimate]	estimate	[low – high estimate]	estimate	[low – high estimate]
EAST ASIA	770 000	[560 000 – 1 000 000]	350 000	[250 000 – 480 000]	760 000	[560 000 – 1 000 000]
China	740 000	[540 000 – 1 000 000]	...	[240 000 – 470 000]	730 000	[540 000 – 1 000 000]
Democratic People's Republic of Korea	...	...	...	...	...	...
Japan	8100	[6300 – 10 000]	6500	[5200 – 8100]	8100	[6300 – 10 000]
Mongolia	<500	[<500 – <1000]	<100	[<100 – <200]	<500	[<500 – <1000]
Republic of Korea	9500	[7000 – 13 000]	5200	[4100 – 6700]	9500	[7000 – 13 000]
OCEANIA	57 000	[50 000 – 64 000]	29 000	[23 000 – 35 000]	54 000	[47 000 – 61 000]
Australia	20 000	[15 000 – 25 000]	13 000	[10 000 – 16 000]	20 000	[15 000 – 25 000]
Fiji	<1000	[<500 – <1000]	<200	[<100 – <500]	<1000	[<500 – <1000]
New Zealand	2500	[2000 – 3200]	1600	[1400 – 2100]	2400	[2000 – 3200]
Papua New Guinea	34 000	[30 000 – 39 000]	14 000	[9400 – 21 000]	31 000	[27 000 – 35 000]
SOUTH AND SOUTH-EAST ASIA	4 100 000	[3 700 000 – 4 600 000]	3 800 000	[3 500 000 – 4 200 000]	4 000 000	[3 600 000 – 4 400 000]
Bangladesh	6300	[5200 – 8300]	1100	[<100 – 2400]	6200	[5100 – 8100]
Bhutan	<1000	[<1000 – 1500]	<200	[<100 – <500]	<1000	[<1000 – 1500]
Cambodia	63 000	[42 000 – 90 000]	92 000	[63 000 – 130 000]	56 000	[38 000 – 82 000]
India	2 400 000	[2 100 000 – 2 800 000]	2 500 000	[2 300 000 – 2 900 000]	2 300 000	[2 000 000 – 2 600 000]
Indonesia	310 000	[200 000 – 460 000]	11 000	[<100 – 34 000]	300 000	[200 000 – 460 000]
Lao People's Democratic Republic	8500	[6000 – 13 000]	<1000	[<100 – 1700]	8300	[5800 – 12 000]
Malaysia	100 000	[83 000 – 120 000]	67 000	[57 000 – 80 000]	100 000	[83 000 – 120 000]
Maldives	<100	[<100 – <100]	<100	[<100 – <100]	<100	[<100 – <100]
Myanmar	240 000	[200 000 – 290 000]	250 000	[190 000 – 310 000]	230 000	[190 000 – 280 000]
Nepal	64 000	[51 000 – 80 000]	60 000	[49 000 – 72 000]	60 000	[48 000 – 75 000]
Pakistan	98 000	[79 000 – 120 000]	39 000	[32 000 – 48 000]	95 000	[76 000 – 120 000]
Philippines	8700	[6100 – 13 000]	1700	[<100 – 4000]	8600	[6000 – 13 000]
Singapore	3400	[2500 – 4400]	2800	[2200 – 3800]	3300	[2400 – 4300]
Sri Lanka	2800	[2100 – 3800]	1300	[<1000 – 1900]	2800	[2100 – 3700]
Thailand	530 000	[420 000 – 660 000]	640 000	[480 000 – 820 000]	520 000	[410 000 – 640 000]
Viet Nam	280 000	[220 000 – 350 000]	140 000	[110 000 – 180 000]	270 000	[220 000 – 350 000]
EASTERN EUROPE AND CENTRAL ASIA	1 400 000	[1 300 000 – 1 600 000]	760 000	[670 000 – 890 000]	1 400 000	[1 200 000 – 1 600 000]
Armenia	1900	[1500 – 2400]	1400	[1100 – 1700]	1900	[1500 – 2300]
Azerbaijan	3600	[2600 – 5200]	1300	[<500 – 1700]	3500	[2500 – 5100]
Belarus	17 000	[13 000 – 20 000]	6300	[5100 – 7800]	16 000	[13 000 – 20 000]
Georgia	3500	[2600 – 4900]	1200	[<100 – 1700]	3400	[2500 – 4800]
Kazakhstan	13 000	[9000 – 19 000]	1800	[<1000 – 3400]	13 000	[8900 – 19 000]
Kyrgyzstan	9800	[6500 – 16 000]	<1000	[<100 – 11 000]	9700	[6400 – 16 000]
Republic of Moldova	12 000	[9900 – 16 000]	12 000	[9900 – 16 000]	12 000	[9800 – 15 000]
Russian Federation	980 000	[840 000 – 1 200 000]	430 000	[350 000 – 550 000]	960 000	[830 000 – 1 100 000]
Tajikistan	9100	[6400 – 13 000]	4100	[3100 – 5300]	8900	[6300 – 12 000]
Ukraine	350 000	[300 000 – 410 000]	290 000	[250 000 – 330 000]	350 000	[300 000 – 410 000]
Uzbekistan	28 000	[18 000 – 46 000]	<1000	[<100 – <100]	28 000	[18 000 – 45 000]
WESTERN AND CENTRAL EUROPE	820 000	[720 000 – 910 000]	630 000	[570 000 – 700 000]	820 000	[720 000 – 910 000]
Austria	15 000	[12 000 – 20 000]	5300	[3900 – 7000]	15 000	[12 000 – 20 000]
Belgium	14 000	[11 000 – 18 000]	12 000	[9500 – 16 000]	14 000	[11 000 – 18 000]
Bulgaria	3800	[2800 – 5200]	1 800	[1300 – 2300]	3800	[2700 – 5200]

ESTIMATED PEOPLE LIVING WITH HIV (continued)

	2001 Adults (15+)		2009 Adult (15–49) prevalence percent		2001 Adult (15–49) prevalence percent	
	estimate	[low – high estimate]	estimate	[low – high estimate]	estimate	[low – high estimate]
EAST ASIA	350 000	[250 000 – 480 000]	0.1	[0.1 – 0.1]	<0.1	[<0.1 – <0.1]
China	...	[240 000 – 470 000]	0.1	[0.1 – 0.1]	...	[<0.1 – 0.1]
Democratic People's Republic of Korea	...	...	...	...	...	...
Japan	6400	[5200 – 8100]	<0.1	[<0.1 – <0.1]	<0.1	[<0.1 – <0.1]
Mongolia	<100	[<100 – <200]	<0.1	[<0.1 – <0.1]	<0.1	[<0.1 – <0.1]
Republic of Korea	5200	[4100 – 6700]	<0.1	[<0.1 – <0.1]	<0.1	[<0.1 – <0.1]
OCEANIA	28 000	[22 000 – 34 000]	0.3	[0.2 – 0.3]	0.2	[0.1 – 0.2]
Australia	13 000	[9900 – 16 000]	0.1	[0.1 – 0.2]	0.1	[0.1 – 0.1]
Fiji	<200	[<100 – <500]	0.1	[0.1 – 0.2]	<0.1	[<0.1 – 0.1]
New Zealand	1600	[1400 – 2100]	0.1	[0.1 – 0.1]	0.1	[0.1 – 0.1]
Papua New Guinea	13 000	[9100 – 19 000]	0.9	[0.8 – 1.0]	0.5	[0.3 – 0.7]
SOUTH AND SOUTH-EAST ASIA	3 700 000	[3 400 000 – 4 100 000]	0.3	[0.3 – 0.3]	0.4	[0.3 – 0.4]
Bangladesh	1100	[<100 – 2300]	<0.1	[<0.1 – <0.1]	<0.1	[<0.1 – <0.1]
Bhutan	<100	[<100 – <500]	0.2	[0.1 – 0.3]	<0.1	[<0.1 – 0.1]
Cambodia	83 000	[58 000 – 110 000]	0.5	[0.4 – 0.8]	1.2	[0.8 – 1.6]
India	2 500 000	[2 200 000 – 2 800 000]	0.3	[0.3 – 0.4]	0.4	[0.4 – 0.5]
Indonesia	11 000	[<100 – 34 000]	0.2	[0.1 – 0.3]	<0.1	[<0.1 – <0.1]
Lao People's Democratic Republic	<1000	[<100 – 1700]	0.2	[0.2 – 0.4]	<0.1	[<0.1 – 0.1]
Malaysia	67 000	[56 000 – 80 000]	0.5	[0.4 – 0.6]	0.4	[0.3 – 0.5]
Maldives	<100	[<100 – <100]	<0.1	[<0.1 – <0.1]	<0.1	[<0.1 – <0.1]
Myanmar	250 000	[190 000 – 310 000]	0.6	[0.5 – 0.7]	0.8	[0.6 – 0.9]
Nepal	57 000	[47 000 – 69 000]	0.4	[0.3 – 0.5]	0.5	[0.4 – 0.6]
Pakistan	39 000	[32 000 – 47 000]	0.1	[0.1 – 0.1]	0.1	[<0.1 – 0.1]
Philippines	1600	[<100 – 3900]	<0.1	[<0.1 – <0.1]	<0.1	[<0.1 – <0.1]
Singapore	2700	[2100 – 3700]	0.1	[0.1 – 0.1]	0.1	[0.1 – 0.1]
Sri Lanka	1300	[<1000 – 1900]	<0.1	[<0.1 – <0.1]	<0.1	[<0.1 – <0.1]
Thailand	610 000	[470 000 – 790 000]	1.3	[1.0 – 1.6]	1.7	[1.3 – 2.1]
Viet Nam	140 000	[110 000 – 170 000]	0.4	[0.3 – 0.5]	0.3	[0.2 – 0.3]
EASTERN EUROPE AND CENTRAL ASIA	750 000	[660 000 – 880 000]	0.8	[0.7 – 0.9]	0.4	[0.4 – 0.5]
Armenia	1400	[1100 – 1700]	0.1	[0.1 – 0.1]	0.1	[0.1 – 0.1]
Azerbaijan	1200	[<500 – 1600]	0.1	[<0.1 – 0.1]	<0.1	[<0.1 – <0.1]
Belarus	6300	[5000 – 7800]	0.3	[0.2 – 0.3]	0.1	[0.1 – 0.1]
Georgia	1200	[<100 – 1700]	0.1	[0.1 – 0.2]	<0.1	[<0.1 – 0.1]
Kazakhstan	1800	[<1000 – 3400]	0.1	[0.1 – 0.2]	<0.1	[<0.1 – <0.1]
Kyrgyzstan	<1000	[<100 – 11 000]	0.3	[0.2 – 0.5]	<0.1	[<0.1 – 0.3]
Republic of Moldova	12 000	[9800 – 16 000]	0.4	[0.4 – 0.6]	0.4	[0.3 – 0.6]
Russian Federation	430 000	[350 000 – 550 000]	1.0	[0.9 – 1.2]	0.5	[0.4 – 0.6]
Tajikistan	4000	[3000 – 5200]	0.2	[0.1 – 0.3]	0.1	[0.1 – 0.1]
Ukraine	290 000	[250 000 – 330 000]	1.1	[1.0 – 1.3]	0.9	[0.8 – 1.1]
Uzbekistan	<1000	[<100 – <100]	0.1	[0.1 – 0.2]	<0.1	[<0.1 – <0.1]
WESTERN AND CENTRAL EUROPE	620 000	[570 000 – 700 000]	0.2	[0.2 – 0.2]	0.2	[0.2 – 0.2]
Austria	5300	[3900 – 7000]	0.3	[0.2 – 0.4]	0.1	[0.1 – 0.2]
Belgium	12 000	[9500 – 16 000]	0.2	[0.2 – 0.3]	0.2	[0.2 – 0.3]
Bulgaria	1800	[1300 – 2300]	0.1	[0.1 – 0.1]	<0.1	[<0.1 – <0.1]

	2009 Women (15+)		2001 Women (15+)		2009 Children (0–14)	
	estimate	[low – high estimate]	estimate	[low – high estimate]	estimate	[low – high estimate]
EAST ASIA	220 000	[160 000 – 300 000]	98 000	[71 000 – 140 000]	8000	[3600 – 13 000]
China	230 000	[160 000 – 300 000]	...	[67 000 – 130 000]	...	...
Democratic People's Republic of Korea	...	...	...	...	...	...
Japan	2700	[2100 – 3400]	2200	[1700 – 2700]	...	...
Mongolia	<200	[<100 – <200]	<100	[<100 – <100]	...	...
Republic of Korea	2900	[2200 – 4000]	1600	[1200 – 2000]	...	...
OCEANIA	25 000	[22 000 – 28 000]	12 000	[9400 – 16 000]	3100	[1500 – 4800]
Australia	6200	[4800 – 7800]	3900	[3100 – 4900]	...	...
Fiji	<200	[<200 – <500]	<100	[<100 – <100]	...	...
New Zealand	<1000	[<1000 – 1000]	<1000	[<500 – <1000]	...	...
Papua New Guinea	18 000	[16 000 – 21 000]	7600	[5100 – 11 000]	3100	[1600 – 4800]
SOUTH AND SOUTH-EAST ASIA	1 400 000	[1 400 000 – 1 700 000]	1 300 000	[1 300 000 – 1 600 000]	150 000	[97 000 – 200 000]
Bangladesh	1900	[1500 – 2400]	<500	[<100 – <1000]	...	...
Bhutan	<500	[<200 – <500]	<100	[<100 – <100]	...	...
Cambodia	35 000	[23 000 – 52 000]	51 000	[34 000 – 71 000]	...	...
India	880 000	[730 000 – 1 000 000]	880 000	[780 000 – 1 000 000]	...	...
Indonesia	88 000	[58 000 – 130 000]	3200	[<100 – 9600]	...	...
Lao People's Democratic Republic	3500	[2400 – 5500]	<500	[<100 – <500]	...	...
Malaysia	11 000	[8600 – 15 000]	6100	[4100 – 8100]	...	...
Maldives	<100	[<100 – <100]	<100	[<100 – <100]	...	...
Myanmar	81 000	[67 000 – 96 000]	67 000	[53 000 – 83 000]	...	...
Nepal	20 000	[16 000 – 25 000]	19 000	[15 000 – 22 000]	...	...
Pakistan	28 000	[23 000 – 35 000]	11 000	[9000 – 13 000]	...	...
Philippines	2600	[1800 – 3900]	<500	[<100 – 1100]	...	...
Singapore	1000	[<1000 – 1300]	<1000	[<1000 – 1100]	...	...
Sri Lanka	<1000	[<500 – <1000]	<500	[<200 – <500]	...	...
Thailand	210 000	[160 000 – 260 000]	220 000	[160 000 – 300 000]	...	...
Viet Nam	81 000	[63 000 – 100 000]	39 000	[31 000 – 50 000]	...	...
EASTERN EUROPE AND CENTRAL ASIA	690 000	[600 000 – 790 000]	330 000	[290 000 – 390 000]	18 000	[8600 – 29 000]
Armenia	<1000	[<500 – <1000]	<500	[<500 – <1000]	...	...
Azerbaijan	2100	[1500 – 3000]	<1000	[<500 – <1000]	...	...
Belarus	8300	[6700 – 10 000]	2300	[1900 – 2900]	...	...
Georgia	1500	[1100 – 2100]	<500	[<100 – <1000]	...	...
Kazakhstan	7700	[5300 – 11 000]	1100	[<1000 – 2000]	...	...
Kyrgyzstan	2800	[1900 – 4700]	<500	[<100 – 3200]	...	...
Republic of Moldova	5100	[4100 – 6600]	3700	[2900 – 4800]	...	...
Russian Federation	480 000	[400 000 – 570 000]	190 000	[160 000 – 250 000]	...	...
Tajikistan	2700	[1900 – 3700]	1100	[<1000 – 1500]	...	...
Ukraine	170 000	[140 000 – 200 000]	130 000	[110 000 – 150 000]	...	...
Uzbekistan	8000	[4900 – 13 000]	<500	[<100 – <100]	...	...
WESTERN AND CENTRAL EUROPE	240 000	[210 000 – 270 000]	180 000	[160 000 – 200 000]	1400	[<1000 – 1800]
Austria	4600	[3500 – 5900]	1600	[1100 – 2100]	...	...
Belgium	4400	[3400 – 5500]	3700	[2900 – 4800]	...	...
Bulgaria	1100	[<1000 – 1500]	<500	[<500 – <1000]	...	...

ESTIMATED PEOPLE LIVING WITH HIV (continued)

	2001 Children (0–14)		2009 Young women (15–24) prevalence (%)		2009 Young men (15–24) prevalence (%)	
	estimate	[low – high estimate]	estimate	[low – high estimate]	estimate	[low – high estimate]
EAST ASIA	2800	[1200 – 5400]	<0.1	[<0.1 – <0.1]	<0.1	[<0.1 – <0.1]
China	…	…	…	[<0.1 – <0.1]	…	[<0.1 – <0.1]
Democratic People's Republic of Korea	…	…	…	…	…	…
Japan	…	…	<0.1	[<0.1 – <0.1]	<0.1	[<0.1 – <0.1]
Mongolia	…	…	<0.1	[<0.1 – <0.1]	<0.1	[<0.1 – 0.1]
Republic of Korea	…	…	<0.1	[<0.1 – <0.1]	<0.1	[<0.1 – 0.1]
OCEANIA	<1000	[<500 – 1600]	0.2	[0.2 – 0.3]	0.1	[0.1 – 0.3]
Australia	…	…	0.1	[<0.1 – 0.1]	0.1	[<0.1 – 0.3]
Fiji	…	…	0.1	[<0.1 – 0.1]	0.1	[<0.1 – 0.3]
New Zealand	…	…	<0.1	[<0.1 – 0.1]	<0.1	[<0.1 – 0.1]
Papua New Guinea	<1000	[<500 – 1500]	0.8	[0.6 – 1.2]	0.3	[0.2 – 0.5]
SOUTH AND SOUTH-EAST ASIA	100 000	[67 000 – 140 000]	0.1	[0.1 – 0.1]	0.1	[0.1 – 0.1]
Bangladesh	…	…	<0.1	[<0.1 – <0.1]	<0.1	[<0.1 – <0.1]
Bhutan	…	…	<0.1	[<0.1 – 0.1]	0.1	[<0.1 – 0.1]
Cambodia	…	…	0.1	[0.1 – 0.3]	0.1	[<0.1 – 0.2]
India	…	…	0.1	[0.1 – 0.2]	0.1	[0.1 – 0.2]
Indonesia	…	…	<0.1	[<0.1 – 0.1]	0.1	[<0.1 – 0.1]
Lao People's Democratic Republic	…	…	0.2	[0.1 – 0.3]	0.1	[0.1 – 0.2]
Malaysia	…	…	<0.1	[<0.1 – <0.1]	0.1	[0.1 – 0.2]
Maldives	…	…	<0.1	[<0.1 – <0.1]	<0.1	[<0.1 – <0.1]
Myanmar	…	…	0.3	[0.2 – 0.3]	0.3	[0.3 – 0.4]
Nepal	…	…	0.1	[0.1 – 0.2]	0.2	[0.1 – 0.6]
Pakistan	…	…	<0.1	[<0.1 – 0.1]	0.1	[<0.1 – 0.2]
Philippines	…	…	<0.1	[<0.1 – <0.1]	<0.1	[<0.1 – <0.1]
Singapore	…	…	<0.1	[<0.1 – 0.1]	<0.1	[<0.1 – 0.2]
Sri Lanka	…	…	<0.1	[<0.1 – <0.1]	<0.1	[<0.1 – <0.1]
Thailand	…	…	…	[0.4 – 0.7]	…	[0.4 – 0.5]
Viet Nam	…	…	0.1	[<0.1 – 0.1]	0.1	[0.1 – 0.1]
EASTERN EUROPE AND CENTRAL ASIA	4000	[2000 – 6100]	0.2	[0.2 – 0.3]	0.1	[0.1 – 0.1]
Armenia	…	…	<0.1	[<0.1 – <0.1]	<0.1	[<0.1 – <0.1]
Azerbaijan	…	…	0.1	[0.1 – 0.1]	<0.1	[<0.1 – 0.1]
Belarus	…	…	0.1	[0.1 – 0.1]	<0.1	[<0.1 – 0.1]
Georgia	…	…	<0.1	[<0.1 – 0.1]	<0.1	[<0.1 – <0.1]
Kazakhstan	…	…	0.2	[0.1 – 0.3]	0.1	[<0.1 – 0.1]
Kyrgyzstan	…	…	0.1	[<0.1 – 0.1]	0.1	[<0.1 – 0.2]
Republic of Moldova	…	…	0.1	[0.1 – 0.1]	0.1	[<0.1 – 0.1]
Russian Federation	…	…	0.3	[0.3 – 0.4]	0.2	[0.1 – 0.2]
Tajikistan	…	…	<0.1	[<0.1 – 0.1]	<0.1	[<0.1 – 0.1]
Ukraine	…	…	0.3	[0.2 – 0.4]	0.2	[0.1 – 0.2]
Uzbekistan	…	…	<0.1	[<0.1 – 0.1]	<0.1	[<0.1 – 0.1]
WESTERN AND CENTRAL EUROPE	2200	[1300 – 3100]	0.1	[<0.1 – 0.1]	0.1	[0.1 – 0.2]
Austria	…	…	0.2	[0.1 – 0.3]	0.3	[0.1 – 0.9]
Belgium	…	…	<0.1	[<0.1 – 0.1]	<0.1	[<0.1 – 0.1]
Bulgaria	…	…	<0.1	[<0.1 – <0.1]	<0.1	[<0.1 – <0.1]

ESTIMATED NEW HIV INFECTIONS

	2009 Adult (15–49) incidence rate		2001 Adult (15–49) incidence rate		2009 Adults + children newly infected	
	estimate	[low – high estimate]	estimate	[low – high estimate]	estimate	[low – high estimate]
EAST ASIA	<0.10	[<0.10 – <0.10]	<0.10	[<0.10 – <0.10]	82 000	[48 000 – 140 000]
China	…	[<0.10 – <0.10]	…	[<0.10 – <0.10]	…	[47 000 – 140 000]
Democratic People's Republic of Korea	…	…	…	…	…	…
Japan	<0.10	[<0.10 – <0.10]	<0.10	[<0.10 – <0.10]	<500	[<200 – <500]
Mongolia	<0.10	[<0.10 – <0.10]	<0.10	[<0.10 – <0.10]	<100	[<100 – <200]
Republic of Korea	<0.10	[<0.10 – <0.10]	<0.10	[<0.10 – <0.10]	<1000	[<500 – 1000]
OCEANIA	<0.10	[<0.10 – <0.10]	<0.10	[<0.10 – <0.10]	4500	[3400 – 6000]
Australia	…	[<0.10 – <0.10]	…	[<0.10 – <0.10]	…	[<1000 – 1500]
Fiji	…	[<0.10 – <0.10]	…	[<0.10 – <0.10]	…	[<100 – <200]
New Zealand	…	[<0.10 – <0.10]	…	[<0.10 – <0.10]	…	[<100 – <200]
Papua New Guinea	<0.10	[<0.10 – 0.13]	0.13	[0.11 – 0.16]	3200	[2100 – 4800]
SOUTH AND SOUTH-EAST ASIA	<0.10	[<0.10 – <0.10]	<0.10	[<0.10 – <0.10]	270 000	[240 000 – 320 000]
Bangladesh	<0.10	[<0.10 – <0.10]	<0.10	[<0.10 – <0.10]	1400	[1000 – 2400]
Bhutan	…	[<0.10 – 0.13]	…	[<0.10 – <0.10]	…	[<200 – <1000]
Cambodia	<0.10	[<0.10 – <0.10]	<0.10	[<0.10 – 0.11]	1700	[<1000 – 4200]
India	<0.10	[<0.10 – <0.10]	<0.10	[<0.10 – <0.10]	140 000	[110 000 – 160 000]
Indonesia	…	[<0.10 – <0.10]	…	[<0.10 – <0.10]	…	[29 000 – 87 000]
Lao People's Democratic Republic	…	[<0.10 – <0.10]	…	[<0.10 – <0.10]	…	[<1000 – 3400]
Malaysia	<0.10	[<0.10 – <0.10]	<0.10	[<0.10 – <0.10]	10 000	[8400 – 13 000]
Maldives	…	[<0.10 – <0.10]	…	[<0.10 – <0.10]	…	[<100 – <100]
Myanmar	<0.10	[<0.10 – <0.10]	<0.10	[<0.10 – <0.10]	17 000	[14 000 – 20 000]
Nepal	<0.10	[<0.10 – <0.10]	<0.10	[<0.10 – <0.10]	4800	[2700 – 7800]
Pakistan	…	[<0.10 – <0.10]	…	[<0.10 – <0.10]	…	[7300 – 15 000]
Philippines	<0.10	[<0.10 – <0.10]	<0.10	[<0.10 – <0.10]	2100	[1200 – 4900]
Singapore	…	[<0.10 – <0.10]	…	[<0.10 – <0.10]	…	[<100 – <500]
Sri Lanka	<0.10	[<0.10 – <0.10]	<0.10	[<0.10 – <0.10]	<500	[<200 – <1000]
Thailand	<0.10	[<0.10 – <0.10]	<0.10	[<0.10 – <0.10]	12 000	[9800 – 15 000]
Viet Nam	…	[<0.10 – <0.10]	…	[<0.10 – <0.10]	…	[16 000 – 38 000]
EASTERN EUROPE AND CENTRAL ASIA	<0.10	[<0.10 – <0.10]	0.14	[0.11 – 0.16]	130 000	[110 000 – 160 000]
Armenia	<0.10	[<0.10 – <0.10]	<0.10	[<0.10 – <0.10]	<500	[<200 – <500]
Azerbaijan	…	[<0.10 – <0.10]	…	[<0.10 – <0.10]	…	[<500 – 1100]
Belarus	<0.10	[<0.10 – <0.10]	<0.10	[<0.10 – <0.10]	1500	[1100 – 2200]
Georgia	<0.10	[<0.10 – <0.10]	<0.10	[<0.10 – <0.10]	<1000	[<500 – 1200]
Kazakhstan	<0.10	[<0.10 – <0.10]	<0.10	[<0.10 – <0.10]	1900	[1200 – 3600]
Kyrgyzstan	<0.10	[<0.10 – 0.22]	<0.10	[<0.10 – <0.10]	2600	[1400 – 6500]
Republic of Moldova	<0.10	[<0.10 – <0.10]	<0.10	[<0.10 – <0.10]	<1000	[<1000 – 1200]
Russian Federation	…	[<0.10 – 0.14]	…	[0.17 – 0.25]	…	[67 000 – 120 000]
Tajikistan	<0.10	[<0.10 – <0.10]	<0.10	[<0.10 – <0.10]	1400	[<1000 – 2300]
Ukraine	…	[<0.10 – 0.12]	…	[0.10 – 0.16]	…	[16 000 – 32 000]
Uzbekistan	…	[<0.10 – <0.10]	…	[<0.10 – <0.10]	…	[3100 – 11 000]
WESTERN AND CENTRAL EUROPE	<0.10	[<0.10 – <0.10]	<0.10	[<0.10 – <0.10]	31 000	[23 000 – 40 000]
Austria	…	[<0.10 – <0.10]	…	[<0.10 – <0.10]	…	[<1000 – 2100]
Belgium	…	[<0.10 – <0.10]	…	[<0.10 – <0.10]	…	[<100 – <500]
Bulgaria	…	[<0.10 – <0.10]	…	[<0.10 – <0.10]	…	[<500 – <1000]

	ESTIMATED NEW HIV INFECTIONS (continued)		ESTIMATED AIDS-RELATED DEATHS			
	2009		**2009**		**2001**	
	Adults newly infected		AIDS-related deaths in adults + children		AIDS-related deaths in adults + children	
	estimate	[low – high estimate]	estimate	[low – high estimate]	estimate	[low – high estimate]
EAST ASIA	81 000	[47 000 – 140 000]	36 000	[25 000 – 50 000]	15 000	[9400 – 28 000]
China	...	[46 000 – 140 000]	26 000	[24 000 – 49 000]	...	[9100 – 28 000]
Democratic People's Republic of Korea	...	...	...	...	...	...
Japan	<500	[<200 – <500]	<100	[<100 – <500]	<100	[<100 – <200]
Mongolia	<100	[<100 – <100]	<100	[<100 – <100]	<100	[<100 – <100]
Republic of Korea	<1000	[<500 – 1000]	<500	[<500 – <1000]	<500	[<100 – <500]
OCEANIA	3700	[2600 – 5300]	1400	[< 1000 – 2400]	<1000	[<500 – 1100]
Australia	...	[<1000 – 1500]	<100	[<100 – <1000]	<100	[<100 – <200]
Fiji	...	[<100 – <200]	<100	[<100 – <100]	<100	[<100 – <100]
New Zealand	...	[<100 – <200]	<100	[<100 – <100]	<100	[<100 – <100]
Papua New Guinea	2400	[1400 – 4100]	1300	[<1000 – 1900]	<1000	[<500 – <1000]
SOUTH AND SOUTH-EAST ASIA	250 000	[220 000 – 300 000]	260 000	[230 000 – 300 000]	230 000	[210 000 – 280 000]
Bangladesh	1400	[<1000 – 2400]	<200	[<100 – <500]	<100	[<100 – <200]
Bhutan	...	[<200 – <1000]	<100	[<100 – <100]	<100	[<100 – <100]
Cambodia	1200	[<200 – 3500]	3100	[<1000 – 5600]	7400	[5000 – 11 000]
India	120 000	[100 000 – 150 000]	170 000	[150 000 – 200 000]	140 000	[120 000 – 170 000]
Indonesia	...	[29 000 – 86 000]	8300	[3800 – 15 000]	<200	[<100 – 1900]
Lao People's Democratic Republic	...	[<1000 – 3100]	<200	[<100 – <500]	<100	[<100 – <100]
Malaysia	10 000	[8400 – 13 000]	5800	[4500 – 7200]	3900	[3000 – 5200]
Maldives	...	[<100 – <100]	<100	[<100 – <100]	<100	[<100 – <100]
Myanmar	16 000	[14 000 – 19 000]	18 000	[13 000 – 23 000]	16 000	[12 000 – 20 000]
Nepal	4300	[2300 – 7200]	4700	[3800 – 5700]	4000	[3200 – 4900]
Pakistan	...	[6700 – 14 000]	5800	[4500 – 7400]	1400	[<1000 – 1900]
Philippines	2100	[1200 – 4800]	<200	[<100 – <500]	<100	[<100 – <500]
Singapore	...	[<100 – <500]	<100	[<100 – <200]	<100	[<100 – <500]
Sri Lanka	<500	[<200 – <1000]	<200	[<100 – <500]	<100	[<100 – <100]
Thailand	12 000	[9500 – 14 000]	28 000	[21 000 – 37 000]	52 000	[39 000 – 68 000]
Viet Nam	...	[15 000 – 37 000]	14 000	[9500 – 20 000]	5500	[3900 – 7500]
EASTERN EUROPE AND CENTRAL ASIA	130 000	[100 000 – 150 000]	76 000	[60 000 – 96 000]	18 000	[14 000 – 23 000]
Armenia	<500	[<200 – <500]	<100	[<100 – <200]	<100	[<100 – <100]
Azerbaijan	...	[<500 – 1100]	<200	[<200 – <500]	<100	[<100 – <100]
Belarus	1500	[1100 – 2200]	<1000	[<500 – <1000]	<200	[<100 – <500]
Georgia	<1000	[<500 – 1200]	<100	[<100 – <200]	<100	[<100 – <200]
Kazakhstan	1900	[1200 – 3600]	<500	[<200 – <1000]	<100	[<100 – <100]
Kyrgyzstan	2600	[1400 – 6500]	<500	[<100 – <500]	<100	[<100 – 3300]
Republic of Moldova	<1000	[<1000 – 1200]	<1000	[<1000 – 1100]	<1000	[<500 – <1000]
Russian Federation	...	[64 000 – 110 000]	...	[35 000 – 65 000]	...	[3000 – 6000]
Tajikistan	1300	[<1000 – 2200]	<500	[<500 – <1000]	<200	[<200 – <500]
Ukraine	...	[16 000 – 32 000]	24 000	[20 000 – 29 000]	13 000	[9400 – 16 000]
Uzbekistan	...	[3100 – 11 000]	<500	[<200 – 1000]	<100	[<100 – <100]
WESTERN AND CENTRAL EUROPE	31 000	[23 000 – 39 000]	8500	[6800 – 19 000]	7300	[5700 – 11 000]
Austria	...	[<1000 – 2100]	<100	[<100 – <100]	<100	[<100 – <100]
Belgium	...	[<100 – <500]	<100	[<100 – <500]	<100	[<100 – <100]
Bulgaria	...	[<500 – <1000]	<200	[<200 – <500]	<100	[<100 – <200]

	ESTIMATED ORPHANS DUE TO AIDS				HIV PREVALENCE (%) IN MOST-AT-RISK GROUPS IN CAPITAL CITY					
	2009 Orphans (0–17) currently living		**2001** Orphans (0–17)		Injecting drug users		Female sex workers		Men who have sex with men	
	estimate	[low – high estimate]	estimate	[low – high estimate]	Year	HIV (%)	Year	HIV (%)	Year	HIV (%)
EAST ASIA	52 000	[35 000 – 78 000]	18 000	[10 000 – 37 000]	...	...	...	...	...	...
China	...	...	...	...	2009	9.3	2009	0.6	2009	5.0
Democratic People's Republic of Korea	...	...	...	...	...	...	...	...	...	...
Japan	...	...	...	...	...	...	...	...	2009	4.0
Mongolia	...	...	...	...	...	...	...	...	2009	1.8
Republic of Korea	...	...	...	...	...	...	...	...	...	...
OCEANIA	6300	[4000 – 10 000]	2700	[1900 – 4400]	...	...	...	...	...	...
Australia	...	...	...	...	2008	1.5	2008	0.1	...	...
Fiji	...	...	...	...	...	...	...	...	...	...
New Zealand	...	...	...	...	2004	0.3	...	...	...	...
Papua New Guinea	...	...	...	...	...	...	2009	7.4	2009	4.4
SOUTH AND SOUTH-EAST ASIA	1 000 000	[820 000 – 1 100 000]	500 000	[420 000 – 620 000]	...	...	...	...	...	...
Bangladesh	...	...	...	...	2007	1.6	2007	0.3	...	...
Bhutan	...	...	...	...	...	...	...	...	...	...
Cambodia	...	...	...	...	2007	24.4	...	...	2005	4.5
India	...	...	...	...	2009	9.2	2009	4.9	2009	7.3
Indonesia	...	...	...	...	2007	52.4	2007	7.8	2007	5.2
Lao People's Democratic Republic	...	...	...	...	...	...	...	...	...	...
Malaysia	...	...	...	...	...	22.1	...	...	2009	3.9
Maldives	...	...	...	...	...	...	...	...	...	...
Myanmar	...	...	...	...	2008	36.3	2008	18.1	2008	28.8
Nepal	...	...	...	...	2009	20.7	2008	2.2	2009	3.8
Pakistan	...	...	...	...	2008	20.8	2009	1.0	...	...
Philippines	...	...	...	...	2009	0.2	2009	0.2	2009	1.0
Singapore	...	...	...	...	...	...	...	...	2009	2.6
Sri Lanka	...	...	...	...	...	...	...	...	2009	0.5
Thailand	...	...	...	...	2009	38.7	2009	2.8	2009	13.5
Viet Nam	...	...	...	...	2009	18.4	2009	3.2	2010	16.7
EASTERN EUROPE AND CENTRAL ASIA	73 000	[59 000 – 91 000]	15 000	[9000 – 22 000]	...	...	...	...	...	...
Armenia	...	...	...	...	...	...	...	...	...	...
Azerbaijan	...	...	...	...	2008	10.3	2008	1.7	2008	1.0
Belarus	...	...	...	...	2009	13.7	2009	6.4	2009	2.7
Georgia	...	...	...	...	2008	2.2	2009	2.0	2007	3.6
Kazakhstan	...	...	...	...	2009	2.9	2009	1.3	2009	0.3
Kyrgyzstan	...	...	...	...	2009	14.3	2009	1.6	...	...
Republic of Moldova	...	...	...	...	...	...	...	...	...	...
Russian Federation	...	...	...	...	2009	15.6	2009	4.5	2009	8.3
Tajikistan	...	...	...	...	2008	17.6	2008	2.8	...	...
Ukraine	...	...	...	...	2009	22.9	...	...	2009	8.6
Uzbekistan	...	...	...	...	2009	11.0	2009	2.2	2009	6.8
WESTERN AND CENTRAL EUROPE	26 000	[22 000 – 42 000]	50 000	[41 000 – 60 000]	...	...	...	...	...	...
Austria	...	...	...	...	2009	4.0	...	...	...	...
Belgium	...	...	...	...	2008	8.7	2009	0.4	2010	5.6
Bulgaria	...	...	...	...	2008	6.8	2008	0.7	2008	3.3

ESTIMATED PEOPLE LIVING WITH HIV

	2009 Adults + Children		2001 Adults + Children		2009 Adults (15+)	
	estimate	[low – high estimate]	estimate	[low – high estimate]	estimate	[low – high estimate]
Croatia	<1000	[<1000 – 1 100]	<1000	[<500 – <1000]	<1000	[<1000 – 1100]
Czech Republic	2000	[1700 – 2300]	1300	[1200 – 1600]	2000	[1700 – 2300]
Denmark	5300	[4000 – 6300]	3300	[2800 – 3800]	5300	[4000 – 6300]
Estonia	9900	[8000 – 12 000]	4700	[3800 – 5700]	9800	[8000 – 12 000]
Finland	2 600	[2200 – 3100]	1600	[1300 – 1900]	2600	[2200 – 3100]
France	150 000	[120 000 – 190 000]	120 000	[100 000 – 140 000]	150 000	[120 000 – 190 000]
Germany	67 000	[56 000 – 75 000]	49 000	[42 000 – 56 000]	67 000	[56 000 – 75 000]
Greece	8800	[7300 – 11 000]	8100	[6800 – 9500]	8800	[7300 – 11 000]
Hungary	3000	[2200 – 3900]	2800	[2100 – 3700]	3000	[2200 – 3900]
Iceland	<1000	[<500 – <1000]	<500	[<500 – <500]	<1000	[<500 – <1000]
Ireland	6900	[5200 – 8700]	4500	[3400 – 5900]	6900	[5200 – 8700]
Israel	7500	[5600 – 9900]	5200	[3900 – 6800]	7500	[5600 – 9900]
Italy	140 000	[110 000 – 180 000]	130 000	[99 000 – 170 000]	140 000	[110 000 – 180 000]
Latvia	8600	[6300 – 12 000]	4700	[3500 – 6 200]	8600	[6300 – 11 000]
Lithuania	1200	[<1000 – 1600]	<1000	[<1000 – <1000]	1200	[<1000 – 1600]
Luxembourg	<1000	[<1000 – 1200]	<1000	[<500 – <1000]	<1000	[<1000 – 1200]
Malta	<500	[<500 – <500]	<500	[<200 – <500]	<500	[<500 – <500]
Netherlands	22 000	[17 000 – 32 000]	18 000	[14 000 – 24 000]	22 000	[17 000 – 32 000]
Norway	4000	[3000 – 5400]	3000	[2300 – 4100]	4000	[3000 – 5400]
Poland	27 000	[20 000 – 34 000]	21 000	[16 000 – 28 000]	27 000	[20 000 – 34 000]
Portugal	42 000	[32 000 – 53 000]	31 000	[24 000 – 41 000]	42 000	[32 000 – 53 000]
Romania	16 000	[12 000 – 20 000]	16 000	[12 000 – 20 000]	15 000	[11 000 – 20 000]
Serbia	4900	[3500 – 7100]	1900	[<500 – 2800]	4900	[3400 – 7100]
Slovakia	<500	[<500 – <500]	<200	[<200 – <500]	<500	[<500 – <500]
Slovenia	<1000	[<500 – <1000]	<500	[<200 – <500]	<1000	[<500 – <1000]
Spain	130 000	[120 000 – 150 000]	120 000	[100 000 – 130 000]	130 000	[120 000 – 150 000]
Sweden	8100	[6100 – 11 000]	6300	[4900 – 8700]	8100	[6100 – 11 000]
Switzerland	18 000	[13 000 – 24 000]	13 000	[9500 – 17 000]	18 000	[13 000 – 24 000]
Turkey	4600	[3400 – 6100]	1700	[1300 – 2300]	4500	[3300 – 6100]
United Kingdom of Great Britain and Northern Ireland	85 000	[66 000 – 110 000]	43 000	[35 000 – 54 000]	85 000	[66 000 – 110 000]
MIDDLE EAST AND NORTH AFRICA	**460 000**	**[400 000 – 530 000]**	**180 000**	**[150 000 – 210 000]**	**440 000**	**[380 000 – 510 000]**
Algeria	18 000	[13 000 – 24 000]	6800	[4900 – 9000]	17 000	[12 000 – 24 000]
Djibouti	14 000	[10 000 – 18 000]	12 000	[9000 – 16 000]	13 000	[9400 – 16 000]
Egypt	11 000	[8400 – 17 000]	3300	[2900 – 5300]	10 000	[8100 – 16 000]
Iran (Islamic Republic of)	92 000	[74 000 – 120 000]	54 000	[45 000 – 65 000]	91 000	[72 000 – 110 000]
Lebanon	3600	[2700 – 4800]	3800	[2900 – 5100]	3400	[2600 – 4600]
Morocco	26 000	[19 000 – 34 000]	14 000	[11 000 – 18 000]	25 000	[19 000 – 33 000]
Oman	1100	[<1000 – 1400]	<500	[<500 – <1000]	1100	[<1000 – 1400]
Qatar	<200	[<100 – <200]	<100	[<100 – <100]	<200	[<100 – <200]
Somalia	34 000	[25 000 – 48 000]	11 000	[<500 – 14 000]	32 000	[23 000 – 46 000]
Sudan	260 000	[210 000 – 330 000]	72 000	[35 000 – 98 000]	250 000	[200 000 – 310 000]
Tunisia	2400	[1800 – 3300]	<1000	[<500 – 1000]	2400	[1700 – 3300]

	2001 Adults (15+)		2009 Adult (15–49) prevalence percent		2001 Adult (15–49) prevalence percent	
	estimate	[low – high estimate]	estimate	[low – high estimate]	estimate	[low – high estimate]
Croatia	<1000	[<500 – <1000]	<0.1	[<0.1 – <0.1]	<0.1	[<0.1 – <0.1]
Czech Republic	1300	[1200 – 1600]	<0.1	[<0.1 – <0.1]	<0.1	[<0.1 – <0.1]
Denmark	3300	[2800 – 3800]	0.2	[0.1 – 0.2]	0.1	[0.1 – 0.1]
Estonia	4700	[3800 – 5700]	1.2	[1.0 – 1.5]	0.6	[0.5 – 0.8]
Finland	1600	[1300 – 1900]	0.1	[0.1 – 0.1]	0.1	[<0.1 – 0.1]
France	120 000	[100 000 – 140 000]	0.4	[0.3 – 0.5]	0.3	[0.3 – 0.4]
Germany	49 000	[42 000 – 56 000]	0.1	[0.1 – 0.2]	0.1	[0.1 – 0.1]
Greece	8000	[6800 – 9500]	0.1	[0.1 – 0.2]	0.1	[0.1 – 0.1]
Hungary	2800	[2100 – 3700]	<0.1	[<0.1 – 0.1]	<0.1	[<0.1 – 0.1]
Iceland	<500	[<500 – <500]	0.3	[0.2 – 0.4]	0.2	[0.2 – 0.3]
Ireland	4500	[3400 – 5900]	0.2	[0.2 – 0.3]	0.2	[0.1 – 0.2]
Israel	5100	[3900 – 6800]	0.2	[0.1 – 0.2]	0.1	[0.1 – 0.2]
Italy	130 000	[99 000 – 170 000]	0.3	[0.2 – 0.3]	0.3	[0.2 – 0.4]
Latvia	4700	[3500 – 6200]	0.7	[0.5 – 0.9]	0.4	[0.3 – 0.5]
Lithuania	<1000	[<1000 – <1000]	0.1	[<0.1 – 0.1]	<0.1	[<0.1 – <0.1]
Luxembourg	<1000	[<500 – <1000]	0.3	[0.2 – 0.4]	0.3	[0.2 – 0.3]
Malta	<500	[<200 – <500]	0.1	[0.1 – 0.1]	0.1	[0.1 – 0.1]
Netherlands	18 000	[14 000 – 24 000]	0.2	[0.1 – 0.3]	0.2	[0.1 – 0.3]
Norway	3000	[2300 – 4100]	0.1	[0.1 – 0.2]	0.1	[0.1 – 0.2]
Poland	21 000	[16 000 – 28 000]	0.1	[0.1 – 0.1]	0.1	[0.1 – 0.1]
Portugal	31 000	[24 000 – 41 000]	0.6	[0.4 – 0.7]	0.5	[0.4 – 0.6]
Romania	16 000	[12 000 – 20 000]	0.1	[0.1 – 0.1]	0.1	[0.1 – 0.2]
Serbia	1900	[<500 – 2700]	0.1	[0.1 – 0.2]	<0.1	[<0.1 – 0.1]
Slovakia	<200	[<200 – <500]	<0.1	[<0.1 – <0.1]	<0.1	[<0.1 – <0.1]
Slovenia	<500	[<200 – <500]	<0.1	[<0.1 – 0.1]	<0.1	[<0.1 – <0.1]
Spain	110 000	[100 000 – 130 000]	0.4	[0.3 – 0.4]	0.4	[0.4 – 0.5]
Sweden	6300	[4900 – 8700]	0.1	[0.1 – 0.2]	0.1	[0.1 – 0.2]
Switzerland	13 000	[9500 – 17 000]	0.4	[0.3 – 0.5]	0.3	[0.2 – 0.4]
Turkey	1700	[1300 – 2300]	<0.1	[<0.1 – <0.1]	<0.1	[<0.1 – <0.1]
United Kingdom of Great Britain and Northern Ireland	43 000	[35 000 – 53 000]	0.2	[0.2 – 0.3]	0.1	[0.1 – 0.2]
MIDDLE EAST AND NORTH AFRICA	**170 000**	**[150 000 – 200 000]**	**0.2**	**[0.2 – 0.3]**	**0.1**	**[0.1 – 0.1]**
Algeria	6700	[4800 – 9000]	0.1	[0.1 – 0.1]	<0.1	[<0.1 – <0.1]
Djibouti	11 000	[8600 – 15 000]	2.5	[1.9 – 3.2]	2.9	[2.2 – 3.9]
Egypt	3200	[2900 – 5300]	<0.1	[<0.1 – <0.1]	<0.1	[<0.1 – <0.1]
Iran (Islamic Republic of)	54 000	[44 000 – 64 000]	0.2	[0.1 – 0.2]	0.1	[0.1 – 0.1]
Lebanon	3700	[2800 – 5000]	0.1	[0.1 – 0.2]	0.2	[0.1 – 0.2]
Morocco	14 000	[10 000 – 18 000]	0.1	[0.1 – 0.2]	0.1	[0.1 – 0.1]
Oman	<500	[<500 – <500]	0.1	[<0.1 – 0.1]	<0.1	[<0.1 – <0.1]
Qatar	<100	[<100 – <100]	<0.1	[<0.1 – <0.1]	<0.1	[<0.1 – <0.1]
Somalia	10 000	[<500 – 13 000]	0.7	[0.5 – 1.0]	0.3	[<0.1 – 0.3]
Sudan	68 000	[34 000 – 89 000]	1.1	[0.9 – 1.4]	0.4	[0.2 – 0.5]
Tunisia	<1000	[<500 – 1000]	<0.1	[<0.1 – 0.1]	<0.1	[<0.1 – <0.1]

ESTIMATED PEOPLE LIVING WITH HIV (continued)

	2009 Women (15+)		2001 Women (15+)		2009 Children (0–14)	
	estimate	[low – high estimate]	estimate	[low – high estimate]	estimate	[low – high estimate]
Croatia	<500	[<500 – <500]	<200	[<200 – <500]	...	...
Czech Republic	<1000	[<1000 – <1000]	<500	[<500 – <500]	...	...
Denmark	1400	[1100 – 1700]	<1000	[<1000 – 1000]	...	...
Estonia	3000	[2400 – 3800]	1400	[1100 – 1700]	...	...
Finland	<1000	[<1000 – <1000]	<500	[<500 – <1000]	...	...
France	48 000	[38 000 – 59 000]	37 000	[31 000 – 44 000]	...	...
Germany	12 000	[11 000 – 14 000]	9000	[7700 – 10 000]	...	...
Greece	2700	[2200 – 3200]	2500	[2100 – 2900]	...	...
Hungary	<1000	[<1000 – 1300]	<1000	[<1000 – 1200]	...	...
Iceland	<200	[<200 – <500]	<100	[<100 – <200]	...	...
Ireland	2000	[1500 – 2600]	1300	[1000 – 1800]	...	...
Israel	2200	[1700 – 2900]	1500	[1200 – 2100]	...	...
Italy	48 000	[36 000 – 61 000]	42 000	[32 000 – 56 000]	...	...
Latvia	2600	[1900 – 3500]	1400	[1000 – 1800]	...	...
Lithuania	<500	[<500 – <500]	<500	[<200 – <500]	...	...
Luxembourg	<500	[<500 – <500]	<200	[<200 – <500]	...	...
Malta	<100	[<100 – <200]	<100	[<100 – <100]	...	...
Netherlands	6900	[5200 – 9700]	5400	[4200 – 7400]	...	...
Norway	1200	[<1000 – 1600]	<1000	[<1000 – 1200]	...	...
Poland	8200	[6200 – 11 000]	6400	[4800 – 8500]	...	...
Portugal	13 000	[9900 – 16 000]	9400	[7300 – 12 000]	...	...
Romania	4700	[3500 – 5900]	4600	[3600 – 5900]	...	...
Serbia	1200	[<1000 – 1600]	<500	[<100 – <1000]	...	...
Slovakia	<100	[<100 – <200]	<100	[<100 – <100]	...	...
Slovenia	<200	[<200 – <500]	<100	[<100 – <100]	...	...
Spain	32 000	[27 000 – 36 000]	28 000	[23 000 – 32 000]	...	...
Sweden	2500	[1900 – 3400]	1900	[1500 – 2700]	...	...
Switzerland	5700	[4100 – 7500]	4000	[3000 – 5200]	...	...
Turkey	1400	[1000 – 1800]	<1000	[<500 – <1000]	...	...
United Kingdom of Great Britain and Northern Ireland	26 000	[20 000 – 32 000]	13 000	[10 000 – 16 000]	...	...
MIDDLE EAST AND NORTH AFRICA	**210 000**	**[180 000 – 240 000]**	**74 000**	**[61 000 – 87 000]**	**21 000**	**[13 000 – 28 000]**
Algeria	5200	[3700 – 7200]	2000	[1500 – 2600]	...	...
Djibouti	7400	[5300 – 9500]	6600	[5000 – 9000]	...	...
Egypt	2400	[2500 – 4900]	<1000	[<1000 – 1600]	...	...
Iran (Islamic Republic of)	26 000	[20 000 – 33 000]	15 000	[12 000 – 18 000]	...	...
Lebanon	1100	[<1000 – 1400]	1100	[<1000 – 1500]	...	...
Morocco	8100	[6000 – 11 000]	4300	[3300 – 5600]	...	...
Oman	<500	[<500 – <500]	<200	[<200 – <200]	...	...
Qatar	<100	[<100 – <100]	<100	[<100 – <100]	...	...
Somalia	15 000	[11 000 – 21 000]	4700	[<200 – 6300]	...	...
Sudan	140 000	[110 000 – 180 000]	39 000	[20 000 – 53 000]	...	...
Tunisia	<1000	[<1000 – 1000]	<500	[<100 – <500]	...	...

	2001 Children (0–14)		2009 Young women (15–24) prevalence (%)		2009 Young men (15–24) prevalence (%)	
	estimate	[low – high estimate]	estimate	[low – high estimate]	estimate	[low – high estimate]
Croatia	...	...	<0.1	[<0.1 – <0.1]	<0.1	[<0.1 – 0.1]
Czech Republic	...	...	<0.1	[<0.1 – <0.1]	<0.1	[<0.1 – 0.1]
Denmark	...	...	0.1	[<0.1 – 0.1]	0.1	[0.1 – 0.1]
Estonia	...	...	0.2	[0.2 – 0.3]	0.3	[0.2 – 0.4]
Finland	...	...	<0.1	[<0.1 – 0.1]	0.1	[<0.1 – 0.2]
France	...	...	0.1	[0.1 – 0.2]	0.2	[0.1 – 0.6]
Germany	...	...	<0.1	[<0.1 – <0.1]	0.1	[0.1 – 0.1]
Greece	...	...	0.1	[<0.1 – 0.1]	0.1	[<0.1 – 0.2]
Hungary	...	...	<0.1	[<0.1 – <0.1]	<0.1	[<0.1 – 0.1]
Iceland	...	...	0.1	[<0.1 – 0.1]	0.1	[<0.1 – 0.4]
Ireland	...	...	0.1	[<0.1 – 0.1]	0.1	[<0.1 – 0.3]
Israel	...	...	<0.1	[<0.1 – 0.1]	0.1	[<0.1 – 0.2]
Italy	...	...	<0.1	[<0.1 – <0.1]	<0.1	[<0.1 – 0.1]
Latvia	...	...	0.1	[0.1 – 0.2]	0.2	[0.1 – 0.2]
Lithuania	...	...	<0.1	[<0.1 – <0.1]	<0.1	[<0.1 – <0.1]
Luxembourg	...	...	0.1	[<0.1 – 0.2]	0.1	[<0.1 – 0.4]
Malta	...	...	<0.1	[<0.1 – <0.1]	<0.1	[<0.1 – 0.1]
Netherlands	...	...	<0.1	[<0.1 – 0.1]	0.1	[<0.1 – 0.3]
Norway	...	...	<0.1	[<0.1 – 0.1]	<0.1	[<0.1 – 0.2]
Poland	...	...	<0.1	[<0.1 – <0.1]	<0.1	[<0.1 – 0.1]
Portugal	...	...	0.2	[0.1 – 0.4]	0.3	[0.1 – 0.9]
Romania	...	...	<0.1	[<0.1 – 0.1]	0.1	[<0.1 – 0.2]
Serbia	...	...	0.1	[<0.1 – 0.1]	0.1	[0.1 – 0.2]
Slovakia	...	...	<0.1	[<0.1 – <0.1]	<0.1	[<0.1 – <0.1]
Slovenia	...	...	<0.1	[<0.1 – 0.1]	<0.1	[<0.1 – 0.1]
Spain	...	...	0.1	[0.1 – 0.1]	0.2	[0.1 – 0.2]
Sweden	...	...	<0.1	[<0.1 – 0.1]	<0.1	[<0.1 – 0.2]
Switzerland	...	...	0.1	[0.1 – 0.2]	0.2	[0.1 – 0.6]
Turkey	...	...	<0.1	[<0.1 – <0.1]	<0.1	[<0.1 – <0.1]
United Kingdom of Great Britain and Northern Ireland	...	...	0.1	[<0.1 – 0.2]	0.2	[0.1 – 0.6]
MIDDLE EAST AND NORTH AFRICA	**7100**	**[3800 – 13 000]**	**0.2**	**[0.2 – 0.3]**	**0.1**	**[0.1 – 0.1]**
Algeria	...	...	<0.1	[<0.1 – 0.1]	0.1	[<0.1 – 0.2]
Djibouti	...	...	1.9	[1.0 – 2.9]	0.8	[0.4 – 1.3]
Egypt	...	...	<0.1	[<0.1 – <0.1]	<0.1	[<0.1 – <0.1]
Iran (Islamic Republic of)	...	...	<0.1	[<0.1 – <0.1]	<0.1	[<0.1 – <0.1]
Lebanon	...	...	<0.1	[<0.1 – 0.1]	0.1	[<0.1 – 0.1]
Morocco	...	...	0.1	[<0.1 – 0.1]	0.1	[<0.1 – 0.3]
Oman	...	...	<0.1	[<0.1 – <0.1]	<0.1	[<0.1 – <0.1]
Qatar	...	...	<0.1	[<0.1 – <0.1]	<0.1	[<0.1 – <0.1]
Somalia	...	...	0.6	[0.4 – 1.1]	0.4	[0.3 – 0.7]
Sudan	...	...	1.3	[0.9 – 1.8]	0.5	[0.4 – 0.7]
Tunisia	...	...	<0.1	[<0.1 – <0.1]	<0.1	[<0.1 – 0.1]

ESTIMATED PEOPLE LIVING WITH HIV (continued)

	2009 Adult (15–49) incidence rate		2001 Adult (15–49) incidence rate		2009 Adults + children newly infected	
	estimate	[low – high estimate]	estimate	[low – high estimate]	estimate	[low – high estimate]
Croatia	...	[<0.10 – <0.10]	...	[<0.10 – <0.10]	...	[<100 – <100]
Czech Republic	...	[<0.10 – <0.10]	...	[<0.10 – <0.10]	...	[<100 – <100]
Denmark	...	[<0.10 – <0.10]	...	[<0.10 – <0.10]	...	[<200 – <500]
Estonia	...	[<0.10 – 0.14]	...	[0.13 – 0.21]	...	[<1000 – 1000]
Finland	...	[<0.10 – <0.10]	...	[<0.10 – <0.10]	...	[<100 – <200]
France	<0.10	[<0.10 – <0.10]	<0.10	[<0.10 – <0.10]	6900	[3900 – 10 000]
Germany	<0.10	[<0.10 – <0.10]	<0.10	[<0.10 – <0.10]	3300	[2500 – 4200]
Greece	...	[<0.10 – <0.10]	...	[<0.10 – <0.10]	...	[<200 – <500]
Hungary	...	[<0.10 – <0.10]	...	[<0.10 – <0.10]	...	[<100 – <1000]
Iceland	...	[<0.10 – <0.10]	...	[<0.10 – <0.10]	...	[<100 – <100]
Ireland	...	[<0.10 – <0.10]	...	[<0.10 – <0.10]	...	[<100 – <500]
Israel	...	[<0.10 – <0.10]	...	[<0.10 – <0.10]	...	[<200 – <500]
Italy	...	[<0.10 – <0.10]	...	...	...	[1700 – 6200]
Latvia	<0.10	[<0.10 – 0.10]	<0.10	[<0.10 – 0.11]	<1000	[<500 – 1200]
Lithuania	<0.10	[<0.10 – <0.10]	<0.10	[<0.10 – <0.10]	<100	[<100 – <200]
Luxembourg	...	[<0.10 – <0.10]	...	[<0.10 – <0.10]	...	[<100 – <100]
Malta	...	[<0.10 – <0.10]	...	[<0.10 – <0.10]	...	[<100 – <100]
Netherlands	...	[<0.10 – <0.10]	...	[<0.10 – <0.10]	...	[<500 – 1100]
Norway	...	[<0.10 – <0.10]	...	[<0.10 – <0.10]	...	[<100 – <500]
Poland	...	[<0.10 – <0.10]	...	[<0.10 – <0.10]	...	[<500 – 1300]
Portugal	...	[<0.10 – <0.10]	...	[<0.10 – <0.10]	...	[<1000 – 2300]
Romania	...	[<0.10 – <0.10]	...	[<0.10 – <0.10]	...	[<500 – 1000]
Serbia	...	[<0.10 – <0.10]	...	[<0.10 – <0.10]	...	[<500 – <1000]
Slovakia	...	[<0.10 – <0.10]	...	[<0.10 – <0.10]	...	[<100 – <100]
Slovenia	...	[<0.10 – <0.10]	...	[<0.10 – <0.10]	...	[<100 – <200]
Spain	...	[<0.10 – <0.10]	...	[<0.10 – <0.10]	...	[2200 – 4100]
Sweden	...	[<0.10 – <0.10]	...	[<0.10 – <0.10]	...	[<100 – <500]
Switzerland	...	[<0.10 – <0.10]	...	[<0.10 – <0.10]	...	[<500 – 1000]
Turkey	...	[<0.10 – <0.10]	...	[<0.10 – <0.10]	...	[<500 – <1000]
United Kingdom of Great Britain and Northern Ireland	...	[<0.10 – <0.10]	...	[<0.10 – <0.10]	...	[1500 – 6000]
MIDDLE EAST AND NORTH AFRICA	<0.10	[<0.10 – <0.10]	<0.10	[<0.10 – <0.10]	75 000	[61 000 – 92 000]
Algeria	...	[<0.10 – <0.10]	...	[<0.10 – <0.10]	...	[1100 – 3700]
Djibouti	0.25	[0.10 – 0.34]	0.29	[0.18 – 0.51]	1300	[<1000 – 1800]
Egypt	...	[<0.10 – <0.10]	...	[<0.10 – <0.10]	...	[<1000 – 2900]
Iran (Islamic Republic of)	...	[<0.10 – <0.10]	...	[<0.10 – <0.10]	...	[5600 – 11 000]
Lebanon	...	[<0.10 – <0.10]	...	[<0.10 – <0.10]	...	[<100 – <500]
Morocco	...	[<0.10 – <0.10]	...	[<0.10 – <0.10]	...	[1200 – 5800]
Oman	...	[<0.10 – <0.10]	...	[<0.10 – <0.10]	...	[<200 – <500]
Qatar	...	[<0.10 – <0.10]	...	[<0.10 – <0.10]	...	[<100 – <100]
Somalia	...	[<0.10 – 0.29]	...	[<0.10 – <0.10]	...	[4200 – 13 000]
Sudan	...	[0.17 – 0.35]	...	[<0.10 – 0.10]	...	[38 000 – 74 000]
Tunisia	...	[<0.10 – <0.10]	...	[<0.10 – <0.10]	...	[<500 – <1000]

	2009 Adults newly infected		ESTIMATED AIDS-RELATED DEATHS 2009 AIDS-related deaths in adults + children		2001 AIDS-related deaths in adults + children	
	estimate	[low – high estimate]	estimate	[low – high estimate]	estimate	[low – high estimate]
Croatia	...	[<100 – <100]	<100	[<100 – <100]	<100	[<100 – <100]
Czech Republic	...	[<100 – <100]	<100	[<100 – <100]	<100	[<100 – <100]
Denmark	...	[<200 – <500]	<100	[<100 – <200]	<100	[<100 – <100]
Estonia	...	[<1000 – 1000]	<500	[<500 – <1000]	<200	[<100 – <200]
Finland	...	[<100 – <200]	<100	[<100 – <100]	<100	[<100 – <100]
France	6800	[3900 – 10 000]	1700	[1400 – 3900]	1200	[<1000 – 3000]
Germany	3300	[2500 – 4200]	<1000	[<1000 – 1900]	<1000	[<500 – <1000]
Greece	...	[<200 – <500]	<500	[<200 – <500]	<500	[<500 – <500]
Hungary	...	[<100 – <100]	<200	[<100 – <200]	<500	[<200 – <500]
Iceland	...	[<100 – <100]	<100	[<100 – <100]	<100	[<100 – <100]
Ireland	...	[<100 – <500]	<100	[<100 – <200]	<100	[<100 – <100]
Israel	...	[<200 – <500]	<100	[<100 – <200]	<100	[<100 – <100]
Italy	...	[1700 – 6200]	<1000	[<1000 – 4100]	1300	[<1000 – 2400]
Latvia	<1000	[<500 – 1200]	<1000	[<500 – <1000]	<200	[<100 – <500]
Lithuania	<100	[<100 – <200]	<100	[<100 – <100]	<100	[<100 – <100]
Luxembourg	...	[<100 – <100]	<100	[<100 – <100]	<100	[<100 – <100]
Malta	...	[<100 – <100]	<100	[<100 – <100]	<100	[<100 – <100]
Netherlands	...	[<500 – 1100]	<100	[<100 – <500]	<100	[<100 – <100]
Norway	...	[<100 – <500]	<100	[<100 – <200]	<100	[<100 – <100]
Poland	...	[<500 – 1300]	<200	[<100 – <1000]	<100	[<100 – <200]
Portugal	...	[<1000 – 2300]	<500	[<100 – 1300]	<500	[<500 – <500]
Romania	...	[<500 – 1000]	<1000	[<500 – 1200]	<500	[<200 – <1000]
Serbia	...	[<500 – <1000]	<200	[<100 – <500]	<500	[<100 – <500]
Slovakia	...	[<100 – <100]	<100	[<100 – <100]	<100	[<100 – <100]
Slovenia	...	[<100 – <200]	<100	[<100 – <100]	<100	[<100 – <100]
Spain	...	[2200 – 4100]	1600	[1200 – 2000]	1800	[1500 – 2100]
Sweden	...	[<100 – <500]	<100	[<100 – <500]	<100	[<100 – <100]
Switzerland	...	[<500 – 1000]	<100	[<100 – <500]	<200	[<100 – <500]
Turkey	...	[<500 – <1000]	<200	[<100 – <500]	<100	[<100 – <200]
United Kingdom of Great Britain and Northern Ireland	...	[<100 – <100]	<1000	[<500 – 1600]	<500	[<200 – <500]
MIDDLE EAST AND NORTH AFRICA	**68 000**	**[55 000 – 84 000]**	**24 000**	**[20 000 – 27 000]**	**8300**	**[6300 – 11 000]**
Algeria	...	[1000 – 3600]	<1000	[<1000 – 1100]	<500	[<200 – <500]
Djibouti	1100	[<500 – 1500]	1000	[<1000 – 1400]	<1000	[<500 – 1400]
Egypt	...	[<1000 – 2700]	<500	[<500 – <1000]	<200	[<100 – <500]
Iran (Islamic Republic of)	...	[5400 – 11 000]	6400	[5200 – 8000]	2000	[1600 – 2600]
Lebanon	...	[<100 – <500]	<500	[<500 – <500]	<500	[<200 – <500]
Morocco	...	[<100 – <100]	1200	[<1000 – 1600]	<1000	[<1000 – 1000]
Oman	...	[<200 – <500]	<100	[<100 – <100]	<100	[<100 – <100]
Qatar	...	[<100 – <100]	<100	[<100 – <100]	<100	[<100 – <100]
Somalia	...	[3700 – 11 000]	1600	[1200 – 2300]	<1000	[<100 – <1000]
Sudan	...	[34 000 – 67 000]	12 000	[9200 – 15 000]	3500	[<1000 – 6700]
Tunisia	...	[<500 – <1000]	<100	[<100 – <200]	<100	[<100 – <100]

	2009 Orphans (0–17) currently living		2001 Orphans (0–17)		HIV PREVALENCE (%) IN MOST-AT-RISK GROUPS IN CAPITAL CITY					
					Injecting drug users		Female sex workers		Men who have sex with men	
	estimate	[low – high estimate]	estimate	[low – high estimate]	Year	HIV (%)	Year	HIV (%)	Year	HIV (%)
Croatia	...	...	...	...	...	...	...	...	...	...
Czech Republic	...	...	...	...	2009	0.1	...	...	2009	2.6
Denmark	...	...	...	...	...	...	...	...	2009	11.8
Estonia	...	...	...	...	2007	62.5	2006	7.7	2007	1.7
Finland	...	...	...	...	2009	0.7	...	...	...	...
France	...	...	...	...	...	...	...	...	...	...
Germany	...	...	...	...	...	...	...	...	...	...
Greece	...	...	...	...	...	...	...	...	...	...
Hungary	...	...	...	...	...	...	...	...	2009	2.6
Iceland	...	...	...	...	...	...	...	...	...	...
Ireland	...	...	...	...	...	...	...	...	...	...
Israel	...	...	...	...	...	...	...	...	...	...
Italy	...	...	...	...	...	...	...	...	...	...
Latvia	...	...	...	...	2007	22.6	...	...	2008	4.0
Lithuania	...	...	...	...	2008	8.0	...	...	...	...
Luxembourg	...	...	...	...	2008	1.8	...	...	...	...
Malta	...	...	...	...	...	...	...	...	...	...
Netherlands	...	...	...	...	...	...	...	...	...	...
Norway	...	...	...	...	...	...	...	...	...	...
Poland	...	...	...	...	...	...	...	...	...	...
Portugal	...	...	...	...	2008	14.0	...	...	...	...
Romania	...	...	...	...	2009	1.1	2009	1.0	2009	4.4
Serbia	...	...	...	...	2008	4.8	...	....	2008	6.1
Slovakia	...	...	...	...	...	...	...	...	...	...
Slovenia	...	...	...	...	...	...	...	...	2009	1.6
Spain	...	...	...	...	2008	19.5	2008	0.9	2008	10.2
Sweden	...	...	...	...	...	...	...	...	...	...
Switzerland	...	...	...	...	2006	10.9	...	...	2007	8.1
Turkey	...	...	...	...	...	...	...	...	...	...
United Kingdom of Great Britain and Northern Ireland	...	...	...	...	...	...	...	...	...	...
MIDDLE EAST AND NORTH AFRICA	96 000	[73 000 – 120 000]	36 000	[22 000 – 63 000]	...	...	...	...	...	...
Algeria	...	...	...	...	...	...	...	...	...	...
Djibouti	...	...	...	...	...	...	2008	20.3	...	...
Egypt	...	...	...	...	...	...	2006	0.9	2006	5.6
Iran (Islamic Republic of)	...	...	...	...	...	...	...	...	...	...
Lebanon	...	...	...	...	...	...	...	...	2008	1.0
Morocco	...	...	...	...	2009	2.1	2009	2.4	...	...
Oman	...	...	...	...	...	...	...	...	...	...
Qatar	...	...	...	...	...	...	...	...	...	...
Somalia	...	...	...	...	...	...	2008	5.5	...	...
Sudan	...	...	...	...	...	...	2008	0.9	...	...
Tunisia	...	...	...	...	2009	3.1	2009	0.4	2009	4.8

ESTIMATED PEOPLE LIVING WITH HIV

	2009 Adults + Children		2001 Adults + Children		2009 Adults (15+)	
	estimate	[low – high estimate]	estimate	[low – high estimate]	estimate	[low – high estimate]
NORTH AMERICA	1 500 000	[1 200 000 – 2 000 000]	1 200 000	[960 000 – 1 400 000]	1 500 000	[1 200 000 – 2 000 000]
Canada	67 000	[56 000 – 78 000]	48 000	[39 000 – 57 000]	67 000	[56 000 – 78 000]
Mexico	220 000	[180 000 – 280 000]	180 000	[150 000 – 210 000]	220 000	[180 000 – 270 000]
United States of America	1 200 000	[930 000 – 1 700 000]	940 000	[730 000 – 1 200 000]	1 200 000	[930 000 – 1 700 000]
CARIBBEAN	240 000	[220 000 – 270 000]	240 000	[210 000 – 270 000]	220 000	[200 000 – 250 000]
Bahamas	6600	[2600 – 11 000]	5900	[3900 – 8500]	6100	[2400 – 11 000]
Barbados	2100	[1800 – 2500]	<1000	[<1000 – 1 000]	2100	[1800 – 2500]
Cuba	7100	[5700 – 8900]	2600	[1900 – 3400]	7000	[5600 – 8800]
Dominican Republic	57 000	[49 000 – 66 000]	54 000	[45 000 – 65 000]	54 000	[45 000 – 62 000]
Haiti	120 000	[110 000 – 140 000]	130 000	[110 000 – 160 000]	110 000	[95 000 – 130 000]
Jamaica	32 000	[21 000 – 45 000]	32 000	[23 000 – 41 000]	31 000	[20 000 – 43 000]
Trinidad and Tobago	15 000	[11 000 – 19 000]	10 000	[7900 – 14 000]	14 000	[11 000 – 19 000]
CENTRAL AND SOUTH AMERICA	1 400 000	[1 200 000 – 1 600 000]	1 100 000	[1 000 000 – 1 300 000]	1 400 000	[1 200 000 – 1 600 000]
Argentina	110 000	[88 000 – 140 000]	80 000	[66 000 – 99 000]	110 000	[87 000 – 140 000]
Belize	4800	[4000 – 5700]	3600	[3000 – 4200]	4400	[3600 – 5300]
Bolivia	12 000	[9000 – 16 000]	12 000	[9100 – 16 000]	11 000	[8400 – 15 000]
Brazil	…	[460 000 – 810 000]	…	[380 000 – 560 000]	…	[450 000 – 800 000]
Chile	40 000	[32 000 – 51 000]	24 000	[19 000 – 31 000]	39 000	[31 000 – 50 000]
Colombia	160 000	[120 000 – 210 000]	210 000	[170 000 – 260 000]	150 000	[120 000 – 200 000]
Costa Rica	9800	[7500 – 13 000]	4400	[3400 – 5900]	9600	[7300 – 12 000]
Ecuador	37 000	[28 000 – 50 000]	36 000	[27 000 – 47 000]	36 000	[27 000 – 49 000]
El Salvador	34 000	[25 000 – 44 000]	25 000	[19 000 – 33 000]	32 000	[24 000 – 42 000]
Guatemala	62 000	[47 000 – 82 000]	31 000	[23 000 – 41 000]	60 000	[45 000 – 79 000]
Guyana	5900	[2700 – 8800]	7800	[5300 – 12 000]	5500	[2400 – 8200]
Honduras	39 000	[26 000 – 51 000]	44 000	[33 000 – 61 000]	37 000	[24 000 – 49 000]
Nicaragua	6900	[5200 – 9100]	3700	[2900 – 4800]	6700	[5000 – 8900]
Panama	20 000	[14 000 – 36 000]	26 000	[17 000 – 50 000]	20 000	[13 000 – 36 000]
Paraguay	13 000	[9800 – 16 000]	9200	[7200 – 13 000]	12 000	[9600 – 16 000]
Peru	75 000	[58 000 – 100 000]	82 000	[65 000 – 100 000]	73 000	[56 000 – 98 000]
Suriname	3700	[2700 – 5300]	3300	[2300 – 4500]	3600	[2700 – 5100]
Uruguay	9900	[8400 – 12 000]	7000	[5900 – 8200]	9600	[8100 – 11 000]
Venezuela	…	…	…	…	…	…

ESTIMATED PEOPLE LIVING WITH HIV (continued)

	2001 Adults (15+)		2009 Adult (15–49) prevalence percent		2001 Adult (15–49) prevalence percent	
	estimate	[low – high estimate]	estimate	[low – high estimate]	estimate	[low – high estimate]
NORTH AMERICA	1 200 000	[950 000 – 1 400 000]	0.5	[0.4 – 0.7]	0.4	[0.4 – 0.5]
Canada	48 000	[39 000 – 57 000]	0.2	[0.1 – 0.3]	0.2	[0.1 – 0.3]
Mexico	180 000	[150 000 – 210 000]	0.3	[0.3 – 0.4]	0.3	[0.2 – 0.4]
United States of America	930 000	[730 000 – 1 200 000]	0.6	[0.4 – 0.8]	0.5	[0.4 – 0.7]
CARIBBEAN	220 000	[200 000 – 250 000]	1.0	[0.9 – 1.1]	1.1	[1.0 – 1.2]
Bahamas	5400	[3400 – 7600]	3.1	[1.2 – 5.4]	3.1	[1.9 – 4.4]
Barbados	<1000	[<1000 – 1000]	1.4	[1.2 – 1.6]	0.5	[0.4 – 0.6]
Cuba	2600	[1900 – 3400]	0.1	[0.1 – 0.1]	<0.1	[<0.1 – 0.1]
Dominican Republic	50 000	[43 000 – 60 000]	0.9	[0.7 – 1.0]	0.9	[0.8 – 1.1]
Haiti	120 000	[100 000 – 140 000]	1.9	[1.7 – 2.2]	2.6	[2.3 – 3.0]
Jamaica	31 000	[22 000 – 39 000]	1.7	[1.1 – 2.5]	1.9	[1.3 – 2.4]
Trinidad and Tobago	10 000	[7800 – 14 000]	1.5	[1.1 – 2.0]	1.2	[0.9 – 1.6]
CENTRAL AND SOUTH AMERICA	1 100 000	[1 000 000 – 1 200 000]	0.5	[0.4 – 0.6]	0.5	[0.4 – 0.5]
Argentina	79 000	[65 000 – 97 000]	0.5	[0.3 – 0.6]	0.4	[0.3 – 0.5]
Belize	3300	[2800 – 3800]	2.3	[2.0 – 2.8]	2.2	[1.9 – 2.6]
Bolivia	11 000	[8600 – 15 000]	0.2	[0.1 – 0.3]	0.2	[0.2 – 0.3]
Brazil	...	[360 000 – 550 000]	...	[0.3 – 0.6]	...	[0.3 – 0.5]
Chile	24 000	[18 000 – 30 000]	0.4	[0.3 – 0.5]	0.3	[0.2 – 0.3]
Colombia	210 000	[160 000 – 260 000]	0.5	[0.4 – 0.7]	0.8	[0.7 – 1.1]
Costa Rica	4400	[3300 – 5800]	0.3	[0.2 – 0.4]	0.2	[0.1 – 0.2]
Ecuador	35 000	[26 000 – 46 000]	0.4	[0.3 – 0.6]	0.5	[0.4 – 0.6]
El Salvador	24 000	[18 000 – 32 000]	0.8	[0.6 – 1.1]	0.8	[0.6 – 1.0]
Guatemala	30 000	[22 000 – 40 000]	0.8	[0.6 – 1.0]	0.5	[0.4 – 0.7]
Guyana	7000	[4600 – 11 000]	1.2	[0.5 – 1.9]	1.4	[0.9 – 2.2]
Honduras	42 000	[31 000 – 57 000]	0.8	[0.5 – 1.0]	1.2	[0.9 – 1.6]
Nicaragua	3600	[2800 – 4700]	0.2	[0.1 – 0.3]	0.1	[0.1 – 0.2]
Panama	25 000	[16 000 – 49 000]	0.9	[0.6 – 1.5]	1.4	[0.9 – 2.7]
Paraguay	9000	[7000 – 12 000]	0.3	[0.2 – 0.4]	0.3	[0.2 – 0.4]
Peru	81 000	[64 000 – 99 000]	0.4	[0.3 – 0.5]	0.5	[0.4 – 0.6]
Suriname	3200	[2300 – 4400]	1.0	[0.7 – 1.4]	1.0	[0.7 – 1.4]
Uruguay	6800	[5800 – 8000]	0.5	[0.4 – 0.6]	0.4	[0.3 – 0.4]
Venezuela	...	...	...	...	...	...

	2009 Women (15+)		2001 Women (15+)		2009 Children (0–14)	
	estimate	[low – high estimate]	estimate	[low – high estimate]	estimate	[low – high estimate]
NORTH AMERICA	390 000	[310 000 – 510 000]	270 000	[220 000 – 320 000]	4500	[4000 – 5800]
Canada	14 000	[12 000 – 16 000]	9 000	[7 000 – 11 000]	...	...
Mexico	59 000	[47 000 – 75 000]	41 000	[33 000 – 49 000]	...	...
United States of America	310 000	[220 000 – 430 000]	210 000	[160 000 – 270 000]	...	...
CARIBBEAN	120 000	[100 000 – 140 000]	120 000	[100 000 – 140 000]	17 000	[8500 – 26 000]
Bahamas	3700	[1500 – 6400]	3300	[2100 – 4600]	...	...
Barbados	<1000	[<1000 – <1000]	<500	[<500 – <500]	...	...
Cuba	2200	[1700 – 2700]	<1000	[<1000 – 1000]	...	...
Dominican Republic	32 000	[26 000 – 37 000]	29 000	[24 000 – 35 000]	...	...
Haiti	67 000	[56 000 – 78 000]	73 000	[61 000 – 87 000]	12 000	[5700 – 18 000]
Jamaica	10 000	[6700 – 14 000]	9900	[7300 – 13 000]	...	...
Trinidad and Tobago	4700	[3500 – 6100]	3300	[2600 – 4300]	...	...
CENTRAL AND SOUTH AMERICA	490 000	[420 000 – 590 000]	370 000	[330 000 – 420 000]	36 000	[25 000 – 50 000]
Argentina	36 000	[28 000 – 45 000]	25 000	[20 000 – 30 000]	...	...
Belize	2600	[2100 – 3100]	1900	[1600 – 2200]	...	...
Bolivia	3600	[2700 – 4800]	3500	[2700 – 4600]	...	...
Brazil	...	[180 000 – 330 000]	...	[140 000 – 210 000]	...	...
Chile	12 000	[9700 – 15 000]	7200	[5500 – 9300]	...	...
Colombia	50 000	[38 000 – 65 000]	65 000	[51 000 – 80 000]	...	...
Costa Rica	2800	[2100 – 3600]	1300	[<1000 – 1700]	...	...
Ecuador	11 000	[8400 – 15 000]	11 000	[8200 – 14 000]	...	...
El Salvador	11 000	[8500 – 14 000]	8000	[6000 – 11 000]	...	...
Guatemala	20 000	[15 000 – 26 000]	9600	[7200 – 13 000]	...	...
Guyana	2800	[1100 – 4200]	3800	[2400 – 5700]	...	...
Honduras	12 000	[7900 – 16 000]	13 000	[9700 – 18 000]	...	...
Nicaragua	2100	[1600 – 2800]	1100	[<1000 – 1400]	...	...
Panama	6300	[4200 – 11 000]	7600	[4900 – 15 000]	...	...
Paraguay	3800	[2900 – 4800]	2700	[2100 – 3700]	...	...
Peru	18 000	[14 000 – 25 000]	15 000	[12 000 – 19 000]	...	...
Suriname	1100	[<1000 – 1600]	<1000	[<1000 – 1300]	...	...
Uruguay	3100	[2600 – 3600]	2100	[1800 – 2500]	...	...
Venezuela	...	...	...	...	...	...

ESTIMATED PEOPLE LIVING WITH HIV (continued)

	2001 Children (0–14)		2009 Young women (15–24) prevalence (%)		2009 Young men (15–24) prevalence (%)	
	estimate	[low – high estimate]	estimate	[low – high estimate]	estimate	[low – high estimate]
NORTH AMERICA	5200	[2900 – 7700]	0.2	[0.1 – 0.3]	0.2	[0.2 – 0.4]
Canada	...	...	0.1	[<0.1 – 0.2]	0.1	[<0.1 – 0.5]
Mexico	...	...	0.1	[0.1 – 0.2]	0.2	[0.1 – 0.2]
United States of America	...	...	0.2	[0.1 – 0.3]	0.3	[0.2 – 0.5]
CARIBBEAN	18 000	[9100 – 27 000]	0.8	[0.6 – 1.0]	0.4	[0.3 – 0.7]
Bahamas	...	...	3.1	[0.8 – 6.6]	1.4	[0.5 – 2.8]
Barbados	...	...	1.1	[0.8 – 1.4]	0.9	[0.7 – 1.1]
Cuba	...	...	0.1	[<0.1 – 0.1]	0.1	[<0.1 – 0.3]
Dominican Republic	...	...	0.7	[0.4 – 0.9]	0.3	[0.1 – 0.4]
Haiti	12 000	[6300 – 19 000]	1.3	[1.0 – 1.8]	0.6	[0.4 – 0.8]
Jamaica	...	...	0.7	[0.3 – 1.4]	1.0	[0.4 – 3.1]
Trinidad and Tobago	...	...	0.7	[0.3 – 1.2]	1.0	[0.4 – 3.3]
CENTRAL AND SOUTH AMERICA	30 000	[20 000 – 42 000]	0.2	[0.1 – 0.3]	0.2	[0.2 – 0.5]
Argentina	...	...	0.2	[0.1 – 0.3]	0.3	[0.1 – 0.8]
Belize	...	...	1.8	[1.4 – 2.7]	0.7	[0.5 – 1.1]
Bolivia	...	...	0.1	[<0.1 – 0.1]	0.1	[<0.1 – 0.3]
Brazil	...	...	...	[0.1 – 0.4]	...	[0.1 – 0.3]
Chile	...	...	0.1	[0.1 – 0.3]	0.2	[0.1 – 0.7]
Colombia	...	...	0.1	[0.1 – 0.3]	0.2	[0.1 – 0.7]
Costa Rica	...	...	0.1	[0.1 – 0.2]	0.2	[0.1 – 0.3]
Ecuador	...	...	0.2	[0.1 – 0.3]	0.2	[0.1 – 0.8]
El Salvador	...	...	0.3	[0.1 – 0.5]	0.4	[0.2 – 1.3]
Guatemala	...	...	0.3	[0.2 – 0.6]	0.5	[0.2 – 1.4]
Guyana	...	...	0.8	[0.2 – 1.5]	0.6	[0.2 – 1.0]
Honduras	...	...	0.2	[0.1 – 0.4]	0.3	[0.1 – 1.1]
Nicaragua	...	...	0.1	[0.1 – 0.1]	0.1	[0.1 – 0.2]
Panama	...	...	0.3	[0.1 – 0.5]	0.4	[0.2 – 1.3]
Paraguay	...	...	0.1	[0.1 – 0.2]	0.2	[0.1 – 0.6]
Peru	...	...	0.1	[0.1 – 0.2]	0.2	[0.1 – 0.3]
Suriname	...	...	0.4	[0.2 – 0.7]	0.6	[0.2 – 2.0]
Uruguay	...	...	0.2	[0.1 – 0.3]	0.3	[0.1 – 1.0]
Venezuela	...	...	...	...	...	...

	2009 Adult (15–49) incidence rate		2001 Adult (15–49) incidence rate		2009 Adults + children newly infected	
	estimate	[low – high estimate]	estimate	[low – high estimate]	estimate	[low – high estimate]
NORTH AMERICA	<0.10	[<0.10 – <0.10]	<0.10	[<0.10 – <0.10]	70 000	[44 000 – 130 000]
Canada	…	[<0.10 – <0.10]	…	[<0.10 – <0.10]	…	[2 300 – 4 300]
Mexico	…	[<0.10 – <0.10]	…	[<0.10 – <0.10]	…	[8800 – 21 000]
United States of America	<0.10	[<0.10 – <0.10]	<0.10	[<0.10 – <0.10]	54 000	[24 000 – 110 000]
CARIBBEAN	<0.10	[<0.10 – <0.10]	<0.10	[<0.10 – 0.11]	17 000	[13 000 – 21 000]
Bahamas	…	[<0.10 – 0.62]	…	[<0.10 – 0.43]	…	[<200 – 1200]
Barbados	…	[<0.10 – 0.16]	…	[<0.10 – 0.13]	…	[<200 – <500]
Cuba	…	[<0.10 – <0.10]	…	[<0.10 – <0.10]	…	[<500 – <1000]
Dominican Republic	<0.10	[<0.10 – <0.10]	<0.10	[<0.10 – 0.10]	3600	[1600 – 5000]
Haiti	0.15	[0.10 – 0.19]	0.19	[0.15 – 0.23]	8800	[6500 – 11 000]
Jamaica	0.13	[<0.10 – 0.27]	0.19	[0.10 – 0.25]	2100	[<1000 – 4200]
Trinidad and Tobago	…	[<0.10 – 0.21]	…	[0.10 – 0.19]	…	[<1000 – 1800]
CENTRAL AND SOUTH AMERICA	<0.10	[<0.10 – <0.10]	<0.10	[<0.10 – <0.10]	92 000	[70 000 – 120 000]
Argentina	<0.10	[<0.10 – <0.10]	<0.10	[<0.10 – <0.10]	7500	[4100 – 11 000]
Belize	0.20	[0.13 – 0.32]	0.30	[0.23 – 0.35]	<500	[<500 – <1000]
Bolivia	…	[<0.10 – <0.10]	…	[<0.10 – <0.10]	…	[<1000 – 1600]
Brazil	…	[<0.10 – <0.10]	…	[<0.10 – <0.10]	…	[18 000 – 70 000]
Chile	…	[<0.10 – <0.10]	…	[<0.10 – <0.10]	…	[1400 – 4300]
Colombia	…	[<0.10 – <0.10]	…	[<0.10 – <0.10]	…	[2800 – 16 000]
Costa Rica	…	[<0.10 – <0.10]	…	[<0.10 – <0.10]	…	[<500 – 1100]
Ecuador	…	[<0.10 – <0.10]	…	[<0.10 – <0.10]	…	[1100 – 6200]
El Salvador	…	[<0.10 – 0.11]	…	[<0.10 – 0.14]	…	[1200 – 4000]
Guatemala	…	[<0.10 – 0.15]	…	[<0.10 – 0.12]	…	[3600 – 11 000]
Guyana	…	[<0.10 – 0.17]	…	[<0.10 – <0.10]	…	[<100 – <1000]
Honduras	…	[<0.10 – <0.10]	…	[<0.10 – 0.13]	…	[<1000 – 3700]
Nicaragua	…	[<0.10 – <0.10]	…	[<0.10 – <0.10]	…	[<500 – 1300]
Panama	…	[<0.10 – 0.11]	…	[<0.10 – 0.14]	…	[<1000 – 2200]
Paraguay	…	[<0.10 – <0.10]	…	[<0.10 – <0.10]	…	[<1000 – 1600]
Peru	…	[<0.10 – <0.10]	…	[<0.10 – <0.10]	…	[2300 – 6700]
Suriname	<0.10	[<0.10 – <0.10]	0.11	[<0.10 – 0.16]	<500	[<100 – <500]
Uruguay	…	[<0.10 – <0.10]	…	[<0.10 – <0.10]	…	[<500 – <1000]
Venezuela	…	…	…	…	…	…

ESTIMATED PEOPLE LIVING WITH HIV *(continued)*

	2009 Adults newly infected		2009 AIDS-related deaths in adults + children		2001 AIDS-related deaths in adults + children	
	estimate	[low – high estimate]	estimate	[low – high estimate]	estimate	[low – high estimate]
NORTH AMERICA	69 000	[43 000 – 120 000]	26 000	[22 000 – 44 000]	30 000	[26 000 – 35 000]
Canada	...	[<1000 – 3800]	<500	[<500 – <1000]	<500	[<500 – <1000]
Mexico	...	[8300 – 20 000]	...	[6400 – 12 000]	...	[9800 – 15 000]
United States of America	54 000	[24 000 – 110 000]	17 000	[13 000 – 36 000]	17 000	[14 000 – 23 000]
CARIBBEAN	15 000	[12 000 – 19 000]	12 000	[8500 – 15 000]	19 000	[16 000 – 23 000]
Bahamas	...	[<100 – 1100]	<500	[<200 – <1000]	<1000	[<500 – <1000]
Barbados	...	[<200 – <500]	<100	[<100 – <100]	<100	[<100 – <100]
Cuba	...	[<500 – <1000]	<100	[<100 – <500]	<200	[<100 – <200]
Dominican Republic	3200	[1300 – 4400]	2300	[1300 – 3400]	3900	[2900 – 5500]
Haiti	7600	[5400 – 10 000]	7100	[5200 – 9400]	12 000	[9200 – 14 000]
Jamaica	2000	[<1000 – 4000]	1200	[<500 – 2100]	2700	[2100 – 3500]
Trinidad and Tobago	...	[<1000 – 1700]	<1000	[<500 – <1000]	<1000	[<500 – <1000]
CENTRAL AND SOUTH AMERICA	87 000	[66 000 – 120 000]	58 000	[43 000 – 70 000]	53 000	[44 000 – 65 000]
Argentina	7400	[4100 – 11 000]	2900	[1600 – 4500]	2800	[1600 – 4100]
Belize	<500	[<500 – <1000]	<500	[<500 – <500]	<500	[<200 – <500]
Bolivia	...	[<500 – 1500]	<1000	[<1000 – 1200]	<1000	[<1000 – 1100]
Brazil	...	[17 000 – 69 000]	...	[2000 – 25 000]	...	[7200 – 24 000]
Chile	...	[1200 – 4000]	...	[<1000 – 2200]	...	[<500 – 1200]
Colombia	...	[2300 – 16 000]	14 000	[11 000 – 18 000]	13 000	[9800 – 17 000]
Costa Rica	...	[<500 – 1000]	<500	[<100 – <1000]	<100	[<100 – <200]
Ecuador	...	[<100 – <100]	2200	[1300 – 3300]	2800	[2100 – 3700]
El Salvador	...	[1000 – 3800]	1400	[<1000 – 2100]	<1000	[<200 – 1100]
Guatemala	...	[3200 – 10 000]	2600	[1600 – 3700]	1500	[1000 – 2100]
Guyana	...	[<100 – <1000]	<500	[<100 – <1000]	<1000	[<1000 – 1300]
Honduras	...	[<1000 – 3400]	2500	[1700 – 3400]	3700	[2800 – 5000]
Nicaragua	...	[<500 – 1300]	<500	[<200 – <500]	<200	[<200 – <500]
Panama	...	[<1000 – 2100]	1500	[<1000 – 3600]	1600	[<1000 – 3200]
Paraguay	...	[<1000 – 1600]	...	[<500 – <1000]	...	[<500 – <1000]
Peru	...	[2100 – 6300]	5000	[3800 – 6600]	6300	[5200 – 7900]
Suriname	<200	[<100 – <500]	<200	[<200 – <500]	<500	[<200 – <500]
Uruguay	...	[<500 – <1000]	...	...	...	...
Venezuela	...	...	...	...	...	...

	2009 Orphans (0–17) currently living		2001 Orphans (0–17)		Injecting drug users		Female sex workers		Men who have sex with men	
	estimate	[low – high estimate]	estimate	[low – high estimate]	Year	HIV (%)	Year	HIV (%)	Year	HIV (%)
NORTH AMERICA	140 000	[110 000 – 180 000]	210 000	[160 000 – 260 000]	...	...	...	...	...	...
Canada	...	...	...	...	2008	12.7	...	...	2008	14.7
Mexico	...	...	...	...	2009	5.0	2009	0.9	2009	10.2
United States of America	...	...	...	...	...	...	...	...	...	...
CARIBBEAN	140 000	[110 000 – 170 000]	100 000	[63 000 – 170 000]	...	...	...	...	...	...
Bahamas	...	...	...	...	...	...	...	...	2009	25.6
Barbados	...	...	...	...	...	...	...	...	...	...
Cuba	...	...	...	...	...	...	2009	0.1	2009	0.7
Dominican Republic	...	...	...	...	...	...	2008	4.8	2004	10.7
Haiti	...	...	...	...	...	...	2009	5.3	...	...
Jamaica	...	...	...	...	...	...	2009	4.9	2007	31.8
Trinidad and Tobago	...	...	...	...	...	...	...	...	...	...
CENTRAL AND SOUTH AMERICA	240 000	[200 000 – 280 000]	190 000	[150 000 – 240 000]	...	...	...	...	...	...
Argentina	...	...	...	...	2008	11.9	2008	1.9	2008	11.8
Belize	...	...	...	...	...	...	...	...	...	...
Bolivia	...	...	...	...	...	...	...	...	2008	11.6
Brazil	...	...	...	...	2009	5.9	...	...	2009	12.6
Chile	...	...	...	...	...	...	...	...	2009	20.3
Colombia	...	...	...	...	...	...	2008	1.6	...	...
Costa Rica	...	...	...	...	...	...	...	...	2009	12.7
Ecuador	...	...	...	...	...	...	...	...	...	...
El Salvador	...	...	...	...	...	...	2009	4.1	2009	9.8
Guatemala	...	...	...	...	...	...	2006	1.0	2006	18.3
Guyana	...	...	...	...	...	...	2009	16.6	2009	19.4
Honduras	...	...	...	...	...	...	2006	2.3	2006	6.6
Nicaragua	...	...	...	...	...	...	...	...	2009	4.2
Panama	...	...	...	...	...	...	...	...	...	...
Paraguay	...	...	...	...	...	...	2008	1.8	2008	9.6
Peru	...	...	...	...	...	...	...	...	2009	10.1
Suriname	...	...	...	...	...	...	...	...	...	...
Uruguay	...	...	...	...	...	...	...	...	2008	9.1
Venezuela	...	...	...	...	...	...	...	...	...	...

Source: Global Report: UNAIDS Report on the Global AIDS Epidemic, 2010.

ONLINE RESOURCES

Tag Key

The tags defined here are used in the entries listed below to denote the information or services provided by each organization or resource cited.

- **Additional Resources:** The Web site contains an area where there are external links, lists of books and/or other media, or any resource that the Web site does not provide onsite.
- **Advocacy:** The Web site features information on how to become politically active in the fight against HIV and AIDS.
- **Clinical Studies:** The Web site contains information about clinical trials and studies for HIV/AIDS.
- **Computer Software:** The Web site has software that is relevant to HIV/AIDS research.
- **Conference Coverage:** The Web site contains either articles, specific documents, or a publication about conferences on the topics of HIV and AIDS.
- **Dietary:** The Web site contains information about living a healthful lifestyle with HIV/AIDS, specifically with regard to diet and nutrition.
- **Donations:** The Web site has a means for those who want to help to contribute financially or volunteer to help with HIV/AIDS research.
- **FAQ/Fact Sheets:** The Web site contains one or both for quick question answering.
- **Guides/Brochures:** The Web site provides guides and/or brochures on topics related

to HIV/AIDS research (either via ordering hard copies or providing downloadable soft copies).

- **Housing Information:** The site has information specifically relating to housing and persons with HIV/AIDS.
- **Medical Rights:** The site contains information about the rights of those with HIV/AIDS.
- **News Articles:** The Web site either contains its own news articles or provides a link to articles.
- **Personal Accounts:** The Web site provides personal accounts either free from the site or through a subscription.
- **Subscription:** The site offers a subscription to its primary publication(s).
- **Testing:** The Web site has information about where you can go locally to get tested for HIV/AIDS.
- **Treatment Information:** The site provides information on how to treat and/or prevent HIV and AIDS.

46664.com

http://www.46664.com
general, nonprofit site, information-based
Tags: Advocacy, FAQ/Fact Sheets, Additional
   Resources

A South African–based HIV/AIDS foundation connected to the Nelson Mandela Foundation. Provides various fund-raisers for Africa-based HIV health care projects. Many famous personalities dedicate time and/or talent to assist the fund-raising.

ACT-UP
http://www.actupny.org
political advocacy site
Tags: News Articles, FAQ/Fact Sheets, Additional Resources, Conference Coverage, Advocacy

This organization is strictly for those looking to become politically active in the HIV/AIDS community. Most of information provided is linked to a policy or current event in the GLBT and HIV/AIDS communities.

AfriAfya (African Network for Health Knowledge Management and Communication)
http://www.afriafya.org
nonprofit site, information-based
Tags: Additional Resources, News Articles

A Web site dedicated to disseminating information from HIV studies and treatment information, health information, and general health information to areas traditionally underserved by information and communication technologies, specifically Kenya and Somalia.

AIDS Action
http://www.aidsaction.org
political site, policy-based
Tags: News Articles, Additional Resources, Advocacy

Their mission statement is for advocacy at the national level, with their goal being to fight until there is a world without AIDS. The site also offers a variety of news articles and publications related to policy action.

AIDS Alliance for Children, Youth & Families
http://www.aids-alliance.org
nonprofit organization, information-based
Tags: News Articles, FAQ/Fact Sheets, Additional Resources, Guides/Brochures

An in-depth resource site focused on providing information about HIV/AIDS with regard to children and families.

AIDS Clinical Trials Group
http://www.actgnetwork.org
nonprofit site, information-based
Tag: Clinical Studies

Must be a member to use this site, but it is free to sign up.

AIDS Clock
http://www.unfpa.org/aids_clock
United Nations site, information-based
Tag: Additional Resources

Statistics by country on the prevalence of AIDS.

AIDS Community Research Initiative of America (ACRIA)
http://www.acria.org
nonprofit database site, information-based
Tags: News Articles, Additional Resources, Donations, Advocacy

Despite a lengthy mission statement and merchandise to help raise funds, this Web site is centered on the ACRIA Update Database. Otherwise, it offers links to other sites and databases, including an engine to search for local trials. For the ACRIA Update Database, click (from the homepage): HIV Health Literacy >> ACRIA Update."

AIDS Education and Training Centers National Resource Center
http://www.aidsetc.org
educational, government site, medicine-based
Tags: News Articles, Treatment Information, Guides/Brochures, Testing

This Web site is focused on disseminating information about all aspects of HIV/AIDS. This includes training materials and curricula for group lectures. Excellent resources for the professional and layperson as well.

AIDS Education Global Information System (AEGIS)
http://www.aegis.com
general, nonprofit site, information-based
Tags: News Articles, Treatment Information, FAQ/Fact Sheets, Additional Resources,

Clinical Studies, Conference Coverage, Donations, Testing, Medical Rights

This Web site is a portal to links but difficult to navigate. To access the AIDSLINE Database, visit http://www.aegis.com/aidsline.

AIDS Foundation of Chicago
http://www.aidschicago.org
information-based, regional, nonprofit site
Tags: Treatment Information, FAQ/Fact Sheets, Additional Resources, Advocacy, Testing

A regional HIV/AIDS education, prevention, and policy group.

AIDS.gov
http://www.aids.gov
http://www.aids.gov/awareness-days/
government site, information-based, education-based
Tags: News Articles, Additional Resources, FAQ/Fact Sheets

A portal Web site from the U.S. Department of Health and Human Services. Provides links to other government sources of information as well as some nonprofit organizations and national awareness days.

AIDSinfo—HIV/AIDS Treatment
http://aidsinfo.nih.gov
general, government site, education-based
Tags: Treatment Information, FAQ/Fact Sheets, Additional Resources, Clinical Studies, Guides/Brochures

This one new link combines both what used to be an AIDS resource sampler and AIDS treatment information. However, it is very informative and run by the U.S. Department of Health and Human Services. Also available in Spanish. For a glossary of HIV/AIDS-related terms, visit http://glossary.hivatis.org.

The AIDS Memorial Quilt
http://www.aidsquilt.org
public site, donation and information-based
Tags: Treatment Information, Additional Resources, Donations, Advocacy

This Web site gives the history of the AIDS Memorial Quilt, which has grown quite large since the late 1980s. Run by the Names Project Foundation, this quilt is a symbol of the fight against AIDS.

AIDS.org
http://www.aids.org
general, public site, education-based, advertisements
Tags: News Articles, Treatment Information, FAQ/Fact Sheets, Personal Accounts, Donations

A very simply designed site but with a wide range of topics to research. There are news articles, treatment information, and other broad topics that lead to a page of links to more specific topics.

AIDSPortugal.com
http://www.aidsportugal.com
general, information-based, nonprofit
Tags: Treatment Information, Guides/Brochures, Additional Resources, News Articles

This Web site provides basic as well as more advanced statistical and medical information in Portuguese. Although much of the information relates to activities in Portugal, there is additional information relevant to other Portuguese-speaking countries, e.g., Brazil.

AIDS Project Los Angeles
http://www.apla.org
general, regional service site, information-based
Tags: News Articles, Treatment Information, FAQ/Fact Sheets, Additional Resources, Clinical Studies, Donations, Testing, Advocacy, Medical Rights

An excellent Web site aiming to increase the quality of life of those living with HIV/AIDS in the Los Angeles area. Sections range from prevention to policy and activism to statistics. For HIV and AIDS services in Los Angeles County, visit http://www.HIVLA.org.

AIDS Research Institute
http://ari.ucsf.edu/home.aspx

general, medical site, university-based

Tags: News Articles, Treatment Information, FAQ/Fact Sheets, Additional Resources, Testing

HIV InSite
http://hivinsite.ucsf.edu/

Center for AIDS Prevention Studies
http://caps.ucsf.edu

AIDS History Project
http://www.library.ucsf.edu/collections/archives/manuscripts/aids

Run by the University of California, San Francisco, this Web site contains information about advances in medical science and HIV/AIDS research. There is also information pertaining to prevention and treatment of HIV/AIDS.

AIDS Resource Foundation for Children
http://www.aidsresource.org
nonprofit organization, foundation-based
Tags: News Articles, Additional Resources, Donations

The group is based on the East Coast of the United States, and the Web site is a vehicle for advertising for events there.

Alternative Medicine Homepage
http://www.pitt.edu/~cbw/hiv.html
university site, information filter–based
Tags: Additional Resources

A portal for alternative medicine relating to HIV.

American Academy of HIV Medicine
http://www.aahivm.org
medical organization, information-based
Tags: News Articles, Treatment Information, Additional Resources, Clinical Studies, Testing

The Web site is not very user friendly, and a lot of the information presented is meant for physicians. However, it offers treatment information in addition to news about upcoming advances in the field of medicine and HIV/AIDS.

American Cancer Society
http://www.cancer.org

Click: Learn About Cancer >> Choose A Cancer Topic >> HIV Infection and AIDS
general, medical association site, education-based
Tags: News Articles, Treatment Information, Clinical Studies, FAQ/Fact Sheets, Additional Resources, Guides/Brochures

A broad general information site that reads like an encyclopedia entry, with the main focus on cancer.

American Civil Liberties Union (ALCU)—HIV/AIDS
http://www.aclu.org/hiv
nonprofit site, advocacy-based
Tags: News Articles, Treatment Information, Additional Resources, Donations, Testing, Advocacy, Housing Information, Medical Rights

The ACLU has a great Web site for getting involved and learning what medical rights one has when diagnosed with HIV and/or AIDS. Also, information is included about what to do when experiencing discrimination associated with HIV/AIDS.

American College of Obstetricians and Gynecologists (ACOG)
http://www.acog.org
Search: HIV/AIDS
general, public site, information/directory-based
Tags: FAQ Fact Sheets, Additional Resources

The Web site's information is directed at females and has some gender-related material regarding HIV under "Women's Issues"; however, the site maintains a links page that can be applicable to anyone.

American Medical Association (AMA)
http://www.ama-assn.org
Search: HIV/AIDS
general, medical site, information-based
Tags: Treatment Information, Additional Resources, Testing, Advocacy

This site has two different places to go for information. The main page is really just two paragraphs that gloss over HIV/AIDS. The second is a student site offering information on how to become active and involved in finding a cure.

American Public Health Association (APHA)

http://www.apha.org
Search: HIV/AIDS
general, medical association site, information-based
Tags: News Articles, Additional Resources, Conference Coverage, Donations, Advocacy

A search for HIV/AIDS leads to a portal listing other Web sites.

American Red Cross

http://www.redcross.org
Search: HIV/AIDS
foundation site, information/donation-based
Tags: News Articles, Treatment Information, Additional Resources, Clinical Studies, Conference Coverage, Donations, Advocacy

General site for the American Red Cross; therefore, a lot of information about other diseases, viruses, and disasters. Information about contributing to HIV prevention as well as materials available for purchase.

amfAR—American Foundation for AIDS Research

http://www.amfar.org
foundation site, information-based
Tags: News Articles, Additional Resources, Donations, Testing

The major purpose of this Web site is to inform the public about the foundation and its constant research in advancing HIV/AIDS awareness, finding a cure, and gathering donations.

Asian AIDS/HIV Information and Archive

http://www.utopia-asia.com/aids.htm
nonprofit site, information filter–based
Tags: Additional Resources.

Region-specific links regarding HIV/AIDS for Asian countries, as well as GLBT information for Asia. Includes safer sex information in Chi-nese, Filipino, French, German, Indonesian, Japanese, Khmer, Malay, Thai, and Vietnamese.

Asian & Pacific Islander Coalition on HIV/AIDS (APICHA)

http://www.apicha.org
nonprofit site, information-based
Tags: News Articles, Additional Resources, Donations, Testing, Medical Rights

This site offers a variety of health care services relating to HIV/AIDS to Asian and Pacific Islanders.

Asian & Pacific Islander Wellness Center

http://www.apiwellness.org
nonprofit site, information-based
Tags: News Articles, Treatment Information, Additional Resources, Donations, Testing, Advocacy

This is a Web site centered on Asian and Pacific Islander cultures. However, it offers general information; it is also supplemented with some additional facts and prevention techniques associated with Asian cultures.

Asia Pacific Leadership Forum on HIV/AIDS and Development

http://www.aplfaids.com
intergovernmental organization, information-based
Tags: Advocacy, Guides/Brochures

Builds leadership in all areas of HIV/AIDS education, public policy, and research. Focuses on the large Asian and Pacific Islands region, stretching from India to Tahiti. Funded by the United Nations in addition to several other countries.

Association of Nurses in AIDS Care

http://www.anacnet.org
association site, information-based
Tags: News Articles, Additional Resources, Clinical Studies, Conference Coverage, Testing

Information for nurses caring for patients with HIV/AIDS as well as announcements related to the organization.

AVERT International AIDS Charity
http://www.avert.org
general, nonprofit site, information-based
Tags: News Articles, Treatment Information, FAQ/Fact Sheets, Personal Accounts, Additional Resources, Guides/Brochures, Testing, Donations, Advocacy

World AIDS Day
http://www.avert.org/world-aids-day.htm

An excellent general information site.

Being Alive
http://www.beingalivela.org
nonprofit site, communal information site
Tags: News Articles, Additional Resources, Personal Accounts, Guides/Brochures, Donations, Testing, Advocacy

HIV/AIDS community support services based in Los Angeles. The site offers a great local link center as well as upcoming community events and ways to volunteer.

Black AIDS Institute
http://www.blackaids.org
general, minority concerns, information-based
Tags: Testing, Donations, Additional Resources, Personal Accounts, Medical Rights, Advocacy

National HIV/AIDS think tank focused solely on AIDS in the African-American community. Offers public policy information, organizational training, advocacy services, and information to individuals and groups.

The Body: The Complete AIDS/HIV Resource
http://www.thebody.com
general, corporate/advertisement site, education-based
Tags: News Articles, Treatment Information, FAQ/Fact Sheets, Additional Resources, Clinical Studies, Conference Coverage

Body Positive and SIDAahora Magazine Archives
http://www.thebody.com/bp/bpix.html

Treatment Action Group (TAG)
http://www.thebody.com/tag/tagpage.html

A very informative site offering links to various sources of information. For example, there is information about how to get involved with clinical trials, drug resistance, and upcoming conferences. This is a highly recommended general information site. A smaller site in Spanish is available.

Canadian AIDS Treatment Information Exchange (CATIE)
http://www.catie.ca
Tags: Treatment Information, FAQ/Fact Sheets, Clinical Studies

A Canadian information site available in both English and French that provides detailed prevention, treatment, and clinical information, and education materials. Ask-an-expert e-mail services are included.

Canadian HIV Trials Network
http://www.hivnet.ubc.ca
health institute site, medicine-based
Tag: Clinical Studies

Clinical study site for Canada. Also available in French.

CDC National Prevention Information Network
http://www.cdcnpin.org
general, government site, education-based
Tags: FAQ/Fact Sheets, Guides/Brochures, Conference Coverage, Testing

Site sponsored by the CDC for the prevention of various diseases, not limited to viruses. The HIV/AIDS section includes a wealth of recent statistics on the spread and prevalence of HIV. Also listed are some commonsense ways for personal prevention. A smaller site in Spanish is included, but many of the statistics and articles have not been translated into Spanish.

CDC WONDER
http://wonder.cdc.gov
database, government site, publication-based
Tags: News Articles, FAQ/Fact Sheets, Additional Resources, Guides/Brochures

The CDC provides an online database for information on all kinds of public health. However, HIV/AIDS is specifically noted on the main page, and a variety of pertinent statistics is included.

Centers for Disease Control and Prevention (CDC)
http://www.cdc.gov/hiv
general, government site, information-based
Tags: News Articles, Treatment Information, FAQ/Fact Sheets, Additional Resources, Clinical Studies, Guides/Brochures, Conference Coverage, Testing

Morbidity and Mortality Weekly Report (MMWR)
http://www.cdc.gov/mmwr

This Web site is another hub for information on HIV/AIDS. From general information to where to go to get tested to conference materials, this site has been one of the better ones for resources from the general guides.

Center of Excellence for Transgender Health
http://transhealth.ucsf.edu
general, transgender health information
Tags: FAQ/Fact Sheets, Additional Resources, Medical Rights, Clinical Studies, Guides/Brochures

University-based information and referral for transgender health issues, with large sections dedicated specifically to HIV/AIDS in the transgender community.

Children With AIDS Project of America
http://www.aidskids.org
nonprofit, adoption information site
Tags: FAQ/Fact Sheets, Additional Resources, Donations, Testing, Housing Information

This site has links and information about becoming the adoptive parent of an abandoned HIV-positive child.

Clinical Trials
http://www.clinicaltrials.gov
government site, medicine based
Tag: Clinical Studies

A clinical trial site sponsored by the government.

Coalition for Positive Sexuality
http://www.positive.org
nonprofit site, sex education–based
Tags: News Articles, Treatment Information, FAQ/Fact Sheets, Additional Resources, Testing, Advocacy

This is a sex education Web site oriented toward teenagers and young adults. The information is not HIV/AIDS specific but relates to many STDs. Some information is available in Spanish.

Critical Path AIDS Project
http://www.critpath.org
activist site, information-based
Tags: News Articles, Treatment Information, Additional Resources, Advocacy, Housing Information, Medical Rights

AIDS Library
Click: AIDS Library

AIDS Glossary
Click: Critical Path AIDS Project >> HIV/AIDS Treatment >> Glossaries

AIDS Law
Click: Critical Path AIDS Project >> Treatment Benefits >> AIDS and the Law

An activist Web site dedicated to HIV/AIDS awareness and erasing the stigma of the virus.

Department of Agriculture: Food Nutrition Information Center
http://fnic.nal.usda.gov
Search: HIV/AIDS
general, government site, health-based
Tags: FAQ/Fact Sheets, Dietary

This site offers copious information about ensuring a healthful diet and working effectively with your body while living with HIV/AIDS.

Department of Health and Human Services (HHS)—AIDS

http://www.aids.gov
general, government site, information-based
Tags: Treatment Information, FAQ/Fact Sheets, Additional Resources, Clinical Studies, Guides/Brochures, Donations, Testing

This site is specific to HIV/AIDS awareness. The sidebar has links that are directly related to the tags, and information is easily accessible.

Department of Veterans Affairs (VA)

http://www.va.gov
Search: HIV/AIDS
general, government site, information-based
Tags: Treatment Information, FAQ/Fact Sheets, Additional Resources, Clinical Studies, Guides/Brochures, Testing

The portal for Veterans Affairs, with pages of general information. However, the VA does a good job of organizing the material and delves a little into the science and biology of the infection.

Deutsche AIDS-Hilfe

http://www.aidshilfe.de/
German, general, public site, education-based
Tags: News Articles, Treatment Information, FAQ/Fact Sheets, Additional Resources

German Web site about HIV/AIDS.

Elizabeth Glaser Pediatric AIDS Foundation

http://www.pedAIDS.org
foundation site, information-based
Tags: News Articles, Treatment Information, Personal Accounts, Additional Resources, Donations, Advocacy

A pediatric HIV/AIDS advocacy site with human-interest stories. It also seeks donations.

European AIDS Treatment Group (EATG)

http://www.eatg.org
information-based, nonprofit, advocacy
Tags: Treatment Information, News Articles, Clinical Studies, Guides/Brochures, Subscription

A European nonprofit organization that advocates for fair and equal treatment across Europe for all HIV-positive people. It provides access to news articles and educational training and works toward a unified European policy with regard to HIV.

FightAIDS@Home

http://www.fightaidsathome.org
research entity site, software-based
Tag: Computer Software

A Web site to assist AIDS research by using a computer program that the user installs. From there the software uses your free space on your computer when idling to help find other medical matches. This is the first computerized medical grid for HIV/AIDS.

Food and Drug Administration (FDA)

http://www.fda.gov
medicinal, government site, information-based
Tags: News Articles, Treatment Information, Additional Resources, Clinical Studies, Testing

There is a lot of pharmaceutical information here: news releases, drug information, and milestones in medical care for HIV/AIDS. However, the additional resources are just links to the other governmen-sponsored Web sites.

Gay and Lesbian Medical Association

http://www.glma.org
Search: HIV/AIDS
foundation site, information-based
Tags: News Articles, Treatment Information, FAQ/Fact Sheets, Additional Resources, Clinical Studies, Conference Coverage, Donations, Testing, Advocacy

Another good general information site. Of note is their extensive archive listing and history of HIV/AIDS in the media.

Gay Men's Health Crisis (GMHC)

http://www.gmhc.org

general, nonprofit site, health-based

Tags: News Articles, Treatment Information, FAQ/Fact Sheets, Additional Resources, Guides/Brochures, Donations, Testing, Advocacy, Housing Information, Medical Rights

Former database site that now provides general information, much of it on living a healthy life with HIV/AIDS.

Global Campaign for Microbicides

http://www.global-campaign.org

nonprofit site, research-based

Tags: Advocacy, Treatment Information, Clinical Studies

International organization created to advocate and work toward the creation and availability of vaginal and rectal microbicides to prevent the spread of HIV.

The Global Fund

http://theglobalfund.org

nonprofit site, foundation site

Tags: News Articles, Additional Resources, Advocacy, Donations

The goal of the group is to provide medicine and increase awareness for three major health issues: HIV/AIDS, tuberculosis, and malaria. The Web site has applications for grants as well as details of fund's current projects.

Grupo de Trabajo sobre Tratamientos del VIH

http://www.gtt-vih.org

Spanish, general, foundation site, education-based

Tags: Treatment Information, FAQ/Fact Sheets, Additional Resources, Donations

Web site, in Spanish, dedicated to improving the quality of life of those living with HIV/AIDS. Offerings include, but are not limited to, legal information, current research and development, and advertising campaigns for prevention.

Harvard AIDS Institute

http://www.aids.harvard.edu

institution site, medical research-based

Tags: News Articles, Clinical Studies, Additional Resources

This Web site concentrates on the advances that Harvard has contributed to the medical field. However, the site is used mainly to inform potential medical students to Harvard about the AIDS Institute for research.

HIV/AIDS Housing—Department of Housing and Urban Development (HUD)

http://www.hud.gov

Search: HIV/AIDS

housing, government site, information-based

Tags: Additional Resources, Housing Information

According to HUD, through their Housing Opportunities for Persons with Aids (HOWPA) program, the goal is to help people with their housing when they encounter rising health costs. However, aside from other links that go to housing information, this Web site is hard to navigate and has no additional HIV/AIDS-related information.

HIV/AIDS—The Office of Minority Health

http://www.omhrc.gov

Search: HIV/AIDS

government database site, information-based

Tag: News Articles

Offers many HIV/AIDS statistics sorted by race.

HIV & AIDS Presentations

http://www.cmeonhiv.com

database site, medical research–based

Tag: News Articles

The site offers many presentations on the advances of research surrounding HIV and AIDS. However, in order to access these file, one is expected to be a professional in the field and register with the site.

HIV/AIDS Programs

http://hab.hrsa.gov

general, government site, policy-based

Tags: News Articles, Treatment Information, Personal Accounts, Additional Resources, Clinical Studies, Donations, Testing, Advocacy

Focused on the Ryan White Program, the Web site contains clear information about where to find HIV/AIDS treatment if you happen to be low-income and uninsured. Also, there are clear links to find current legislation about HIV/AIDS.

HIV and Hepatitis.com

http://www.hivandhepatitis.com

general, public site, education-based, advertisements

Tags: News Articles, Treatment Information, FAQ/Fact Sheets, Additional Resources, Clinical Studies, Conference Coverage, Testing

This Web site is an excellent starting source for someone trying to find information on HIV/AIDS. Front and center are up-to-date news articles. Also includes information about its spread around the world, prevention/treatment information, and several other outlets to answer HIV/AIDS inquiries. Includes news about other communicable diseases.

HIV Databases

http://hiv-web.lanl.gov

government database site

Tag: News Articles

An easy-to-navigate site of HIV databases. The four database types are related to sequencing, resistance, immunology, and vaccine trials.

HIV i-Base

http://www.i-base.info

medicinal, activist site, medicine-based

Tags: Treatment Information, Conference Coverage, Guides/Brochures, FAQ/Fact Sheets, Additional Resources

HIV i-Base is a great resource for those who want to find out more about HIV/AIDS. Unlike most other general sites, this one is geared toward those seeking to understand treatment.

It describes medical theories in understandable terms. In addition, it offers coverage of a variety of other issues related to living with HIV/AIDS, such as drug addiction and opioid dependence.

HIV Travel

http://www.hivtravel.org

foundation site, information- and policy-based

Tags: News Articles, Additional Resources, Advocacy

Excellent, up-to-date site on the travel laws for those living with HIV/AIDS. Information is organized by nation or level of restriction. Also offers pertinent news articles.

INSIGHT

http://insight.ccbr.umn.edu

research site

Tags: Clinical Studies, Treatment Information, Additional Resources

Highlights the work of INSIGHT (International Network for Strategic Initiatives in Global HIV Trials). Multinational research studies on the treatment and management of HIV as well as other viral infections.

Institute for Traditional Medicine

http://www.itmonline.org

nonprofit site, medicinal information-based

Tags: Treatment Information, Additional Resources, Dietary

A general introduction to alternative medicine. The links are for specific diseases and how to combat them naturally.

International AIDS Economics Network

http://www.iaen.org/index.html

informational database site

Tags: News Articles, Personal Accounts

This Web site is designed exclusively for economists and policy makers involved in the fight against AIDS. It provides a database that offers a variety of publications, records, and tools related to HIV/AIDS and economics.

International AIDS Vaccine Initiative

http://www.iavi.org

political site, medical research-based

Tags: News Articles, Treatment Information, Additional Resources, Clinical Studies, Conference Coverage, Donations, Testing, Advocacy

This Web site is focused on HIV/AIDS vaccination research. No or limited information about other types of treatment and prevention.

International Association of Physicians in AIDS Care

http://www.iapac.org

information-based, nonprofit site

Tags: Treatment Information, Conference Coverage

This Web site promotes a professional association for physicians involved in the treatment of AIDS/HIV. Membership is required to view the information.

International Council of AIDS Service Organizations (ICASO)

http://www.icaso.org

humanitarian site, information-based

Tags: News Articles, Treatment Information, Additional Resources, Donations, Advocacy

Another Web site focused on the relief effort in Africa with the goal of improving human rights and better access to HIV prevention and care.

International Treatment Preparedness Coalition

http://www.itpcglobal.org

international, information-based

Tags: Treatment Information, Advocacy, Medical Rights, Conference Coverage, News Articles

Advocacy group that seeks global access to treatment, prevention, and access to basic medical care for all people who are HIV positive, through treatment education, community building, and small grants to local groups.

Joint United Nations Programme on HIV/AIDS (UNAIDS)

http://www.unaids.org

policy- and information-based

Tags: Advocacy, Conference Coverage, Guides/Brochures

This site documents the global effect of HIV by focusing on government policy and social practices. Its additional resources include details of individual country responses to the HIV epidemic. The Web site is offered in four Western languages; however, documents originate in English, and the translation project is ongoing.

Kaiser Family Foundation—HIV/AIDS Research

http://www.kff.org/hivaids

foundation site, information-based

Tags: Treatment Information, Additional Resources, FAQ/Fact Sheets, Guides/Brochures, Donations, Testing, Advocacy

This is an offshoot of the VA Web site. It contains a lot of detailed information and fact sheets pertaining to race, age, and gender. Also, there are many links to additional Web sites offering further information.

Lambda Legal: HIV

http://www.lambdalegal.org

Click: Our Work >> Issues >> HIV

independent site, policy-based

Tags: News Articles, Treatment Information, FAQ/Fact Sheets, Additional Resources, Advocacy, Medical Rights

A legal site dedicated to HIV and LGBT issues. It offers up-to-date information about recent rulings and pending cases as well.

Médecins Sans Frontières/Doctors Without Borders (MSF-USA)

http://doctorswithoutborders.org/news/issue.cfm?id=2392

humanitarian site, information-based

Tags: News Articles, Treatment Information, Additional Resources, Donations, Testing

The Doctors Without Borders page related specifically to HIV/AIDS. The Web site also offers many articles and up-to-date news regarding the fight against the disease and the spread of the virus.

Minority AIDS Project

http://www.map-usa.org
nonprofit site, charity-based
Tags: Treatment Information, Personal Accounts, Additional Resources, Testing, Housing Information, Medical Rights

Christian-based activism site dedicated to improving the quality of life of those living with HIV/AIDS. The Web site offers no direct services, but the charity is based in Los Angeles.

National AIDS Treatment Advocacy Project (NATAP)

http://www.natap.org
political, nonprofit site, information-based
Tags: News Articles, Treatment Information, Additional Resources, Clinical Studies, Conference Coverage, Donations, Testing, Advocacy

There are links to several news articles connected to specific topics beyond HIV and AIDS, including hepatitis B and C and conferences, in addition to information concerning ways to get involved in HIV/AIDS advocacy.

National Association of People with AIDS (NAPWA)

http://www.napwa.org
nonprofit site, information-based
Tags: Additional Resources, Conference Coverage, Donations, Advocacy

Promotional site for the oldest AIDS organization network in the nation. This Web site promotes the group's activities as well as other conferences and events but offers little general information about the virus.

National Cancer Institute (NCI)

http://www.cancer.gov
Search: HIV/AIDS
medical, government site, information-based

Tags: Treatment Information, FAQ/Fact Sheets, Additional Resources, Clinical Studies, Guides/Brochures, Conference Coverage, Testing

There is testing and clinical trial information on this Web site; however, information is related to cancer and HIV, with cancer the central focus.

National Center for Health Statistics

http://www.cdc.gov/nchs
general statistical, information-based
Tags: FAQ/Fact Sheets, Guides/Brochures, Additional Resources

A governmental Web site dedicated to all statistics about health problems, deaths, disease, and health behavior in the United States.

National Center for HIV, STD, and TB Prevention

http://www.cdc.gov/nchstp
general, information-based, prevention
Tags: FAQ/Fact Sheets, Guides/Brochures, Testing

A government Web site that provides access to prevention information about HIV as well as sexually transmitted infections and tuberculosis.

National Criminal Justice Reference Service (NCJRS)

http://www.ncjrs.gov
Search: HIV/AIDS
criminal justice information-based, government site
Tags: Treatment Information, Medical Rights

This site has information concerning people with HIV/AIDS and their rights in court/jail/prison, including medical care and treatment options.

National Gay and Lesbian Task Force

http://thetaskforce.org
Click: Health & HIV/AIDS
political, foundation site, policy-based
Tags: News Articles, FAQ/Fact Sheets, Additional Resources, Conference Coverage, Donations, Advocacy

This site focuses on political issues sponsored by the National Gay and Lesbian Task Force. It has some good statistics about HIV/AIDS in relation to the GLBT community.

National Hemophilia Foundation

http://www.hemophilia.org
Click: Blood and Product Safety >> HIV/AIDS
nonprofit, information-based
Tags: FAQ/Fact Sheets, Conference Coverage, Treatment Information.

A national organization for people with blood coagulation disorders and for clinicians who work with them.

National Human Genome Research Institute Glossary

http://www.genome.gov/glossary.cfm
government site, information-based
Tags: FAQ/Fact Sheets, Additional Resources

This is a general glossary related to DNA and other genetic terms and is not specific to HIV/AIDS.

National Institute for Mental Health (NIMH)

http://www.nimh.nih.gov
Search: HIV/AIDS
research, government site, information-based
Tag: Clinical Studies

Information on this site is related to mental health problems and disorders associated with HIV/AIDS.

National Institutes of Health (NIH)

http://www.nih.gov
Search: HIV/AIDS
Search provides articles and links for
National Institute of Allergy and Infectious Diseases (NIAID)
National Institute on Drug Abuse (NIDA)
National Institute on Aging (NIA)
National Institute on Alcohol Abuse and Alcoholism (NIAAA)
National Institute for Dental and Craniofacial Research (NIDCR)

Institute of Neurological Disorders and Stroke (NINDS)
Office of Aids Research (OAR)
Office of Medical Application and Research (OMAR)

database, government site, information-based
Tags: News Articles, Treatment Information, FAQ/Fact Sheets, Guides/Brochures, Conference Coverage, Testing

HIV Vaccine Glossary

http://www.niaid.nih.gov/factsheets/
GLOSSARY.htm

National Center for Complementary and Alternative Medicine

http://www.nccam.nih.gov

General information and database articles from subsidiaries of the National Institutes of Health.

National Latino AIDS Awareness Day

http://www.nlaad.org
general, information-based, nonprofit site
Tags: Personal Accounts, Advocacy

An organization promoting awareness and education of Latinos in the United States about HIV.

National Minority AIDS Council

http://www.nmac.org
general, minority concerns, information-based
Tags: FAQ/Facts Sheets, Conference Coverage, Advocacy, Additional Resources

An organization based on training and educating people of color to address developments in the HIV/AIDS field. Provides treatment and research guidance, publications, and public policy information.

National Native American AIDS Prevention Center

http://www.nnaapc.org
nonprofit site, information-based
Tags: News Articles, Treatment Information, FAQ/Fact Sheets, Additional Resources, Donations, Testing

This Web site is directed toward the Native American community. It offers good general information as well as Native American–specific statistics.

National Pediatric AIDS Network (NPAN)
http://www.npan.org
general, nonprofit site, information-based
Tags: News Articles, Treatment Information, FAQ/Fact Sheets, Personal Accounts, Additional Resources, Clinical Studies, Conference Coverage, Donations, Testing, Advocacy, Housing Information, Medical Rights

An excellent Web site with a spectrum of information relating to pediatric HIV/AIDS. This includes, but is not limited to, preconception care, legal issues, young adult care, and issues in schools. The scope of information available cannot be completely detailed here. This site is recommended for those seeking information regarding any aspect of pediatric HIV/AIDS.

North American Syringe Exchange Network
http://www.nasen.org/index.html
medical- and information-based
Tags: Treatment Information, Additional Resources

Web site offering some information about the limited syringe exchange locations.

Office of Justice Programs—HIV/AIDS Victim Service
http://www.ojp.gov
Search: HIV/AIDS
government site, policy-based
Tags: News Articles, Treatment Information, Additional Resources, Medical Rights

Web site offering information about the rights of HIV/AIDS patients who have been the victim of a crime.

OneWorld AIDSRadio
http://www.aidschannel.org
OneWorld affiliate database site, information-based
Tags: News Articles, Additional Resources

This is an offshoot of the OneWorld Web site that provides news articles and streaming radio.

Pasteur Institute, Paris
http://www.pasteur.fr/recherche
French, public site, science-based
Tag: Additional Information

Web site of the world-famous institute and all of its research. Pages are available in English.

Physicians for Human Rights
http://physiciansforhumanrights.org
Click: What We Do >> Global Health Action Campaign
political, activist site, humanitarian-based
Tags: News Articles, Treatment Information, Guides/Brochures, Donations, Advocacy, Medical Rights

This Web site advocates for humane treatment of patients and has specific papers related to HIV/AIDS.

POZ Magazine
http://www.poz.com
magazine site, advertising, information-based
Tags: News Articles, Treatment Information, FAQ/Fact Sheets, Additional Resources, Guides/Brochures, Conference Coverage, Testing, Subscriptions

This magazine is very informative when it comes to HIV/AIDS. There are fact sheets, FAQs, and articles for those at every stage of the disease and for others looking to help.

Project Inform
http://www.projectinform.org
nonprofit site, information-based
Tags: News Articles, Treatment Information, Additional Resources, Guides/Brochures, Donations, Testing, Advocacy

A large number of news articles under such specific topics as hepatitis and bone marrow issues, in addition to HIV/AIDS are available for reading. The site also offers a phone service for those living with HIV/AIDS who have specific questions about their own treatment and experience.

San Francisco AIDS Foundation

http://www.sfaf.org
general, nonprofit site, information-based
Tags: News Articles, Treatment Information,
FAQ/Fact Sheets, Additional Resources,
Donations, Testing, Advocacy, Housing
Information, Medical Rights

Bulletin of Experimental Treatments for AIDS (BETA)

Click: AIDS INFO >> Bulletin of Experimental Treatment for AIDS

A now general site with a weath of information. One of the most complete and focused sites of a nonprofit organization.

Secretariat of the Pacific—HIV

http://www.spc.int/hiv
nonprofit site, information-based
Tags: News Articles, Treatment Information,
FAQ/Fact Sheets, Additional Resources,
Guides/Brochures, Advocacy

The Web site is dedicated to improving the quality of life of those in the Pacific who suffer from HIV/AIDS and other STIs.

Social Security Administration (SSA)

http://www.ssa.gov
Search: HIV/AIDS
financial aid, government site,
information-based
Tags: FAQ/Fact Sheets, Additional Resources,
Guides/Brochures, Medical Rights

Web site pertaining to HIV/AIDS-related disabilities and those individuals eligible to receive disability benefits, as outlined by their fact sheet and applications.

Southern Africa AIDS Information Dissemination Service

http://www.safaids.net/
general, nonprofit site, information-based
Tags: Treatment Information, FAQ/Fact Sheets,
Additional Resources, Guides/Brochures,
Testing

General information Web site relating to the coverage of HIV/AIDS in the southern African region.

STOP AIDS

http://www.stopAIDS.org
nonprofit site, information-based
Tags: News Articles, Treatment Information,
Additional Resources, Donations, Testing,
Advocacy, Dietary

This Web site and group, based in San Francisco, cater to the people living in the Bay Area, although the organization also sponsors a program that reaches out nationwide. A list of community groups to get involved with is included.

TreatHIV

http://www.treathiv.com
medicinal, corporate site, medicine-based
Tags: Treatment Information, Clinical Studies,
Additional Resources

A general information site on HIV/AIDS run by GlaxoSmithKline.

Treatment Action Campaign

http://www.tac.org.za
nonprofit site, information-based
Tags: Treatment Information, FAQ/Fact Sheets,
Additional Resources, Donations, Advocacy

An advocacy group seeking to improve the access to medicine for those with HIV/AIDS in Africa. Along with information about their specific goals, they provide some general information about the virus as well.

Treatment Action Group (TAG)

http://aidsinfonyc.org/tag
political, medicinal, policy-based
Tags: News Articles, Additional Resources,
Advocacy, Medical Rights

The site offers some avenues for advocacy, but it is dominated by advertising, making it harder to navigate its informational sections.

U.S. National Library on Medicine (NLM)
http://gateway.nlm.nih.gov/gw/Cmd
Search: HIV/AIDS
general, government site, information-based
Tags: News Articles, Treatment Information,
    Clinical Studies, Conference Coverage, Testing

Search function for the National Library of Medicine. Searches for HIV or AIDS returned thousands of results in journals, news articles, and other government databases.

WebMD HIV and AIDS Health Center
http://www.webmd.com/hiv-aids/default.htm
medicinal, public site, education-based,
    advertisements
Tags: News Articles, Treatment Information,
    FAQ/Fact Sheets, Additional Resources,
    Testing

A popular destination site for general health issues and related questions that has an informative section on HIV/AIDS. However, information seems to be based on popular questions and is good primarily for a quick overview of the subject; it does not offer very in-depth information on any particular area.

World AIDS Day
http://www.worldaidsday.org
foundation site, information-based

Tags: News Articles, Treatment Information,
    FAQ/Fact Sheets, Guides/Brochures, Confer-
    ence Coverage, Donations, Testing, Advocacy

The Web site of Worlds AIDS Day, promoting outreach and education and providing general information about the virus.

World Health Organization (WHO)
http://www.who.int/hiv/en
United Nations division, information-based
Tags: News Articles, FAQ/Fact Sheets, Addi-
    tional Resources, Advocacy

The goal of the Web site is to disseminate information about the HIV/AIDS pandemic, in addition to providing aid to UN Member States to help them with both treatment and prevention practices.

Yahoo! Health: AIDS/HIV Directory
http://dir.yahoo.com/Health/
    Diseases_and_Conditions/AIDS_HIV
general, search engine site, directory-based
Tag: Additional Resources

A section of the Yahoo! Health Directory. A more refined search engine that leads to sites with information about HIV/AIDS as a medical crisis and not to donations and blogs about HIV/AIDS. Many of the sites listed in this section can be found here.

INDEX

Note: **Boldface** page numbers indicate extensive treatment of a topic.

fosamprenavir **118–119,** 256
    dosage of 118
    drug interactions of 92, 107, 115,
       118–119, 181
    side effects of 119
foscarnet
    for herpes simplex infection 133
    for HHV-6 and HHV-7 infection 151
    for retinal necrosis 312
FPV. *See* fosamprenavir
France 313, 314
French Guiana 63
French National Agency for Research
    on AIDS 75
French Polynesia 234–235
FTC. *See* emtricitabine
fumagillin, for microsporidiosis 213
fungal infections 236. *See also* specific
    infections
fusin. *See* CXCR4 protein
fusion inhibitors. *See* entry inhibitors
Fuzeon. *See* enfuvirtide

G

gag proteins, drugs targeting 51, 203
Gallo, Robert 143, 303, 305
ganciclovir
    for cytomegalovirus 88
    for HHV-6 and HHV-7 infection 151
    interaction with didanosine 94
    for multicentric Castleman disease
      153
    for retinal necrosis 312
Gardasil 167
garlic supplements 118, 181, 221
gay men. *See* men who have sex with
    men
Gay Men's Health Crisis (GMHC) 16,
    23
gay-related immune disorder (GRID)
    65
generic drugs 34, 100–101, 106, 187,
    243, 289–290
Geneva definition 321
genital herpes. *See* herpes simplex virus
genital infections, and risk of HIV
    transmission 280–281
genital warts (HPV) **164–167**
genotypic testing 55, 259
Georgia (Europe) 105
Germany
    Global Fund donations by 121
    HIV infection rate in 314
Ghana 74, 243
gift 47
gift giver 47
Gilead Sciences 39, 108–109, 179, 274,
    293
Gladstone Institute of Virology 226
GlaxoSmithKline Pharmaceuticals 27,
    113, 118, 185, 291, 324

Global Alliance for Vaccines and
    Immunizations 308
Global Campaign for Microbicides 211
Global Fund to Fight AIDS,
    Tuberculosis, and Malaria (Global
    Fund) xiii, **120–121,** 242, 299, 308
global gag order 244
Global HIV Vaccine Enterprise 308
glucose-6-phosphate dehydrogenase
    (G6PD) deficiency 201
GMHC. *See* Gay Men's Health Crisis
Goosby, Eric 242
gorillas 161
gp41 112
gp120 112, 163, 307
granulocyte(s) 53–54, 154–155
granulocyte-macrophage colony-
    stimulating factor (GM-CSF), for
    leishmaniasis 194
grapefruit juice, interactions of 202,
    259, 266
Greece 314
Greenland 229, 231
GRID. *See* gay-related immune disorder
growth factors 155
GSK-572. *See* dolutegravir
GS-9137. *See* elvitegravir
GS-9350 109
Guam 234–235
Guatemala 99, 187, 188
Guinea-Bissau 267
gummas 272–273
Guyana 61, 63, 243
gynecological issues 318–319

H

HAART. *See* highly active antiretroviral
    therapy
Haemophilus influenzae 44, 303
Haiti 61–62, 243
Haitian immigrants 12, 162
Health and Human Services,
    Department of (HHS) 3, 64, 80, 171,
    243, 249, 303
health care workers 15, 247, 287
health insurance 11, 230
Health Resources and Services
    Administration 21
heart disease 55, 208
Heckler, Margaret 143, 303
helper T cells 155
hematocrit 53
hemoglobin 53
hemophilia
    and hepatitis C 129
    and HIV **122–123,** 282
hepatitis, definition of 123, 129
hepatitis A vaccine 302
hepatitis B **123–129**
    acute 126
    chronic 126

co-infection with hepatitis D 126
co-infection with HIV 125–126
diagnosis of 124–126
jaundice in 54, 124
prevention of 127–128
risk factors for 127–128
seroconversion in 126
symptoms of 124–126
transmission of 124, 127
treatment of 126–127, 185, 186,
    274–275, 293
vaccine against 124, 128, 301, 302,
    303
hepatitis B core antibody (anti-HBc)
    125
hepatitis B e antibody (anti-HBe) 125
hepatitis B e antigen (HBeAg) 125
hepatitis B immune globulin 128
hepatitis B surface antibody (anti-HB)
    125
hepatitis B surface antigen (HBsAg)
    124–125
hepatitis C **129–132**
    acute 129
    chronic 129–130
    diagnosis of 130
    jaundice in 54, 129
    prevention of 131
    risk factors for 131
    symptoms of 129–130
    treatment of 130–131
hepatitis D 126
herbal medicine 26
heroin. *See* injection drug use(r)
herpes simplex virus **132–134**
    diagnosis of 133
    prevention of 133–134
    risk factors for 133–134
    symptoms of 132–133
    treatment of 133
    type 1 (oral) 132
    type 2 (genital) 132
herpes viruses, human
    HHV-5. *See* cytomegalovirus
    HHV-6 and HHV-7 **151–152**
    HHV-8 **152–153**
herpes zoster 310–312
herpes zoster vaccine 301
HHS. *See* Health and Human Services,
    Department of
high-density lipoprotein (HDL) 55
highly active antiretroviral therapy
    (HAART) **134–135,** 159–160
    access to xiii–xiv, 10
    in African Americans 11
    assistance program for 21
    in children 72
    effectiveness of 134
    parents and pricing for 98–102
    for prevention of opportunistic
      infections 237